Disorders of Gut-Brain Interaction

Hiroshi Kaneko • Toshimi Chiba
Shin Fukudo • Kotaro Maeda
Hiroto Miwa
Editors

Disorders of Gut-Brain Interaction

Diagnosis and Treatments for DGBI

Springer

Editors
Hiroshi Kaneko
Division of Internal Medicine
Hoshigaoka Maternity Hospital
Nagoya, Aichi, Japan

Shin Fukudo
Department of Behavioral Medicine,
Graduate School of Medicine,
Research Center for Accelerator
and Radioisotope Science
Tohoku University
Sendai, Japan

Japanese Red Cross Ishinomaki Hospital
Ishinomaki, Japan

Hiroto Miwa
Kawanishi City Medical Center
Kawanishi, Hyogo, Japan

Toshimi Chiba
Division of Internal Medicine,
Department of Oral Medicine
Iwate Medical University
Morioka, Japan

Kotaro Maeda
Medical Corporation
Himawariseishinnkai Oumeimai
Hospital
Ome, Tokyo, Japan

ISBN 978-981-95-6973-1 ISBN 978-981-95-6974-8 (eBook)
https://doi.org/10.1007/978-981-95-6974-8

Translation from the Japanese language edition: "Kinousei Shoukakan Shikkan no Shindan to Chiryo - Shinkei Shoukakibyougaku heno Shoutai" by Hiroshi Kaneko et al., © Asakura Publishing Co., Ltd 2024. Published by Asakura Publishing Co., Ltd. All Rights Reserved.

This Springer imprint is published by the registered company Springer Nature Singapore Pte Ltd.
The registered company address is: 152 Beach Road, #21-01/04 Gateway East, Singapore 189721, Singapore

Foreword

The publication of this textbook on disorders of gut-brain interaction constitutes a landmark in the field of neurogastroenterology and motility. The esteemed and internationally recognized authors have assembled a comprehensive treatise covering the entire gastrointestinal tract from the esophagus to the anorectum with focused sections on the esophagus, stomach and duodenum, small bowel and colon, and anorectum. Each section has a very important introduction of the anatomy, physiology, and control mechanisms, particularly peptides, in each section of the gut.

The organization of each anatomical section provides sections on mechanisms, diagnostic tests followed by discussions of the diverse disorders from a practice perspective. Importantly, these sections include not only the disorders of function that are encompassed under the general classification of DGBI but also the diseases where the mechanisms are far clearer or there are objective motility disorders. This is exemplified by the inclusion in the esophageal section of conditions like functional heartburn (a DGBI) as well as achalasia (a definite motility disorder) and esophageal scleroderma or in the stomach and duodenum section by coverage of functional dyspepsia and gastroparesis, or in the anorectum section by inclusion of dyssynergic defecation as well as rectal prolapse.

The coverage of diagnostic testing is comprehensive. For example, there are four chapters on different methods to measure gastric emptying, and two chapters on assessment of gastric sensitivity using drink test (non-invasive) or barostat measurements, the latter requiring an intragastric balloon inflated with air under constant pressure by means of an electronically controlled barostat. Similarly, small bowel and colon sections incorporate measurements of contractions, transit, cine-MRI, and intestinal permeability, and the section on anorectum appraises anorectal motor, sensory, nerve conduction, electromyography, defecography, and balloon expulsion tests.

Each section also includes case discussions which clearly draw on the experience of the authors in their respective areas of expertise to provide the reader with education from practical perspective.

Section X appropriately groups the practical findings on clinical examination focusing on the role of psychosomatic etiology, as well as the physical findings in the abdomen and on digital rectal examination. It also covers the different modalities of treatments for the DGBI or motility disorders focusing on psychotherapy or behavioral therapy as well as pharmacological approaches, including Kampo formula treatment, which is a holistic approach that combines traditional Japanese herbal medicine with other therapeutic methods designed to address the whole person, not just the symptoms of an illness.

After the general introductory chapters, each subsequent "topic" chapter text itself covers introductory concepts, etiology and pathophysiology, clinical diagnostic criteria including symptoms, findings on testing including endoscopy and relevant motility or sensory tests, the diverse clinical syndromes or manifestations, and treatment, culminating in important take-home messages as well as relevant references. Illustrations and figures complement the text.

The appendix is an interesting section that provides the reader with opportunities to self evaluate their road to expertise and the format based on questions on each topic area followed by the provision of answers rounds out the educational value of this multi-author textbook.

Michael Camilleri, MD, DSc
Professor of Medicine
Pharmacology and Physiology
Mayo Clinic
Rochester, MN, USA
camilleri.michael@mayo.edu

Preface to the English Edition

The Japanese book, *Diagnosis and Treatment of Functional Gastrointestinal Disorders: An Introduction to Neurogastroenterology*, originally published by Asakura Publishing Co., Ltd., has been selected as a recommended reference for the certification exam for specialists in functional gastrointestinal disorders by the Japanese Society of Neurogastroenterology and Motility. Recognizing its significance, we have decided to translate it into English under the title *Disorders of Gut-Brain Interaction: Diagnosis and Treatments for DGBI*.

Various academic groups dedicated to the advancement of neurogastroenterology exist worldwide, particularly under the leadership of the Rome Foundation, focusing on disorders of gut-brain interaction (DGBI) and gastrointestinal motility disorders across Europe, the Americas, and Asia. Despite the growing body of research in this field, comprehensive textbooks on DGBI and motility disorders remain surprisingly scarce. While some notable works have been published in regions such as Southeast Asia, India, Belgium, and the United Kingdom, their overall number is still limited.

Neurogastroenterology has a distinct historical background, yet the number of healthcare professionals engaged in its research and education remains relatively small in Japan. DGBI represents a paradigm shift in understanding chronic gastrointestinal symptoms and associated psychological distress in the absence of organic disease, emphasizing the interplay between the gut and the brain. While this concept has evolved primarily from Western research, its importance is increasingly recognized in Japan, where original contributions to the field are steadily growing.

Given this context, we strongly believe that publishing this textbook in English will allow us to share Japan's expertise in DGBI research with a global audience of healthcare professionals. Furthermore, we hope that this translation will help raise important questions and contribute to the continued development of this field. We are grateful to Asakura Publishing for granting permission to translate the original work and to Springer for accepting the English edition for publication.

The authors of this book are among Japan's leading researchers and clinicians in neurogastroenterology. They have made great efforts to ensure that the translation maintains the accuracy of the original medical terminology while adopting expressions that are internationally accepted. Additionally, they have provided supplementary explanations where necessary to enhance the book's accessibility for a global audience. Nevertheless, we recognize the inherent challenges of translation, and we would greatly appreciate any constructive feedback from our readers.

A deeper understanding of patients with chronic or recurrent gastrointestinal symptoms—including those who have not yet sought medical attention—will facilitate timely intervention, potentially reducing healthcare costs and improving overall quality of life. We sincerely hope that this book will serve as a valuable reference for both clinical practice and research.

Finally, we would like to express our heartfelt gratitude to the many experts who contributed to the translation and publication of this book.

Nagoya, Japan Hiroshi Kaneko
Morioka, Japan Toshimi Chiba
Ishinomaki, Japan Shin Fukudo
Ome, Japan Kotaro Maeda
Kawanishi, Japan Hiroto Miwa

Preface (Original Japanese Textbook)

Gastrointestinal diseases are broadly categorized as either "organic gastrointestinal diseases," such as infections and tumors, which are visible, or "functional gastrointestinal disorders (FGIDs)/disorders of gut-brain interaction (DGBI)," where the morphological abnormalities that explain the symptoms are difficult to detect. In Japan, it has made remarkable progress in examinations for detecting morphological abnormalities, typified by endoscopy, and many world-leading textbooks are available on this subject. In contrast, invisible FGIDs/DGBI, such as irritable bowel syndrome and functional dyspepsia, significantly impact quality of life and socioeconomic activity, exerting substantial biological, psychological, and social effects. In Western gastroenterology, FGIDs/DGBI have long been recognized as a primary focus of neurogastroenterology. In Japan, these disorders are also becoming more important due to growing public demand for a more holistic approach to healthcare that prioritizes quality of life and treats the "person with illness." Although FGIDs/DGBI are increasingly covered in medical education, many practitioners struggle to meet patient needs adequately. This may be due to a lack of clear etiology and treatment methods for these invisible illnesses, their limited impact on life prognosis and insufficient knowledge. In other words, a gap in understanding between patients and healthcare providers is problematic.

The gut is often referred to as the "little brain" or "second brain," and the concept of the brain-gut axis has recently received more attention. Specifically, the close relationship with gut-brain peptides in gastrointestinal motility has been clarified, and the relationship between the nerves involved in gut-brain peptides and psychosomatic medicine is also being elucidated. Furthermore, it has been suggested that gut microbiota may be involved in the gut-brain interactions. However, there are hardly any textbooks on FGIDs/DGBI in Japan. Against this backdrop, this book has been compiled to bring together knowledge on FGIDs/DGBI, which have diverse etiologies and pathologies, and to provide clinically useful content.

This book is organized into twelve chapters, each designed to provide a comprehensive understanding of neurogastroenterology and FGIDs/DGBI. Part 1 serves as an introduction, outlining the scope and objectives of the book. Parts 2 through 9 cover the major regions of the gastrointestinal tract—the esophagus, stomach and duodenum, small bowel and colon, and anorectum. Each region is presented in two formats: the Basic Edition and the Practical Edition. The Basic Edition summarizes anatomy, physiology and motility testing relevant to gastrointestinal function, while the Practical Edition focuses on FGIDs/DGBI, detailing concepts, epidemiology, etiology, pathophysiology, diagnostic criteria and tests, differential diagnosis, complications, and treatment. A distinctive feature of the Practical Edition is the inclusion of case discussions, which aim to foster a multifaceted understanding of patients through real-world examples. Part 10, titled *Practical Treatment*, addresses cross-cutting clinical topics such as psychosomatic medicine, abdominal physical examination findings, management of refractory abdominal pain, family medicine approaches, and Kampo (Japanese herbal) therapy. Part 11, *New Perspectives on Disorders of Gut-Brain Interaction*, introduces emerging concepts and recent advances in this rapidly evolving field. *Appendix: The Road to Expertise—Toward Becoming a Medical Specialist*, uses a question-and-answer format with explanatory notes to reinforce key knowledge and deepen understanding of the diseases and principles discussed throughout the book. This textbook integrates case-based learning within the Practical Editions and includes a “Topics” section highlighting essential updates for specialists. With approximately 260 color figures, 80 tables, and 340 illustrations, the book aims to make neurogastroenterology accessible and clinically relevant for learners and practitioners alike.

Finally, we would like to express our heartfelt gratitude to all the authors, editors, and staff at Asakura Shoten.

Nagoya, Japan	Hiroshi Kaneko
Morioka, Japan	Toshimi Chiba
Ishinomaki, Japan	Shin Fukudo
Ome, Japan	Kotaro Maeda
Kawanishi, Japan	Hiroto Miwa

Contents

Part IX Anorectum, Practical Edition

Part X Practical Treatment

Contributors

Tatsuya Abe Department of Proctology, Kunimoto Hospital, Anorectal Surgery, Asahikawa, Japan

Shuhei Agawa Department of Internal Medicine, Division of Gastroenterology, Nippon Medical School, Tokyo, Japan

Junichi Akiyama Division of Gastroenterology and Hepatology, National Center for Global Health and Medicine, Tokyo, Japan

Haruka Amitani Department of Psychosomatic Internal Medicine, Kagoshima University Graduate School of Medical and Dental Sciences, Kagoshima, Japan

Makoto Arai Department of Gastroenterology, Tokyo Women's Medical University Yachiyo Medical Center, Yachiyo, Japan

Akihiro Asakawa Department of Psychosomatic Internal Medicine, Kagoshima University Graduate School of Medical and Dental Sciences, Kagoshima, Japan

Toshimi Chiba Division of Internal Medicine, Department of Oral Medicine, Iwate Medical University, Morioka, Japan

Yasuhiro Fujiwara Osaka Metropolitan University, Osaka, Japan

Shin Fukudo Department of Behavioral Medicine, Graduate School of Medicine, Research Center for Accelerator and Radioisotope Science, Tohoku University, Sendai, Japan

Japanese Red Cross Ishinomaki Hospital, Ishinomaki, Japan

Yoshikazu Fukui Department of Human Sciences, Faculty of Letters, Konan University, Kobe, Japan

Mikihiko Fukunaga Department of Psychosomatic Medicine, Naniwa Ikuno Hospital, Osaka, Japan

Yasushi Funaki Department of Gastroenterology, Aichi Medical University School of Medicine, Nagakute, Japan

Department of Gastroenterology, Aichi Medical University Medical Center, Okazaki, Japan

Seiji Futagami Department of Internal Medicine, Division of Gastroenterology, Nippon Medical School, Tokyo, Japan

Akiko Fuyuki Department of Palliative Care, Shin-yurigaoka General Hospital, Kawasaki, Japan

Ken Haruma Department of General Internal Medicine, Kawasaki Medical School General Medical Center, Okayama, Japan

Jiro Hata Department of General Medicine, Kawasaki Medical School, Kurashiki, Japan

Mariko Hojo Department of Gastroenterology, Juntendo University Faculty of Medicine, Tokyo, Japan

Yuko Homma Department of Surgery, Division of Gastroenterological, General and Transplant Surgery, Jichi Medical University, Shimotsuke, Japan

Michio Hongo Tohoku University, Sendai, Japan

Hiroko Hosaka Department of Gastroenterology and Hepatology, Gunma University Graduate School of Medicine, Maebashi, Japan

Eikichi Ihara Department of Medicine and Bioregulatory Science, Graduate School of Medical Sciences, Kyushu University, Fukuoka, Japan

Katsunori Iijima Gastroenterology, Akita University Graduate School of Medicine, Akita, Japan

Masahiko Inamori Department of Medical Education, Yokohama City University of School of Medicine, Yokohama, Japan

Masatomo Ishioh Department of General Medicine, Asahikawa Medical University, Asahikawa, Japan

Katsuhiko Iwakiri Department of Gastroenterology, Nippon Medical School, Graduate School of Medicine, Tokyo, Japan

Kazuhiro Kamada Department of Gastroenterology, Matsushita Memorial Hospital, Moriguchi, Japan

Tomoari Kamada Department of Health Care Medicine, Kawasaki Medical School General Medical Center, Okayama, Japan

Takeshi Kamiya Department of Medical Innovation, Nagoya City University Graduate School of Medical Sciences, Gastroenterology, Internal Medicine, Regulatory Science, Nagoya, Japan

Motoyori Kanazawa Department of Behavioral Medicine, Tohoku University Graduate School of Medicine, Sendai, Japan

Hiroshi Kaneko Division of Internal Medicine, Hoshigaoka Maternity Hospital, Nagoya, Japan

Kunio Kasugai Aichi Medical University Department of Gastroenterology, Nagakute, Japan

Department of Gastroenterology, Aichi Medical University Medical Center, Okazaki, Japan

Mototsugu Kato Public Interest Foundation, Gastroenterology, Sapporo, Japan

Hidetoshi Katsuno Department of Surgery, Fujita Health University Okazaki Medical Center, Okazaki, Japan

Noriyuki Kawami Department of Gastroenterology, Nippon Medical School, Graduate School of Medicine, Tokyo, Japan

Takaomi Kessoku Department of Palliative Medicine and Gastroenterology, International University Health and Welfare Narita Hospital, Narita, Japan

Department of Gastroenterology, International University Health and Welfare Graduate School of Medicine, Narita, Japan

Department of Gastroenterology and Hepatology, Yokohama City University Graduate School of Medicine, Yokohama, Japan

Keiji Koda Surgery Unit, Coloproctology Center Takano Hospital, Kumamoto, Japan

Tomoyuki Koike Division of Gastroenterology, Tohoku University Graduate School of Medicine, Sendai, Japan

Shigeto Koizumi Gastroenterology, Koizumi Hospital, Akita, Japan

Shiko Kuribayashi Department of Gastroenterology and Hepatology, Gunma University Graduate School of Medicine, Maebashi, Japan

Joji Kuromizu Department of Anorectal Surgery and Anorectal Physiology, Matsushima Hospital, Coloproctology Center, Yokohama, Japan

Hiroaki Kusunoki Junpukai Health Maintenance Center Kurashiki, Okayama, Japan

Takatsugu Machida Department of Psychosomatic Medicine, Tohoku Rosai Hospital, Sendai, Japan

Tomomi Machida Department of Psychosomatic Medicine, Tohoku Rosai Hospital, Sendai, Japan

Kotaro Maeda Medical Cooperation Himawariseishinkai Oumeimai Hospital, Ome, Tokyo, Japan

Noriaki Manabe Division of Endoscopy and Ultrasonography, Department of Clinical Laboratory Medicine, Kawasaki Medical School, Okayama, Japan

Tatsuhiro Masaoka Kawasaki Municipal Hospital, Kawasaki, Japan

Masashi Matsushima Department of Internal Medicine (Gastroenterology), Tokai University School of Medicine, Isehara, Japan

Hiroshi Mihara Department of Educational Development, Center for Medical Education and Department of General Medicine, Faculty of Medicine, Sapporo Medical University, Sapporo, Japan

Toshiki Mimura Division of Gastroenterological, General and Transplant Surgery, Department of Surgery, Jichi Medical University, Shimotsuke, Japan

Hiroto Miwa Kawanishi City Medical Center, Hyogo, Kawanishi, Japan

Takeshi Mizukami Department of Endoscopy Center, NHO Kurihama Medical and Addiction Center, Yokosuka, Japan

Mitsuru Moriya Health Sciences University of Hokkaido, Sapporo, Japan

Akihito Nagahara Department of Gastroenterology, Juntendo University Faculty of Medicine, Tokyo, Japan

Yuji Naito Department of Human Immunology and Nutrition Science, Kyoto Prefectural University of Medicine, Kyoto, Japan

Miwako Nakano Yoshikawa Kids Clinic, Tokyo, Japan

Suzuki Children's Clinic, Urawa, Japan

Toshihiro Noake Kurume Coloproctology Center, Coloproctology, Kurume, Japan

Taisuke Nomura NOMURA Internal and Psychosomatic Medicine, Sendai, Japan

Tsukasa Nozu Asahikawa Medical University, Asahikawa, Japan

Naotaka Ogasawara Department of Gastroenterology, Aichi Medical University School of Medicine, Nagakute, Japan

Department of Gastroenterology, Aichi Medical University Medical Center, Okazaki, Japan

Hidenori Ohkubo Gastroenterology Division, Sagami Rinkan Hospital, Sagamihara, Japan

Hirokuni Okumi Okumi Clinic, Ihoukai Medical Association, PsychoSomatic Medicine, Gastroenterology, Japanese Traditional (Kampo) Medicine, Osaka, Japan

Toshikatsu Okumura Asahikawa Medical University, Asahikawa, Japan

Tadayuki Oshima Department of Gastroenterology, Okazaki City Medical Association, Public Health Center, Okazaki, Japan

Department of Gastroenterology and Metabolism, Nagoya City University Graduate School of Medical Science, Nagoya, Japan

Masahiro Saito Division of Gastroenterology, Tohoku University Graduate School of Medicine, Sendai, Japan

Ryuji Sakakibara Neurology Clinic Tsudanuma and Dowakai Chiba Hospital, Funabashi, Japan

Ken Sato Hirosaki University, Health Service Center/Graduate School of Gastroenterology, Hematology and Clinical Immunology, Hirosaki, Japan

Akiko Shiotani Department of Gastroenterology and Hepatology, Kawasaki Medical School, Kurashiki, Japan

Hidekazu Suzuki Division of Gastroenterology and Hepatology, Department of Internal Medicine, Tokai University School of Medicine, Isehara, Japan

Tomoko Takahashi Kameda Medical Center, Chiba, Japan

Shota Takano Department of Functional Anorectal Disorder, Coloproctology Center, Takano Hospital, Kumamoto, Japan

Hiroshi Takeda Gastroenterology, Caress Memorial Hospital, Sapporo, Japan

Faculty of Pharmaceutical Sciences, Hokkaido University, Sapporo, Japan

Fumio Tanaka Department of Gastroenterology, Osaka Metropolitan University Graduate School of Medicine, Osaka, Japan

Kazunari Tominaga Department of Gastroenterology, Osaka Gyomeikan Hospital, Osaka, Japan

Toshihiko Tomita Department of Gastroenterology, Faculty of Medicine, Hyogo Medical University, Nishinomiya, Japan

Osamu Tsuchida Division of Psychosomatic Medicine, Functional Gastrointestinal Disorders, Saiseikai Iizuka-kaho Hospital, Iizuka, Japan

Shingo Tsujinaka Tohoku Medical and Pharmaceutical University, Sendai, Japan

Akira Uehara Uehara Clinic, Sapporo, Japan

Yoshihisa Urita Urita Clinic, General Medicine, Aomori, Japan

Sayuri Yamamoto Department of General Medicine & Gastroenterology, Aichi Medical University, Nagakute, Japan

Takatsugu Yamamoto Division of Gastroenterology, Department of Medicine, Teikyo University School of Medicine, Tokyo, Japan

Part I

Introduction

1 Overview of Disorders of Gut-Brain Interaction (DGBI) 1: Neurogastroenterology and Rome Diagnostic Criteria

Shin Fukudo

Abstract

Neurogastroenterology is the field of study that investigates how the bidirectional relationship between the nervous system and the gastrointestinal tract contributes to human health and disease. The largest components of the nervous system are the brain and spinal cord, which constitute the central nervous system (CNS). The gastrointestinal tract contains the enteric nervous system (ENS), which regulates gastrointestinal sensation and motility. The autonomic nervous system (ANS) mediates between the CNS and ENS, linking the brain and gut through neural pathways. Furthermore, physiologically active substances such as hormones and cytokines, as well as immune cells, are secreted or increased primarily by both the nervous system and the gastrointestinal tract and affect whole body via systemic circulation. Disorders of gut-brain interaction (DGBI) are internationally diagnosed with Rome IV or coming Rome V criteria and defined as disorders characterized by chronic or recurrent gastrointestinal symptoms that are not attributable to detectable organic disorders on routine clinical testing. DGBI are being addressed through a multidisciplinary approach involving gastrointestinal physiology, brain imaging, immunology, microbiology, genetics, clinical epidemiology, and biopsychosocial medicine. These disorders are expected to occupy an increasingly important position in the field of gastroenterology and general medicine.

Keywords

Central nervous system (CNS) · Enteric nervous system (ENS) · Autonomic nervous system (ANS) · Brain-gut interactions · Disorders of gut-brain interaction (DGBI) · Neurogastroenterology · Rome IV criteria · Rome V criteria · Multi-dimensional clinical profile (MDCP) · Quality of life (QOL)

1 Introduction

Neurogastroenterology is the field of study that investigates how the bidirectional relationship between the nervous system and the gastrointestinal tract contributes to human health and disease. The largest components of the nervous system are the brain and spinal cord, which constitute the central nervous system (CNS) [1].

S. Fukudo (✉)
Department of Behavioral Medicine, Graduate School of Medicine, Research Center for Accelerator and Radioisotope Science, Tohoku University, Sendai, Japan

Japanese Red Cross Ishinomaki Hospital, Ishinomaki, Japan
e-mail: shin.fukudo.c6@tohoku.ac.jp

H. Kaneko et al. (eds.), *Disorders of Gut-Brain Interaction*,
https://doi.org/10.1007/978-981-95-6974-8_1

Within the gastrointestinal organs themselves, neurons and glial cells are also present. In particular, the gastrointestinal tract contains the enteric nervous system (ENS), which regulates gastrointestinal sensation and motility [2]. The autonomic nervous system (ANS) mediates between the CNS and ENS, linking the two through neural pathways [3]. Furthermore, physiologically active substances such as hormones and cytokines, as well as immune cells, are secreted or increased primarily by both the nervous system and the gastrointestinal tract and affect whole body via systemic circulation. These substances influence not only adjacent and nearby organs but also induce functional changes—and in some cases, morphological alterations—in both systems [4].

The Rome Foundation was established to standardize the diagnostic criteria for functional gastrointestinal disorders (FGIDs) on an international level. With the advancement of scientific understanding as described above, it is now recommended that the term "neurogastroenterological diseases" or "disorders of gut-brain interaction (DGBI)" be used to describe this group of conditions [5]. Currently, based on accumulated research findings, the diagnostic criteria are being revised from Rome IV to Rome V. This article outlines the global trends in neurogastroenterology (Table 1.1).

Table 1.1 Disorders of Gut-Brain Interaction (DGBI)

A. Functional Esophageal Disorders
A1. Functional chest pain
A2. Functional heartburn
A3. Reflux hypersensitivity
A4. Globus
A5. Functional dysphagia
B. Functional Gastroduodenal Disorders
B1. Functional dyspepsia
B1a. Postprandial distress syndrome (PDS)
B1b. Epigastric pain syndrome (EPS)
B2. Belching disorders
B2a. Excessive supragastric belching
B2b. Excessive gastric belching
B3. Nausea and vomiting disorders
B3a. Chronic nausea vomiting syndrome (CNVS)
B3b. Cyclic vomiting syndrome (CVS)
B3c. Cannabinoid hyperemesis syndrome (CHS)
B4. Rumination syndrome
C. Functional Bowel Disorders
C1. Irritable bowel syndrome (IBS)
IBS with predominant constipation (IBS-C)
IBS with predominant diarrhea (IBS-D)
IBS with mixed bowel habits (IBS-M)
IBS unclassified (IBS-U)
C2. Functional constipation
C3. Functional diarrhea
C4. Functional abdominal bloating/distention
C5. Unspecified functional bowel disorder
C6. Opioid-induced constipation
D. Centrally Mediated Disorders of Gastrointestinal Pain
D1. Centrally mediated abdominal pain syndrome (CAPS)
D2. Narcotic bowel syndrome (NBS)
Opioid-induced GI hyperalgesia

(continued)

Table 1.1 (continued)

E. Functional Gallbladder and Sphincter of Oddi Disorders
E1. Biliary pain
E1a. Functional gallbladder disorder
E1b. Functional biliary sphincter of Oddi disorder
E2. Functional pancreatic sphincter of Oddi disorder
F. Functional Anorectal Disorders
F1. Fecal incontinence
F2. Functional anorectal pain
F2a. Levator ani syndrome
F2b. Unspecified functional anorectal pain
F2c. Proctalgia fugax
F3. Functional defecation disorders
F3a. Inadequate defecatory propulsion
F3b. Dyssynergic defecation
G. Functional Gastrointestinal Disorders: Neonates and Toddlers
G1. Infant regurgitation
G2. Rumination syndrome
G3. Cyclic vomiting syndrome (CVS)
G4. Infant colic
G5. Functional diarrhea
G6. Infant dyschezia
G7. Functional constipation
H. Childhood Functional Gastrointestinal Disorders: Child/Adolescent
H1. Functional nausea and vomiting disorders
H1a. Cyclic vomiting syndrome
H1b. Functional nausea and functional vomiting
H1b1. Functional nausea
H1b2. Functional vomiting
H1c. Rumination syndrome
H1d. Aerophagia
H2. Functional abdominal pain disorders
H2a. Functional dyspepsia
H2a1. Postprandial distress syndrome (PDS)
H2a2. Epigastric pain syndrome (EPS)
H2b. Irritable bowel syndrome (IBS)
H2c. Abdominal migraine
H2d. Functional abdominal pain—NOS
H2d1. Childhood functional abdominal pain syndrome
H3. Functional defecation disorders
H3a. Functional constipation
H3b. Non-retentive fecal incontinence

Based on Rome IV Criteria. Adapted with permission from: Drossman and Hasler [5]. Elsevier
Note: These are not rare or obscure diagnoses internationally. They are frequently encountered in routine internal medicine practice. All of these disorders have established diagnostic criteria. For details, refer to Rome IV

2 What Are the Rome Diagnostic Criteria?

DGBIs are defined as disorders characterized by chronic or recurrent gastrointestinal symptoms that are not attributable to detectable organic disorders on routine clinical testing [5]. The prototypical example is irritable bowel syndrome (IBS) [6]. The core symptoms of IBS are abdominal pain and associated alterations in bowel habits, yet colonoscopy typically reveals no abnormalities [6]. Because these disorders cannot be diagnosed through specific biomarkers, diagnostic practices varied across countries and among clinicians, hindering the identification of distinct pathophysiological mechanisms [7].

This situation began to change at the 1988 World Congress of Gastroenterology in Rome [5]. At that time, international diagnostic guidelines for IBS were proposed and published the following year. Once IBS was clearly defined, it became necessary to define related but distinct disorders. For example, diarrhea without abdominal pain or discomfort is not IBS; it is defined as functional diarrhea. Similarly, constipation without abdominal pain or discomfort is not IBS; it is defined as functional constipation. These disorders fall under the category of functional bowel disorders. Once these were clearly delineated, it also became necessary to define disorders that resemble functional bowel disorders but originate in different parts of the gastrointestinal tract. For instance, abdominal pain without altered bowel habits is not a functional bowel disorder and should be diagnosed as functional abdominal pain syndrome.

Thus, the multinational Rome committee was formed, and the first international diagnostic criteria—known as the Rome criteria—were announced in 1990 and published in 1992 [8]. A comprehensive textbook followed in 1994 [5]. This marked the beginning of a global movement to standardize FGID diagnostic criteria, leading to the publication of the Rome II criteria in 1999 [9]. These criteria gained international acceptance and significantly advanced the diagnosis, treatment, research, and drug development for FGIDs.

The Rome III criteria were published in 2006 [10]. Since then, it has become standard practice to specify the version of the Rome criteria used when discussing FGIDs. The Rome IV criteria were published in 2016 [5, 11], with participation from Japanese committee members [12]. Rome committee commonly decided to refer the disorders as DGBI. Rome IV criteria will be revised to Rome V criteria in 2026.

3 Characteristics of the Rome Diagnostic Criteria

The representative DGBIs include six adult disorders—esophageal disorders, gastroduodenal disorders, bowel disorders, centrally mediated gastrointestinal pain disorders, biliary tract and sphincter of Oddi disorders, and anorectal disorders—as well as two pediatric disorders—neonatal/infant and child/adolescent disorders—making a total of eight categories [5]. All of these disorders now have internationally standardized diagnostic criteria. As a result, the previous inconsistencies in diagnosis across countries and among clinicians have largely been resolved.

4 Features of Rome IV

Rome IV was published in the journal *Gastroenterology* and also released as a comprehensive textbook series (Fig. 1.1). While many readers may think of Rome IV as a collection of diagnostic criteria, it is in fact a comprehensive knowledge system encompassing both basic and clinical research findings accumulated through the revisions of Rome I, II, and III (Table 1.2). Therefore, it is important to understand the full scope of the Rome IV framework (Fig. 1.2).

The introduction of the Rome criteria has significantly advanced the field. In particular, research on IBS has progressed rapidly, as evidenced by the increasing number of publications [13]. IBS is highly prevalent in developed countries and is slightly more common in women. Although IBS is a benign condition, it impairs patients' quality of life (QOL) and requires

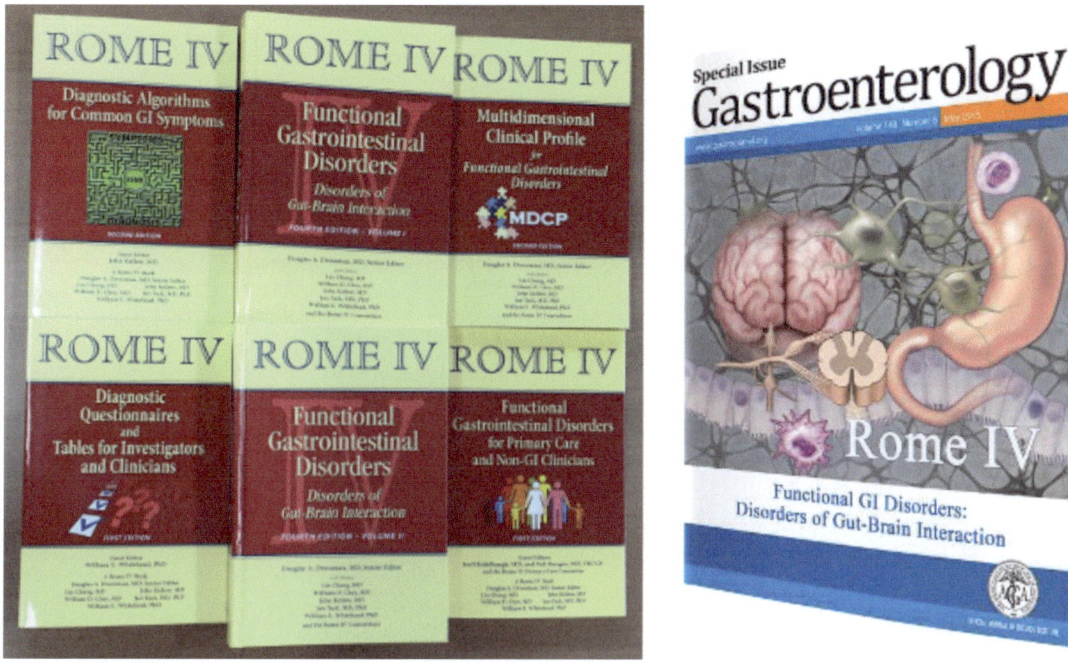

Fig. 1.1 Rome IV textbook (left) and *Gastroenterology* edition (right)

Table 1.2 Chapters of Rome IV

1. The Functional Gastrointestinal Disorders and the Rome IV Process
2. Fundamentals of Neurogastroenterology—Basic Science
3. Fundamentals of Neurogastroenterology—Physiology/Motility-Sensation
4. Intestinal Microenvironment and Functional GI Disorders
5. Pharmacological, Pharmacokinetic and Pharmacogenomic Aspects of Functional GI Disorders
6. Age, Gender, Women's Health and the Patient
7. Multi-cultural Aspects of Functional Gastrointestinal Disorders
8. Biopsychosocial Aspects of Functional Gastrointestinal Disorders
9. Functional Esophageal Disorders
10. Functional Gastroduodenal Disorders
11. Functional Bowel Disorders
12. Centrally Mediated Disorders of Gastrointestinal Pain
13. Functional Gallbladder and Sphincter of Oddi Disorders
14. Functional Anorectal Disorders
15. Childhood Functional Gastrointestinal Disorders: Neonate/Toddler
16. Childhood Functional Gastrointestinal Disorders: Child/Adolescent
17. Design of Treatment Trials for Functional Gastrointestinal Disorders
18. Development and Validation of the Rome IV Diagnostic Questionnaire
19. History of Functional GI Disorders and the Rome Foundation

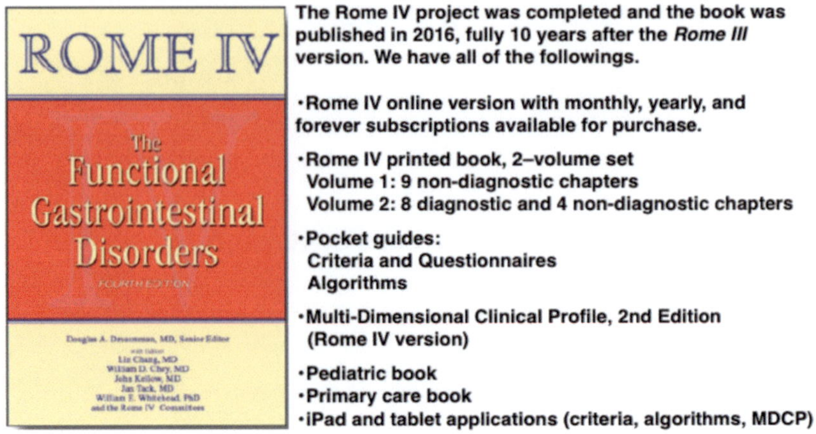

Fig. 1.2 Rome IV online version, questionnaires, and diagnostic algorithms

appropriate care. While the pathogenesis of IBS remains unclear, it is known to occur following recovery from infectious enteritis (post-infectious IBS). The pathophysiology of IBS emphasizes the gut-brain axis, particularly the relationship between central and gastrointestinal functions. The key mechanisms include (1) abnormal gastrointestinal motility, (2) visceral hypersensitivity, and (3) psychological disturbances. Additional contributing factors include (4) low grade inflammation of the mucosa, (5) increased mucosal permeability, (6) gut microbiota, (7) diet, (8) stress, (9) autonomic-endocrine interactions, (10) central nervous system responses, and (11) genetic factors. These findings are now being applied not only to other DGBI but also to other disease groups.

Accurate epidemiological studies based on Rome IV have been conducted globally, revealing a worldwide prevalence of 4.1% for IBS and 40.3% for DGBIs overall [14].

One notable example of progress in DGBI research is the use of patient-reported outcomes (PROs) and psychometric tools to quantify symptoms, which has led to the development of new therapeutic approaches. The diagnosis and treatment of IBS are guided by national and international clinical practice guidelines, including those published by the Japanese Society of Gastroenterology [6]. Diagnosis is based on the Rome IV criteria. In the first stage of treatment, pharmacotherapy targeting the gastrointestinal tract is combined with general integrative care with emphasis of good physician-patient relationship. If this is ineffective, the second stage involves the use of antidepressants, although some cases respond well to Kampo (traditional Japanese) medicine. If pharmacotherapy is ineffective, the third stage involves brain-gut behavioral therapies such as cognitive behavioral therapy. This approach aligns with the multi-dimensional clinical profile (MDCP) (Fig. 1.3).

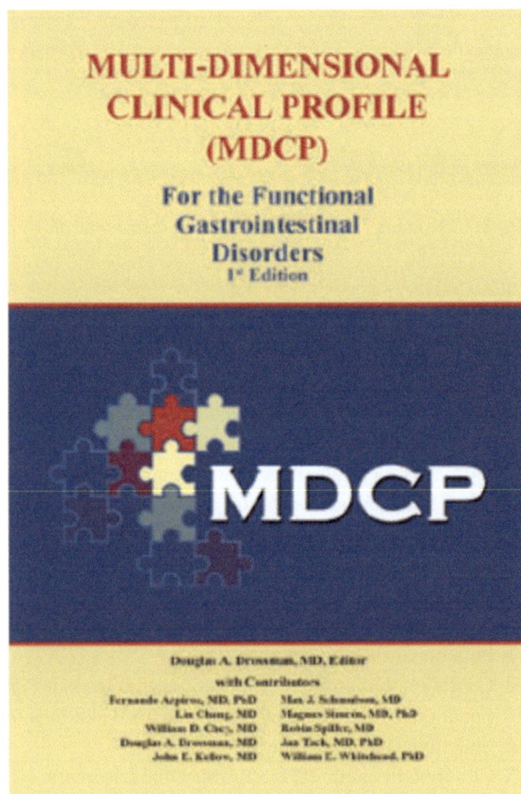

Fig. 1.3 Multi-Dimensional Clinical Profile (MDCP)

MDCP categorizes each DGBI patient as follows:

Category A: Rome diagnosis

Category B: Additional clinically useful diagnoses (e.g., IBS-D [with predominant diarrhea] or IBS-C [with predominant constipation])

Category C: Impact of the disorder on the individual (mild, moderate, severe)

Category D: Psychosocial factors (e.g., depression, anxiety)

Category E: Physiological test findings (e.g., gastrointestinal manometry, barostat) and biological markers (e.g., mucosal permeability, gut microbiota)

Treatment is tailored according to these findings (Table 1.3).

Table 1.3 Clinical Application of MDCP (Multi-Dimensional Clinical Profile)

Category A. IBS
Category B.
General Modifiers
Functional Somatic Syndromes (e.g., fibromyalgia, chronic fatigue)
Narcotic Bowel Syndrome
Fatigue, sleep disturbance
Clinical Modifiers
Post-infectious
Postprandial symptoms
FODMAP sensitivity
Stool pattern: IBS-D, IBS-C, IBS-M, IBS-U
With urgency
With fecal incontinence
With pain predominance
Frequent vs. sporadic symptoms
With bloating
IBD-IBS overlap
Category C. Disease severity: none / mild / moderate / severe
Category D. Psychosocial influences
Anxiety, depression
Suicidal ideation
Abuse and trauma (including partner abuse)
Pain
Somatic symptoms associated with distress and health concerns
Drug or alcohol abuse
Category E.
Wall structure and activity: Manometry, MRI
Movement of contents: Radiopaque markers, scintigraphy, SmartPill, MRI
Sensitivity: Barostat
Evidence of inflammation: Histology, calprotectin, perfusion/diffusion, cytokines, mRNA
Other analytical techniques (disease-specific): Permeability, fecal tryptase, microbiota (HITChip)

5 Conclusion

DGBI, including IBS, are currently being addressed through a multidisciplinary approach involving gastrointestinal physiology, brain imaging, immunology, microbiology, genetics, clinical epidemiology, and biopsychosocial medicine. These disorders are expected to occupy an increasingly important position in the field of gastroenterology and general medicine.

Competing Interests The author(s) has no competing interests to declare that are relevant to the content of this manuscript.

References

1. Kandel ER, et al. Principles of neural science. 6th ed. New York: McGraw-Hill; 2021.
2. Christensen J, et al. A guide to gastrointestinal motility. Bristol: John Wright; 1983.
3. Fukudo S. IBS: autonomic dysregulation in IBS. Nat Rev Gastroenterol Hepatol. 2013;10:569–71.
4. Fukudo S. Hypothalamic-pituitary-adrenal axis in gastrointestinal physiology. In: Johnson LR, editor. Physiology of the gastrointestinal tract. 5th ed. Amsterdam: Elsevier; 2012. p. 795–815.
5. Drossman DA, Hasler WL. Rome IV—Functional GI disorders: disorders of gut-brain interaction. Gastroenterology. 2016;150:1257–61.
6. Fukudo S, et al. Evidence-based clinical practice guidelines for irritable bowel syndrome 2020. J Gastroenterol. 2021;56:193–217.
7. Whitehead WE, et al. Irritable bowel syndrome: definition of the syndrome and relation to other disorders. In: Whitehead WE, Schuster MM, editors. Gastrointestinal disorders: behavioral and physiological basis for treatment. Orlando: Academic; 1985. p. 155–209.
8. Thompson WG, et al. Functional bowel disease and functional abdominal pain. Gastroenterol Int. 1992;5:75–91.
9. Thompson WG, et al. Functional bowel disorders and functional abdominal pain. Gut. 1999;45(Suppl II):II43–7.
10. Longstreth GF, et al. Functional bowel disorders. Gastroenterology. 2006;130:1480–91.
11. Lacy BE, et al. Bowel disorders. Gastroenterology. 2016;150:1393–407.
12. Francisconi CF, et al. Multicultural aspects in functional gastrointestinal disorders (FGIDs). Gastroenterology. 2016;150:1344–54.
13. Thompson WG. The road to Rome. Gastroenterology. 2006;130:1552–6.
14. Sperber AD, et al. Worldwide prevalence and burden of functional gastrointestinal disorders, results of Rome Foundation global study. Gastroenterology. 2021;160:99–114.e3.

2 Overview of Disorders of Gut-Brain Interaction (DGBI) 2: The Evolving Role of Functional Gastrointestinal Disorders and Gastrointestinal Motility Disorders in Gastroenterology

Hiroshi Kaneko and Toshimi Chiba

Abstract

Functional Gastrointestinal Disorders (FGIDs) or Disorders of Gut-Brain Interaction (DGBI) are characterized by abdominal symptoms without detectable structural abnormalities that could explain the symptoms. Since FGIDs are not life-threatening, they have historically been given limited attention in Japan. However, their impact on patients' quality of life and social productivity has gained increasing recognition. Over the past three decades, a growing body of evidence has enhanced our understanding of FGIDs, leading to the development of effective therapeutic strategies. This chapter explains changes in symptom perception over time, gastrointestinal motility function test, brain-gut hormones and their functions, changes in transition of academic activities, and positioning of FGIDs defined by Rome IV criteria. The first conference of the Japanese Society of Neurogastroenterology was held in 2002, aimed to develop a new field of research called "neurogastroenterology." The diseases discussed in this book are centered around FGID/DGBI, with surrounding diseases primarily focused on gastrointestinal motility disorders (GIMDs). Recently, drugs targeting gut-brain hormone pathways have been developed for diabetes treatment, GIP/GLP-1 receptor agonists, which have appetite suppression as a side effect "physiological action." Advancements in gastrointestinal function tests have contributed to the understanding of pathophysiology and diagnosis. Further development of Neurogastroenterology, the study of FGID and related disorders, is expected in the future.

Keywords

Functional gastrointestinal disorders (FGIDs) · Disorders of gut-brain interaction (DGBI) · Gastrointestinal motility disorders (GIMDs) · Gastrointestinal Motility Function Test · Brain-Gut Hormones · Rome IV criteria · Neurogastroenterology

H. Kaneko (✉)
Division of Internal Medicine, Hoshigaoka Maternity Hospital, Nagoya, Japan
e-mail: hkaneko@fujita-hu.ac.jp

T. Chiba
Division of Internal Medicine, Department of Oral Medicine, Iwate Medical University, Morioka, Japan
e-mail: toschiba@iwate-med.ac.jp

H. Kaneko et al. (eds.), *Disorders of Gut-Brain Interaction*,
https://doi.org/10.1007/978-981-95-6974-8_2

1 Introduction

Significant advancements have been made in the diagnostic techniques for diseases associated with structural abnormalities, such as peptic ulcers, gastric cancer, inflammatory bowel disease, and colorectal cancer, in Japan. Gastrointestinal contrast imaging and gastrointestinal endoscopy are recognized as being at the forefront of global practice. However, clinical gastroenterology in Japan has traditionally placed a stronger emphasis on morphological diagnosis, with less attention paid to the functional aspects of the gastrointestinal tract.

In clinical practice, many patients presenting with chronic or recurrent abdominal pain as their primary complaint are diagnosed with irritable bowel syndrome (IBS). Additionally, more than half of those reporting epigastric pain or postprandial fullness are diagnosed with functional dyspepsia (FD). Both IBS and FD are classified as functional gastrointestinal disorders (FGIDs) or, more recently, disorders of gut-brain interaction (DGBI). These conditions are characterized by abdominal symptoms without detectable structural abnormalities that could explain the symptoms.

Functional dyspepsia was recognized as a reimbursable diagnosis in 2013, with the release of acotiamide—the only medication currently approved for FD under the national health insurance system in Japan. In clinical practice, FD patients were previously classified under the reimbursable diagnosis of "chronic gastritis (with associated upper abdominal complaints)." While this conventional diagnosis remains common, FD requires confirmation of the absence of mucosal abnormalities through endoscopic examination, reflecting the morphology-centric approach of Japanese gastroenterology.

Since FGIDs are not life-threatening, they have historically been given limited attention in Japan. However, their impact on patients' quality of life and social productivity has gained increasing recognition. Over the past three decades, a growing body of evidence has enhanced our understanding of FGIDs, leading to the development of effective therapeutic strategies.

This textbook focuses on FGIDs in the absence of morphological abnormalities and related gastrointestinal motility disorders (GIMDs), exploring their pathophysiology, diagnosis, and treatment strategies.

2 The Gap with Clinical Practice

In real-world clinical practice, among patients complaining of chronic heartburn, only a minority exhibit mucosal damage confirmed by endoscopy, such as erosive esophagitis or esophageal ulcers. The majority are diagnosed with non-erosive reflux disease (NERD). While a definitive diagnosis of NERD requires the presence of gastroesophageal reflux, in practice, NERD is often diagnosed when endoscopy reveals no mucosal injury and there is a positive response to acid-suppressive therapy.

NERD can be further classified based on esophageal pH and impedance monitoring results into two subgroups: those with confirmed excessive reflux of gastric contents (narrowly defined or true NERD) and those without excessive reflux, categorized as reflux hypersensitivity or functional heartburn [1].

In the treatment of functional gastrointestinal disorders (FGIDs), while gastrointestinal-targeted medications are typically the first-line therapy, psychosomatic approaches and psychotropic drugs (including anxiolytics and antidepressants) are recommended when symptoms do not improve. A survey targeting certified physicians in internal medicine in Japan revealed that 25.1% of doctors prescribed anxiolytics and 12.2% prescribed antidepressants for patients with functional dyspepsia (FD) [2]. Additionally, primary care physicians often emphasize psychological factors as a major cause of irritable bowel syndrome (IBS) [3].

However, many patients resist the interpretation of their condition as "psychological" and are reluctant to accept psychotropic medications. Clinicians need to be aware of this disconnect between their own understanding and the patient's perspective. Recognizing this gap is crucial to enhancing patient satisfaction, which is often used as an outcome measure in clinical research, despite the time constraints and practical challenges of routine clinical care.

3 Changes in Symptom Perception over Time

Epigastric pain and epigastric discomfort are common chief complaints (main worry) encountered in clinical practice. For patients experiencing chronic or recurrent symptoms, upper gastrointestinal endoscopy is often performed. When endoscopy does not reveal any mucosal abnormalities that explain the symptoms, a diagnosis of functional dyspepsia (FD) is made. However, in reality, treatment is typically provided under the reimbursable diagnosis of "chronic gastritis." [2]

Figure 2.1 illustrates the evolution in how dyspeptic symptoms without macroscopic mucosal abnormalities have been classified over time [4]. In the past, upper gastrointestinal barium studies were used to diagnose organic lesions, such as ulcerative or neoplastic conditions, as well as functional disorders like gastric ptosis and gastric spasm. The advent of advanced upper gastrointestinal endoscopy enabled direct mucosal observation, making it easier to diagnose chronic gastritis (endoscopic gastritis) based on findings of redness, swelling, and erosion.

At the same time, chronic gastritis with symptoms but without mucosal abnormalities—equivalent to symptomatic gastritis or today's FD—was also recognized. In 1988, a working group of the American Gastroenterological Association proposed the term *non-ulcer dyspepsia (NUD)* to describe a chronic condition involving upper gastrointestinal symptoms (including heartburn) in the absence of peptic ulcers. During this period, the prevailing theory attributed NUD primarily to gastrointestinal motility disorders.

From the late 1990s, research on the relationship between *Helicobacter pylori* (HP) and FD gained traction. NUD had a reflux-type subtype, but since *Rome II*, reflux-type dyspepsia has been classified separately as *gastroesophageal reflux disease (GERD)*. Additionally, the introduction of the concept of *visceral hypersensitivity* led to the inclusion of reflux hypersensitivity in *Rome IV*.

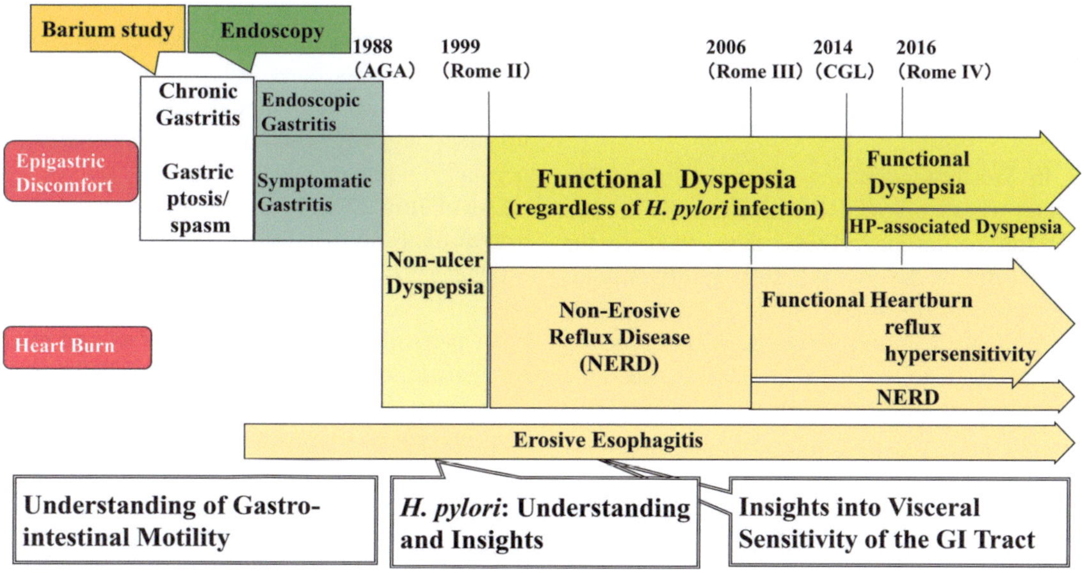

Fig. 2.1 Evolution of clinical diagnostic terminology for upper gastrointestinal symptoms. NUD non-ulcer dyspepsia, NERD non-erosive reflux disease, HP *Helicobacter pylori*, AGA American Gastroenterological Association, Rome Rome Committee, CGL clinical practice guidelines

For patients with positive HP infection, eradication therapy is the first-line treatment. If symptoms resolve following HP eradication, the condition is classified as *HP-associated dyspepsia*. The prokinetic agent *acotiamide*, effective for symptoms such as postprandial fullness, epigastric bloating, and early satiety in FD, was designated a first-line treatment in the 2021 *Clinical Guidelines for the Management of Functional Dyspepsia*.

Further changes in the understanding of FD, including its pathophysiology and therapeutic approaches, are anticipated as research and drug development continue to evolve.

4 Evolution of Gastrointestinal Motility Function Test

Figure 2.2 illustrates the historical progression of gastrointestinal motility function tests [5]. These tests for evaluating smooth muscle function can be broadly categorized into four groups:

1. Measurement of intraluminal pressures
2. Direct assessment of the movement of ingested contents
3. Evaluation of physiological and physical changes associated with content transit
4. Functional assessment except smooth muscle activity

In Western countries, micro-balloon techniques were employed as early as the 1950s [6]. Electrogastrography (EGG) dates back to the 1922 work of Alvarez [7], followed by studies by Sarna, Stern, Koch, Duthie [8], Hongo and Chen. Gastric motility was first observed by Beaumont, who studied a traumatic gastric fistula, and in 1833, he reported that emotions affected both acid secretion and gastric motility [9]. This observation can be considered one of the early reports in the field of Gastroenterological Psychosomatic Medicine. Later, in the 1960s, pressure radiotelemetry capsules were introduced [10], and from the 1970s to 1980s, gastrointestinal pressure measurement [11–13] and direct assessment of the movement of ingested materials became possible [14–16]. In the field of rectal and anal sphincter function test, pressure measurement techniques were reported in the late 1960s [17], and in the 1980s, defecography was introduced [18]. The 1990s saw reports on the use of barostats for the stomach and rectum [19, 20], leading to the introduction of concepts such as sensory dysfunction and visceral hypersensitivity in gastrointestinal disorders. High-resolution manometry (HRM) established normal pressure values for the rectum and anal canal [21].

Esophageal motility test, in particular, advanced significantly in 2000 with the development of esophageal topography and the adoption of high-resolution esophageal manometry, revealing new pathophysiological insights [22]. In 2008, the *Chicago Classification* was introduced [23], with the most recent *4th edition* classifying esophageal motility disorders into *Disorders of EGJ Outflow* and *Disorders of Peristalsis*, and a flowchart based on clinical findings is shown [24]. Additionally, 24-hour esophageal multicahnnel intraluminal impedance pH (MII-pH) monitoring have enabled the assessment of reflux types (liquid or gas) and the correlation between impedance changes (retrograde or antegrade) and symptoms [25].

The evaluation of visceral perception using evoked potentials dates back to the 1970s. In 2000, Kanazawa and Fukudo reported a method for assessing hypersensitivity in functional dyspepsia (FD) [26].

As of July 2025, insurance coverage for gastrointestinal motility test in Japan is limited to esophageal manometry, esophageal pH monitoring, and anorectal manometry. Manometry for other parts of the gastrointestinal tract and tests for gastric emptying using ^{13}C-labeled compounds or colonic transit time with radiopaque markers are not approved. Ultrasound-based gastric emptying tests and cine-MRI for small and large bowel motility are also excluded from coverage. Future research into FGIDs/DGBI will benefit from techniques like electroencephalography, single-photon emission computed tomography (SPECT), and functional magnetic resonance imaging (fMRI) [27, 28].

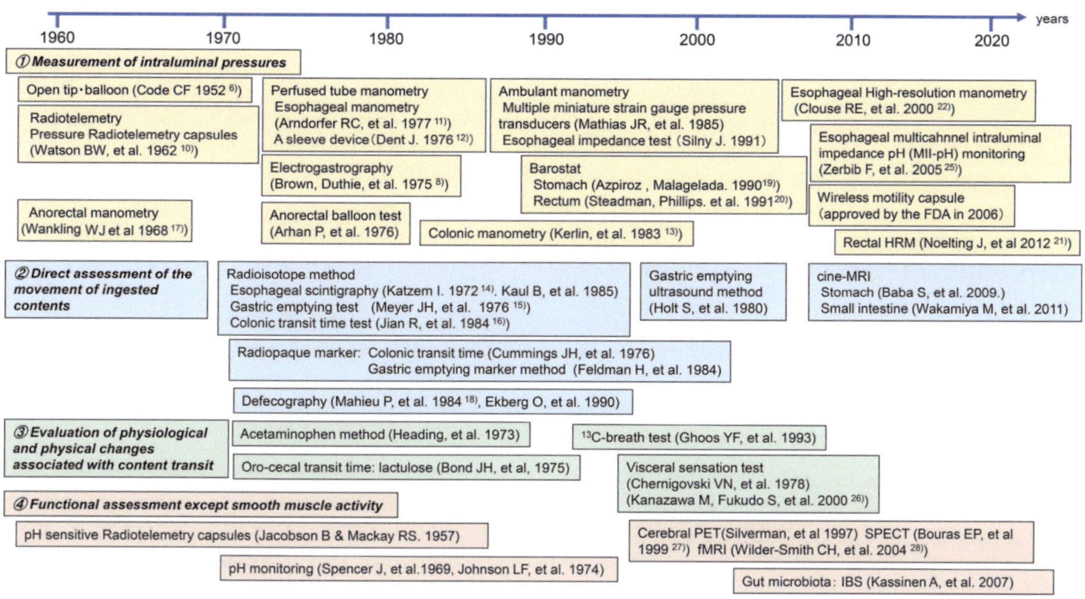

Fig. 2.2 Historical development of gastrointestinal motility function test. (Arhan P, et al. *Journal of Applied Physiology*. 1976;41:677–682, Baba S, et al. *Gastroenterology and Hepatology*. 2009;24:1401–1406, Bond JH, et al. *Journal of Laboratory and Clinical Medicine*. 1975;85:546–555, Chernigovskii VN, et al. *Neuroscience and Behavioral Physiology*. 1978;9:273–282, Cummings JH, et al. *American Journal of Clinical Nutrition*. 1976;29:1468–1473, Ekberg O, et al. *Radiology*. 1985;155:45–48, Feldman M, et al. *Gastroenterology*. 1984;87:895–902, Ghoos YF, et al. *Gastroenterology*. 1993;104:1640–1647, Heading RC, et al. *British Journal of Pharmacology*. 1973;47:415–421, Holt S, et al. *Digestive Diseases and Sciences*. 1990;35:1345–1351, Johnson LF, et al. *American Journal of Gastroenterology*. 1974;62:325–332, Kaul B, et al. *Scandinavian Journal of Gastroenterology*. 1986;21:31–34, Kassinen A, et al. *Gastroenterology*. 2007;133:24–33, Mackey RS, Jacobson B. *Nature*. 1957;179:1239–1240, Mathias JR, et al. *Gastroenterology*. 1985;88:101–107, Silverman DH, et al. *Gastroenterology*. 1997;112:64–72, Spencer J. *British Journal of Surgery*. 1969;56:912–914, Silny J. *Journal of Gastrointestinal Motility*. 1991;3:151–162, Wakamiya M, et al. *Japanese Magnetic Resonance Imaging*. 2011;33:1235–1240)

5 Brain-Gut Hormones

Enteroendocrine cells (EECs), dispersed throughout the gastrointestinal tract, make up approximately 1% of all mucosal cells. They respond to luminal stimuli, such as pH levels and nutrients like sugars and lipids, by secreting specific gut-brain hormones that regulate gastrointestinal motility, appetite, and hormone secretion (Table 2.1). Since the discovery of *secretin* in 1902, many hormones first identified in the gut were later found to exist in the brain as well, leading to their classification as *brain- gut hormones* (or alternatively, *gut hormones* or *gut peptides*). In the 1980s, numerous studies on gastrointestinal hormones were promoted, and among them, research on motilin-induced motility during the fasting period was led by Japan. Ghrelin, discovered in 1999, which has appetite-enhancing effects, is mainly found in the X/A--like cells of the gastric body, and its content is high in the intestines. As a result, the intestines have been referred to as the “second brain” or “little brain,” and embryologically, the intestines can be considered to have a central role. Currently, more than 20 types of brain-gut hormones are known, with roles in nutrition, digestion, absorption, and insulin secretion regulation. It has also been found that they play a role in regulating anxiety and depression. In recent years, the gut microbiota has been found to be deeply involved not only in intestinal diseases but also in cardiovascular diseases, kidney diseases, neurological disorders, neurodevelopmental disorders, and mental illnesses. In other words, the interaction

Table 2.1 Major enteroendocrine cell types, their localization, and functions

Cell type	Hormones produced	Localization	Primary functions
A	Ghrelin, Nesfatin	Stomach	Appetite regulation, growth hormone secretion
D	Somatostatin	Stomach, intestine	Inhibition of acid and insulin secretion
EC	Serotonin	Small and large intestine	Appetite regulation, gastrointestinal motility
G	Gastrin	Stomach	Stimulation of gastric acid secretion
I	Cholecystokinin	Proximal small intestine	Appetite regulation, bile secretion, GI motility
K	GIP (Glucose-dependent Insulinotropic Polypeptide)	Proximal small intestine	Insulin secretion
L	GLP-1, GLP-2, PYY, Oxyntomodulin	Terminal ileum, colon, rectum	Insulin secretion, appetite regulation, GI motility
M	Motilin	Small and large intestine	Gastrointestinal motility
N	Neurotensin	Ileum	Gastrointestinal motility
P	Leptin	Stomach	Appetite regulation
S	Secretin	Duodenum, small and large intestine	Pancreatic exocrine secretion (bicarbonate)

Adapted from: Laurila S, et al. "Pleiotropic Effects of Secretin: A Potential Drug Candidate in the Treatment of Obesity?" *Frontiers in Endocrinology (Lausanne)*. 2021;12:737686; Sun L-J, et al. "Gut hormones in microbiota-gut-brain cross-talk." *Chinese Medical Journal*. 2020;133:826–833

Abbreviations: *EC* enterochromaffin cells, *GIP* glucose-dependent insulinotropic polypeptide, *GLP* glucagon-like peptide, *PYY* peptide YY

between the gut microbiota, the intestines, and the brain is gaining attention.

From a therapeutic perspective, only a few of these hormones were available for clinical use until recently. Thyrotropin-releasing hormone (TRH) preparations, approved in 1978, have been used for spinocerebellar degeneration and prolonged consciousness disorders, while somatostatin analogs, introduced in 1989, are used to manage gastrointestinal symptoms in hormone-producing tumors and palliative care for gastrointestinal obstruction. More recently, drugs targeting gut-brain hormone pathways have been developed for diabetes treatment, including *GLP-1 receptor agonists (approved in 2021)* and *GIP/GLP-1 receptor agonists (approved in 2023)*. Notably, these medications have *appetite suppression* as a side effect (or physiological action).

6 The Transition of Academic Activities in Japan (Fig. 2.3)

The Japan Internatioinal Society of Gastroinetestinal Motility (JISGM; President: Takeshi Miwa, followed by Michio Hongo) was established in July 2008 as a related research association of the Japanese Gastroenterological Society, inheriting the "Gastrointestinal Motility Research Society," which had been active for about 6 years under the Japanese Society of Gastroenterology. The society aims to promote both basic and clinical research on gastrointestinal motility, while fostering the exchange of knowledge both domestically and internationally. It also strives to contribute to the improvement of human health and welfare. Annual meetings have been held every spring since the first meeting in April 2009. A heated debate also took place

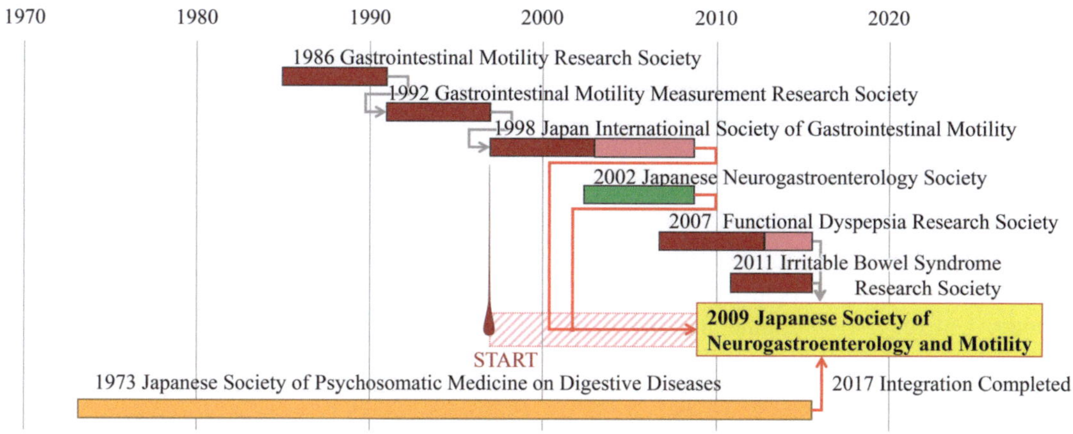

Fig. 2.3 Evolution of academic activity in Japan. (Modified with permission from Professor Michio Hongo, Tohoku University (Emeritus))

regarding whether the Japanese term for FD should be "functional dyspepsia" or "functional gastrointestinal disorder (in Japanese)."

The Japanese Society of Neurogastroenterology (President: Takeshi Miwa, later Nobuhiro Sato) focuses on the new perspective of the correlation between gastrointestinal and neurological functions, aiming to analyze the mechanisms of onset, progression, and healing of both functional and organic gastrointestinal diseases, as well as providing integrated understanding. The goal is to contribute to the clarification and treatment of gastrointestinal diseases. The first conference, held in October 2002, aimed to develop a new field of research called "neurogastroenterology." The proceedings, titled *Gastrointestinal Motility: Pursuing Invisible Gastrointestinal Diseases*, were published by Medical Review (Editors-in-Chief: Nobuhiro Sato; Editorial Board: Jun Kawano, Shigeru Harasawa, Michio Hongo, Kei Matsueda).

The Japanese Society of Psychosomatic Medicine on Digestive Diseases (JSPSMDD), originally the Gastrointestinal PSM Research Society (founded by Masayoshi Namiki), was launched in March 1973, holding biannual meetings in conjunction with the Japanese Society of Gastroenterology. Its purpose was to explore psychosomatic issues in gastrointestinal diseases and contribute to the development and improvement of clinical medicine. At the 44th meeting in 1994, Michio Hongo, former President of the Japanese Society of Neurogastroenterology and Motility, presented a topic on "Gastrointestinal Psychosomatic Disease—The Aspect of Functional Abnormalities," which was the same year the first edition of the Rome Criteria was published. Afterward, research presentations unraveling FGIDs from the perspective of brain-gut interaction and psychosomatic medicine became central. Starting from the 70th meeting in 2008, the society established the "Namiki Award" in honor of the late Professor Masayoshi Namiki, Emeritus Professor at Asahikawa Medical University, which is awarded to particularly outstanding oral presentations and contributes to the development of young researchers.

In April 2009, the Japanese Neurogastroenterology Society and JISGM merged to form the Japanese Society of Neurogastroenterology and Motility. The goal is to analyze the mechanisms of onset, progression, and healing of both functional and organic diseases of the gastrointestinal and nervous systems from the perspective of their functional correlations, and through integrated understanding, to contribute to the elucidation and treatment of gastrointestinal and neurological pathologies. The 11th conference of the Japanese Society of Neurogastroenterology and Motility was held in September 2009. Additionally, in 2017, the previously separate research societies for functional dyspepsia (FD), JSPSMDD, and IBS were integrated into one unified entity.

7 Positioning of Functional Gastrointestinal Disorders (FGID) Defined by Rome IV Criteria and Related Disorders

The concept of functional gastrointestinal disorders (FGIDs) is driven by the understanding that these conditions involve both motility and perception. Unlike gastrointestinal motility disorders (GIMDs), the concept of functional diseases requires the involvement of central mechanisms, particularly when peripheral hypersensitivity alone cannot explain the symptoms. DGBI (Disorders of Gut-Brain Interaction) can be understood as a concept that includes the involvement of central functions for conditions that cannot be explained by peripheral hypersensitivity.

The diseases discussed in this book are centered around "Functional Gastrointestinal Disorders: FGID" (also referred to as Disorders of Gut-Brain Interaction: DGBI in Rome IV), with surrounding diseases primarily focused on gastrointestinal motility disorders (GIMD), as illustrated in Fig. 2.4. "Functional Gastrointestinal Disorders (DGBI in Rome IV)" are conditions where no significant morphological abnormalities are seen at the macro level, and symptoms are thought to arise due to interactions between the gut and the brain. On the other hand, diseases that present some abnormal findings on simple X-rays, CT scans, gastrointestinal endoscopy, or gastrointestinal imaging tests, and where gastrointestinal motility dysfunction is recognized, are categorized as "Gastrointestinal Motility Disorders (GIMD)."

Non-erosive gastroesophageal reflux disease (NERD), non-cardiac chest pain, rectocele, and rectal prolapse are not considered GIMD, but are included in this book as peripheral disorders of FGID, considering clinical practices.

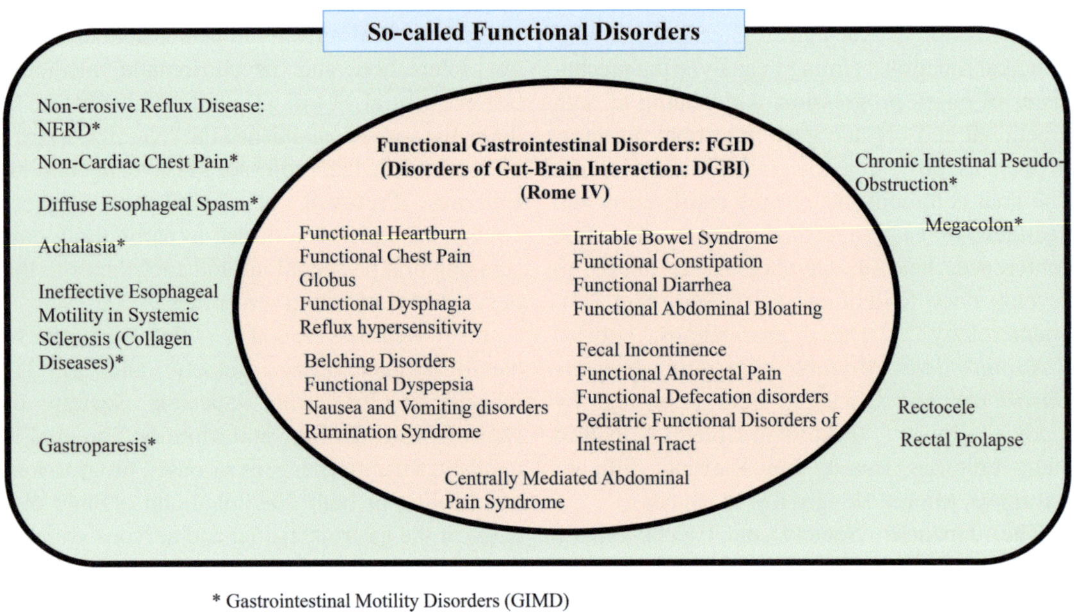

Fig. 2.4 Functional gastrointestinal disorders and related conditions covered in this text book

8 Summary

FGID is defined by the Rome criteria, which have been updated through revisions. There has been a shift toward using the term "Gut-Brain Interaction Disorders (DGBI)" or brain-gut interaction diseases in the diagnosis. Additionally, advancements in gastrointestinal function tests have contributed to the understanding of pathophysiology and diagnosis. While neurogastroenterology, the study of FGIDs and related disorders, has flourished in Europe and the USA, the history of this field is still relatively short in Japan, and further development is expected in the future.

Competing Interests The author(s) has no competing interests to declare that are relevant to the content of this manuscript.

References

1. Aziz Q. Gastroenterology. 2016;150:1368–79.
2. Kaneko H, et al. J Neurogastroenterol Motil. 2014;20:94–103.
3. Mujagic Z, et al. Eur J Gastroenterol Hepatol. 2017;29:651–6.
4. Kaneko H. Psychosom Gastroenterol. 2014;21:28–32. (in Japanese)
5. Kumar D, Wingate DL, editors. An illustrated guide to gastrointestinal motility. 2nd Edition. Churchill Livingstone, London, UK; 1993. p. 165–318.
6. Code CF. Am J Med. 1952;13:328–51.
7. Alvarez WC. JAMA. 1922;78:1116–8.
8. Brown BH, et al. Med Biol Eng. 1975;13:97–103.
9. Haubrich WS. Gastroenterology. 1999;116:14. (Original: Beaumont W. New York: Plattsburgh, 1833)
10. Watson BW, et al. Gut. 1962;3:181–6.
11. Arndorfer RC, et al. Gastroenterology. 1977;73:23–7.
12. Dent J. Gastroenterology. 1976;71:263–7.
13. Kerlin P, et al. Aust NZ J Med. 1983;13:591–3.
14. Katzem I. AJR Am J Roentgenol. 1972;115:681–9.
15. Meyer JH, et al. Am J Dig Dis. 1976;21:296–304.
16. Jian R, et al. Gut. 1984;25:728–31.
17. Wankling WJ, et al. Gut. 1968;9:457–60.
18. Mahieu P, et al. Gastrointest Radiol. 1984;9:253–61.
19. Azpiroz F, et al. Gastroenterology. 1990;98:1193–8.
20. Steadman CJ, et al. Gastroenterology. 1991;101:37 3–81.
21. Noelting J, et al. Am J Gastroenterol. 2012;107:15 30–6.
22. Clouse RE, et al. Am J Gastroenterol. 2000;95:2 720–30.
23. Kahrilas PJ, et al. J Clin Gastroenterol. 2008;42:6 27–35.
24. Yadlapati R, et al. Neurogastroenterol Motil. 2020;33:e 14058.
25. Zerbib F, et al. Aliment Pharmacol Ther. 2005;22:10 11–21.
26. Kanazawa M, et al. Neurogastroenterol Motil. 2000;12:87–94.
27. Bouras EP, et al. Am J Physiol. 1999;277:G687–94.
28. Wilder-Smith CH, et al. Gut. 2004;53:1595–601.

Part II

Esophagus, Basic Edition

Esophagus, Anatomy, Physiology of Gastrointestinal Motility, Peptides

3

Takatsugu Yamamoto

Abstract

This review provides an integrated overview of esophageal anatomy and the physiology of gastrointestinal motility, as well as the role of ion channels in digestive function. The esophagus is a muscular tube that connects the pharynx to the stomach and facilitates the transport of food via coordinated peristaltic movements. Gastrointestinal motility is regulated by complex neural and hormonal mechanisms to ensure the proper propulsion and mixing of contents within the digestive tract. Recent studies have revealed that ion channels play a critical role in modulating motility, sensation and other esophageal functions. Understanding the interplay between anatomical structures and the role of ion channels is essential for comprehending normal gastrointestinal function and the pathophysiology of motility disorders. This review highlights recent advances in this area of research.

Keywords

Anatomy · Nervous system · Motility · Upper esophageal sphincter · Lower esophageal sphincter · Visceral sensation · Ion channel

T. Yamamoto (✉)
Division of Gastroenterology, Department of Medicine, Teikyo University School of Medicine, Tokyo, Japan
e-mail: ymmt@med.teikyo-u.ac.jp

1 Anatomy of the Esophagus

The esophagus is a muscular, tubular organ approximately 25 cm in length, extending from the pharynx to the stomach. It originates at the inferior margin of the cricoid cartilage, corresponding to the level of the sixth cervical vertebra, traverses the esophageal hiatus of the diaphragm, and terminates at the gastric cardia around the level of the eleventh to twelfth thoracic vertebrae.

Anatomically, the esophagus is divided into three regions: cervical, thoracic, and abdominal. The cervical esophagus (Ce), measuring approximately 5–6 cm, extends from the inferior border of the cricoid cartilage to the superior margin of the sternum. Situated anterior to the vertebral column and posterior to the trachea, it is closely associated with vital neurovascular structures. The recurrent laryngeal nerve courses between the trachea and esophagus, while the common carotid arteries, internal jugular veins, and vagus nerves lie bilaterally.

The thoracic esophagus (Te), approximately 15–18 cm in length, spans from the upper border of the sternum to the diaphragm and is further subdivided into three segments: the upper thoracic esophagus (Ut) near the tracheal bifurcation, the middle thoracic esophagus (Mt), and the lower thoracic esophagus (Lt). This segment descends posterior to the trachea and heart, gradually shifting from the right to the

H. Kaneko et al. (eds.), *Disorders of Gut-Brain Interaction*,
https://doi.org/10.1007/978-981-95-6974-8_3

left of the descending aorta, and enters the abdominal cavity through the esophageal hiatus anterior to the aorta.

The abdominal esophagus (Ae), the shortest segment, extends 2–3 cm from the esophageal hiatus to the gastric cardia.

When empty, the esophagus appears flattened in the anteroposterior dimension but dilates to accommodate ingested material. Three physiological constrictions are observed along its course: the upper esophageal constriction, located approximately 15 cm from the incisors at the pharyngoesophageal junction (also referred to as the cricopharyngeal constriction), results from the contraction of the lower pharyngeal constrictor muscle anchored to the cricoid cartilage; the aortic constriction, approximately 25 cm from the incisors, where the esophagus is compressed by the aortic arch and left main bronchus; and the diaphragmatic constriction, approximately 40 cm from the incisors, where the esophagus traverses the diaphragm. These constrictions are common sites for the impaction or delayed passage of ingested material [1].

2 Structure of the Esophageal Wall

The esophageal wall, measuring approximately 4–5 mm in thickness, exhibits a concentric, layered organization characteristic of hollow viscera. From the lumen outward, it comprises the mucosa, submucosa, muscularis propria, and adventitia.

The mucosa consists of three components: the stratified squamous epithelial lining, adapted to withstand mechanical stress; the lamina propria, composed of loose connective tissue rich in capillaries and lymphatic vessels; and the muscularis mucosae, a thin layer of smooth muscle demarcating the boundary between the mucosa and submucosa.

The submucosa contains loose connective tissue interwoven with elastic fibers, blood vessels, lymphatics, nerves, and the intrinsic esophageal glands. Neural elements, including the submucosal (Meissner's) plexus, are implicated in regulating muscularis mucosae motility and glandular secretion.

The muscularis propria is notably more developed than in other regions of the gastrointestinal tract, especially the outer longitudinal muscle layer. The upper esophagus is composed predominantly of striated muscle, transitioning to smooth muscle distally. Interposed between the inner circular and outer longitudinal muscle layers is the myenteric (Auerbach's) plexus, which coordinates esophageal motility.

Unlike most gastrointestinal organs, the esophagus lacks a serosal covering; instead, its outer surface is enveloped by an adventitia composed of connective tissue that loosely anchors it to adjacent structures.

A distinctive feature of the esophagus is the presence of specialized sphincters at both ends. The upper esophageal sphincter (UES) functions primarily through the synergistic action of the lower pharyngeal constrictor and cricopharyngeal muscles, controlling the entry of material into the esophagus. The lower esophageal sphincter (LES), formed by thickened circular smooth muscle fibers and augmented by the diaphragmatic crura, maintains a resting pressure of approximately 20 mmHg over a 4 cm segment. This sphincter prevents gastroesophageal reflux under resting conditions and relaxes during swallowing to permit the passage of food into the stomach [2].

3 Blood Supply and Lymphatic Drainage of the Esophagus

The arterial blood supply to the esophagus is segmentally distributed. The upper third receives blood from the inferior thyroid arteries, branches of the thyrocervical trunk originating from the subclavian arteries. The middle third is vascularized by esophageal branches arising from the thoracic aorta, whereas the lower third is supplied by branches of the left gastric artery, itself a branch of the celiac trunk.

Venous drainage parallels the arterial supply. Blood from the upper third drains into the inferior thyroid veins, from the middle third into the azygos and hemiazygos veins, and from the lower third into the left gastric vein. Notably, anastomotic connections between the azygos system and the portal circulation via the left gastric vein create a potential collateral pathway.

In conditions of portal hypertension, such as liver cirrhosis, increased portal pressure diverts blood through these anastomoses into the systemic circulation. As a consequence, submucosal veins in the distal esophagus become dilated, leading to the formation of esophageal varices, which are prone to life-threatening hemorrhage.

4 Nervous System of the Esophagus

The nervous system of the digestive tract comprises extrinsic sensory nerves, including sympathetic and parasympathetic fibers, with their neuronal bodies located outside the tract. Sympathetic innervation consists of adrenergic neurons that terminate via preganglionic fibers within the enteric plexuses, exerting their effects there. Parasympathetic innervation is mediated by cholinergic neurons, which form synapses within these plexuses. Gastrointestinal motility is regulated by the interplay between adrenergic inhibitory nerves and cholinergic excitatory nerves.

In the esophagus, parasympathetic innervation is primarily provided by the vagus nerve, composed of afferent fibers that transmit information to the central nervous system (entering the nucleus of the solitary tract) and efferent fibers arising from the dorsal motor nucleus of the medulla oblongata. The vagus nerves descend dorsally to the bronchi, traveling along the esophagus to the abdominal cavity. Within the esophagus, they branch into several trunks to form the esophageal plexus, which also communicates with sympathetic fibers, notably from the greater splanchnic nerve [2].

The upper and lower regions of the esophagus exhibit distinct patterns of innervation. The muscle layer of the upper esophagus consists of striated muscle, primarily innervated by lower motor neurons originating from the nucleus ambiguus and the facial motor nucleus of the brainstem. Acetylcholine serves as the neurotransmitter responsible for contraction in this region. Electrical stimulation of the vagus nerve induces simultaneous contractions in both the proximal and distal esophagus. Bilateral central transection of the vagus nerve abolishes peristalsis, whereas unilateral transection preserves it, suggesting extensive cross-innervation within the esophageal wall. Although inhibitory innervation was once thought to be absent in the striated muscle region, recent studies have identified its presence [3].

By contrast, the muscle layer of the middle and lower esophagus is composed of smooth muscle. Movement in these regions is governed not only by central mechanisms but also by the intrinsic enteric nervous system within the gut wall. Neurons originating in the dorsal motor nucleus of the vagus nerve act through postganglionic fibers to initiate and propagate primary peristaltic waves. Electrical stimulation of the vagus nerve in the smooth muscle portion elicits peristaltic waves with a distinct time lag between proximal and distal contractions, in contrast to the simultaneous contraction observed in the striated portion. Notably, peristaltic waves can still be induced by electrical stimulation of the esophagus even after extrinsic nerve inputs are severed, implicating a significant role for intrinsic neural circuits. Furthermore, direct stimulation of the smooth muscle layer can generate peristaltic waves independently of neural control, as demonstrated by experiments using pharmacologic blockade. In the smooth muscle region, acetylcholine serves as the primary excitatory neurotransmitter, while nitric oxide (NO) functions as the principal inhibitory mediator. Other neurotransmitters, including substance P, vasoactive intestinal peptide (VIP), and adenosine triphosphate (ATP), have also been implicated. Dual innervation by excitatory and inhibitory nerves leads to initial relaxation followed by contraction upon vagal stimulation, contributing to the observed time lag in peristaltic propagation [4].

In addition to extrinsic sensory nerves, the digestive tract possesses an intrinsic nervous system comprising the myenteric plexus, located between the longitudinal and circular muscle layers, and the submucosal plexus, which is involved in regulating mucosal function. These plexuses are interconnected via neural anastomoses and operate in concert.

5 Movement of Upper Esophageal Sphincter

UES exhibits sphincter function through coordinated movement among related muscle groups. It shows high pressure over approximately 4 cm at rest, referred to as the upper esophageal high-pressure zone. Its primary roles are to prevent air inflow into the esophagus during inspiration when intrathoracic pressure becomes negative and to prevent reflux of contents into the pharyngolarynx during peristalsis.

UES is significantly involved in swallowing. Swallowing is divided into three phases: the oral phase (first phase), where the bolus is voluntarily transferred from the oral cavity to the pharynx; the pharyngeal phase (second phase), where the bolus is involuntarily transferred through the relaxed UES to the upper esophagus; and the esophageal phase (third phase), where the bolus is transferred through the LES into the stomach. During the pharyngeal phase, the following processes occur: (1) the tongue pushes the bolus into the oropharynx, (2) the soft palate closes the nasopharynx, and the epiglottis begins to tilt downward, (3) the soft palate approaches the tongue root, the contraction of the superior pharyngeal constrictor muscle closes the oropharyngeal cavity, the airway is closed by the epiglottis, and the UES relaxes, (4) the bolus enters the esophagus.

The lower pharyngeal constrictor muscle and cricopharyngeal muscle, which form the UES, perform delicate and precise coordinated movements with muscles related to the pharyngeal phase, such as the suprahyoid muscles (geniohyoid, mylohyoid, digastric), extrinsic tongue muscles (styloglossus, hyoglossus), soft palate muscles, and middle pharyngeal constrictor muscle controlling pharyngeal movement. This complex movement is executed as a swallowing reflex in the swallowing center, primarily located in the nucleus ambiguus and solitary nucleus of the medulla oblongata. Stimulation of the swallowing reflex induction site by the bolus activates the central pattern generator (CPG). The CPG triggers patterned swallowing reflexes in the motor nervous system executing swallowing movements and also acts on the respiratory center to cause temporary cessation of breathing during swallowing [5].

6 Movement of Esophageal Body

In the esophageal body, peristalsis occurs when the intestinal tract stretches due to food. Contraction on the oral side and relaxation on the anal side occur, causing a contraction wave to move from the oral side to the anal side, thereby moving the contents towards the anus. When the smooth muscle of the intestinal tract is excited, the peristaltic movement is transmitted continuously through nerve stimulation or intercellular gap junctions.

In the esophagus, the primary stimulus for peristalsis is swallowing, and the peristaltic wave that occurs with swallowing is called the primary peristaltic wave. During swallowing, the contraction of the pharynx causes the UES to relax, allowing the bolus to enter the esophagus, and the bolus is then transported towards the stomach by the peristaltic wave. The LES relaxes during swallowing, facilitating the entry of the bolus into the stomach. The transmission speed of the primary peristaltic wave is 2.5–5 cm/sec, faster in the middle esophagus and slightly slower in the upper and lower esophagus. The average pressure is higher in the lower esophagus, averaging around 70 mmHg [6]. The transmission speed and contraction pressure are influenced by the quantity, nature, and temperature of the bolus; larger quantities slow the transmission speed and increase the contraction pressure [7]. Secondary peristaltic waves are those induced by stimuli such as the stretching of the esophageal wall, unrelated to swallowing.

Contraction of the esophageal longitudinal muscle shortens the esophagus, simultaneously increasing the lumen diameter and volume. The increase in diameter lowers the local internal pressure, suppressing the rise in internal pressure during circular muscle contraction. The longitudinal muscle is innervated by the vagus nerve, with acetylcholine as the primary neurotransmitter. Additionally, the involvement of substance P released from capsaicin-sensitive neurons has been reported [8, 9].

7 Movement of Lower Esophageal Sphincter

The LES maintains a higher resting pressure compared to other parts of the esophagus, preventing the reflux of food and gastric acid into the esophagus (see figure 1 in GI Motility Online, "Sphincter mechanisms at the lower end of the esophagus," Mittal & Goyal, May 2006; https://doi.org/10.1038/gimo14). Both myogenic and neurogenic elements are involved, with high resting membrane potential and significant depolarization in the muscle cells, and clear intercellular signaling pathways [4]. The lower esophageal sphincter is innervated similarly to the lower esophagus, with dual innervation by excitatory and inhibitory systems via postganglionic nerves. Additionally, the interdigestive migrating myoelectrical contraction (IMMC) originates from the LES [10]. IMMC involves strong contraction waves that start from the LES and propagate through the stomach to the anal side of the small intestine, lasting about 20 minutes after a resting period of approximately 70–80 minutes. IMMC is regulated by the gastrointestinal hormone motilin and is thought to prepare the digestive tract for the next intake of food by clearing intestinal contents towards the anus.

The diaphragmatic crura surround the esophagogastric junction, working together with the lower esophageal sphincter to perform sphincter functions. The diaphragm is composed of striated muscle and is innervated by the phrenic nerve. When abdominal pressure rises rapidly, the diaphragmatic crura contract quickly, increasing the pressure at the esophagogastric junction and preventing reflux. The diaphragmatic crura relax along with the contraction of the esophageal longitudinal muscle in response to swallowing or stretching of the esophageal wall.

The LES relaxes in response to swallowing or pharyngeal stimulation. Relaxation begins within 2 seconds after swallowing and lasts for about 6–10 seconds until the peristaltic wave reaches the LES. After relaxation, a post-relaxation contraction occurs for about 10 seconds [11]. In addition to swallowing, LES relaxation can be induced by vagal nerve stimulation or stretching of the esophageal body, with nitric oxide (NO) being the primary neurotransmitter involved.

LES relaxation can also be induced by gastric distension, a phenomenon unrelated to swallowing known as transient lower esophageal sphincter relaxation (TLESR), which is considered the mechanism of belching. TLESR is defined by the following criteria: (1) no swallowing before or after the onset of LES relaxation, (2) LES pressure decreases by more than 1 mmHg/sec, (3) complete relaxation within 10 seconds of the onset of LES relaxation, and (4) minimum LES pressure during relaxation is less than 2 mmHg [12]. During TLESR, the lower esophageal sphincter relaxes simultaneously with the relaxation of the diaphragmatic crura and contraction of the longitudinal muscle, shortening the esophagus and opening the esophagogastric junction. TLESR lasts longer than LES relaxation associated with swallowing, typically 10–45 seconds, and is related to gastric acid reflux. Most gastroesophageal reflux in healthy individuals is associated with this phenomenon [13]. TLESR is induced by vagal nerve stimulation, with NO involved in the relaxation of the lower esophageal sphincter and diaphragmatic crura. Additionally, drugs such as γ-aminobutyric acid (GABA) agonists, glutamate, cannabinoid receptor agonists, cholecystokinin A receptor antagonists, atropine, and morphine have been reported to reduce the frequency of TLESR by mechanisms such as decreased sensitivity of pressure receptors to gastric distension, inhibition of the dorsal motor nucleus of the vagus nerve, and inhibition of motor neurons in the esophageal wall [4].

8 Transmission of Visceral Sensation and Ion Channels

Afferent sensory stimuli from the digestive tract to the central nervous system are transmitted via sensory neurons of the spinal nerves and neurons of the spinal dorsal horn, through the contralateral spinothalamic tract and spinal reticular tract to the thalamus, and projected to the somatosensory area, insula, and prefrontal cortex. Central nervous system excitation activates inhibitory systems, suppressing visceral perception through endogenous opioids, noradrenaline, and serotonin neurons. Additionally, direct physical and chemical stimulation of the digestive tract mucosa activates the vagal afferent pathway, triggering the synthesis of various neurotransmitters in the brain [14].

Recently, various ion channels have been shown to play important roles in the physiology and pathology of visceral sensation transmission, particularly in pain onset. These channels have attracted attention as therapeutic and drug development targets. Among them, transient receptor potential (TRP) channels are expressed not only in nerve cells but also in the epithelial cells of the digestive tract mucosa.

In the esophageal mucosa, epithelial cells express calcium-sensing receptors (CaSR), protease-activated receptors (PAR2), epithelial sodium channels (ENaC), acid-sensing ion channels (ASIC), and TRP channels. TRP channels are non-selective cation channels with six transmembrane domains. TRPV1 (TRP vanilloid 1) was cloned in 1997 as a temperature-sensitive TRP channel. TRPV1 is hypothesized to function as a pain receptor, leading to the discovery of other TRP channel superfamily members. Currently, the TRP channel superfamily in mammals includes 28 members divided into six subfamilies: ankyrin (TRPA1), canonical (TRPC1–7), melastatin (TRPM1–8), mucolipin (TRPML1–3), polycystin (TRPP1–3), and vanilloid (TRPV1–6). These channels are present in almost all cells in the body, including the digestive tract, and are implicated in maintaining homeostasis and the onset of various diseases, although many aspects remain unclear [15].

In the digestive tract, multiple TRP channels are expressed in nerves and mucosal epithelial cells. TRPV1 activation occurs due to temperature, acid, and capsaicin, with these stimuli perceived as pain via extrinsic sensory nerves derived from the vagus nerve of the stomach and esophagus. Regarding high-temperature stimuli, the activation temperature threshold for TRPV1 is about 43 °C, above body temperature. However, during inflammation, TRPV1 sensitization by inflammation-related mediators released from the injury site lowers the temperature threshold, causing activation and pain at normal body temperature. Additionally, TRPV1 activation increases intracellular Ca^{2+} concentration, releasing calcitonin gene-related peptide (CGRP) and substance P, which enhance vasodilation and vascular permeability. This mechanism is hypothesized to contribute to symptom onset in functional gastrointestinal disorders. In functional dyspepsia, increased TRPV1 responsiveness to capsaicin has been reported. In patients with gastroesophageal reflux disease (GERD), excessive TRPV1 expression in the esophageal mucosa is suggested to cause hypersensitivity to acid reflux [15].

TRPA1 is primarily expressed in extrinsic sensory nerves and is activated by noxious cold stimuli below 17 °C, food components like wasabi, and inflammation-related mediators. TRPA1 and TRPV1 interact to increase sensory nerve sensitivity. Allyl isothiocyanate, a TRPA1 agonist, activates mechanical stimulus transmission via sensory and pelvic nerves, with this response absent in TRPA1 gene-deficient animals, suggesting its role in visceral sensation to mechanical stimuli. TRPA1 is also expressed in non-neuronal cells like epithelial and enterochromaffin (EC) cells, implicating its involvement in gastric emptying [16].

TRPV4 is expressed not only in extrinsic sensory nerves but also in esophageal epithelial cells, influencing a wide range of functions, including mechanical stimuli and wound healing. TRPV4-regulating drugs are expected to be effective in treating heart failure, respiratory diseases, gastrointestinal diseases, arthritis, and other conditions [17].

GERD is a multifactorial disease triggered by gastric acid, mechanical stimuli, and thermal stimuli, with ion channel changes reported to influence its development. TRPV2 is highly expressed in the enteric nervous system and is suggested to be involved in esophageal motility. Particularly in the lower esophageal sphincter (LES), TRPV2 expression is thought to cause NO-mediated relaxation, leading to acid reflux. TRPC is expressed in the vagus nerve, enteric nervous system, smooth muscle cells, and interstitial cells of Cajal, suggesting some involvement. Additionally, TRPM4 and TRPV2 are sensitized by inflammation-related mediators released from specialized mast cells infiltrating the digestive tract, resulting in nerve activation and further mast cell activation, indicating an interaction [18]. TRPV3 and TRPM5 are also highly expressed in the digestive tract, although their details remain unclear, warranting further investigation.

9 Summary

This chapter provided an overview of the anatomy and physiology of esophageal motility. It covers the fundamental knowledge of esophageal movement. Ion channels, which have recently gained attention and are accumulating information, are currently being actively researched, and future research outcomes are anticipated.

Competing Interests The author(s) has no competing interests to declare that are relevant to the content of this manuscript.

References

1. Ito T, revised by Takano H. Esophagus. In: Anatomy lecture, 3rd ed. Nanzando; 2012. p. 282–5. (in Japanese).
2. Supervised by Honma K. General principles of digestion and absorption. In: Standard physiology. 9th ed. Igaku-Shoin; 2019. p. 830–49. (in Japanese).
3. Kallmunzer B, et al. Enteric co-innervation of striated muscle fibres in human oesophagus. Neurogastroenterol Motil. 2008;29:597–610.
4. Kuribayashi Y, et al. Understanding gastrointestinal contraction function for gastrointestinal disorders; Esophageal motility. J Jpn Soc Gastroenterol. 2021;118:114–25. (in Japanese)
5. Supervised by Honma K. Ingestion and transport of food. In: Standard physiology, 9th ed. Igaku-Shoin; 2019. p. 850–4. (in Japanese).
6. Hollis JB, et al. Effect of dry swallows and wet swallows of different volumes on esophageal peristalsis. J Appl Physiol. 1975;38:1161–4.
7. Ren J, et al. Determinants of intrabolus pressure during esophageal peristatic bolus transport. Am J Phys. 1993;264:G407–13.
8. Sugarbaker DJ, et al. Swallowing induces sequential activation of esophageal longitudinal smooth muscle. Am J Phys. 1984;247:G515–9.
9. Cris J, et al. Role of substance P nerves in longitudinal smooth muscle contractions of the esophagus. Am J Phys. 1986;250:G336–43.
10. Dent J, et al. Interdigestive phasic contractions of the human lower esophageal sphincter. Gastroenterology. 1983;84:453–60.
11. Mittal RK, et al. Characteristics of lower esophageal sphincter relaxation induced by pharyngeal stimulation with minute amounts of water. Gastroenterology. 1996;111:378–84.
12. Holloway RH, et al. Criteria for objective definition of transient lower esophageal sphincter relaxation. Am J Phys. 1995;268:G128–33.
13. Dodds WJ, et al. Mechanisms of gastroesophageal reflux in patients with reflux esophagitis. N Engl J Med. 1982;307:1547–52.
14. Kanazawa M, et al. Changes in the central nervous system - brain-gut axis brain function imaging in functional gastrointestinal disorders. J Jpn Soc Gastroenterol. 2013;102:17–24. (in Japanese)
15. Boudaka A, et al. Physiological and pathological significance of esophageal TRP channels: special focus on TRPV4 in esophageal epithelial cells. Int J Mol Sci. 2022;23(9):4550.
16. Guarino MPL, et al. Increased TRPV1 gene expression in esophageal mucosa of patients with non-erosive and erosive reflux disease. Neurogastroenterol Motil. 2010;22:746–52.
17. Ueda T, et al. TRPV4 channel is a novel regulator of intracellular Ca2+ in human esophageal epithelial cells. Am J Physiol Gastrointest Liver Physiol. 2011;301:G138–47.
18. van Diest SA, et al. Relevance of mast cell-nerve interactions in intestinal nociception. Biochim Biophys Acta. 2012;1822:74–84.

4 Esophageal Motility Test, Esophageal Manometry

Shiko Kuribayashi

Abstract

Esophageal manometry evaluates the motility of the esophageal body and the swallow-related relaxation of the esophagogastric junction (EGJ) to diagnose esophageal motility. There are two pressure measurement systems: water-perfused system and intraluminal transducer system. Conventional manometry measuring pressures at several sites of the esophagus used to be performed. Nowadays high-resolution manometry (HRM) measuring pressures at 1–2 cm apart is a gold standard to evaluate esophageal motility. Location of the EGJ is changed with respiration; therefore, a single sensor cannot measure pressure of the EGJ continuously. The sleeve sensor which has a 6 cm pressure-sensitive membrane using the water-perfused system is developed to measure pressure of the EGJ continuously. E-sleeve function with HRM allows measuring pressure of the EGJ continuously.

The Chicago Classification is a systematical classification of esophageal motility disorders. There are several parameters evaluating esophageal motility: integrated relaxation pressure (IRP) for swallow-related EGJ relaxation, distal contractile integral (DCI) for esophageal contraction vigor, contractile front velocity (CFV) for velocity of peristalsis, and distal latency (DL) for latency between swallow and the time peristalsis reaches the distal esophagus. When there is a large break in peristalsis, CFV cannot assess the velocity of peristalsis precisely. Thus, CFV is no longer used, and DL is used to evaluate presence of spasm in the Chicago Classification v4.0.

Keywords

Esophageal motility · Esophageal manometry · Sleeve sensor · Conventional manometry · High-resolution esophageal manometry · Chicago classification

S. Kuribayashi (✉)
Department of Gastroenterology and Hepatology, Gunma University Graduate School of Medicine, Maebashi, Japan
e-mail: shikokuri@gunma-u.ac.jp

H. Kaneko et al. (eds.), *Disorders of Gut-Brain Interaction*,
https://doi.org/10.1007/978-981-95-6974-8_4

1 Esophageal Motility

Esophageal manometry evaluates the motility of the esophageal body and the swallow-related relaxation of the esophagogastric junction (EGJ), diagnosing esophageal motility disorders.

1.1 Motility of the Esophageal Body

After swallowing, a peristaltic contraction propagates from the top to the bottom of the esophagus, known as the primary peristalsis (Fig. 4.1). In contrast, a peristalsis can occur independently of swallowing, referred to as secondary peristalsis, which is induced by distension stimuli. Primary peristalsis is basically evaluated to diagnose esophageal motility disorders, although abnormalities in secondary peristalsis could be found.

1.2 Motility of the Esophagogastric Junction

The EGJ, comprising the lower esophageal sphincter (LES) and the diaphragmatic crura, typically forms a high-pressure zone preventing gastric contents from refluxing (Fig. 4.1). After swallowing, the EGJ transiently relaxes, allowing the bolus propelled by the primary peristalsis to enter the stomach (Fig. 4.2). In achalasia, this swallow-related relaxation of the EGJ is impaired.

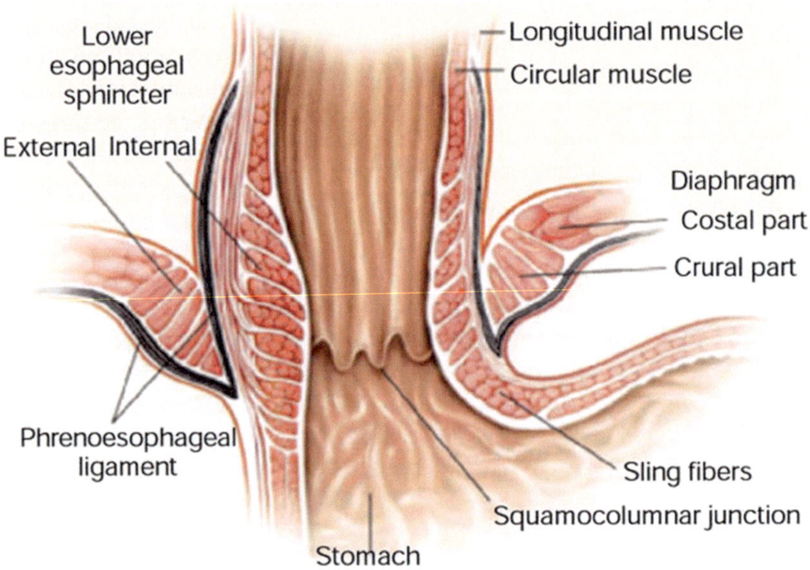

Fig. 4.1 Structure of the esophagus and primary peristalsis detected by esophageal manometry. (GI Motility online (May 2006) | https://doi.org/10.1038/gimo14)

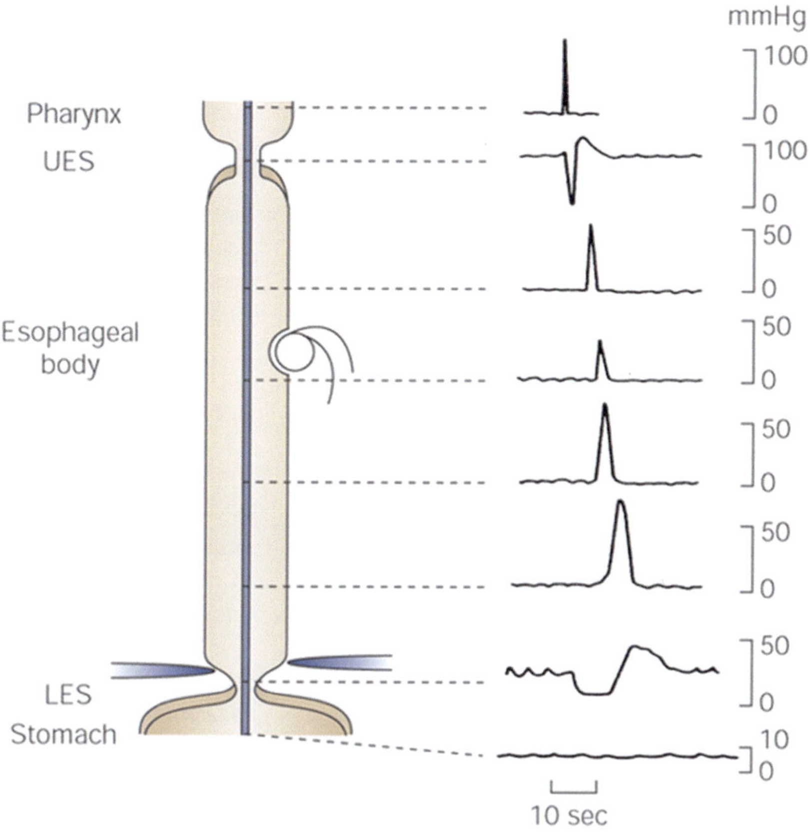

Fig. 4.2 Structure of the sleeve sensor. (Kenji Tsuneoka et al., *Upper Gastrointestinal Motility Disorders: Pathophysiology and Treatment*, Bunkodo; 1985 (in Japanese)). In the water-perfused system, a small amount of water flows through the catheter, and the pressure preventing the water flow is measured. A sleeve sensor (dent sleeve) with a pressure-sensitive membrane is attached to the catheter, and water flows beneath the pressure-sensitive membrane to measure the maximum pressure applied to it

2 Methods of Esophageal Manometry

Esophageal manometry can be performed using the water-perfused system or the intraluminal solid-state transducer system. Each system has its advantages and disadvantages. Traditionally, the water-perfused system was widely used, but recently, the intraluminal transducer system has become mainstream.

2.1 Water-Perfused System

This system measures the force preventing the outflow of water from side holes in a thin polyvinyl tube. The catheter consists of bundled thin tubes, each with an outlet positioned at different locations. Water is injected via a pump, and the pressure is measured by a transducer attached to the pump. Although pressures in 3–5 locations in the esophageal body, EGJ, and stomach are measured in the conventional manometry, water-perfused high-resolution manometry is also performed. For pharyngeal pressure, either side holes in the pharyngeal region or electromyography can be used to evaluate swallowing. This system allows the use of sleeve sensors (discussed later) and is cost-effective. Additionally, air or liquid can be injected into the esophagus through unused tubes to evaluate reflexive esophageal motility and perception. This system is usually performed in the supine position to avoid measurement errors due to height differences between the transducer and side holes; thus, the issue should be considered if esophageal manometry is performed in the upright position using this system.

2.2 Intraluminal Transducer System

This system directly attaches transducers to the catheter to measure pressure, unaffected by water or gravity. However, the transducers are fragile and expensive. Continuous measurement of the EGJ, whose location fluctuates with respiration, requires a sleeve sensor, which cannot be used with the intraluminal transducer system. E-sleeve function measures the highest pressure. Recently, high-resolution esophageal manometry (HRM) with transducers placed at 1 cm intervals has developed the e-sleeve function, enabling continuous EGJ measurement.

3 Methods for Measuring Esophagogastric Junction Pressure

3.1 Sleeve Sensor

Due to respiratory-related positional changes, single-point pressure measurement cannot continuously measure the EGJ pressure. The sleeve sensor (Dentsleeve), with a 6 cm silicone membrane, was developed to continuously measure the EGJ. Water flows beneath the pressure-sensitive membrane, allowing pressure measurement at any point on the membrane, recording the maximum pressure (Figs. 4.3 and 4.4). Esophageal pressure is referenced to atmospheric pressure, while EGJ pressure is referenced to gastric pressure.

3.2 E-sleeve Function

The intraluminal transducer system cannot use the sleeve sensor, which does not allow to measure the EGJ pressure continuously. However, in HRM, selecting the maximum pressure between sensors positioned at the EGJ effectively substitutes the sleeve sensor function (e-sleeve function), enabling continuous EGJ measurement (Fig. 4.5).

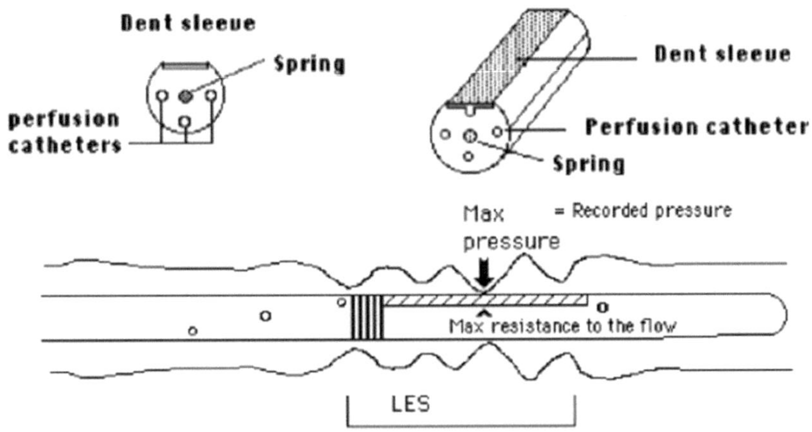

Fig. 4.3 Respiratory variation of LES and measurement principle using a sleeve sensor. (Guidelines for the Diagnosis of Esophageal Motility Disorders (in Japanese)). The LES position changes proximally during expiration and distally during inspiration. Due to these respiratory-induced positional changes, single-point pressure measurement cannot continuously measure LES pressure. Using a sleeve sensor with a 6 cm pressure-sensitive membrane allows continuous LES pressure measurement despite respiratory movements

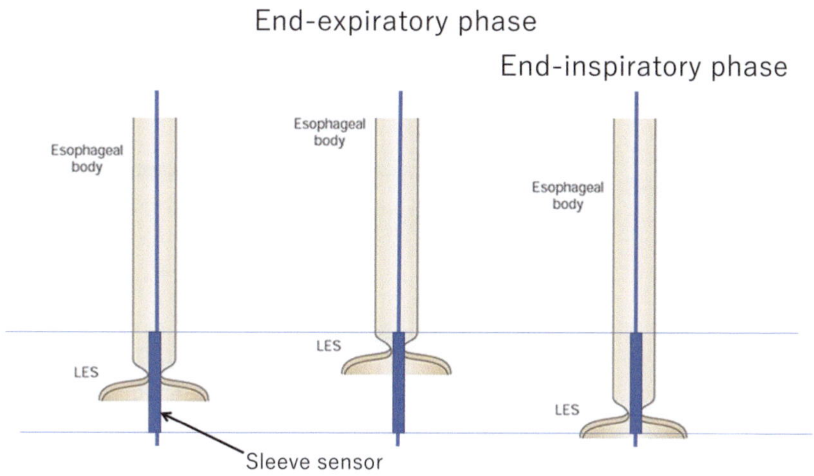

Fig. 4.4 Respiratory movement of LES and measurement principle using the e-sleeve function. (Guidelines for the Diagnosis of Esophageal Motility Disorders (in Japanese)). Pressure sensors are placed at 1 cm intervals, and the maximum pressure at each interval is calculated, enabling continuous LES pressure measurement

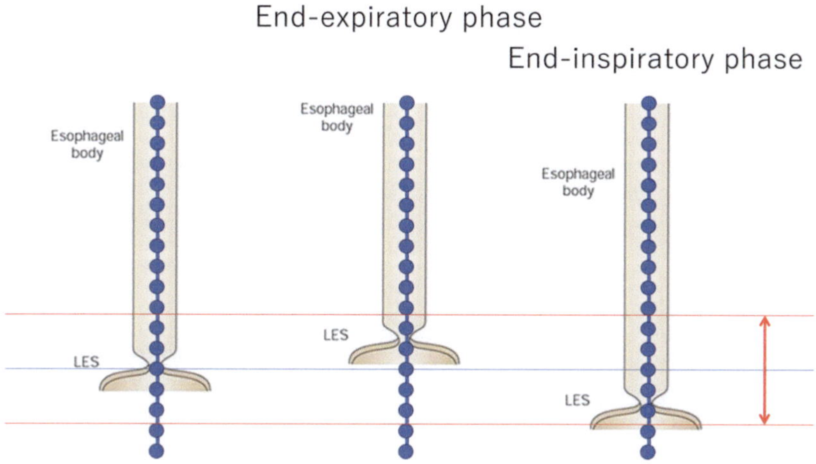

Fig. 4.5 Pressure changes at the esophagogastric junction. (GI Motility online (May 2006) | https://doi.org/10.1038/gimo14). Pressure sensors are inserted into the stomach and gradually withdrawn, showing pressure increases at the esophagogastric junction. Compared to intragastric and intraesophageal pressures, the LES exhibits high pressure, allowing identification of the LES location

4 Practical Aspects of Esophageal Manometry

4.1 Conventional Esophageal Manometry

Traditionally, esophageal manometry measured pressures at several locations in the esophagus to evaluate motility, with the water-perfused system being the gold standard due to the use of the sleeve sensor. Positioning the sleeve sensor at the EGJ requires inserting the catheter deeply into the stomach and pulling it back through the esophagus while measuring pressure changes (pull-through method). Pressure increases at the EGJ and decreases in the esophagus (Fig. 4.6). During inspiration, gastric pressure reflecting abdominal pressure increases, while esophageal pressure reflecting intrathoracic pressure decreases (Fig. 4.6). The point where pressure changes from increasing to decreasing during pull-through is called the respiratory inversion point (RIP) or pressure inversion point (PIP) (Fig. 4.7). The pull-through method includes rapid pull-through (Fig. 4.8), in which breathing is stopped, and the catheter is pulled out quickly,

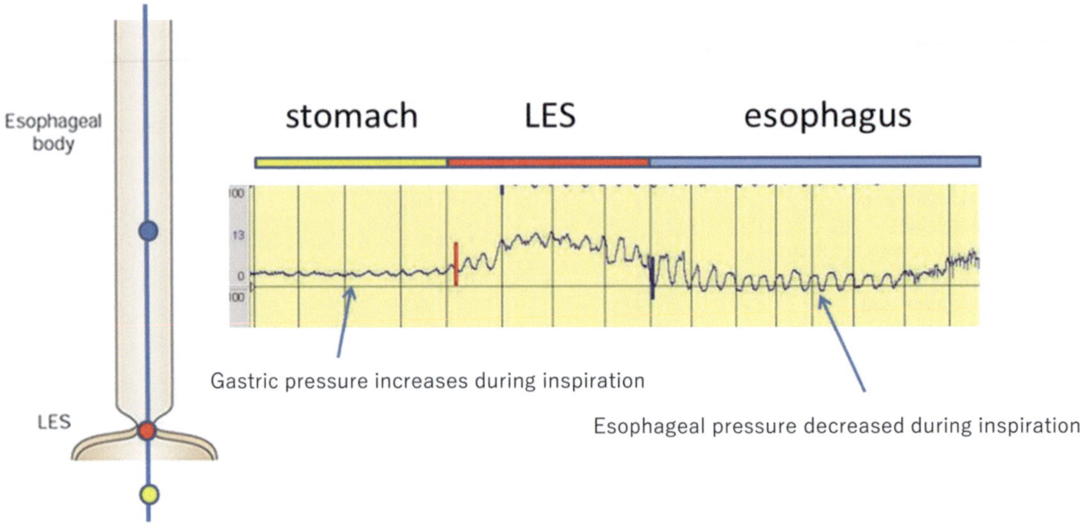

Fig. 4.6 Explanation of the Respiratory Inversion Point. (GI Motility online (May 2006) | https://doi.org/10.1038/gimo14). Pressure changes at the esophagogastric junction are shown as the pressure sensor is gradually withdrawn from the stomach. In the stomach, intraluminal pressure reflects abdominal pressure and increases during inspiration, while in the esophagus, intraluminal pressure reflects intrathoracic pressure and decreases during inspiration. As the pressure sensor is gradually withdrawn from the stomach to the esophagus, the point of pressure change is identified, known as the respiratory inversion point (RIP)

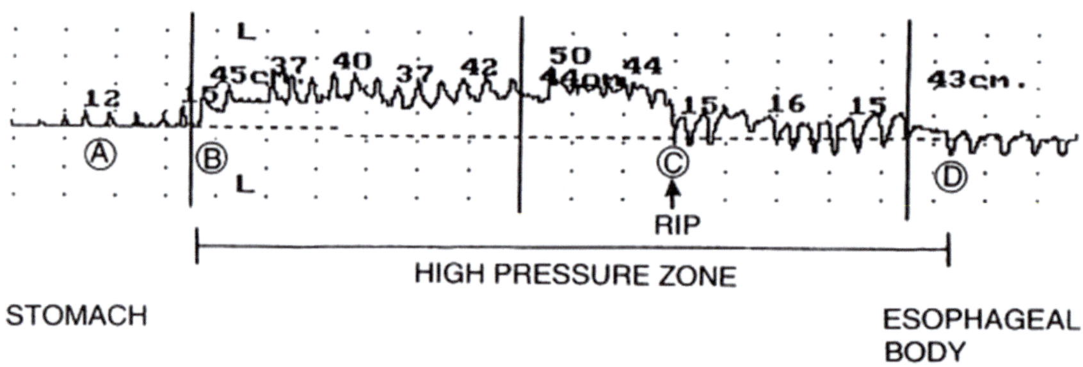

Fig. 4.7 Rapid pull-through method. (GI Motility online (May 2006) | https://doi.org/10.1038/gimo14). The catheter is withdrawn rapidly while the subject holds their breath during expiration, measuring LES pressure. This method allows measurement of LES position and pressure

while station pull-through (Fig. 4.9), in which the catheter is pulled out slowly with breathing. Identifying the EGJ position from pressure changes requires experience and can be challenging for beginners. Esophageal pressure is displayed as waveforms similar to electroencephalograms, making peristaltic wave evaluation difficult for those unfamiliar with esophageal manometry (Fig. 4.10).

Conventional esophageal manometry evaluates EGJ relaxation during swallowing, amplitude and velocity of primary peristalsis, and simultaneous contractions. EGJ pressure fluctuates with respiration, and the end-expiratory pressure is considered the EGJ resting pressure. An EGJ resting pressure below 5 mmHg is abnormal. EGJ relaxation during swallowing is normal if the minimum pressure is below 7 mmHg and

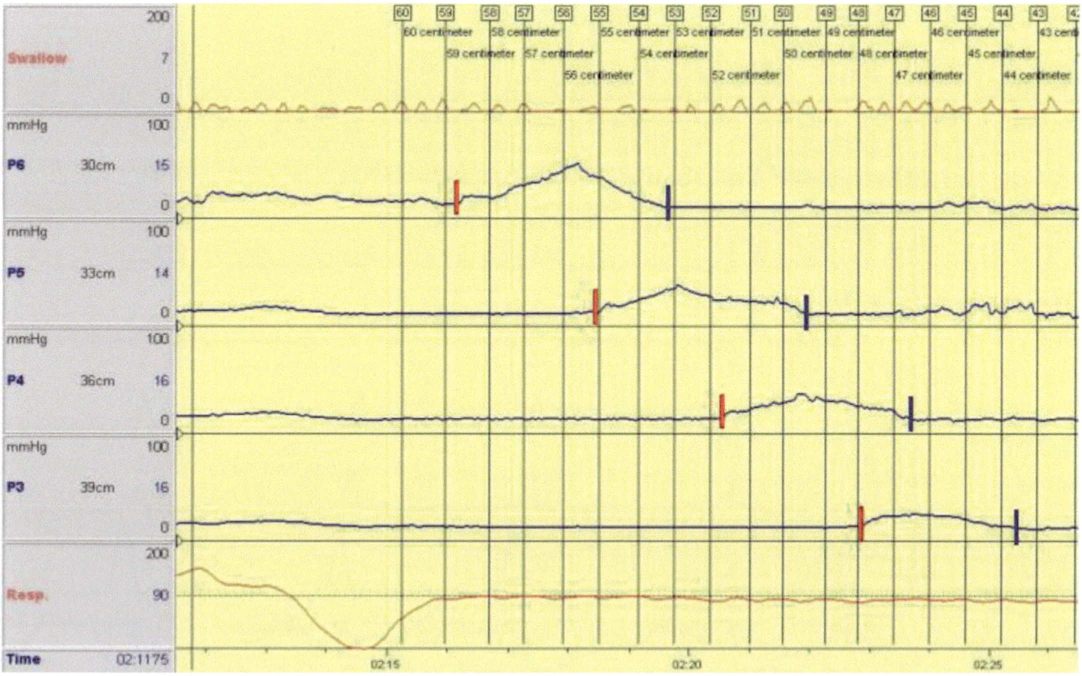

Fig. 4.8 Station pull-through method. (GI Motility online (May 2006) | https://doi.org/10.1038/gimo14). The catheter is slowly withdrawn without breath-holding, measuring intraluminal pressure. This method measures respiratory-induced pressure variations, identifying LES position, LES pressure, and the respiratory inversion point (RIP)

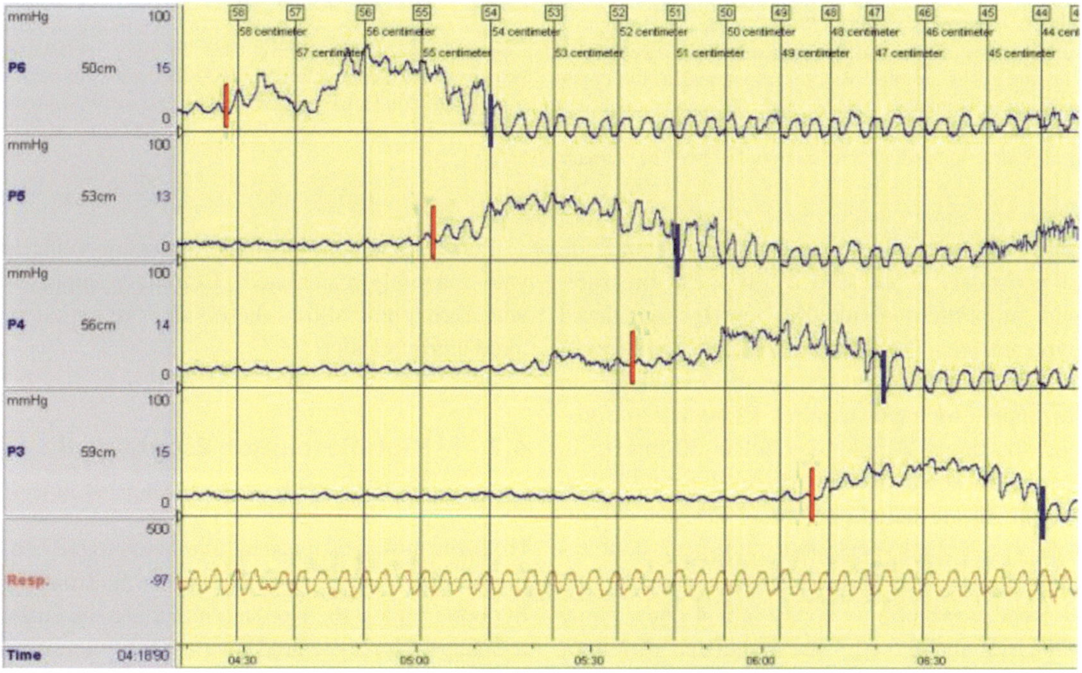

Fig. 4.9 Pressure representation using line traces in conventional manometry. Primary peristalsis propagate from the upper to the lower esophagus following pharyngeal contraction during swallowing. LES pressure decreases after swallowing (LES relaxation) and increases upon arrival of the peristalsis

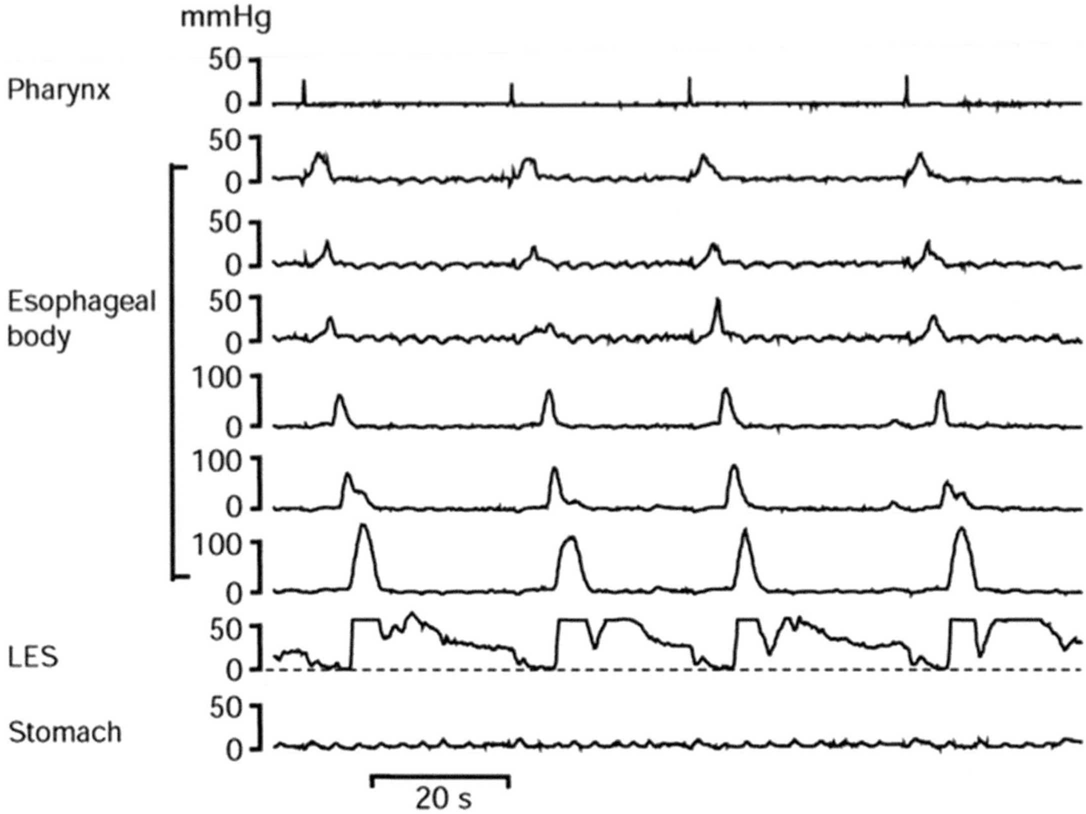

Fig. 4.10 Pressure representation using topographic color contour plots in HRM (Frontispiece 1). High pressure is shown in red, and low pressure in blue. Two high-pressure zones are observed, corresponding to the upper esophageal sphincter (UES) and the esophagogastric junction (EGJ), respectively. Swallowing induces pharyngeal contraction and UES relaxation, followed by primary peristalsis propagating from the upper to the lower esophagus. EGJ pressure decreases after swallowing. The Chicago Classification evaluates primary peristalsis velocity (CFV), contraction vigor (DCI), latency of deglutitive inhibition (DL), and EGJ relaxation after swallowing (IRP)

relaxation time is less than 8 seconds. Amplitude of peristalsis is assessed by the peak pressure, with amplitudes above 180 mmHg considered hypertensive. The lower esophagus requires a peristaltic amplitude of at least 30 mmHg, and the upper esophagus requires 12 mmHg to transport the bolus. Amplitudes below 30 mmHg in the lower esophagus are hypotensive, and below 10 mmHg are failed peristalsis. Peristalsis typically has a single peak, but multi-peak contractions (more than three phases) are abnormal. Normal propagation velocity is 2–4 cm/s, while velocities above 6 cm/s are associated with poor clearance.

Peristaltic amplitude and propagation velocity was manually calculated. Computer input of waveforms now allows these values to be calculated automatically.

4.2 High-Resolution Esophageal Manometry

High-resolution esophageal manometry (HREM) measures pressures at 1–2 cm intervals from the hypopharynx to the stomach including the entire esophagus. It is now gold standard for diagnosing esophageal motility disorders, often using the intraluminal transducer method. Although HRM can be performed using the water-perfused system, the influence of injected water could be a problem. In addition, the height between a catheter hole and the introducer affect pressure values, which should be considered to evaluate esophageal motility in different body positions. The upper esophageal sphincter (UES) and EGJ could be identified when the catheter is inserted into the stomach, while the catheter must be positioned precisely so that the sleeve sensor can detect the EGJ pressure in conventional manometry. However, catheter positioning must be adjusted to measure the UES pressure for swallowing and the gastric pressure for evaluating the EGJ pressure. Conventional manometry displayed pressure waveforms as traces similar to electroencephalograms, while HRM can transform pressure into a topographic color contour, making detection of overall pressure changes easier than pressure waveforms (Fig. 4.11).

HRM software automatically calculates parameters of primary peristalsis. EGJ relaxation is evaluated using the minimum pressure during any 4-second period within the 10 seconds following swallowing (integrated relaxation pressure: IRP). Contractile strength is assessed using contractile vigor above 20 mmHg along time and the distance spanning the transition zone and proximal border of the EGJ (distal contractile integral: DCI). Initially, velocity of peristalsis was evaluated by the slope of the tangent line to

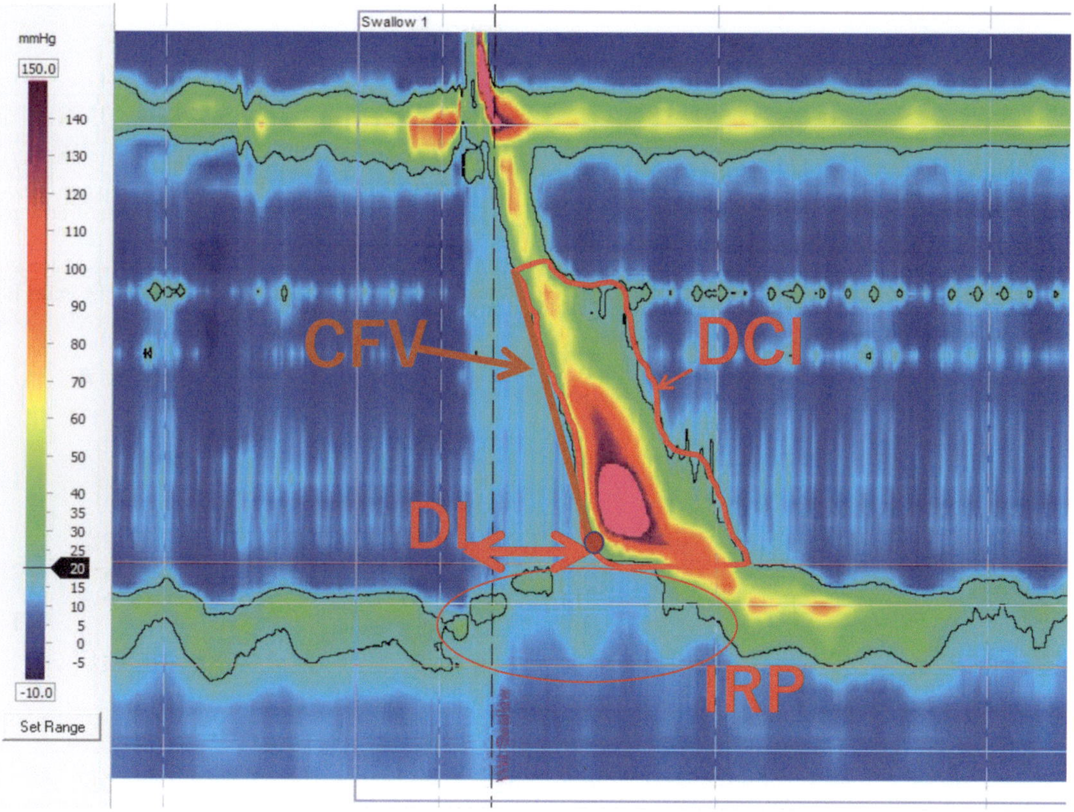

Fig. 4.11 Standard protocol in Chicago Classification v4.0. The upper panel shows the standard protocol in the supine position, and the lower panel shows the standard protocol in the upright position. *Upper panel:* Supine Position—After catheter insertion, the subject lies supine, adapts for 60 seconds, performs three deep breaths, and undergoes a 30-second baseline measurement. This is followed by ten 5 mL water swallows and multiple rapid swallows. *Lower panel:* Upright Position—After the supine examination, the subject changes to an upright position, adapts for 60 seconds, performs three deep breaths, and undergoes a 30-second baseline measurement. This is followed by five 5 mL water swallows and a rapid drink challenge

the initial portion of the contraction (between transition zone and the contractile deceleration point) (contractile front velocity: CFV). However, CFV may not accurately assess waves with significant breaks, so distal latency (DL), the time from the onset of swallow to the contractile deceleration point, is now used. Cutoff values for these parameters vary with different HRM systems. Cutoff values in ManoScan™ report IRP below 15 mmHg, DCI below 100 mmHg as failed, below 450 mmHg as ineffective, above 8000 mmHg as hypercontractile, and DL below 4.5 seconds as premature.

5 Standard Protocol

Esophageal manometry evaluates primary peristalsis with 5 mL water swallows. Even healthy individuals may have failed peristalsis or ineffective swallow, necessitating evaluation of at least 10 water swallows. Dry swallow is no longer assessed in the standard protocol of the Chicago classification. The standard protocol for Chicago Classification v3.0 involved 10 water swallows in the supine position [1]. However, EGJ relaxation cannot be evaluated adequately in the supine assessment alone, and healthy individuals may have ineffective swallows more than 50% of 10 water swallows. Therefore, Chicago Classification v4.0 includes evaluations in both supine (Fig. 4.11(A)) and upright positions (Fig. 4.11(B)), along with provocative tests [2].

Take-Home Message
Subjects often repeatedly swallow due to catheter discomfort. If a second swallow occurs immediately after the first, peristalsis of the first swallow is inhibited by the second (deglutitive inhibition). Therefore, it is crucial to instruct subjects not to swallow multiple times during a single water swallow and exclude data from multiple swallows during analysis.

Competing Interests The author(s) has no competing interests to declare that are relevant to the content of this manuscript.

References

1. Kahrilas PJ, et al. The Chicago Classification of esophageal motility disorders, v3.0. Neurogastroenterol Motil. 2015;27:160–74.
2. Yadlapati R, et al. Esophageal motility disorders on high-resolution manometry: Chicago classification version 4.0(c). Neurogastroenterol Motil. 2020;33:e14058.

Esophageal Motility Test, High-Resolution Impedance Oesophageal Manometry

5

Shiko Kuribayashi

Abstract

High-resolution impedance manometry (HRIM) measures both intraluminal pressure and impedance. Bolus retention and distensibility can be evaluated by HRIM. HRIM is performed to assess esophageal motility and swallow function. Esophageal bolus retention is evaluated with parameters, such as bolus flow time (BFT) and esophageal impedance integral (EII) ratio. EII ratio may be a better indicator for assessment of esophageal bolus retention than esophagram. Esophageal distention could be evaluated by pressure-flow analysis or distention-contraction profile using HRIM. Pharyngeal HRIM can evaluate meso-pharyngeal contraction and upper esophageal sphincter relaxation during swallow, which allows assessment of swallow function.

HRIM during post-prandial periods can detect rumination, supra-gastric belching and excessive transient lower esophageal sphincter. HRIM is a better method to assess rumination syndrome, excessive supra-gastric belching than impedance monitoring alone.

Keywords

High-resolution impedance manometry · Bolus flow time · Esophageal impedance integral ratio · Pressure-flow analysis · Distention-contraction profile · Post-prandial high-resolution impedance manometry · Pharyngeal high-resolution manometry impedance

1 Esophageal High-Resolution Impedance Manometry

High-resolution manometry (HRM) has become the standard for evaluating esophageal manometry. Many HRM systems, such as ManoScan™ with 36-channel solid-state sensors and 18 impedance channels, can measure both pressure and impedance. High-resolution impedance manometry (HRIM) measures impedance at 18 locations at 2 cm intervals (Fig. 5.1). By measuring both pressure and impedance, HRIM can evaluate bolus movement and cross-sectional area (CSA) of the lumen, demonstrating the utility of HRIM in these assessments.

S. Kuribayashi (✉)
Department of Gastroenterology and Hepatology, Gunma University Graduate School of Medicine, Maebashi, Japan
e-mail: shikokuri@gunma-u.ac.jp

H. Kaneko et al. (eds.), *Disorders of Gut-Brain Interaction*,
https://doi.org/10.1007/978-981-95-6974-8_5

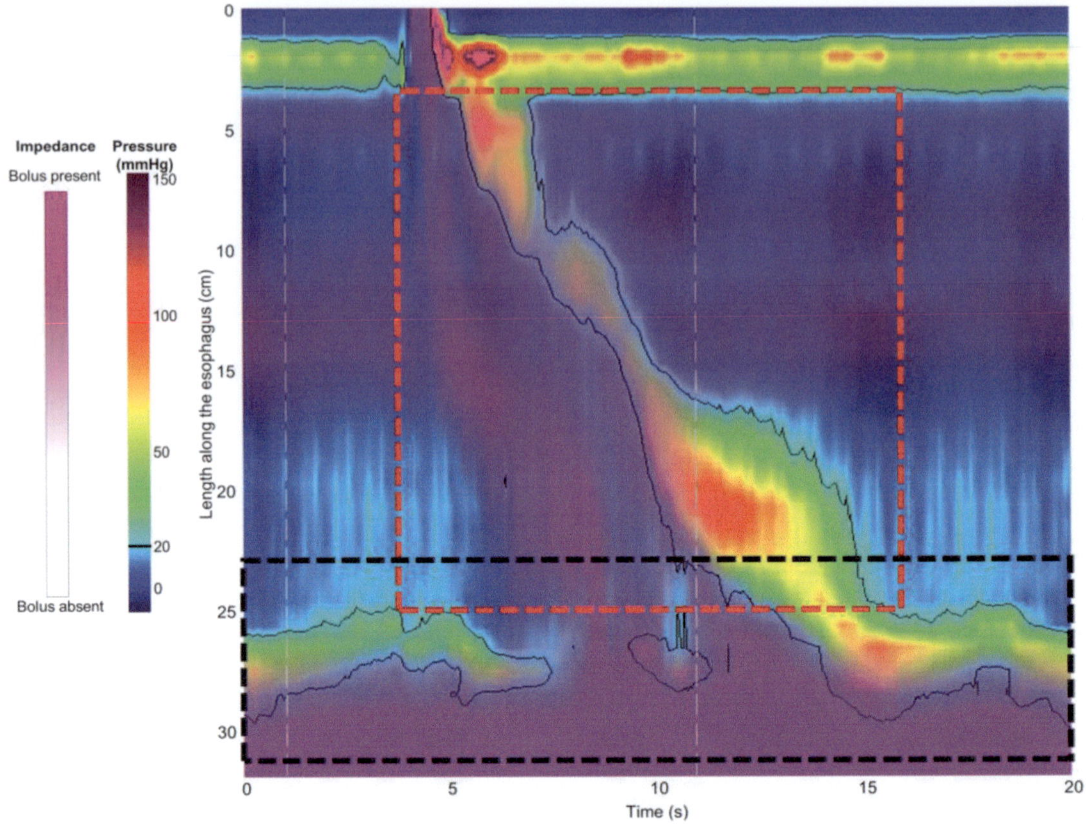

Fig. 5.1 Primary peristalsis and bolus dynamics detected by high-resolution impedance manometry [3]. Pressure and impedance measured by high-resolution impedance manometry are displayed in color plot, with high pressure in red, low pressure in blue, low impedance in purple, and high impedance in white. The bolus entering the esophagus with swallowing is transported through the esophagus by the primary peristalsis and enters the stomach

2 Evaluation of Bolus Retention

2.1 Examination Protocol

After catheter placement, a 2-minute baseline measurement is performed, followed by ten 5 mL swallows of 0.45% saline in the supine position and five swallows in the upright position.

2.2 Evaluation Items for Esophageal Bolus Retention

(i) Esophageal impedance integral (EII) Ratio: The vertical axis spans from the lower edge of the upper esophageal sphincter (UES) to the upper edge of the esophagogastric junction (EGJ). The horizontal axis spans from the onset of UES relaxation during swallowing to the end of the primary peristalsis or 12 seconds after UES relaxation. The esophageal impedance integral (EII) is measured before (Z1) and after (Z2) the primary peristalsis. The EII ratio is calculated as EII-Z2/EII-Z1, with higher values indicating greater bolus retention in the esophagus (Fig. 5.2).

(ii) Bolus Flow Time (BFT): BFT is measured by positioning three impedance and three manometry signals through the EGJ at 1-cm intervals with the distal signals positioned within the hiatus as identified by crural contractions. The bolus presence time (BPT) at the EGJ is determined as the time from which the impedance dropped to 90% of the

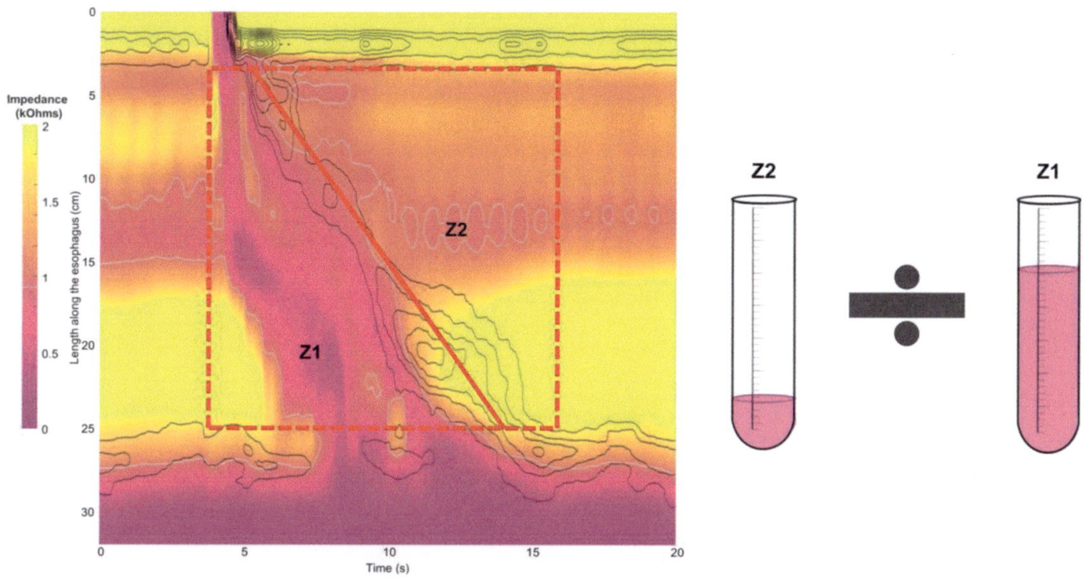

Fig. 5.2 EII ratio [2]. Pressure is displayed as isobars contour, with low impedance in pink and high impedance in yellow. The area before the primary peristalsis is Z1, and the area after the primary peristalsis is Z2. The esophageal impedance integral (EII) is calculated as impedance value × length × time for each area, and the EII ratio is calculated as EII-Z2/EII-Z1

nadir until the impedance returned to 50% of the impedance baseline. The BFT is derived as the sum of all periods during the BPT when a flow-permissive pressure gradient (i.e., when the esophageal pressure is greater than both the crural and intragastric pressure signals) was present. If the impedance drop is not greater than 50% at each axial location and/or a flow-permissive pressure gradient is not achieved, the BFT is considered to be zero (Fig. 5.3). Lower BFT values indicate impaired bolus passage.

(iii) Impedance Ratio (IR): Similar to the EII ratio, the vertical axis spans from the lower edge of the UES to the upper edge of the EGJ, and the horizontal axis spans from the onset of UES relaxation during swallowing to the end of the primary peristaltic wave or 12 seconds after UES relaxation. The impedance ratio (IR) is calculated as the minimum impedance value divided by the impedance value at maximum pressure at each location (Fig. 5.4). Higher IR values indicate greater bolus retention in the esophagus.

2.3 Utility of Each Parameter

Studies comparing these parameters in patients without major esophageal motility disorders found that the EII ratio most accurately reflected esophageal bolus retention [2]. Additionally, comparisons of BFT, integrated relaxation pressure (IRP), EGJ resting pressure, and EGJ contractile integral (EGJ-CI) with treatment outcomes for achalasia found that BFT best reflected treatment efficacy [3]. Furthermore, comparisons of EII ratio and esophagography findings with achalasia treatment outcomes found that the EII ratio better reflected treatment efficacy than esophagography [4]. Thus, HRIM is useful for evaluating esophageal bolus retention.

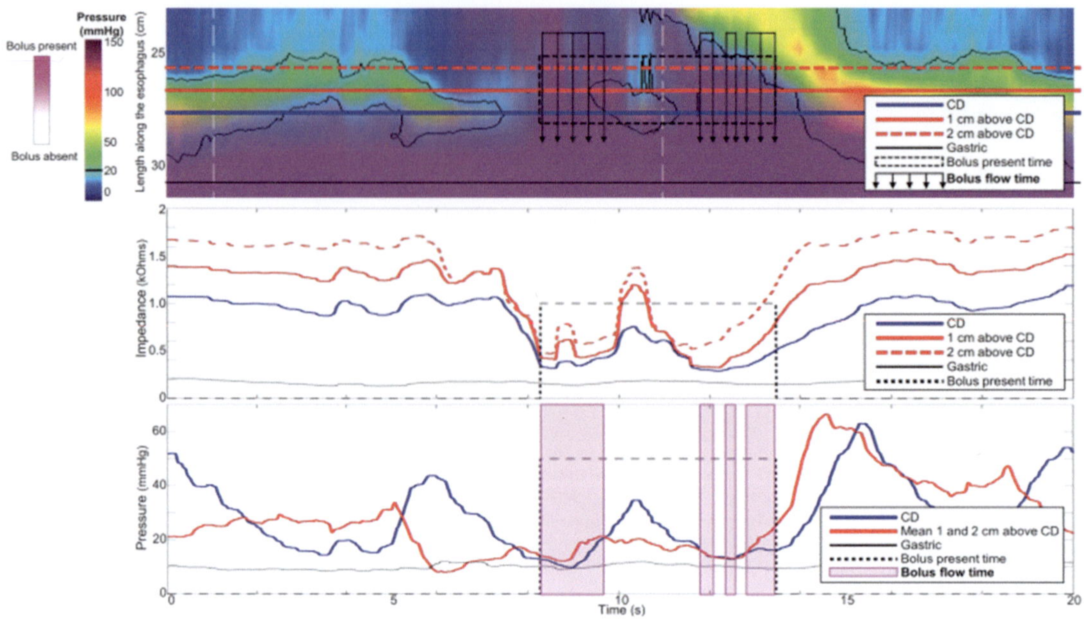

Fig. 5.3 Bolus flow time [2]. *Top*: Changes in pressure and impedance at the esophagogastric junction after swallowing, measured by high-resolution impedance manometry. The position of the diaphragmatic crura (CD) is shown by a blue solid line, 1 cm oral side of the diaphragmatic crura by a red solid line, 2 cm oral side by a red dotted line, and the gastric pressure measurement site by a black solid line. The time the bolus is present at the esophagogastric junction is enclosed by a black dotted line, and the bolus flow time is indicated by a downward arrow. *Middle*: Pressure changes at the diaphragmatic crura (blue solid line), 1 cm oral side (red solid line), 2 cm oral side (red dotted line), and gastric pressure (black solid line) are displayed as pressure traces. The time the bolus is present at the esophagogastric junction is enclosed by a black dotted rectangle. *Bottom*: Diaphragmatic crura pressure is shown by a blue solid line, the average pressure of 1 cm and 2 cm oral side by a red solid line, and gastric pressure by a black solid line. The time the bolus is present at the esophagogastric junction is enclosed by a black dotted rectangle. When the pressure above the diaphragmatic crura is higher than the diaphragmatic crura pressure, a downward pressure gradient is created, allowing the bolus to flow from the esophagus into the stomach. This time is enclosed by a pink rectangle as the bolus flow time

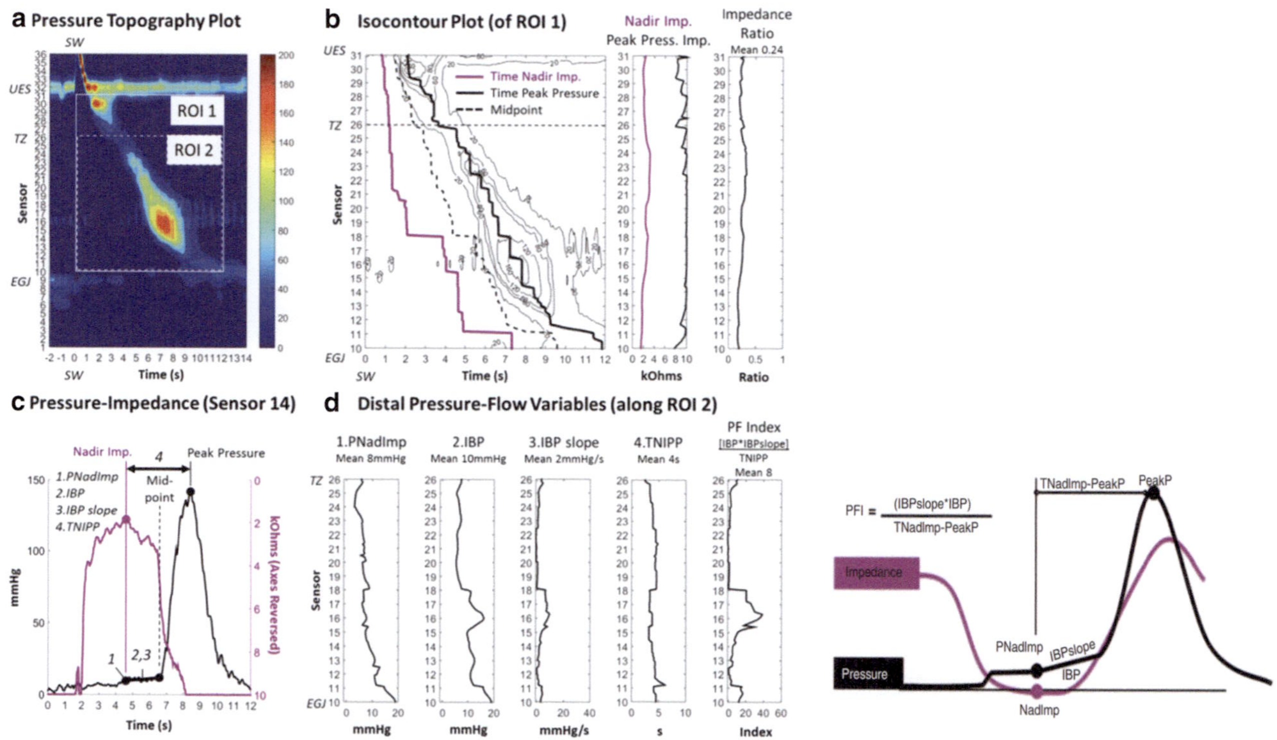

Fig. 5.4 Pressure flow analysis [2]. (**a**) Pressure changes in a healthy individual after swallowing 5 mL of saline, displayed in color. Two regions of interest (ROI) are defined: ROI 1 from the lower edge of the upper esophageal sphincter to the upper edge of the esophagogastric junction, and ROI 2 from the transition zone to the upper edge of the esophagogastric junction. (**b**) *Left*: Pressure of the primary peristaltic wave is shown as isobars, with the location and time of the lowest impedance indicated by a purple solid line, the location and time of the highest pressure by a black solid line, and the midpoint between the lowest impedance and highest pressure by a black dotted line. The lowest impedance indicates the timing of bolus distension, and the highest pressure indicates the maximum contraction. (**b**) *Middle*: Impedance values at each location. (**b**) *Right*: Impedance ratio, calculated as the impedance value at the lowest impedance divided by the impedance value at the highest pressure. (**c**) Impedance and pressure measured by sensor 14. Impedance values from the start of swallowing (0 s) to 12 seconds are shown by a purple solid line, and pressure by a black solid line. Impedance is inverted for display, with the lowest value at the top. This figure shows a representative example of the four main parameters calculated: PNadImp (pressure at nadir impedance), IBP (intrabolus pressure), IBP slope (pressure change gradient from nadir impedance to midpoint between nadir impedance and maximum pressure), and TNIPP (time from nadir impedance to peak pressure). (**d**) Values of each parameter shown in C for each sensor in ROI 2 and their averages. The pressure flow (PF) index is calculated as IBP × IBP slope / TNIPP. At the lower position of sensor 18, IBP significantly increases, and TNIPP shortens, indicating a passage obstruction at the esophagogastric junction, causing localized pressure increase in the esophageal body due to retained bolus. *Right Figure*: Schematic of C and PFI (PF index)

3 Evaluation of Esophageal Distensibility

3.1 Pressure-Flow Analysis

(i) Examination Protocol: After resting for 10 minutes with the head elevated at 30°, the subject swallows 5 mL and 10 mL of 0.9% saline, 5 mL and 10 mL of 450 K cPs viscous, and 2 cm^2 and 4 cm^2 solid food five times each (Fig. 5.4) [1]. However, protocols vary among studies, and ten 5 mL 0.45% saline swallows in the supine position and five in the upright position were performed in a study with comparisons of pressure-flow metrics with EII ratio and BFT [2].

(ii) Pressure-Flow Metrics: When a bolus passes through the esophagus, impedance becomes lowest when the esophagus is most distended. Pressure-flow metrics include PNadImp (pressure at nadir impedance), intrabolus pressure (IBP), IBP slope (time from nadir impedance to midpoint between nadir impedance and maximum pressure), and TNIPP (time from nadir impedance to maximum pressure). The pressure-flow index (PFI) is calculated as (IBP × IBP slope) / TNIPP (Fig. 5.4). PFI correlates with dysphagia symptoms [5].

3.2 Distension-Contraction Profile

(i) Examination Protocol: After catheter insertion, the subject swallows 10 mL of 0.5 N saline warmed to 37 °C eight to ten times in the Trendelenburg position (−15° head-down). This differs from the standard Chicago Classification protocol, particularly in position and swallow volume. The Trendelenburg position is preferred to prevent swallowed air from affecting CSA evaluation [6].

(ii) Utility of Distension-Contraction Profile: Comparisons between nutcracker esophagus patients and healthy individuals found that nutcracker esophagus patients had higher peristaltic amplitudes, smaller CSA during bolus passage, and faster bolus transit (Fig. 5.5) [7]. Evaluations of distension-contraction profiles in patients with dysphagia but normal HRM findings showed smaller CSA during bolus passage compared to healthy individuals [8]. Thus, abnormalities in distensibility, not just contraction, may cause dysphagia.

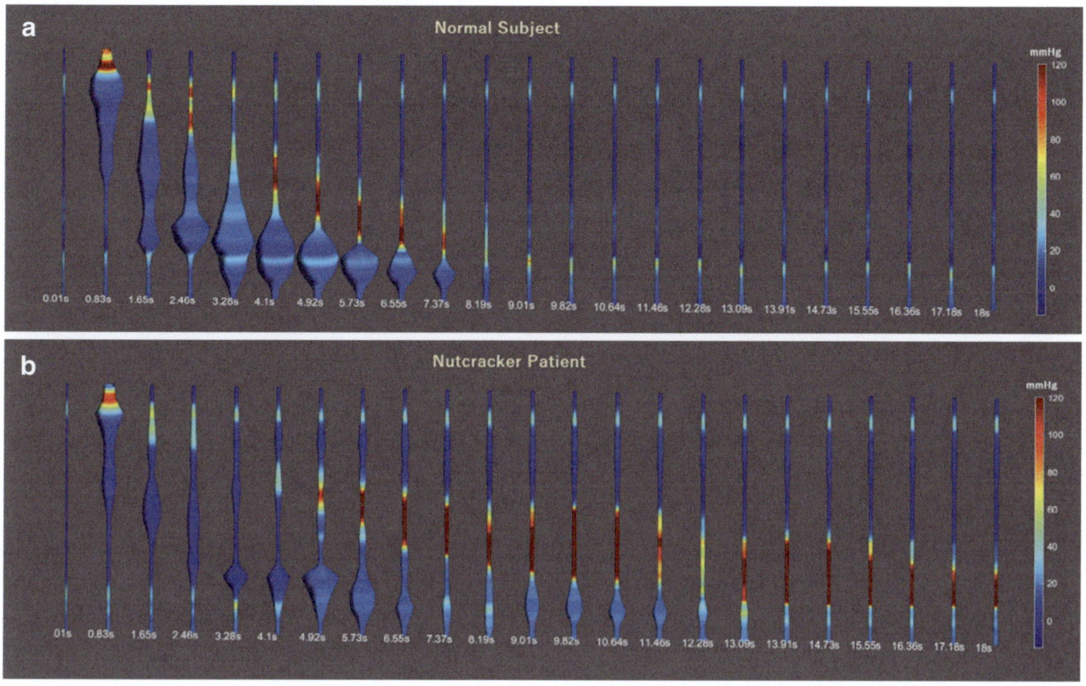

Fig. 5.5 Differences in distension-contraction profiles between healthy individuals and nutcracker esophagus patients [7]. Pressure is displayed in color, with high pressure in red and low pressure in blue. Bolus-induced esophageal distension is shown over time. Nutcracker esophagus patients have faster bolus transit to the lower esophagus, smaller bolus-induced esophageal distension, and fragmented distension (mixed areas of distension and non-distension) compared to healthy individuals

4 Evaluation with Post-prandial Period

4.1 Examination Protocol

Chicago Classification v4.0 introduces HRIM protocols with meal challenges, observing esophageal motility for at least 10 minutes after consuming 200 g of soft solid food or a symptom-inducing meal [9].

4.2 Evaluation Items

(i) Presence of Motility abnormalities: Abnormal esophageal motility is typically not observed after meal challenges in healthy subjects. Healthy individuals may have transient lower esophageal relaxation (TLESR) during post-prandial state (Fig. 5.6), with up to four TLESR events in 10 minutes after meal intake considered normal in Chicago Classification v4.0 [9].

(ii) Rumination: Rumination is the regurgitation of undigested food from the stomach back up into the mouth. HRIM can detect that gastric contents reflux into the mouth through the UES (Fig. 5.7). HRIM defines rumination is defined as more than 30 mmHg gastric pressure increase from the baseline pressure with anterograde pressure gradient, followed by gastric contents refluxing into the pharynx through the UES within 10 seconds without nausea [10]. Rumination syndrome is a condition in which rumination is chronically observed. Absence of rumination in 10 minutes post-prandial period is considered normal in Chicago Classification v4.0 [9].

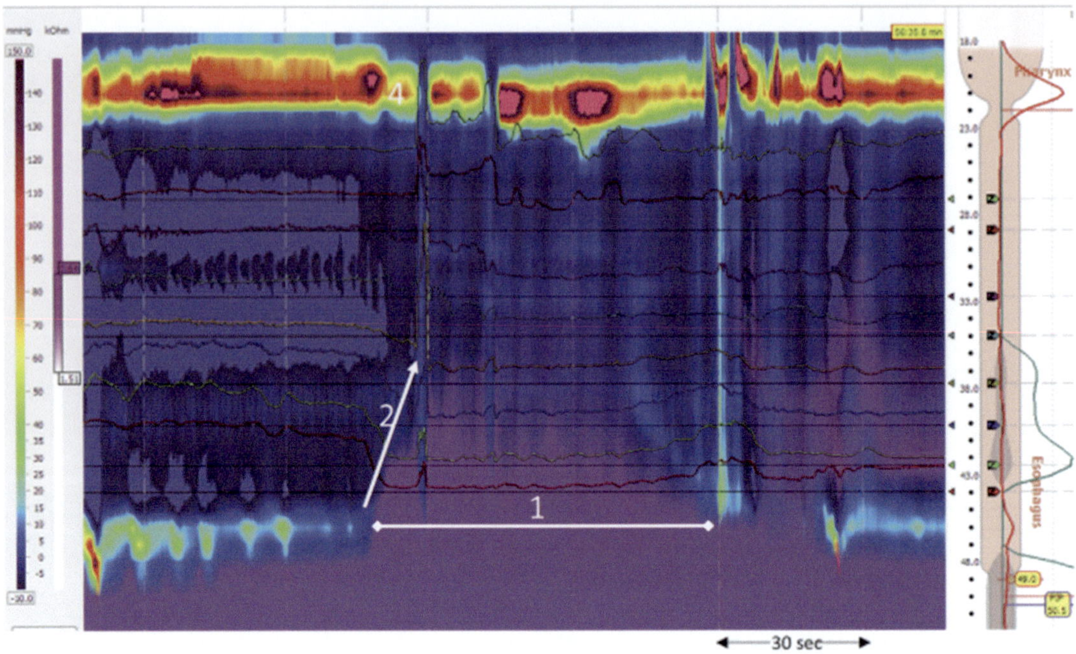

Fig. 5.6 Transient lower esophageal sphincter relaxation and gastroesophageal reflux detected by high-resolution impedance manometry [10]. Relaxation of the esophago-gastric junction for more than 10 seconds is observed (arrow 1), with gastric contents refluxing into the esophagus (arrow 2)

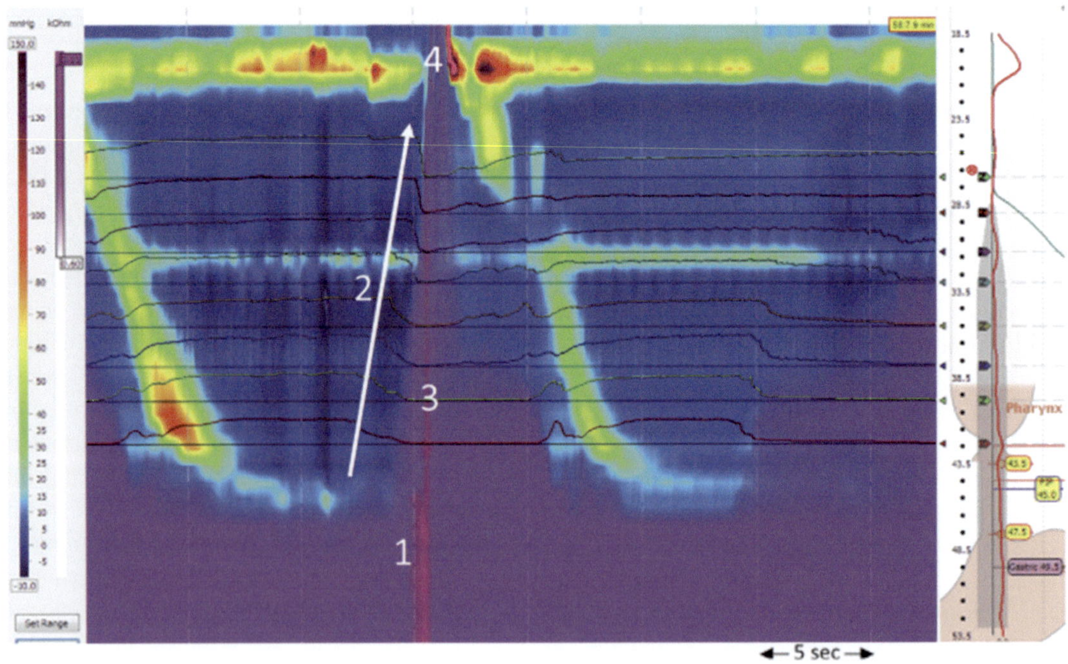

Fig. 5.7 Example of rumination [10]. Gastric pressure increases by more than 30 mmHg from baseline (arrow 1), gastric contents reflux to the upper esophageal sphincter (arrow 2), esophageal pressure increases due to reflux (arrow 3), and upper esophageal sphincter relaxation is observed (arrow 4)

(iii) Supra-Gastric Belching: There are two types of belching: gastric belching is when air rises from the stomach into the mouth. On the other hand, air from the esophagus rising into the oral cavity is called supra-gastric belching. Supra-gastric belching is observed frequently in patients with excessive supra-gastric belching [11]. HRIM is defined as a phenomenon in which air enters the esophagus with relaxation of the UES, followed immediately by expulsion of air from the esophagus, accompanied by contraction of the EGJ or negative intrathoracic pressure, or both (Fig. 5.8) [10]. Although supra-gastric belching can be detected by conventional impedance monitoring, HRIM can detect relaxation of the UES and changes in intrathoracic pressure when supra-gastric belching occurs [10]. According to the Chicago Classification v4.0, the absence of supra-gastric belching during the 10-minute postprandial period is considered normal [9].

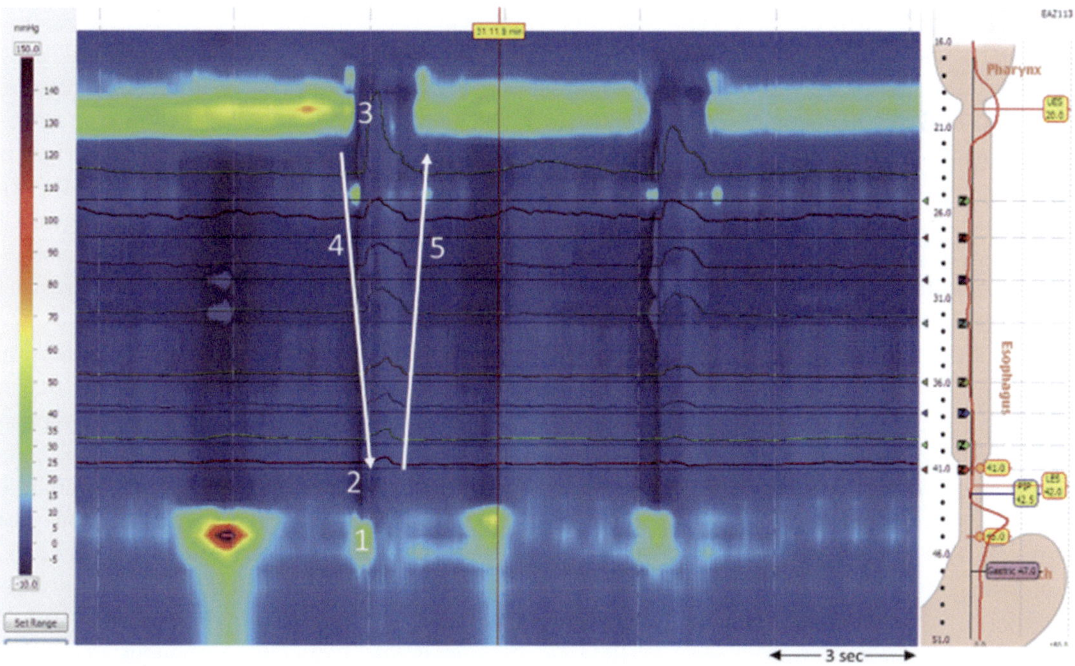

Fig. 5.8 Example of supra-gastric belch [10]. Contraction of the esophagogastric junction (1) increases negative intrathoracic pressure (2), leading to relaxation of the upper esophageal sphincter (3). Impedance values increase from proximal to distal (arrow 4) and then decrease from distal to proximal (arrow 5)

4.3 Utility of HRIM During Post-prandial Period

HRIM with a solid refluxogenic test meal in 94 patients unresponsive to proton pump inhibitors (PPI) found abnormalities in 76%: with 42% exhibiting supra-gastric belching, 20% rumination, and 14% excessive TLESR events [10]. Comparisons of pots-prandial HRIM and impedance-pH monitoring found higher diagnostic accuracy and inter-rater reliability for impedance-pH monitoring, but post-prandial HRIM detected supra-gastric belching and rumination more frequently [12]. These studies differed from Chicago Classification v4.0, conducting studies 20–90 minute post-prandial periods, with abnormalities defined as more than six TLESR events/hour, more than two supra-gastric belching events/hour, and more than one rumination event/hour.

5 Evaluation of Pharyngolaryngeal Function

Videofluoroscopic studies are the gold standard for evaluating pharyngolaryngeal and UES function during swallowing, which can evaluate presence of aspiration as well as swallowing function. Recently, HRM has been used for assessment of swallowing. Moreover, combining HRM with impedance measurements (pharyngeal high-resolution manometry impedance: P-HRM-I) allows assessment of distensibility, demonstrating utility in diagnosing pharyngolaryngeal function abnormalities.

5.1 Examination Protocol

The High-Resolution Pharyngeal Manometry (HRPM) International Working Group proposes recommended protocols [13]. HRM systems should have at least ten solid-state sensors at 1 cm intervals, with impedance measured at 2 cm intervals if available. Catheter insertion follows the same nasal route as esophageal HRM, with nasal anesthesia. After catheter placement, it takes 5 minutes for accommodation before testing. The subject keeps in the upright position with the head straight, and test boluses of 5 or 10 mL (sometimes 20 mL) are injected via syringe, with at least three swallows, adjusted as needed.

5.2 Evaluation Items

The HRPM International Working Group recommends evaluating eight parameters across three elements [13].

(i) Pharyngeal Luminal Contraction Pressure: Similar to Chicago Classification for esophageal motility disorders, contraction vigor is evaluated using contractile integral (CI), with 4 parameters including pharyngeal CI (PhCI), velopharyngeal CI (VCI), mesopharyngeal CI (MCI), and hypopharyngeal CI (HCI) (Fig. 5.9).

(ii) Hypopharyngeal Intrabolus Distension Pressure: Evaluates pressure changes due to bolus using hypopharyngeal intrabolus pressure (Fig. 5.10).

(iii) UES Relaxation and Opening: Similar to esophageal Chicago Classification for esophageal motility disorders, UES relaxation is evaluated using integrated relaxation pressure (IRP). While EGJ IRP is assessed over a continuous or non-continuous 4-second period (4 s-IRP), UES IRP is evaluated over non-continuous 0.20–0.25 second intervals. Due to positional changes of UES during swallowing, IRP using e-sleeve functionality provides a more accurate assessment of UES relaxation than single-point pressure measurement. Additional recommended parameters include UES relaxation time and UES maximum admittance (UES MaxAd), with admittance being the reciprocal of impedance (Fig. 5.10).

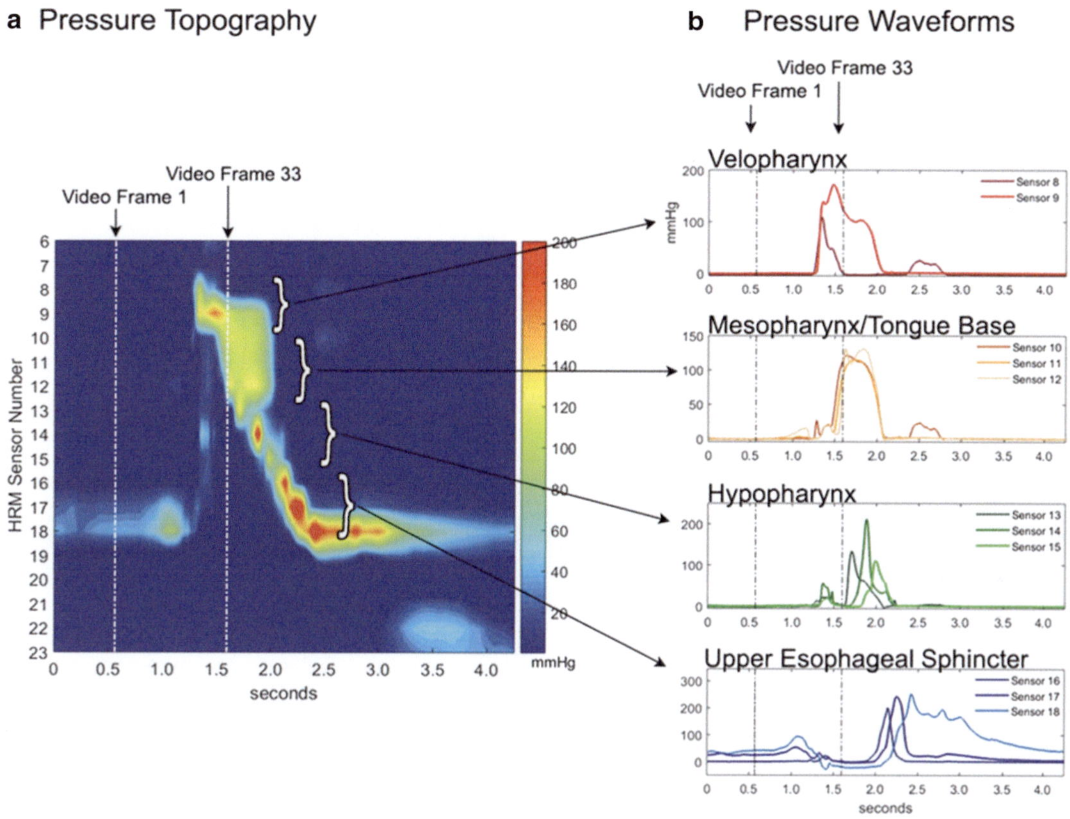

Fig. 5.9 Pressure changes in the pharynx after swallowing 10 mL of barium [13]. Swallowing induces pressure changes propagating from the velopharynx to the mesopharynx/tongue base and hypopharynx. The upper esophageal sphincter (UES) initially relaxes, followed by the contraction wave propagating through the pharynx to the UES. Panel A displays pressure in color, while panel B shows pressure changes at each location as pressure traces

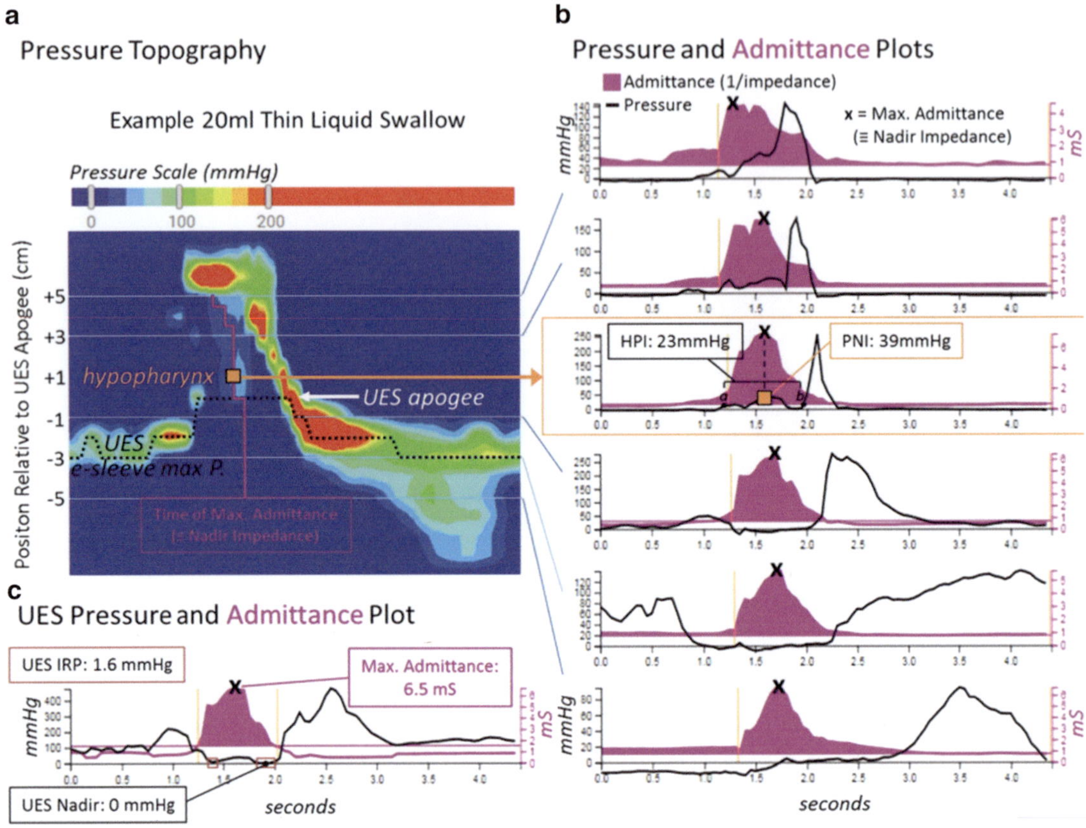

Fig. 5.10 Pressure and impedance changes during swallowing detected by high-resolution pharyngeal impedance manometry [13]. (**a**) Pressure changes in the pharynx and UES after swallowing 20 mL of barium, displayed in color. Pharyngeal contraction and UES relaxation are observed post-swallowing. (**b**) Pressure changes (black solid line) and admittance (pink) at each location. Admittance values are calculated as the reciprocal of impedance. X indicates the maximum admittance (lowest impedance), representing maximum bolus-induced distension at each location. Pressure at nadir impedance (PNI) is measured 1 cm oral side of the highest point of the UES, serving as a validated marker of pharyngeal flow resistance (orange rectangle). Other markers include the average hypopharyngeal contraction pressure above 20 mmHg (hypopharyngeal pressure increment, HPI)

5.3 Utility of P-HRM-I

High IBP and low UES MaxAd indicate abnormal UES relaxation. Normal values for these parameters are established, and P-HRM-I is useful to assess age-related changes of swallowing function and treatment efficacy. Additionally, pharyngeal pressurization patterns are useful for evaluating UES relaxation, classified into type 1 (pan pressurization), type 2 (distal compartmentalized pressurization), and type 3 (transient pressurization) (Fig. 5.11) [14]. Only 9% of patients without pressurization had abnormal UES relaxation, while 70–80% of patients with types 1 and 2, and 30% of patients with type 3 had abnormal UES relaxation. Cutoff values in this study were high UES IRP >8 mmHg, high IBP >25 mmHg, and low UES MaxAd <3.7 mS. Additionally, low pharyngeal contraction pressure is also important as well as UES relaxation in dysphagia, with low peak pressure <61 mmHg considered abnormal, as shown in the diagnostic flowchart (Fig. 5.12).

Take-Home Message

Impedance measurements involve electrical resistance, so distilled or tap water cannot accurately measure impedance values. Therefore, saline should be used for esophageal HRM-impedance measurements.

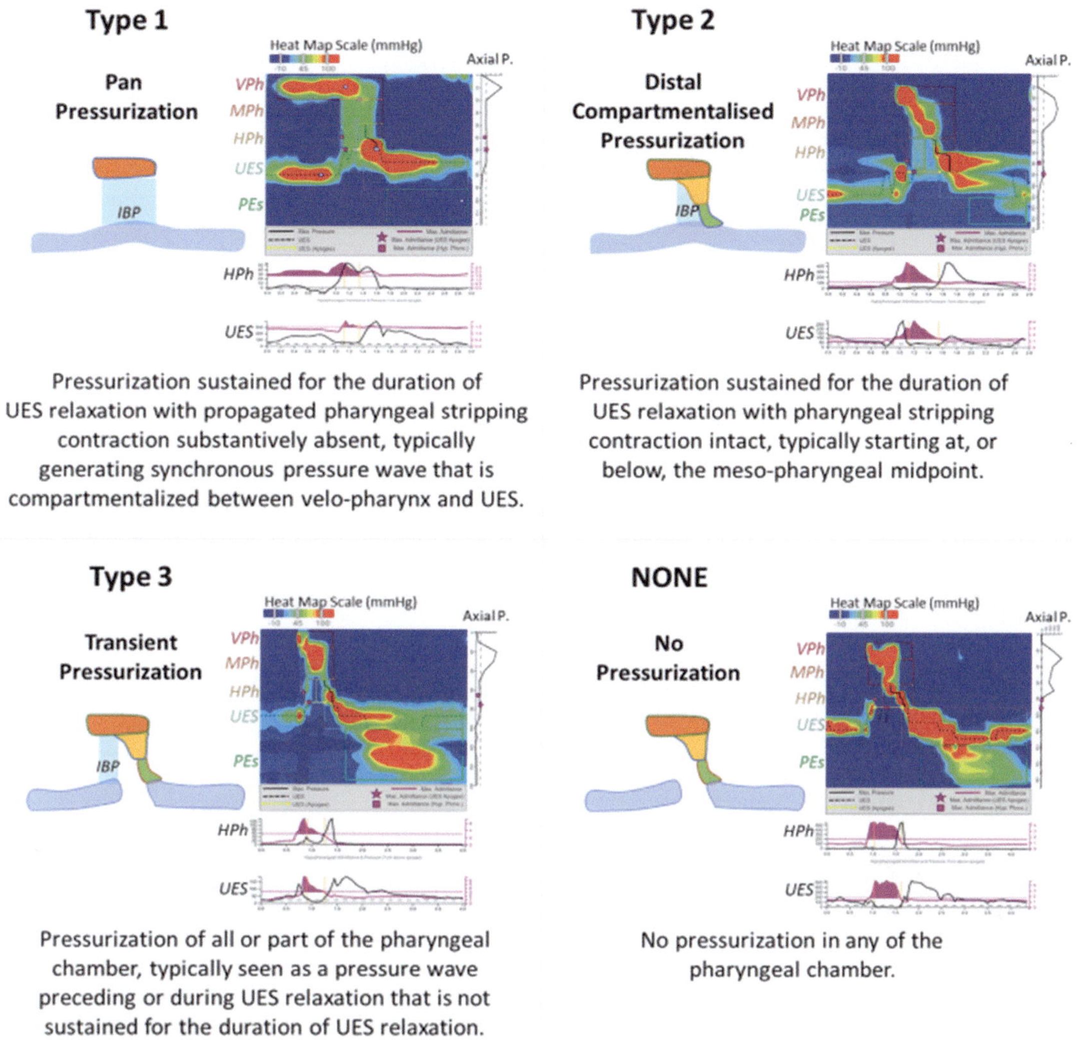

Fig. 5.11 Patterns of pharyngeal pressurization observed in high-resolution pharyngeal manometry [13]. *Type 1*: Sustained pressure increase between the velopharynx and UES during UES relaxation, with minimal propagation of pharyngeal contraction. *Type 2*: Propagating contraction starting from the middle or lower mesopharynx, with sustained pressure increase between the velopharynx and UES during UES relaxation. *Type 3*: Transient pressure increase in the pharynx before or during UES relaxation, without sustained pressure increase during UES relaxation. *NONE*: No pressurization observed in the pharynx

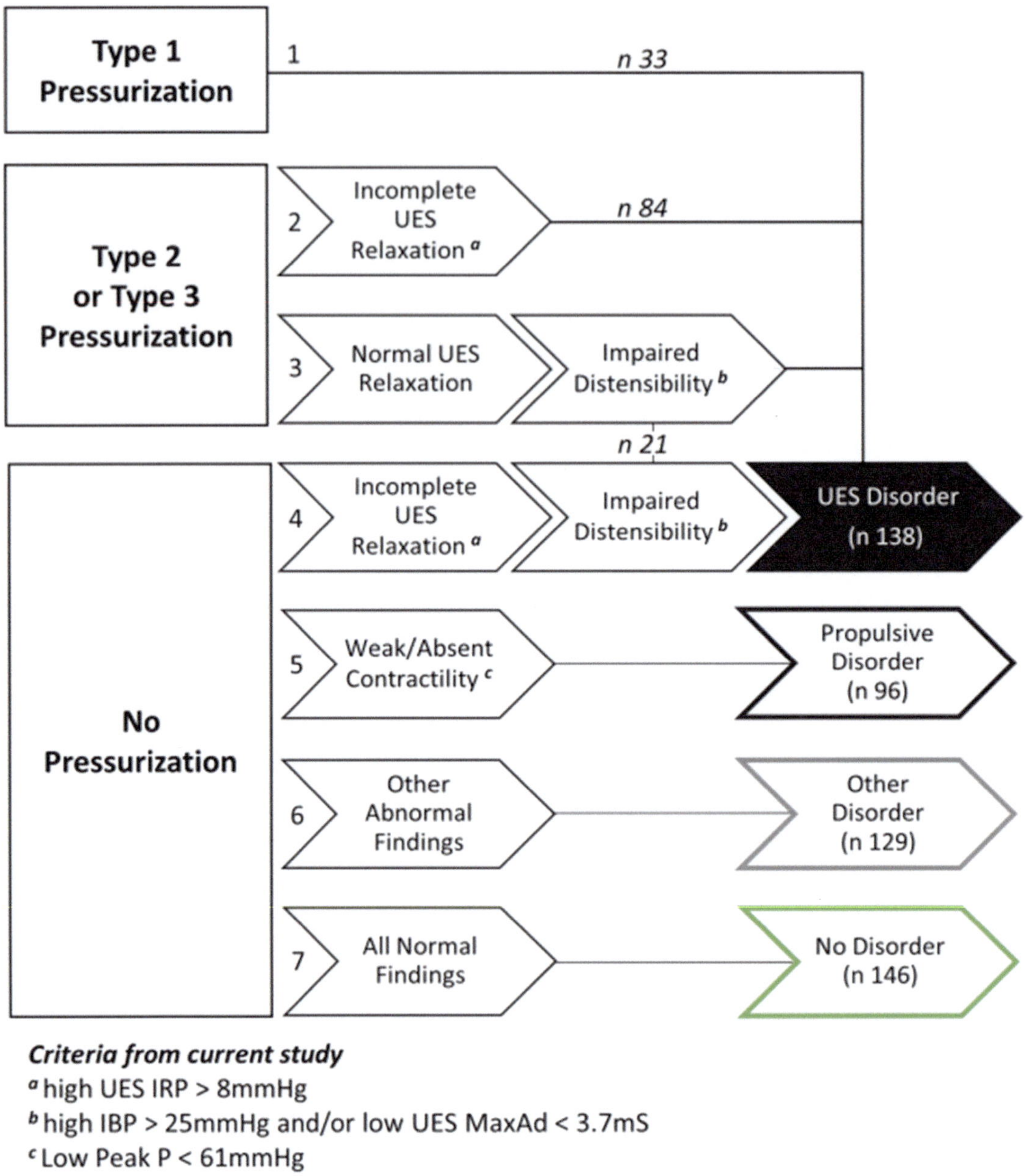

Fig. 5.12 Schematic of upper esophageal sphincter disorders [13]. *Level 1*: Type 1 pressure increase suggests UES disorder, not observed in healthy individuals. *Level 2*: Type 2 or 3 pressure increase suggests incomplete UES relaxation or distension disorder if UES relaxation is maintained. *Level 4*: No pressure increase suggests incomplete UES relaxation or distension disorder. *Level 5*: Weak or absent contraction suggests propulsion disorder. *Level 6*: Other abnormal findings suggest other disorders. *Level 7*: All normal findings suggest no disorder

Competing Interests The author(s) has no competing interests to declare that are relevant to the content of this manuscript.

References

1. Omari T, et al. Impedance as an adjunct to manometric testing to investigate symptoms of dysphagia: what it has failed to do and what it may tell us in the future. United European Gastroenterol J. 2014;2:355–66.
2. Carlson DA, et al. High-resolution impedance manometry parameters enhance the esophageal motility evaluation in non-obstructive dysphagia patients without a major Chicago Classification motility disorder. Neurogastroenterol Motil. 2017;29(3).
3. Carlson DA, et al. High-resolution impedance manometry metrics of the esophagogastric junction for the assessment of treatment response in achalasia. Am J Gastroenterol. 2016;111:1702–10.
4. Carlson DA, et al. Improved assessment of bolus clearance in patients with achalasia using high-resolution impedance manometry. Clin Gastroenterol Hepatol. 2018;16:672–680 e1.
5. Nguyen NQ, et al. Automated impedance-manometry analysis detects esophageal motor dysfunction in patients who have non-obstructive dysphagia with normal manometry. Neurogastroenterol Motil. 2013;25(238–245):e164.
6. Zifan A, et al. Measurement of peak esophageal luminal cross-sectional area utilizing nadir intraluminal impedance. Neurogastroenterol Motil. 2015;27:971–80.
7. Zifan A, et al. Distension-contraction profile of peristalsis in patients with nutcracker esophagus. Neurogastroenterol Motil. 2021;33:e14138.
8. Mittal RK, et al. Abnormal esophageal distension profiles in patients with functional dysphagia: a possible mechanism of dysphagia. Gastroenterology. 2021;160:1847–1849 e2.
9. Yadlapati R, et al. Esophageal motility disorders on high-resolution manometry: Chicago classification version 4.0(c). Neurogastroenterol Motil. 2020;33:e14058.
10. Yadlapati R, et al. Postprandial high-resolution impedance manometry identifies mechanisms of nonresponse to proton pump inhibitors. Clin Gastroenterol Hepatol. 2018;16:211–218 e1.
11. Stanghellini V, et al. Gastroduodenal disorders. Gastroenterology. 2016;150:1380–92.
12. DeLay K, et al. Diagnostic yield and reliability of postprandial high-resolution manometry and impedance-pH for detecting rumination and supragastric belching in PPI non-responders. Neurogastroenterol Motil. 2021;33:e14106.
13. Omari TI, et al. High-resolution pharyngeal manometry and impedance: protocols and metrics—recommendations of a High-Resolution Pharyngeal Manometry International Working Group. Dysphagia. 2020;35:281–95.
14. Omari T, et al. Using high-resolution manometry impedance to diagnose upper esophageal sphincter and pharyngeal motor disorders. Neurogastroenterol Motil. 2023;35:e14461.

6 Esophageal Motility Test, New Testing Methods Such as EndoFLIP

Junichi Akiyama and Hiroko Hosaka

Abstract

EndoFLIP is a novel diagnostic tool for evaluating esophageal motility and distensibility, especially in cases where high-resolution manometry (HRM) results are inconclusive. Unlike HRM, which measures pressure at contact points within the esophagus, EndoFLIP uses a balloon catheter and impedance planimetry to assess the esophageal lumen's cross-sectional area (CSA) and pressure in real-time. This allows for the evaluation of esophagogastric junction (EGJ) distensibility and esophageal contraction patterns through a procedure called FLIP panometry. The examination is typically performed during sedated endoscopy and includes stepwise balloon inflation while monitoring the EGJ distensibility index (EGJ-DI) and contractile responses. The FLIP Panometry Classification system combines EGJ opening and contraction pattern analysis to categorize motility disorders. FLIP panometry provides a well-tolerated method that can complement, or in some cases be an alternative to HRM, for evaluating esophageal motility disorders.

Keywords

EndoFLIP · FLIP panometry · EGJ distensibility index (EGJ-DI) · Contractile response · Esophageal motility

1 EndoFLIP

1.1 Introduction

Esophageal motility disorders have traditionally been diagnosed through esophagography, which visually captures esophageal movements. However, the advent of esophageal manometry, which allows for quantitative and objective evaluation, has significantly advanced the field of diagnostics. Currently, high-resolution manometry (HRM) is the gold standard for a more detailed assessment.

Manometry, including HRM, involves measuring the pressure within the esophageal lumen over time using a catheter with pressure sensors. This test evaluates the transport function of food and liquids through the esophagus and investigates the causes of symptoms such as chest pain due to hypercontraction. However, some patients report a sensation of obstruction or chest pain despite normal HRM results. This may be because HRM can only capture the

J. Akiyama (✉)
Division of Gastroenterology and Hepatology, National Center for Global Health and Medicine, Tokyo, Japan

H. Hosaka
Department of Gastroenterology and Hepatology, Gunma University Graduate School of Medicine, Maebashi, Japan

H. Kaneko et al. (eds.), *Disorders of Gut-Brain Interaction*,
https://doi.org/10.1007/978-981-95-6974-8_6

pressure at the points where the sensor catheter contacts the esophageal wall or within closed spaces, potentially failing to accurately assess the state of the esophageal lumen. Additionally, HRM cannot evaluate the distensibility of the esophagus when food or liquids enter. This article provides an overview of EndoFLIP, a diagnostic method developed to assess esophageal distensibility.

1.2 What Is FLIP?

FLIP (functional luminal imaging probe) is a new device that uses impedance planimetry to simultaneously measure the cross-sectional area (CSA) and pressure within the gastrointestinal lumen. The catheter, equipped with multiple impedance electrodes, is covered by a balloon, and a specialized pump controls the rate and volume of fluid injected into the balloon (Fig. 6.1) [1].

The current diagnostic device using FLIP, known as EndoFLIP, includes 8 cm (with 16 sensors at 0.5 cm intervals) and 16 cm (with 16 sensors at 1 cm intervals) diagnostic balloon catheters, as well as therapeutic catheters for balloon dilation procedures. This article discusses the diagnostic procedure using the 16 cm diagnostic catheter.

The FLIP 1.0 module converts impedance information into CSA and displays the measurements in real-time 3D. The FLIP 2.0 or FLIP 300 module evaluates the distensibility of the esophagogastric junction (EGJ) and the contraction patterns of the esophageal body induced by balloon inflation, known as FLIP panometry (Fig. 6.1).

FLIP is particularly useful in cases where HRM results are inconclusive, for assessing the therapeutic effects of achalasia treatment, for intraoperative adjustments during fundoplication for GERD and esophageal motility disorders, and for evaluating strictures in eosinophilic esophagitis.

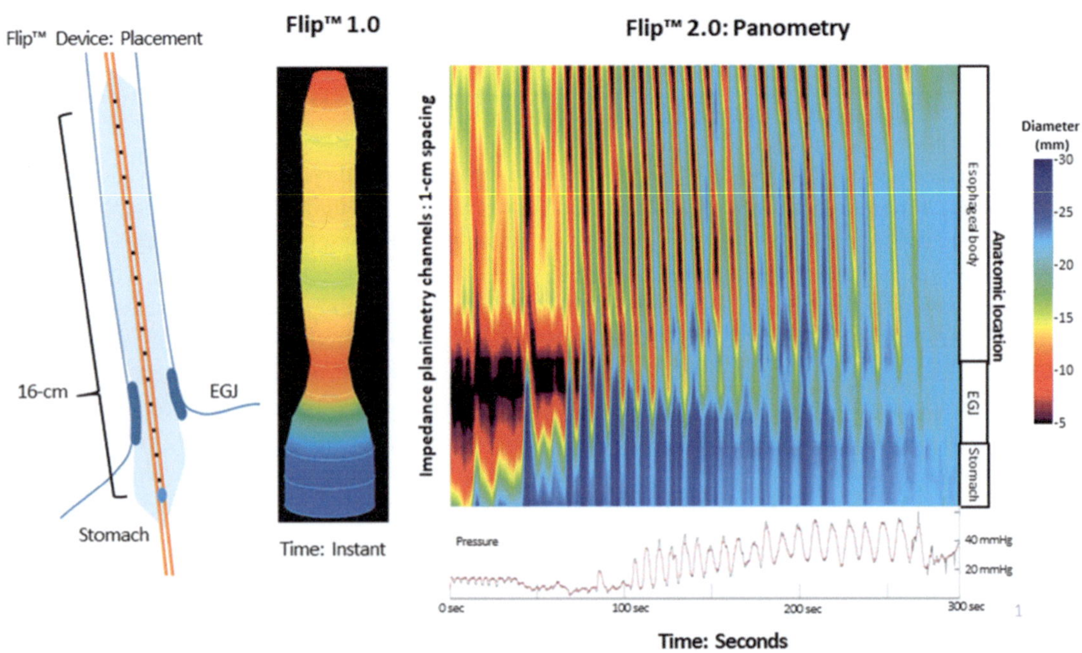

Fig. 6.1 FLIP device placement through the EGJ and the correlating FLIP 1.0 images using a 3-dimensional rendering of the esophageal lumen created by cross-sectional area measurements at 1 cm intervals for the 16-cm catheter and 0.5 cm in the 8-cm catheter. The FLIP 2.0 panometry uses FLIP topography to provide a space-time domain representation of diameter changes that represent contraction and distention of the esophageal lumen. EGJ esophagogastric junction, FLIP functional lumen imaging probe. (Adopted from Savarino E, *Am J Gastroenterol* 2020;115:1786–1796)

1.3 Examination Protocol

FLIP is performed on the same day as upper gastrointestinal endoscopy (EGD), following these steps:

1. Under Sedation, the Patient Was Placed in the Left Lateral Decubitus Position
(Exclude organic diseases via endoscopy, clean and aspirate esophageal residues, and confirm the distance from the incisors to the EGJ.)
2. Insert the FLIP balloon orally, and vertical placement may be confirmed by identifying the EGJ as the narrowed area ("waist" on FLIP display) above the gastric cavity at a fill volume of 40 mL and ideally should include 2 cm of the distal portion in the gastric cavity.
3. The standard FLIP panometry study protocol was agreed on to involve sequential FLIP filling to 50 mL, 60 mL, and 70 mL, holding each fill volume for at least 30 seconds.
4. During the examination, observe the contraction patterns of the esophageal body induced by balloon inflation and obtain the EGJ distensibility index (EGJ-DI) at 60 mL and the maximum EGJ diameter at 70-mL fill volume.

1.4 FLIP Panometry Analysis

FLIP panometry analysis is based on the distensibility of the EGJ and the contraction patterns of the esophageal body induced by balloon inflation. The initial classifications of FLIP panometry include the 2020 consensus by Savarino et al. [1] and the 2021 multicenter study by Carlson et al. [2], which have been further refined to develop the FLIP Panometry Classification version 2.0 in 2025 [3].

1.4.1 Evaluation of EGJ Distensibility [3]

The distensibility of the esophagogastric junction (EGJ) is evaluated using two indices: the EGJ distensibility index (EGJ-DI) and the EGJ diameter. EGJ-DI is calculated as CSA/pressure (mm^2/mmHg) at the narrowest CSA point of the EGJ during balloon inflation at 60 mL. The EGJ diameter is the maximum EGJ diameter at 70-mL fill volume (Fig. 6.2). The EGJ opening is classified into three categories: normal EGJ opening (NEO) with maximum EGJ diameter $\geq$16 mm and EGJ-DI at 60 mL $\geq$2.0 mm^2/mmHg, reduced EGJ opening (REO) with maximum EGJ diameter <12 mm and EGJ-DI at 60 mL <2.0 mm^2/mmHg, and inconclusive EGJ opening with all cases in between NEO and REO.

1.4.2 Evaluation of Esophageal Body Contraction Patterns Induced by Balloon Inflation [3]

Normally, esophageal distension stimuli induce secondary peristaltic waves in the esophagus, which are peristaltic waves not associated with swallowing. Balloon inflation with FLIP also induces secondary peristaltic waves. The reduction in CSA displayed by FLIP indirectly evaluates esophageal contraction.

Esophageal contractile activity can be defined by a transient decrease in diameter, represented by the color variation on a scale of red being low diameter and blue being high diameter, and further defined by direction (antegrade or retrograde) or other morphologic appearance (Fig. 6.3). Contraction features and patterns may be noted at specific volumes, whereas the contractile response category reflects an overall assessment of the aggregate of fill volumes of 50, 60, and 70 mL (Fig. 6.1). A normal cadence includes a rate of 6 ± 3 contractions per minute at a regular rhythm, although abnormal cadence can be represented by rapid or slow rate and variations in rhythm from irregular to sporadic.

The key contraction patterns (Fig. 6.3) and categories (Fig. 6.4) reflect a nonlinear spectrum of function related to secondary peristalsis and the esophageal contractile response to distention. A hierarchical approach, informed by the presence of specific contraction features and patterns, can be applied to determine the contractile response categories (Figs. 6.3, 6.4, and 6.5). Repetitive antegrade contractions or multiple distinct antegrade contractions define a "normal" response. On the other side of the spectrum is an

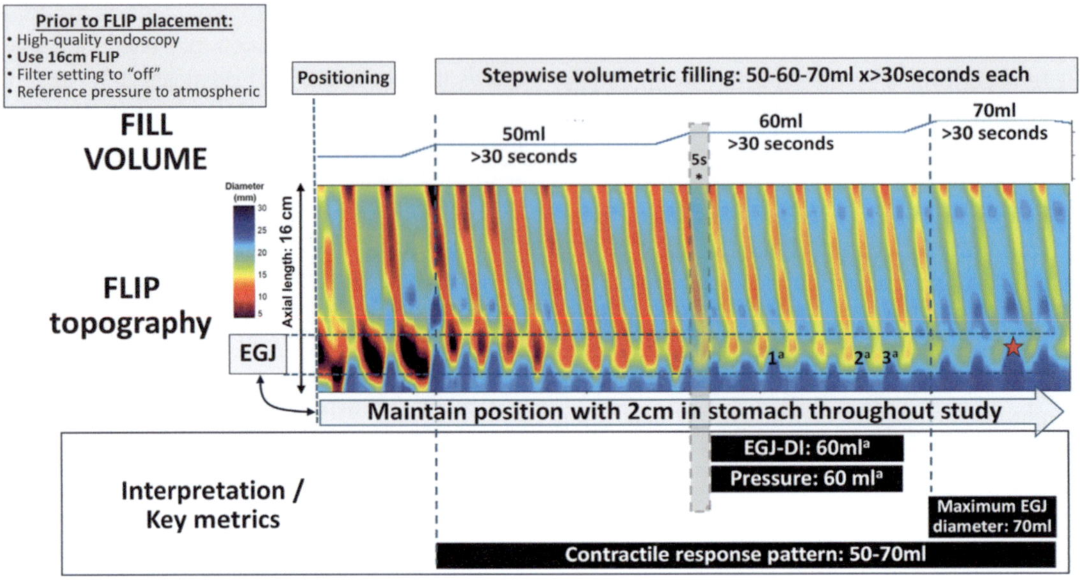

Fig. 6.2 The FLIP panometry study protocol. Key components and steps of the FLIP panometry study protocol are illustrated. Key metrics are made relative to the FLIP fill volumes during the standardized filling protocol. *The first 5 seconds after filling to 60 mL should be omitted from the EGJ-DI measurement to avoid incorporating filling-associated effects in the metric. [a]Then, the EGJ-DI is measured at 3 points of greatest EGJ opening diameter (1[a] -2[a] -3[a]), applying the median value of the 3 measures to classify EGJ opening. The associated pressure at times of EGJ-DI measures should also be noted and median value applied. The maximum EGJ diameter is measured at the time of greatest EGJ opening during the 70-mL fill volume (red star). (Adopted from Carlson DA, *Gastroenterol* 2025;168:1114–1127)

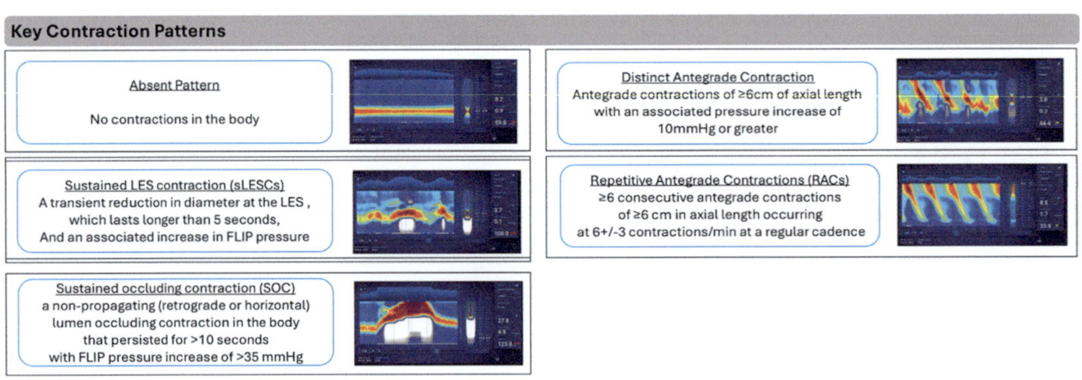

Fig. 6.3 FLIP panometry key contraction patterns. (Adopted from Carlson DA, *Gastroenterol* 2025;168:1114–1127)

"absent" contractile response or a "spastic" contractile response (Fig. 6.4). Key spastic patterns, which are often irregular and associated with higher vigor, include sustained LES contractions and sustained occluding contractions (SOCs) (Fig. 6.3), and are associated with spastic motility disorders, such as type III achalasia. For cases not meeting clear spastic, normal, or absent contractile response criteria, pressure can separate cases into "diminished" contractile response (low pressure), or "disordered" contractile response (high pressure).

Category	Morphology	Cadence	Vigor	Key Patterns	Example
Spastic Contractile Response	Retrograde Horizontal	Irregular Sporadic	Consider with Pressure increase of >35 mmHg	SOC's sLESc's	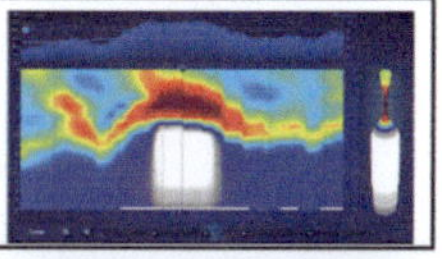
Disordered Contractile Response	Variable	Variable	>40 mmHg at 60 at EGJ-DI Consider with Pressure increase of >35 mmHg		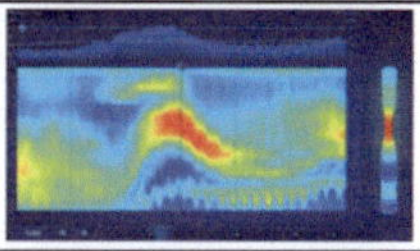
Normal Contractile Response	Antegrade	Repetitive or Inconsistent Normal Rate	Variable	RAC's, Multiple Distinct Antegrade Contractions	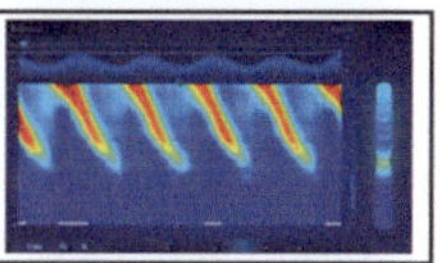
Diminished Contractile Response	Variable	Variable	< 40 mmHg at 60 at EGJ-DI		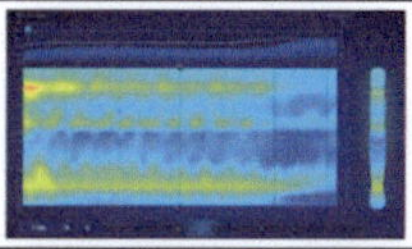
Absent Contractile Response	Absent at all fill volumes	N/A	Often < 40 mmHg at 60 at EGJ-DI	Absent Pattern	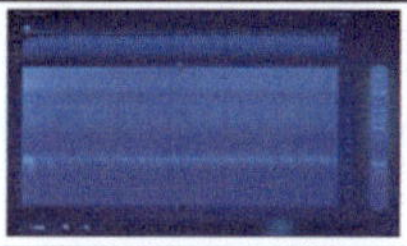

Fig. 6.4 Contractile response categories. Each contractile response category is demonstrated with an example representative image, features based on morphology, cadence and vigor, and the associated key pattern. (Adopted from Carlson DA, *Gastroenterol* 2025;168:1114–1127)

1.4.3 FLIP Panometry Classification

The EGJ opening classification (Fig. 6.2) and the contractile response categories (Figs. 6.3, 6.4, and 6.5) were jointly applied to designate a FLIP panometry motility classification, version 2.0 (Fig. 6.6).

A major motor disorder is unlikely in the setting of a "normal" FLIP panometry classification. "Diminished" or "absent" contractile response with reduced esophageal opening supports the diagnosis of a disorder of EGJ outflow. A "spastic" or "inconclusive" FLIP panometry classification should prompt further workup, such as with HRM and/or timed barium esophagram with tablet.

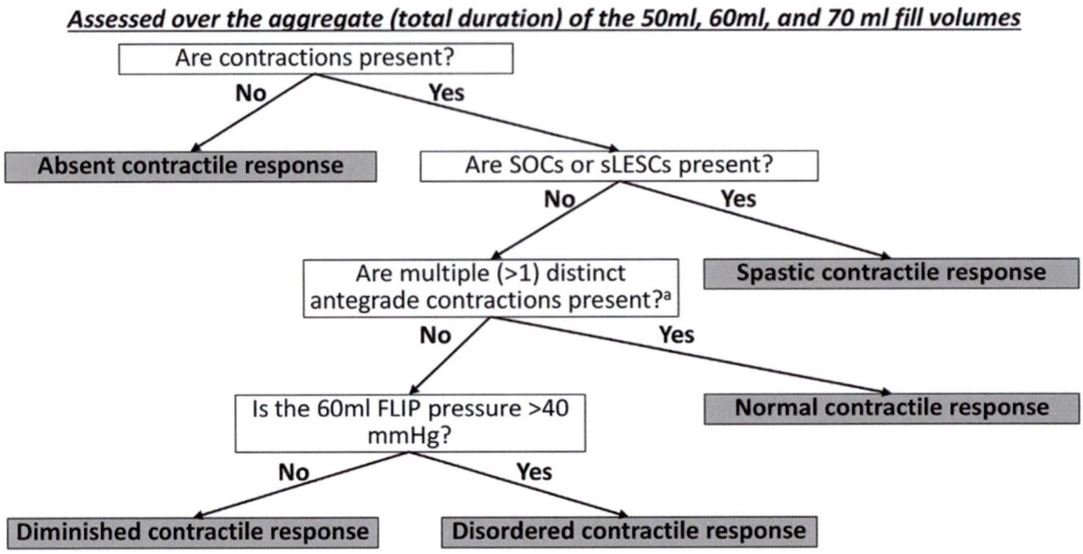

Fig. 6.5 A hierarchical approach to classifying the FLIP panometry contractile response category. Presence (or absence) or key contractile features (in addition to the pressure taken with the EGJ-DI during the 60-mL fill volume) can be applied to classify the contractile response. a Presence of more than 1 distinct antegrade contraction defined the normal contractile response, which did not require that distinct antegrade contractions occur in the repetitive antegrade contraction (RAC) pattern. (Adopted from Carlson DA, *Gastroenterol* 2025;168:1114–1127)

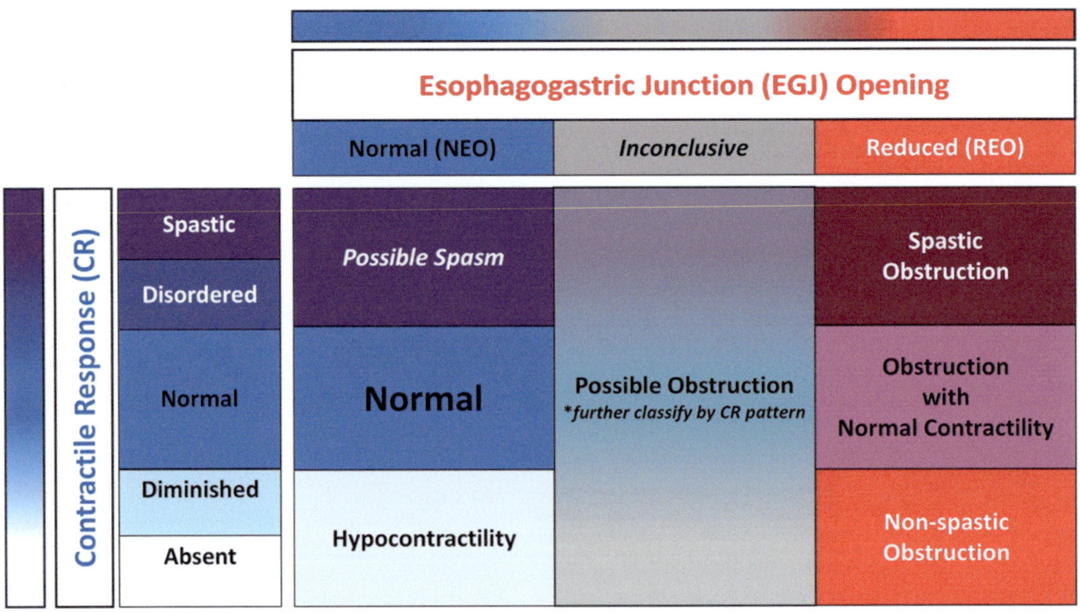

Fig. 6.6 The FLIP Panometry Motility Classification, version 2.0. The Dallas consensus incorporated the contractile response (CR) and EGJ opening categories to classify esophageal motility with FLIP panometry. *With inconclusive EGJ opening, which suggests "possible obstruction," the motility classification should be further described with the contractile response category. These esophageal motility classifications should be applied in the context of the patient's history and endoscopy findings to help guide clinical management. *With inconclusive EGJ opening, which suggests "possible obstruction," the motility classification should be further described with the contractile response category. (Adopted from Carlson DA, *Gastroenterol* 2025;168:1114–1127)

1.5 Advantages of FLIP

FLIP is performed under sedation following endoscopy, making it well-tolerated by patients. Unlike HRM, which requires contact with the catheter's pressure sensors to detect pressure, FLIP can identify esophageal motility disorders even in cases where HRM fails to detect abnormalities due to poor distensibility and lack of significant pressure increase. Reports indicate that FLIP identified esophageal motility disorders in nearly 30% of cases where HRM did not [4]. Additionally, FLIP can assess the loss of esophageal wall distensibility in eosinophilic esophagitis and the progression of distensibility with age and disease duration, although it is difficult to assess poor esophageal wall distensibility due to long-term inflammation and fibrosis, such as eosinophilic esophagitis, with HRM (Fig. 6.5) [5, 6].

FLIP is also useful for evaluating the effectiveness of medications for esophageal motility disorders and for intraoperative adjustments during treatments for esophageal motility disorders and GERD, such as balloon dilation, myotomy, or fundoplication, to set appropriate luminal diameters [7].

1.6 Conclusion

FLIP panometry can evaluate esophageal motility in response to sustained esophageal distention at the time of sedated endoscopy. This assessment can be applied to improve the diagnostic yield of endoscopy and direct immediate intervention (such as dilation), or direct the need for additional complementary evaluation.

Take-Home Message

FLIP, a new diagnostic method for esophageal motility disorders, simultaneously measures the cross-sectional area and pressure within the gastrointestinal lumen. EndoFLIP can evaluate the distensibility of the esophagogastric junction (EGJ) and the contraction patterns of the esophageal body induced by balloon inflation. FLIP panometry provides a well-tolerated method that can complement, or in some cases be an alternative to HRM, for evaluating esophageal motility disorders.

Competing Interests The author(s) has no competing interests to declare that are relevant to the content of this manuscript.

References

1. Savarino E, et al. Use of the functional lumen imaging probe in clinical esophagology. Am J Gastroenterol. 2020;115(11):1786–96.
2. Carlson DA, et al. Classifying esophageal motility by FLIP panometry: a study of 722 subjects with manometry. Am J Gastroenterol. 2021;116(12):2357–66.
3. Carlson DA, et al. A standardized approach to performing and interpreting functional lumen imaging probe panometry for esophageal motility disorders: the Dallas Consensus. Gastroenterology. 2025;168(6):1114–27 e5.
4. Carlson DA, et al. Evaluating esophageal motility beyond primary peristalsis: assessing esophagogastric junction opening mechanics and secondary peristalsis in patients with normal manometry. Neurogastroenterol Motil. 2021;33(10):e14116.
5. Menard-Katcher C, et al. Influence of age and eosinophilic esophagitis on esophageal distensibility in a pediatric cohort. Am J Gastroenterol. 2017;112(9):1466–73.
6. Kwiatek MA, et al. Mechanical properties of the esophagus in eosinophilic esophagitis. Gastroenterology. 2011;140(1):82–90.
7. Hsing LC, et al. The predictive value of intraoperative esophageal functional luminal imaging probe panometry in patients with achalasia undergoing peroral endoscopic myotomy: a single-center experience. J Neurogastroenterol Motil. 2022;28(3):474–82.

7 Esophageal Motility Test, Esophagram

Shiko Kuribayashi

Abstract

Esophagram allows for the observation of the movement of the bolus within the esophagus as well as esophageal motility. Esophagram can be performed at many institutes and is useful for detecting esophageal motility and evaluating treatment efficacy. Timed barium esophagram (TBE) is useful for quantitative evaluation of esophageal motility. In addition, morphology and degree of dilation of the esophagus can be assessed by not esophageal manometry but esophagram, which are associated with treatment outcome. The sensitivity of detecting esophageal motility disorders is higher when solid objects or foods are ingested in combination with liquids than when liquids are ingested alone. Usefulness of esophagram with barium tablet, marshmallow, and onigiri is reported.

Keywords

Esophagram · Timed barium esophagram · Barium tablet · Marshmallow · Onigiri

S. Kuribayashi (✉)
Department of Gastroenterology and Hepatology, Gunma University Graduate School of Medicine, Maebashi, Japan
e-mail: shikokuri@gunma-u.ac.jp

1 Esophagram

Esophagram allows for the observation of not only esophageal motility but also the movement of the bolus within the esophagus. Although esophageal manometry is performed for the diagnosis of esophageal motility disorders, the availability of institutes capable of conducting this test is limited. In contrast, esophagram can be performed at many institutes and is useful for detecting esophageal motility disorders and evaluating treatment efficacy.

The "bird's beak" appearance at the esophagogastric junction in achalasia (Fig. 7.1) and the "corkscrew" appearance in diffuse esophageal spasm (Fig. 7.2) can be observed. These are qualitative evaluations, with diagnostic sensitivity reported to be 56–69% [1].

For quantitative evaluation of esophagram, the timed barium esophagram (TBE) is standardly performed. Additionally, the utility of swallowing evaluation in the prone position has been reported as a new quantitative assessment [2]. When barium is ingested in the prone position and the esophageal transit time exceeds 40 seconds, normal primary peristalsis are not observed on high-resolution manometry (HRM), and the odds ratio for abnormal primary peristalsis is six times higher compared to patients with transit times less than 40 seconds.

H. Kaneko et al. (eds.), *Disorders of Gut-Brain Interaction*,
https://doi.org/10.1007/978-981-95-6974-8_7

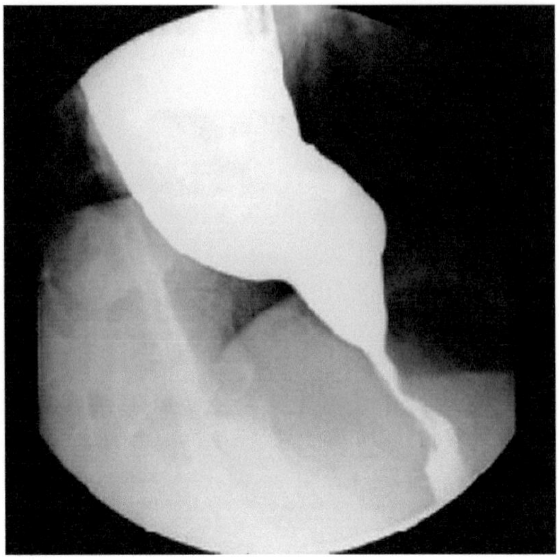

Fig. 7.1 Esophagram findings in esophageal achalasia (https://radiologyspot.weebly.com/b.html). The "bird's beak" appearance at the esophagogastric junction is observed in patients with esophageal achalasia

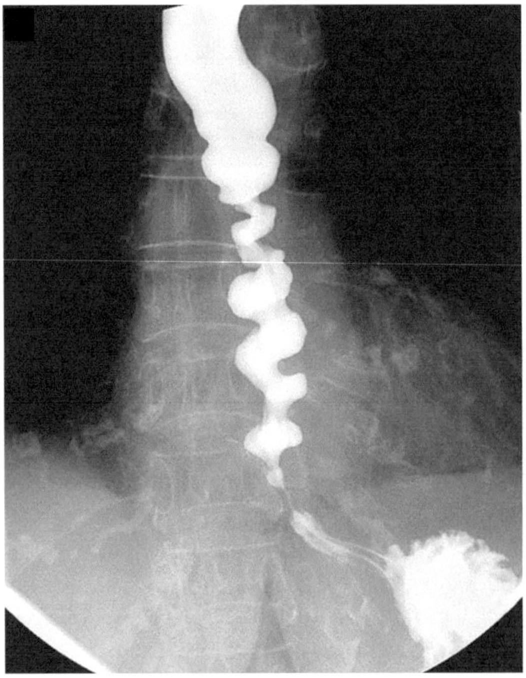

Fig. 7.2 Esophagram findings in diffuse esophageal spasm (https://radrounds.com/radiology-case-images-teaching-file/diffuse-esophageal-spasm/#google_vignette). The "corkscrew" appearance is observed

2 Timed Barium Esophagram (TBE)

2.1 Protocol

A low-density barium sulfate (45 weight/volume%) (100–200 mL) is ingested over 30–40 seconds, and images are taken in the right anterior oblique position at 1 minute, 2 minutes, and 5 minutes post-ingestion to measure the width and height of the barium retained in the esophagus [3, 4]. However, the amount of barium and ingestion time are not standardized. A review summarizing the methods and utility of TBE mentions ingestion of 100–250 mL over 15–20 seconds [5]. Recently, it has been recommended to use 8 ounces (236 mL) of barium for the test [1, 6, 7]. In healthy individuals, no barium retention is observed at 1 minute and 5 minutes post-ingestion [8].

2.2 Evaluation Method and Utility

The achalasia guidelines of the International Society for Diseases of the Esophagus (ISDE) recommend performing TBE for the evaluation of disease state and treatment efficacy, rather than qualitative evaluation through esophagram [4].

(i) Detection of Esophageal Motility Disorders

In a study evaluating untreated achalasia, esophagogastric junction outflow obstruction (EGJOO), and non-achalasia dysphagia patients diagnosed using high-resolution manometry (HRM), the height of barium retained in the esophagus at 1 minute post-ingestion *of 8 ounces (236 mL)* was 5 cm, with a sensitivity of 94% and specificity of 71% for differentiating untreated achalasia from other disorders (EGJOO and non-achalasia dysphagia). Additionally, in this study, the sensitivity was 85% and specificity was 86% when 2 cm of barium retention was observed at 5 minutes post-ingestion. Therefore, it is proposed to use 5 cm at 1 minute and 2 cm at 5 minutes post-ingestion as cutoff values for barium retention in the esophagus [6].

(ii) Post-treatment Evaluation

In a study investigating the relationship between symptoms before and after pneumatic dilation (PD) and the height of barium retained at 5 minutes post-ingestion in TBE, 30% of patients with more than 90% symptom improvement had less than 50% reduction in barium height post-treatment compared to pre-treatment [8]. In cases where temporary symptom improvement was achieved but no improvement in barium retention was observed post-treatment, 90% of patients experienced symptom recurrence within 12 months [9]. Furthermore, 77% of patients who showed improvement in both symptoms and barium retention post-treatment maintained symptom improvement for 6 years, whereas none of the patients who showed temporary symptom improvement but no improvement in barium retention maintained symptom improvement for 6 years [9]. Another study found that patients with barium height less than 5 cm at 5 minutes post-ingestion after PD had a significantly lower need for re-treatment (hazard ratio 0.80, 95% confidence interval: 0.66–0.97) [10].

Comparing TBE and esophageal manometry findings, a study of 41 achalasia patients found that TBE evaluation of barium height >5 cm at 5 minutes post-ingestion was more useful for predicting treatment efficacy than lower esophageal sphincter (LES) pressure >10 mmHg [11]. In achalasia patients treated with PD or laparoscopic Heller myotomy (LHM), 13 patients with barium height ≥5 cm at 5 minutes post-ingestion had residual symptoms in 7 cases (54%) and symptom improvement in 6 cases (46%) [12]. Among the 7 patients with residual symptoms, 6 had post-treatment integrated relaxation pressure (IRP) >15 mmHg, while 4 of the 6 patients with symptom improvement had IRP <15 mmHg. Among the 12 patients with barium height <5 cm at 5 minutes post-ingestion post-treatment, 9 showed symptom improvement and IRP <15 mmHg, 1 showed no symptom improvement and IRP >15 mmHg, and 2 showed IRP <15 mmHg but no symptom improvement. In such cases, evaluating the distensibility of the esophagogastric junction may be useful.

There are two methods for post-treatment evaluation using TBE: assessing changes in barium retention before and after treatment and evaluating the amount of barium retained post-treatment. In achalasia patients treated with PD, LHM, or per-oral endoscopic myotomy (POEM), a study comparing the change in barium height at 5 minutes post-ingestion before and after treatment and the absolute amount of barium retained post-treatment found that when the amount of barium retained post-treatment decreased by more than 3% compared to pre-treatment, the sensitivity of treatment efficacy was 60% and specificity was 99%. In contrast, when the barium height at 5 minutes post-ingestion was >5 cm, the sensitivity was 70% and specificity was 75%, indicating that evaluating the change in barium retention before and after treatment better reflected treatment efficacy [13]. Another study comparing the change in barium height at 5 minutes post-ingestion before and after treatment and the absolute amount of barium retained post-treatment in achalasia patients treated with PD or POEM found that when the barium height at 5 minutes post-ingestion decreased by more than 38% compared to pre-treatment, the sensitivity of treatment efficacy was 100% and specificity was 65%. In contrast, when the barium height at 5 minutes post-ingestion was >5 cm, the sensitivity was 75% and specificity was 45%, indicating that evaluating the change in barium retention before and after treatment was useful for predicting treatment efficacy [14].

3 Radiographic Classification (Evaluation of Morphology and Degree of Dilation)

(i) Protocol

The 4th edition of the Japanese descriptive rules for achalasia of the esophagus states, "Ingest 100 mL of 100 weight/volume% barium sulfate as quickly as possible and take images at 1 minute post-ingestion" [15].

(ii) Morphology Types of the Esophagus

The 1st to 3rd editions of the Japanese descriptive rules for achalasia of the esophagus classified the morphology of the esophagus into three types: spindle type, flask type, and sigmoid type. However, the pathophysiological differences between spindle type and flask type are not clear, and these types are not distinguished in Western countries. On the other hand, the degree of deviation and meandering of the upper esophagus may affect treatment outcomes in sigmoid type, and the 4th edition classifies expansion into two types: straight type (St type) and sigmoid type (Sg type) [15]. In cases where the esophagus deviates markedly to the right and presents an L-shape, it is classified as advanced sigmoid type (aSg type) (Fig. 7.3). TBE is considered more useful than esophageal manometry for evaluating these morphology types of the esophagus [4]. Additionally, when the esophagus is meandering, it is often difficult to insert the catheter from the esophagogastric junction into the stomach during esophageal manometry.

(iii) Degree of Dilation

The 4th edition of the Japanese descriptive rules for achalasia of the esophagus classifies the degree of esophageal dilation based on the maximum esophageal transverse diameter (*d*) perpendicular to the long axis of the esophagus. Grade I is defined as $d < 3.5$ cm, Grade II as $3.5 \leq d < 6.0$ cm, and Grade III as $d \geq 6.0$ cm (Fig. 7.4) [15]. Additionally, the descriptive rules list the following as supplementary items: meandering of the upper thoracic esophagus, leftward meandering of the esophagus, coexistence of diaphragmatic diverticulum (pulsion diverticulum), and coexistence of esophageal cancer (location, size, depth of invasion).

(iv) Differences in Treatment Outcomes by Radiographic Classification

In a study of nine patients with Grade III esophageal dilation (esophageal diameter > 7 cm)

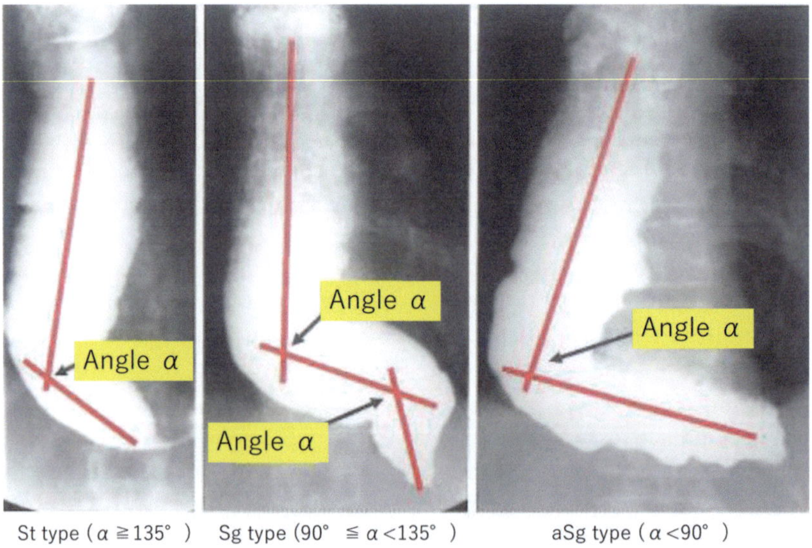

Fig. 7.3 Morphological classification of esophageal achalasia. (From the 4th edition of the Japanese descriptive rules for achalasia of the esophagus). Esophageal achalasia is classified based on the presence or absence of esophageal flexion observed in esophagram into straight type (St type) and sigmoid type (Sg type). In cases where the esophagus deviates markedly to the right and presents an L-shape, it is classified as advanced sigmoid type (aSg type)

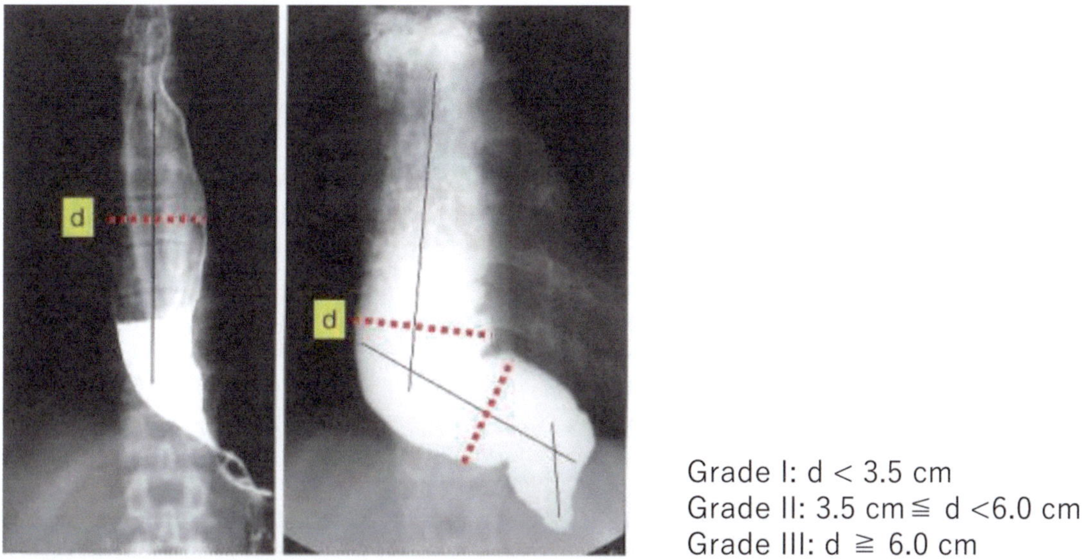

Fig. 7.4 Classification of esophageal dilation in esophageal achalasia. (From the 4th edition of the Japanese descriptive rules for achalasia of the esophagus). The degree of esophageal dilation is classified based on the maximum esophageal transverse diameter (*d*) perpendicular to the long axis of the esophagus: Grade I ($d < 3.5$ cm), Grade II ($3.5 \leq d < 6.0$ cm), and Grade III ($d \geq 6.0$ cm)

who underwent pneumatic dilation (PD) using a 35 mm balloon, the procedure was performed without complications, and symptom improvement was achieved in all cases for at least 12 months [16]. Additionally, long-term outcomes of PD indicated that esophageal dilation was not a factor for poor treatment outcomes [17]. However, in general, patients with marked esophageal dilation and meandering often experience recurrence shortly after temporary improvement with PD.

A study summarizing the long-term outcomes of laparoscopic Heller myotomy (LHM) for sigmoid type (Sg type) achalasia reported that 71% of patients maintained symptom improvement (Eckardt score < 3) 9 years postoperatively, and no re-treatment was necessary. Although treatment outcomes were significantly worse compared to non-Sg type patients, good treatment outcomes were still achieved in Sg type patients [18].

Initially, advanced sigmoid type (aSg type) was excluded from the indications for per-oral endoscopic myotomy (POEM) [19]. However, subsequent studies including aSg type demonstrated good treatment outcomes regarding safety and efficacy [20]. A prospective study evaluating the treatment outcomes of POEM in 31 Sg type patients reported an efficacy rate of 96.8%, with symptom improvement also observed in three aSg type patients [21]. However, a multicenter study summarizing the treatment outcomes of POEM in 1826 patients from 12 institutes worldwide reported a significantly higher incidence of mucosal injury and intraoperative and postoperative complications in Sg type patients [22]. Therefore, the POEM clinical guidelines states, "POEM for sigmoid type requires advanced skills and should be performed with sufficient experience" [23].

4 Esophagram Using Solid Objects and Solid Foods

1. Barium Tablet

A 13 mm barium tablet is ingested to observe its passage from the esophagus to the stomach. In a study evaluating untreated achalasia, esophagogastric junction outflow obstruction (EGJOO), and non-achalasia dysphagia patients diagnosed using HRM, the diagnostic accuracy for untreated achalasia improved from 79.5% to 100%, and the diagnostic accuracy for EGJOO improved from 48.9% to 60% by combining the evaluation with a 13 mm tablet in combination with the standard TBE [6]. Based on these results, the American College of Gastroenterology (ACG) guidelines recommend combining the evaluation with a 13 mm barium tablet in addition to the standard TBE using low-concentration barium sulfate [7].

2. Marshmallow

Marshmallows coated with barium sulfate have been used during esophagram to investigate the cause of dysphagia. In a study of 37 patients with no abnormalities detected by upper gastrointestinal endoscopy, esophagram using only barium sulfate, or conventional esophageal manometry, esophagram using a 5 cm^3 marshmallow revealed dysphagia in 89% of patients, compared to 9% with barium sulfate alone, suggesting nonspecific esophageal motility disorders in these patients [24]. In a study comparing HRM and esophagram using marshmallows for preoperative evaluation of esophageal motility in gastroesophageal reflux disease (GERD), 3 out of 18 patients who had marshmallows pass through the esophagogastric junction developed postoperative dysphagia, with a positive predictive value of 0.833 for the absence of postoperative dysphagia when marshmallows passed through. Additionally, 23 out of 27 patients with abnormal HRM findings did not have marshmallows pass through, with a negative predictive value of 0.767 for abnormal HRM findings. In this study, half-sized marshmallows were used, and the tests were performed not only in the upright position but also in the supine and Trendelenburg positions [25].

3. Onigiri (Rice Ball)

The utility of esophagram using onigiri has been reported from Japan [26]. First, 10 mL of 100 weight/volume% liquid barium is ingested, and if it does not pass through the esophagogastric junction, it is classified as OL4. Then, a 10 g onigiri coated with barium powder is chewed 15 times and swallowed. If it passes through the esophagogastric junction, it is classified as OL0; if it does not pass but passes with additional swallowing, it is classified as OL1; if it passes with the addition of 10 mL of liquid barium, it is classified as OL2; and if it does not pass even with the addition of liquid barium, it is classified as OL3 (Fig. 7.5). The proportion of patients with

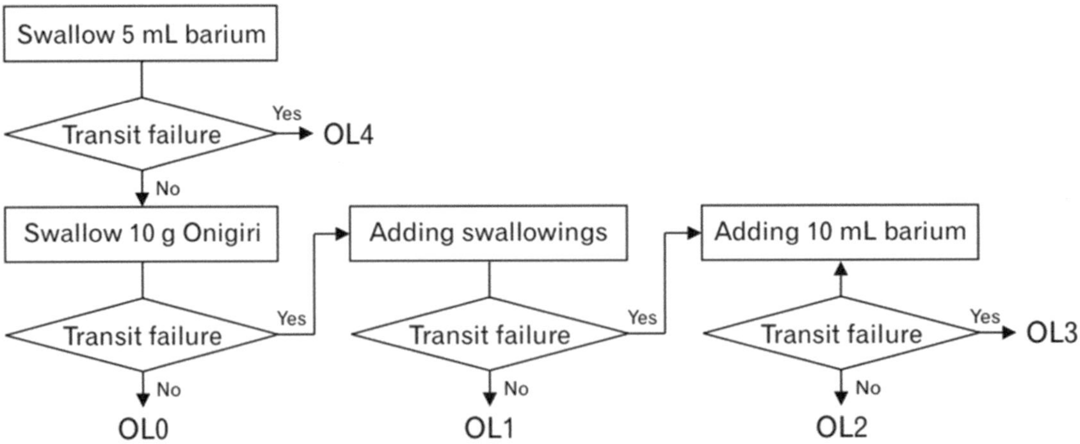

Fig. 7.5 Diagnostic flowchart for esophagram using onigiri [26]. First, 5 mL of 100 weight/volume% liquid barium is ingested. If it does not pass through the esophagogastric junction, it is classified as OL4. Then, a 10 g onigiri coated with barium powder is chewed 15 times and swallowed. If it passes through the esophagogastric junction, it is classified as OL0; if it does not pass but passes with additional swallowing, it is classified as OL1; if it passes with the addition of 10 mL of liquid barium, it is classified as OL2; and if it does not pass even with the addition of liquid barium, it is classified as OL3

esophageal motility disorders detected by HRM was 32.3% for OL0, 50.0% for OL1, 88.0% for OL2, and 100% for OL3 and OL4. The sensitivity and specificity for detecting esophageal motility disorders by HRM with OL1 or higher findings were 87.3% and 61.3%, respectively, and it is proposed to use OL1 as the cutoff for detecting esophageal motility disorders.

Take-Home Message

Although frontal images are often taken, it is better to take images in the first oblique position (right anterior oblique) to avoid overlapping the esophagus and spine, which makes observation difficult. Additionally, since barium is used in esophagram, a laxative should be prescribed after the examination.

Competing Interests The author(s) has no competing interests to declare that are relevant to the content of this manuscript.

References

1. Patel DA, et al. Esophageal motility disorders: current approach to diagnostics and therapeutics. Gastroenterology. 2022;162:1617–34.
2. Razia D, et al. Association of bolus transit time on barium esophagram with esophageal peristalsis on high-resolution manometry and nonobstructive dysphagia. J Clin Gastroenterol. 2022;56:748–55.
3. de Oliveira JM, et al. Timed barium swallow: a simple technique for evaluating esophageal emptying in patients with achalasia. Am J Roentgenol. 1997;169:473–9.
4. Zaninotto G, et al. The 2018 ISDE achalasia guidelines. Dis Esophagus. 2018:31.
5. Neyaz Z, et al. How to perform and interpret timed barium esophagogram. J Neurogastroenterol Motil. 2013;19:251–6.
6. Blonski W, et al. Timed barium swallow: diagnostic role and predictive value in untreated achalasia, esophagogastric junction outflow obstruction, and non-achalasia dysphagia. Am J Gastroenterol. 2018;113:196–203.
7. Gyawali CP, et al. ACG clinical guidelines: clinical use of esophageal physiologic testing. Am J Gastroenterol. 2020;115:1412–28.
8. Vaezi MF, et al. Assessment of esophageal emptying post-pneumatic dilation: use of the timed barium esophagram. Am J Gastroenterol. 1999;94:1802–7.
9. Vaezi MF, et al. Timed barium oesophagram: better predictor of long term success after pneumatic dilation in achalasia than symptom assessment. Gut. 2002;50:765–70.
10. Farhoomand K, et al. Predictors of outcome of pneumatic dilation in achalasia. Clin Gastroenterol Hepatol. 2004;2:389–94.
11. Rohof WO, et al. Esophageal stasis on a timed barium esophagogram predicts recurrent symptoms in patients with long-standing achalasia. Am J Gastroenterol. 2013;108:49–55.
12. Nicodeme F, et al. A comparison of symptom severity and bolus retention with Chicago classification esophageal pressure topography metrics in patients with achalasia. Clin Gastroenterol Hepatol. 2013;11:131–7.
13. Blonski W, et al. Timed barium swallow for assessing long-term treatment response in patients with achalasia: absolute cutoff versus percent change —a cross-sectional analytic study. Neurogastroenterol Motil. 2021;33:e14005.
14. Sanagapalli S, et al. The timed barium swallow and its relationship to symptoms in achalasia: analysis of surface area and emptying rate. Neurogastroenterol Motil 2020;32:e13928.
15. Japan Esophageal Society. Guidelines for the management of esophageal achalasia. 4th ed. Kinbara Publishing; 2012. (in Japanese).
16. Khan AA, et al. Massively dilated esophagus in achalasia: response to pneumatic balloon dilation. Am J Gastroenterol. 1999;94:2363–6.
17. Ghoshal UC, et al. Long-term follow-up after pneumatic dilation for achalasia cardia: factors associated with treatment failure and recurrence. Am J Gastroenterol. 2004;99:2304–10.
18. Salvador R, et al. Laparoscopic Heller-Dor is an effective long-term treatment for end-stage achalasia. Surg Endosc. 2023;37:1742–8.
19. Inoue H, et al. Peroral endoscopic myotomy (POEM) for esophageal achalasia. Endoscopy. 2010;42:265–71.
20. Inoue H, et al. Per-oral endoscopic myotomy: a series of 500 patients. J Am Coll Surg. 2015;221:256–64.
21. Li QL, et al. Clinical impact of submucosal tunneling endoscopic resection for the treatment of gastric submucosal tumors originating from the muscularis propria layer (with video). Surg Endosc. 2015;29:3640–6.
22. Haito-Chavez Y, et al. Comprehensive analysis of adverse events associated with per oral endoscopic myotomy in 1826 patients: an international multicenter study. Am J Gastroenterol. 2017;112:1267–76.
23. Inoue H, et al. POEM clinical guidelines. Gastroenterological Endoscopy. 2018;60:1251–71. (in Japanese)
24. Meshkinpour H, et al. Unexplained dysphagia: viscous swallow-induced esophageal dysmotility. Dysphagia. 1996;11:125–8.
25. Caudell CW, et al. Can the marshmallow esophagram replace high-resolution manometry as an appropriate screening for esophageal motility prior to anti-reflux surgery? Am J Surg. 2022;224:1366–9.
26. Hamada S, et al. Onigiri esophagography as a screening test for esophageal motility disorders. J Neurogastroenterol Motil. 2022;28:43–52.

Part III

Esophagus, Practical Edition

Diagnosis and Treatment of DGBI of the Esophagus, Introduction

8

Toshimi Chiba

Abstract

According to the Rome IV criteria, FGIDs in the esophageal region include Functional Chest Pain, Functional Heartburn, Reflux Hypersensitivity, Globus, and Functional Dysphagia. Esophageal motility testing is performed using high-resolution manometry (HRM) to systematically evaluate esophageal motility disorders. The Chicago Classification, now in its fourth version, provides a diagnostic flow diagram of esophageal motility disorders. The practical section of this chapter addresses functional heartburn, non-cardiac chest pain, globus, functional dysphagia/dysphagia, followed by NERD/reflux hypersensitivity, GIMD including achalasia, diffuse esophageal spasm (DES), and esophageal motility abnormalities associated with scleroderma and collagen diseases.

Keywords

Functional Chest Pain · Functional Heartburn · Reflux Hypersensitivity · Globus · Functional Dysphagia · Symptom index · Symptom association probability · Non-Erosive Reflux Disease · Chicago Classification

T. Chiba (✉)
Division of Internal Medicine, Department of Oral Medicine, Iwate Medical University, Morioka, Japan
e-mail: toschiba@iwate-med.ac.jp

1 Diagnosis and Treatment of Functional Esophageal Disorders

1.1 Introduction

The primary symptoms associated with the esophagus include heartburn, chest pain, and dysphagia. The manifestation of these symptoms involves swallowing function, upper esophageal sphincter (UES) pressure, esophageal primary peristaltic waves, lower esophageal sphincter (LES) pressure, and the reflux of gastric contents, with psychological factors also playing a role.

Functional Gastrointestinal Disorders (FGIDs) are conditions based on unexplained symptoms. According to the Rome IV criteria, FGIDs in the esophageal region are 5 of classified as Functional Esophageal Disorders (A). These include Functional Chest Pain (A1), Functional Heartburn (A2), Reflux Hypersensitivity (A3), Globus (A4), and Functional Dysphagia (A5). These disorders are characterized by the absence of gastroesophageal reflux disease (GERD), eosinophilic esophagitis, or major esophageal motility disorders [1]. The causes of Non-Cardiac Chest Pain (NCCP) (A1) often include esophageal motility disorders such as nutcracker esophagus, nonspecific esophageal motility disorders, diffuse esophageal spasm, hypertensive LES, and achalasia. These conditions are caused by gastrointestinal motility disorders (GIMD). Other cases are classified as

H. Kaneko et al. (eds.), *Disorders of Gut-Brain Interaction*,
https://doi.org/10.1007/978-981-95-6974-8_8

functional chest pain. Functional Heartburn (A2) and Reflux Hypersensitivity (A3) are conditions associated with gastroesophageal reflux disease (GERD) and are diagnosed using impedance esophageal pH monitoring to assess reflux and the symptom index (SI) and symptom association probability (SAP) indices to assess symptom association. Globus (A4) and Functional Dysphagia (A5) are diagnosed based on primary symptoms according to the Rome IV criteria. However, clear differentiation in clinical practice can be difficult, and overlap with other FGIDs should be considered. Non-Erosive Reflux Disease (NERD) is characterized by heartburn symptoms induced by acid reflux.

Currently, esophageal motility testing is performed using high-resolution manometry (HRM), an intraluminal catheter-based technique with pressure measurement sites placed 1 cm apart, to systematically evaluate esophageal motility disorders. The Chicago Classification, now in its fourth version, provides a diagnostic flow diagram of esophageal motility disorders [2] (Fig. 8.1).

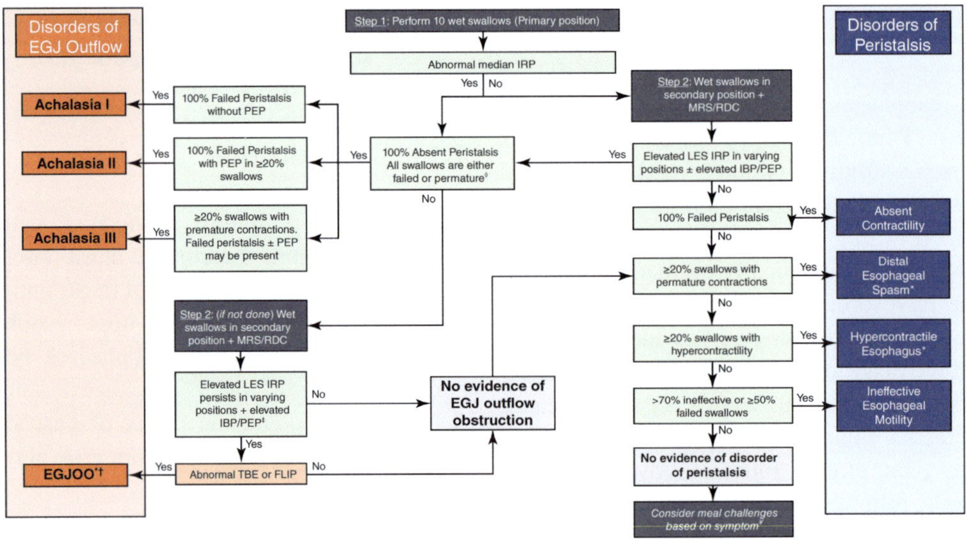

Fig. 8.1 Chicago Classification 4.0 Hierarchical Classification Scheme. (Adapted with permission from: Yadlapati et al. [2]. Wiley). This flow diagram represents a conceptual model of a state of-the-art algorithm that defines the flow process of how the CCv4.0 diagnosis is generated within the constructs of the various phases of the protocol. In this conceptual model, the current protocol allows for some flexibility if the diagnosis is conclusive with 10 swallows in either the primary supine or upright position and allows for a sequenced progression of the protocol to help confirm or rule out the diagnosis. This flow diagram represents the optimal flow process; however exceptions will exist based on the fact that some cutoffs are arbitrary and that the model assumes that a motility expert or a highly qualified motility technician or nurse is performing the protocol and analysis. *Denote manometric patterns of unclear clinical relevance. A clinically relevant conclusive diagnosis requires additional information which may include clinically relevant symptoms and/or supportive testing (as detailed in the document). †Patients with EGJ obstruction and presence of peristaltic swallows would fulfill strict criteria for EGJOO and may have features suggestive of achalasia or other patterns of peristalsis defined by criteria for disorders of peristalsis: EGJOO with spastic features, EGJOO with hypercontractile esophagus, EGJOO with ineffective motility, or EGJOO with no evidence of disordered peristalsis. ‡RDC, solid test swallows, and/or pharmacologic provocation with amyl nitrite or cholecystokinin (if available) can be instituted here to assess for obstruction. ◊Patients previously defined absent contractility based on 10 swallows in the primary position may have achalasia if the IRP is elevated in the alternate position, with the RDC, and/or with MRS. These cases should be considered inconclusive for type I or II achalasia as appropriate and evaluated further with TBE/FLIP. ¥If no evidence of a disorder of peristalsis or EGJ outflow in a patient with high probability of a missed EGJOO, a solid test meal can be added to rule out an obstructive pattern; if abnormal then possibility of a mechanical obstruction should be readdressed. In a patient with regurgitation or belching, postprandial high-resolution impedance monitoring can be used to assess for rumination/belching disorder. IRP integrated relaxation pressure, MRS multiple rapid swallow, RDC rapid drink challenge, LES lower esophageal sphincter, IBP intrabolus pressurization, PEP panesophageal pressurization, EGJ esophagogastric junction: EGJOO EGJ outflow obstruction, TBE timed barium esophagram, FLIP functional lumen imaging probe

The practical section of this chapter addresses functional heartburn, non-cardiac chest pain, globus, functional dysphagia/dysphagia, followed by NERD/reflux hypersensitivity, GIMD including achalasia, diffuse esophageal spasm (DES), and esophageal motility abnormalities associated with scleroderma and collagen diseases.

Competing Interests The author(s) has no competing interests to declare that are relevant to the content of this manuscript.

References

1. Aziz Q, et al. Esophageal disorders. Gastroenterology. 2016;150:1368–79.
2. Yadlapati R, et al. Esophageal motility disorders on high-resolution manometry: Chicago classification version 4.0©. Neurogastroenterol Motil. 2021;33:e14058.

Diagnosis and Treatment of DGBI of the Esophagus, Functional Heartburn

9

Noriaki Manabe

Abstract

Functional heartburn (FH) is defined as retrosternal burning despite normal esophageal acid exposure on 24-hour pH monitoring and absence of major esophageal motor disorders or mucosal abnormalities like erosive esophagitis, Barrett's esophagus, or eosinophilic esophagitis on endoscopy. This condition is often misdiagnosed as proton pump inhibitor (PPI)-resistant gastroesophageal reflux disease (GERD), leading to unnecessary long-term PPI use. Studies show FH accounts for 21–39% of patients with PPI-resistant heartburn, highlighting its prevalence in clinical practice. Unlike non-erosive reflux disease (NERD), FH does not involve acid as a primary cause, suggesting a different visceral hypersensitivity mechanism. Patients with FH often exhibit generalized gastrointestinal visceral hypersensitivity and a higher comorbidity with anxiety and other emotional disorders, indicating central processing abnormalities of sensory signals. Brain imaging studies reveal distinct neural activation patterns in FH patients compared to healthy individuals and GERD patients during esophageal stimulation. Diagnosis involves careful history taking to differentiate from other gastric symptoms, endoscopy with biopsy to rule out other esophageal diseases, and 24-hour impedance-pH monitoring to assess reflux and symptom association. Treatment aims to improve symptoms and quality of life and includes lifestyle modifications (though evidence is limited for FH specifically), neuromodulators, and psychological interventions. PPIs are generally ineffective unless there is overlapping GERD. Surgical or endoscopic anti-reflux procedures should be avoided in FH due to poor outcomes. While FH typically does not lead to long-term organic complications, it significantly impairs patients' quality of life. Future research is needed to establish long-term clinical courses and optimal treatments for this common condition.

Keywords

Functional heartburn · GERD · Esophageal hypersensitivity · Neuromodulators · pH-impedance monitoring

1 Concept

Functional heartburn is defined as a condition characterized by a burning sensation behind the sternum similar to gastroesophageal reflux dis-

N. Manabe (✉)
Division of Endoscopy and Ultrasonography, Department of Clinical Laboratory Medicine, Kawasaki Medical School, Okayama, Japan
e-mail: n_manabe@med.kawasaki-m.ac.jp

H. Kaneko et al. (eds.), *Disorders of Gut-Brain Interaction*,
https://doi.org/10.1007/978-981-95-6974-8_9

ease (GERD), but without abnormal esophageal acid exposure on 24-hour pH monitoring, major esophageal motility disorders on high-resolution esophageal manometry, or erosive esophagitis, Barrett's esophagus, or eosinophilic esophagitis on esophageal mucosal biopsy during endoscopy [1]. In other words, acid suppression therapy is generally ineffective for functional heartburn, and anti-reflux surgery, including endoscopic treatment, should be avoided. Functional heartburn, if not evaluated with functional tests such as 24-hour pH monitoring, may be misdiagnosed as proton pump inhibitor (PPI)-resistant GERD, leading to unnecessary long-term acid suppression therapy, making it a condition that requires careful attention in daily clinical practice.

2 Epidemiology

The frequency of functional heartburn varies depending on whether the patients are seen by primary care physicians, gastroenterologists, or are PPI-resistant cases. It also varies depending on the type of tests used to exclude GERD (PPI test, 24-hour pH monitoring, 24-hour impedance-pH testing, etc.), requiring careful consideration. Therefore, it is challenging to investigate the prevalence of functional heartburn in primary care settings. Zerbib et al. reported that among patients with PPI-resistant heartburn, 21–39% met the criteria for functional heartburn based on 24-hour impedance-pH monitoring [2], indicating that 1/4 to 1/2 of PPI-resistant GERD patients have functional heartburn, making it highly prevalent in daily clinical practice. A prospective study of 366 refractory heartburn patients among U.S. veterans also reported that 99 patients (27%) had functional heartburn based on esophageal function tests such as 24-hour impedance-pH monitoring, 23 patients (6%) had non-GERD esophageal diseases, and 7 patients (2%) had esophageal motility disorders, indicating a high proportion of functional heartburn among refractory heartburn patients.

3 Etiology and Pathophysiology

Previous esophageal acid perfusion tests have shown that non-erosive reflux disease (NERD) patients experience heartburn symptoms when acid is perfused into the esophagus, whereas functional heartburn patients do not, indicating that acid is not involved in the etiology of this condition [3]. Studies on the distribution of afferent nerves in the esophageal mucosa have shown that functional heartburn, unlike NERD, exhibits a nerve distribution similar to that of healthy volunteers, suggesting the involvement of nociceptive mechanisms similar to other functional gastrointestinal disorders [4]. Balloon distension tests have demonstrated that functional heartburn patients exhibit visceral hypersensitivity in both the esophagus and rectum, suggesting generalized visceral hypersensitivity in the gastrointestinal tract [5]. Additionally, functional heartburn patients have been reported to have a high prevalence of anxiety disorders and other affective disorders, suggesting the involvement of abnormalities in the central processing of sensory signals [6].

Regarding the central processing of sensory signals from the periphery, studies on cerebral evoked potentials during esophageal balloon distension in functional heartburn patients have shown shorter latencies and larger amplitudes of the N1, P1, and N2 waves. Recent advances in brain functional imaging diagnostic devices such as positron emission tomography (PET) and functional magnetic resonance imaging (fMRI) have elucidated the brain regions involved in processing sensations such as heartburn when the esophagus is stimulated (Fig. 9.1) [7]. Functional gastrointestinal disorders, such as irritable bowel syndrome (IBS), often worsen with stress, and functional heartburn is no exception, with heartburn symptoms closely related to stress. In patients with GERD, auditory stress from noise and loud sounds, as well as stress from sleep deprivation, has been shown to enhance esopha-

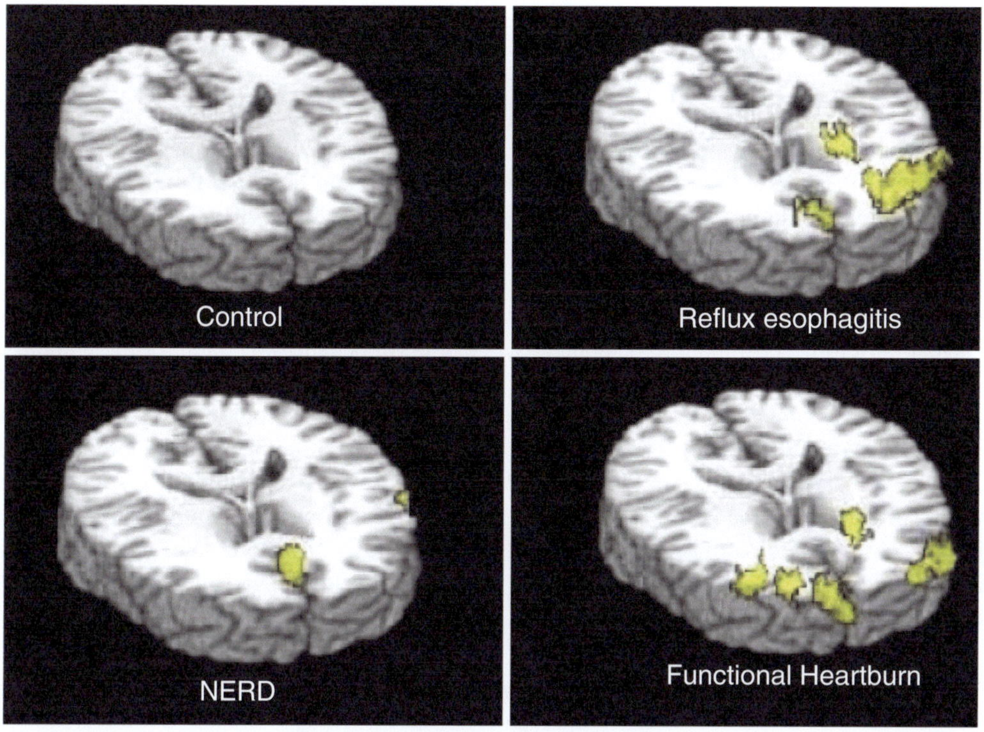

Fig. 9.1 Differences in Brain Responses to Esophageal Acid Stimulation in Healthy Individuals, Reflux Esophagitis, NERD, and Functional Heartburn (fMRI). (Adapted from Reference [7]). Brain processing during esophageal stimulation involves the prefrontal cortex, anterior cingulate cortex, and insula. Additionally, this brain processing differs among healthy individuals, reflux esophagitis, NERD, and functional heartburn

geal acid sensitivity. Various life stresses are related to the worsening of heartburn symptoms, and studies have reported that depression is associated with more frequent medication for heartburn symptoms. Furthermore, comparisons of psychosocial status between functional heartburn and GERD patients have shown that functional heartburn patients exhibit stronger somatization of psychological stress. Wang et al. investigated the relationship between psychological factors and heartburn symptoms using fMRI, showing that functional heartburn patients exhibit esophageal hypersensitivity and different brain activity regions when the esophagus is stimulated, with psychological factors more closely influencing symptom onset compared to GERD patients [7].

4 Diagnostic Criteria and Examination

Today, the diagnostic criteria for NERD, reflux hypersensitivity (heartburn induced by physiological gastroesophageal reflux episodes), and functional heartburn have been redefined by the Rome IV criteria, which provide stricter diagnostic criteria and reduce confusion between true GERD/NERD and functional heartburn [8]. The mechanisms of heartburn other than gastroesophageal reflux, represented by functional heartburn, are thought to contribute to the decreased efficacy of PPI therapy in heartburn patients [9].

The first step in diagnosing functional heartburn is taking a medical history. Generally, patients may present with epigastric pain, indigestion, abdominal bloating, and other symptoms as "heartburn," requiring careful history taking [10]. The clinical symptoms of functional heartburn are similar to those of GERD, so the diagnosis should be considered when heartburn symptoms do not improve or worsen with PPI therapy.

Next, endoscopy is performed to exclude other esophageal and gastric diseases such as esophageal stricture, eosinophilic esophagitis, drug-induced esophagitis, Barrett's esophagus, and cancer in patients with insufficient response to PPI therapy (Fig. 9.2) [11]. Generally, the prevalence of erosive esophagitis in PPI-resistant heartburn patients is less than 10%, and the prevalence of eosinophilic esophagitis does not exceed 8%, although the frequency is low [12]. To adhere to the definition of functional heartburn, esophageal mucosal biopsies should be performed as needed to definitively exclude eosinophilic esophagitis.

Many refractory heartburn patients who do not respond to PPI therapy have normal results on endoscopy and esophageal biopsy, necessitating 24-hour impedance-pH monitoring to evaluate the degree of gastroesophageal reflux. According to recent consensus statements, patients not previously diagnosed with GERD should undergo pH or impedance-pH monitoring without acid suppression therapy to establish baseline reflux levels [1]. High-resolution esophageal manometry is necessary for esophageal motility disorders, but mild esophageal motility disorders such as ineffective esophageal motility do not preclude the diagnosis of functional heartburn if GERD is excluded. Additionally, adding impedance information to pH monitoring allows detection of

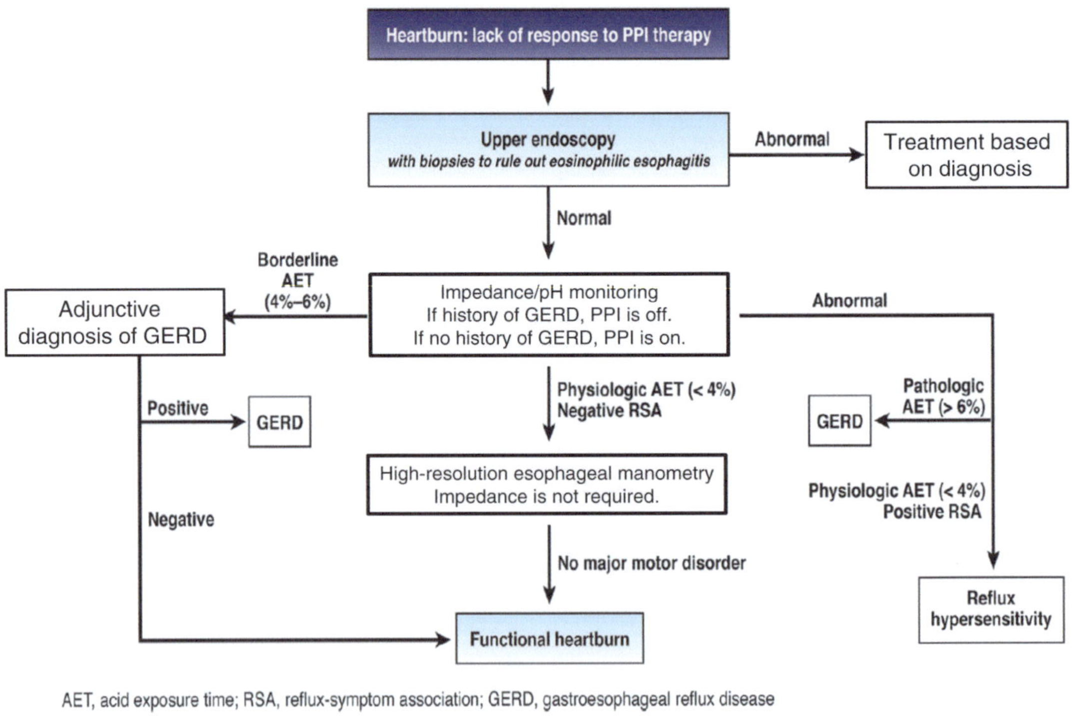

Fig. 9.2 Diagnostic Flowchart for Persistent Heartburn Symptoms Despite Appropriate Acid Suppression Therapy [11]. In Step 1, a biopsy is performed during endoscopy to exclude eosinophilic esophagitis. In Step 2, impedance-pH monitoring is conducted without acid suppression therapy in patients with no history of GERD, and during acid suppression therapy in patients with a history of GERD. Functional heartburn is diagnosed when there is no esophageal mucosal damage on endoscopy, no major motility disorders on high-resolution esophageal manometry, and normal esophageal acid exposure time (less than 4%)

weakly acidic reflux episodes, enabling more accurate correlation between symptoms and reflux episodes and characterization of reflux episodes.

Esophageal acid exposure time is considered abnormal if it exceeds 6% and normal if it is below 4%. When esophageal acid exposure time is normal, symptom index (SI) and symptom association probability (SAP) are used to differentiate functional heartburn from reflux hypersensitivity. SI is a simple parameter that determines the proportion of symptoms related to reflux, with values above 50% considered positive. SAP is calculated by dividing the 24-hour measurement period into 2-minute intervals, recording the presence or absence of symptoms and reflux events, creating a 2 × 2 table, and using Fisher's exact test to calculate the p-value, with SAP calculated as $(1.0 - p) \times 100$ (%). SAP is an evaluation method that considers both reflux events and symptoms, with values above 95% considered positive, although the calculation is labor-intensive. These two indices (SI and SAP) are complementary, but neither is 100% reliable, and their correlation may be questioned depending on symptom frequency and reflux occurrence.

In refractory heartburn, if endoscopy, esophageal acid exposure time are normal, SI and SAP are both negative, functional heartburn can be definitively diagnosed. Conversely, if both SI and SAP are positive, reflux hypersensitivity can be diagnosed. However, if there is a discrepancy between SI and SAP results, there is currently no consensus on which result should be prioritized [13]. Additionally, patients with a history of GERD and persistent heartburn symptoms despite PPI therapy should consider impedance-pH monitoring under double-dose PPI therapy to detect weakly acidic reflux. In such cases, impedance-pH monitoring during PPI therapy can establish the relationship between symptoms and acid or weakly acidic reflux in 10% and 30–40% of patients, respectively. If esophageal acid exposure time is normal and SI and SAP are both negative for acid and weakly acidic reflux, the diagnosis is a combination of GERD and functional heartburn.

When esophageal acid exposure time is between 4% and 6%, or if there is a discrepancy in SI and SAP results, or if impedance/pH monitoring results are borderline or inconclusive, additional measurement criteria may be useful. Low mean nocturnal baseline impedance (MNBI) (<2292 ohms) is cited as a permeability marker of esophageal mucosa altered by reflux, useful in distinguishing patients with reflux-related symptoms from those with functional heartburn. The proportion of swallows following reflux episodes in impedance-pH monitoring, known as post-reflux swallow-induced peristaltic wave (PSPW), reflects primary peristalsis induced by reflux episodes. A normal PSPW index (>0.61) may be useful in distinguishing functional heartburn from GERD patients, but further investigation is needed.

5 Differential Diagnosis and Complications

Important conditions to be differentiated and excluded include gastrointestinal cancers such as gastric and pancreatic cancer, as well as inflammatory esophageal diseases such as GERD, drug-induced esophagitis, and eosinophilic esophagitis. Additionally, other disease groups such as reflux hypersensitivity and esophageal motility disorders must also be considered. Before making a final diagnosis of functional heartburn, it is crucial to exclude systemic diseases such as thyroid disorders and various collagen diseases. Conditions that frequently coexist with functional heartburn include functional dyspepsia, irritable bowel syndrome (IBS), depression, anxiety disorders, and sleep disorders.

6 Treatment

It is important to consider functional heartburn as a separate condition from GERD, requiring multifaceted management. Therefore, whether functional heartburn occurs alone or overlaps with GERD, it is unlikely to improve without appropriate management of altered visceral per-

Table 9.1 Therapeutic options for functional heartburn

Therapeutic options
Lifestyle modifications
Improved sleep experience
Pharmacotherapy
Tricyclic antidepressants
Selective serotonin reuptake inhibitors
Tegaserod
Histamine 2 receptor antagonists
Melatonin
Alternative/complementary medicine
Acupuncture
Psychological intervention
Hypnotherapy

ception and the aforementioned psychological stress. The treatment goals for functional heartburn are (1) symptom improvement, ideally symptom resolution, (2) prevention of symptom recurrence, and (3) improvement of health-related quality of life (QOL). The main treatment methods include (1) lifestyle modifications, (2) pharmacotherapy with neuromodulators, (3) alternative and complementary medicine, and (4) psychological and psychiatric interventions (Table 9.1) [11]. Some functional heartburn patients may require more than one of these treatment methods for symptom control.

6.1 Lifestyle Modifications

It has been confirmed that the frequency of sleep disorders increases with the severity and frequency of heartburn. Additionally, stress, including sleep deprivation, is suggested to be associated with esophageal hypersensitivity or its exacerbation [14], and improving sleep quality may positively impact the alleviation of functional heartburn symptoms, although evidence is limited. While there is evidence that avoiding certain foods and physical activities that trigger heartburn symptoms is beneficial for GERD patients, there is currently no established evidence that lifestyle modifications are effective for functional heartburn patients.

6.2 Pharmacotherapy

Acid suppression therapy, including PPIs, is ineffective unless GERD overlaps with functional heartburn. However, if overlap with GERD is confirmed by upper gastrointestinal endoscopy or 24-hour impedance-pH monitoring, PPI therapy should be maintained while adding treatment for functional heartburn. Neuromodulators, which alter nerve function without acting as neurotransmitters, have central and minor peripheral effects on esophageal pain and have been tried in non-cardiac chest pain patients. They are classified into (1) tricyclic antidepressants, (2) selective serotonin reuptake inhibitors (SSRIs), (3) serotonin modulators (agonists and antagonists), and (4) serotonin-norepinephrine reuptake inhibitors.

Table 9.2 shows the neuromodulators tried for functional heartburn [11]. In a double-blind placebo-controlled trial evaluating the effect of 25 mg/day of imipramine for 8 weeks in patients with functional heartburn and reflux hypersensitivity, there was no difference in heartburn improvement, but significant improvement in QOL was observed. Fluoxetine (not approved by the Japanese Ministry of Health, Labour and Welfare and not listed or sold as a prescription drug in Japan) is the only SSRI evaluated for functional heartburn, showing improvement in heartburn symptoms. In a double-blind placebo-controlled trial using tegaserod (a 5-HT_4 agonist removed from the market in 2007 due to potential cardiovascular adverse effects), improvement in heartburn symptoms and esophageal sensory thresholds was observed. Ranitidine, a histamine-2 receptor antagonist, has been shown to have pain-modulating effects by reducing chemoreceptor sensitivity to esophageal acid perfusion [15]. Melatonin, which regulates visceral pain in the gastrointestinal tract, has been proven effective in various functional pain syndromes and significantly improves QOL in functional heartburn patients [16]. Although clinical trials evaluating the efficacy of neuromodulators in functional heartburn are limited, these results

Table 9.2 Neuromodulator trials in functional heartburn

Class	Drug	Dose	No. of subjects	Outcome	Study type
TCA	Imipramine	25 mg/d	83	No difference than placebo in symptom relief	RCT
				Improved QOL	
SSRI	Fluoxetine	20 mg/d	144	Improvement in percentage of heartburn-free days	RCT
Serotonin agonist ($5\text{-}HT_4$)	Tegaserod	6 mg bid	42	Decreased frequency of heartburn, regurgitation, and distress	RCT
H_2RA	Ranitidine	150 mg	18	Decrease in esophageal sensitivity	RCT
Miscellaneous anxiolytics, sedatives, and hypnotics	Melatonin	6 mg bid	60	Improved GERD-HRQOL	RCT

bid twice per day, *H_2RA* histamine 2 receptor antagonist, *HRQOL* health-related quality of life, *QOL* quality of life, *RCT* randomized controlled trial, *SSRI* selective serotonin reuptake inhibitor, *TCA* tricyclic antidepressant

suggest that neuromodulators play a therapeutic role as first-line drugs for functional heartburn. Currently, there are no large-scale studies evaluating the efficacy of alternative and complementary therapies for functional heartburn. However, very small-scale studies have shown that hypnotherapy tends to improve heartburn symptoms, anxiety, and QOL.

On the other hand, normal preoperative esophageal acid exposure time has been shown to be a risk factor for poor prognosis after surgical intervention [17], and anti-reflux surgery or endoscopic treatment for GERD should be avoided in functional heartburn patients.

7 Prognosis

True GERD and functional heartburn can overlap, and 24-hour impedance-pH monitoring may miss abnormalities in esophageal acid exposure due to diurnal variation [18]. Therefore, even in patients considered to have functional heartburn, long-term complications of GERD, such as Barrett's esophagus and gastrointestinal strictures, may be identified. However, these are considered very rare cases, and the prognosis for most functional heartburn patients should focus on the significant reduction in QOL rather than organic complications. Like other functional gastrointestinal disorders, functional heartburn does not typically lead to long-term complications, but the significant reduction in patient QOL necessitates targeted treatment [19].

8 Conclusion

The lack of heartburn symptom relief or only partial relief despite optimal treatment is an important starting point for considering a diagnosis of functional heartburn. Functional tests are reliable diagnostic methods for identifying the mechanisms of heartburn symptoms and providing precise individualized medical care [20]. During treatment, ineffective therapies such as acid suppression therapy should be discontinued while neuromodulators are administered. However, as neuromodulators are not covered by insurance for functional heartburn, careful explanation and administration are required. Despite being a common condition encountered in daily practice, there is currently no evidence on the long-term course and prognosis of functional heartburn, necessitating future studies on the long-term clinical course and treatment methods in a large number of cases.

Take-Home Message

Among refractory heartburn patients with persistent symptoms despite appropriate treatment, there is a high likelihood of functional heartburn.

Conducting 24-hour impedance-pH monitoring in these patients allows for a more objective understanding of their condition.

Competing Interests The author(s) has no competing interests to declare that are relevant to the content of this manuscript.

References

1. Aziz Q, et al. Functional esophageal disorders. Gastroenterology. 2016;150:1368–79.
2. Zerbib F, et al. Clinical, but not oesophageal pH-impedance, profiles predict response to proton pump inhibitors in gastro-oesophageal reflux disease. Gut. 2012;61:501–6.
3. Weijenborg PW, et al. Esophageal acid sensitivity and mucosal integrity in patients with functional heartburn. Neurogastroenterol Motil. 2016;28:1649–54.
4. Nikaki K, et al. Esophageal mucosal innervation in functional heartburn: closer to healthy asymptomatic subjects than to non-erosive reflux disease patients. Neurogastroenterol Motil. 2019;31:e13667.
5. Freede M, et al. Comparison of rectal and esophageal sensitivity in women with functional heartburn. Gastroenterol Nurs. 2016;39:348–58.
6. de Bortoli N, et al. Functional heartburn overlaps with irritable bowel syndrome more often than GERD. Am J Gastroenterol. 2016;111:1711–7.
7. Wang K, et al. Differences in cerebral response to esophageal acid stimuli and psychological anticipation in GERD subtypes—an fMRI study. BMC Gastroenterol. 2011;11:28.
8. Zhang M, et al. The Rome IV versus Rome III criteria for heartburn diagnosis: a comparative study. United European Gastroenterol J. 2018;6:358–66.
9. Hillman L, et al. A review of medical therapy for proton pump inhibitor nonresponsive gastroesophageal reflux disease. Dis Esophagus. 2017;30:1–15.
10. Manabe N, et al. Differences in recognition of heartburn symptoms between Japanese patients with gastroesophageal reflux, physicians, nurses, and healthy lay subjects. Scand J Gastroenterol. 2008;43:398–402.
11. Fass R, et al. AGA clinical practice update on functional heartburn: expert review. Gastroenterology. 2020;158:2286–93.
12. Abe N, et al. Long-term outcomes of combination of endoscopic submucosal dissection and laparoscopic lymph node dissection without gastrectomy for early gastric cancer patients who have a potential risk of lymph node metastasis. Gastrointest Endosc. 2011;74:792–7.
13. Bennett MC, et al. Chronic cough is associated with long breaks in esophageal peristaltic integrity on high-resolution manometry. J Neurogastroenterol Motil. 2018;24:387–94.
14. Fass R, et al. The effect of auditory stress on perception of intraesophageal acid in patients with gastroesophageal reflux disease. Gastroenterology. 2008;134:696–705.
15. Rodriguez-Stanley S, et al. A single dose of ranitidine 150 mg modulates oesophageal acid sensitivity in patients with functional heartburn. Aliment Pharmacol Ther. 2004;20:975–82.
16. Basu P, et al. The effect of melatonin in functional heart-burn: a randomized, placebo-controlled clinical trial. Op J Gastroenterol. 2014;2014:56–61.
17. Khajanchee YS, et al. Outcomes of antireflux surgery in patients with normal preoperative 24-hour pH test results. Am J Surg. 2004;187:599–603.
18. Penagini R, et al. Inconsistency in the diagnosis of functional heartburn: usefulness of prolonged wireless pH monitoring in patients with proton pump inhibitor refractory gastroesophageal reflux disease. J Neurogastroenterol Motil. 2015;21:265–72.
19. Josefsson A, et al. Oesophageal symptoms are common and associated with other functional gastrointestinal disorders (FGIDs) in an English-speaking Western population. United European Gastroenterol J. 2018;6:1461–9.
20. Katzka DA, et al. Phenotypes of gastroesophageal reflux disease: where Rome, Lyon, and Montreal meet. Clin Gastroenterol Hepatol. 2020;18:767–76.

10 Diagnosis and Treatment of Motility Disorder of the Esophagus, Non-Cardiac Chest Pain

Yasushi Funaki, Naotaka Ogasawara, and Kunio Kasugai

Abstract

Non-cardiac chest pain (NCCP) is epidemiologically common among cases of chest pain, and most causes of NCCP originate from esophageal disorders within the spectrum of gastrointestinal diseases. Among these, functional esophageal disorders hold an important clinical position, with key symptoms including heartburn, chest pain, and dysphagia. These disorders involve overlapping conditions such as esophageal motility disorders, gastroesophageal reflux disease (GERD), and NCCP. For diagnosis, it is essential first to rule out structural diseases of the upper gastrointestinal tract and ischemic heart disease. Subsequently, diagnostic tests such as esophagography, esophageal manometry, and 24-hour esophageal impedance-pH monitoring are necessary. The mechanism of pain in NCCP is thought to involve a lowered pain threshold. Emotional stress, such as anxiety, and psychosocial factors also contribute to the condition, often leading to delays in diagnosis and treatment. Therefore, while appropriate pharmacological treatment tailored to each individual pathology is essential, a psychosomatic approach similar to that used in treating functional somatic syndromes and chronic pain is also recommended.

Keywords

Noncardiac chest pain · Gastroesophageal reflux disease · Esophageal motility disorders · Pain hypersensitivity · 24-hour esophageal impedance-pH monitoring

1 Concept

Chest pain is well-known as a symptom of cardiovascular diseases such as angina pectoris, myocardial infarction, and aortic dissection, as well as respiratory diseases such as vascular disorders of pulmonary origin, pneumothorax, and pulmonary embolism. However, when patients present with chest pain and detailed examinations reveal no organic disease, and cardiovascular examinations show no abnormalities, the condition is collectively referred to as non-cardiac chest pain (NCCP) [1].

Y. Funaki (✉) · N. Ogasawara · K. Kasugai
Department of Gastroenterology, Aichi Medical University School of Medicine, Nagakute, Japan

Department of Gastroenterology, Aichi Medical University Medical Center, Okazaki, Japan
e-mail: momomaru@aichi-med-u.ac.jp

H. Kaneko et al. (eds.), *Disorders of Gut-Brain Interaction*,
https://doi.org/10.1007/978-981-95-6974-8_10

2 Epidemiology

NCCP recurrents episode of pain below the sternum similar to angina pectoris, despite not being cardiac in origin. It is epidemiologically more frequent among chest pains, with a prevalence of approximately 25% in Western countries and 19% in Asia (China) among patients presenting with chest pain [2]. Gender differences indicate that female NCCP patients are more likely to visit emergency departments, although there is no gender difference in the intensity of chest pain [2]. NCCP is frequently encountered in daily clinical practice, with an annual prevalence of about 25% [3], accounting for 2–5% of emergency patients in hospitals [4]. Due to the chief complaint of chest pain, patients are often examined by cardiologists, and even after cardiac chest pain is excluded at the initial visit, most patients continue to be treated by cardiologists or primary care physicians. Only a small number of patients are referred to gastroenterologists for detailed examination, indicating a need for awareness reform among healthcare providers regarding the pathophysiology of NCCP.

3 Etiology and Pathophysiology

The etiology of NCCP includes gastrointestinal diseases, respiratory diseases, musculoskeletal disorders, and psychogenic factors (Table 10.1), with 20–60% of cases attributed to esophageal diseases [5]. Gastroesophageal reflux disease (GERD) accounts for approximately 50–60% of NCCP cases, making it the most frequent cause [1]. Conversely, chest pain is a representative atypical symptom of GERD. The Montreal Definition, a global definition of GERD, includes the term "reflux chest pain syndrome," indicating that GERD can cause chest pain indistinguishable from cardiac pain such as angina pectoris [6]. In Western countries, where the proportion of GERD patients among NCCP cases is high, GERD patients frequently visit emergency departments. Due to the similarity between chest pain caused by myocardial ischemia, which requires urgent treatment and is life-threatening, and chest pain caused by GERD, significant healthcare costs are spent on managing chest pain cases in emergency care, and there is high

Table 10.1 Causes of non-cardiac chest pain

Category	Subcategory	Example conditions
Gastrointestinal disorders	Esophageal disorders	Gastroesophageal reflux disease (GERD)
Esophageal motility disorders		
Eosinophilic esophagitis		
Esophageal cancer		
Esophageal rupture due to forceful vomiting		
Functional esophageal disorders		
	Gastrointestinal disorders	Gastric/duodenal ulcer, perforation
Functional dyspepsia		
Intestinal obstruction		
	Biliary disorders	Gallstones, cholecystitis, acute cholangitis
Respiratory disorders		Pneumothorax, asthma, lung cancer, pleuritis, pneumonia
Musculoskeletal/neurological disorders		Musculoskeletal pain, rib fractures, intercostal neuralgia
Psychogenic		Somatoform disorder

interest in NCCP. In Japan, the proportion of GERD among NCCP cases in emergency departments is lower compared to Western countries [7], likely due to lower GERD prevalence and a lower proportion of severe reflux esophagitis cases. Additionally, there is a difference in recognition regarding chest pain caused by GERD, and there are many cases where "NCCP due to GERD" is not diagnosed. With the decrease in *Helicobacter pylori* infection rates and the Westernization of dietary habits, the number of GERD cases, including reflux esophagitis, has been increasing in Japan, and the importance of GERD in emergency care is expected to increase in the future.

Esophageal motility disorders are the second most common cause of NCCP after GERD, with approximately 30% of NCCP patients without GERD having esophageal motility disorders [8]. Common esophageal motility disorders causing NCCP include nutcracker esophagus with abnormally high primary peristaltic waves (14.8%), nonspecific esophageal motility disorders (10.8%), diffuse esophageal spasm (3%), high-pressure lower esophageal sphincter (LES) (1.2%), and achalasia (0.6%) [8]. Nutcracker esophagus is diagnosed when LES relaxation is normal, peristaltic waves are normal, but the average peristaltic wave height exceeds 180 mmHg. Typical cases present with chest pain accompanied by high wave heights during swallowing. Approximately half of these esophageal motility disorder patients have abnormal gastric acid reflux, and the relationship between these disorders and GERD is being investigated. The Rome criteria, an international standard for functional gastrointestinal disorders, classify functional chest pain of presumed esophageal origin as one type of NCCP, defining it as occurring the symptoms at least once a week and excluding major organic esophageal motility disorders such as GERD, eosinophilic esophagitis, organic obstruction, achalasia, diffuse esophageal spasm, jackhammer esophagus, and absent peristalsis [9]. Although the frequency is unclear, cohort studies report that 32–35% of NCCP patients correspond to functional esophageal chest pain [10]. The cause of symptom onset is not clear, but peripheral and central hypersensitivity are likely involved [11].

GERD and esophageal motility disorders, functional esophageal diseases in the broad sense encountered in daily clinical practice, overlap with each other (Fig. 10.1). Considering this, the pathophysiology of esophageal-origin NCCP is discussed. The mechanism of esophageal-origin chest pain is not fully understood, but it is thought that afferent sensory signals from the esophagus and heart are transmitted to the same dorsal spinal nerves, and chemical receptor stimulation by gastric acid or abnormal esophageal contractions (spasms) caused by gastric acid reflux, as well as mechanical receptor stimulation within the esophagus, may cause chest pain. However, in patients who complain of chest pain due to acid injection into the esophagus, abnormal esophageal motility is rarely observed during acid injection. This suggests that the pain is caused by chemoreceptor stimulation, which is the cause of most NCCP due to GERD. One mechanism of NCCP pain is presumed to be a decrease in pain threshold, i.e., pain hypersensitivity. The mechanism of pain hypersensitivity involves abnormalities at the peripheral or central level. Peripheral sensory receptors in the esophagus include chemical receptors sensing acid, mechanical receptors sensing distension, and temperature receptors sensing heat [12]. Peripheral mechanisms of visceral hypersensitivity in NCCP involve significant roles for mechanical and chemical receptors. Central mechanisms involve the role of the central nervous system in processing visceral sensory information and visceral pain hypersensitivity. Brain imaging studies have shown that non-painful sensations from esophageal balloon distension are associated with the insular cortex, primary somatosensory cortex, and operculum, while painful sensations are associated with activation of the right anterior insular cortex and anterior cingulate cortex. These brain regions, such as the insular cortex and anterior cingulate cortex, are known to recognize unpleasant experiences like pain through the medial spinal thalamic tract and spinal reticular thalamic tract, and are associated with emotional instability in NCCP patients. The high prevalence of anxiety in

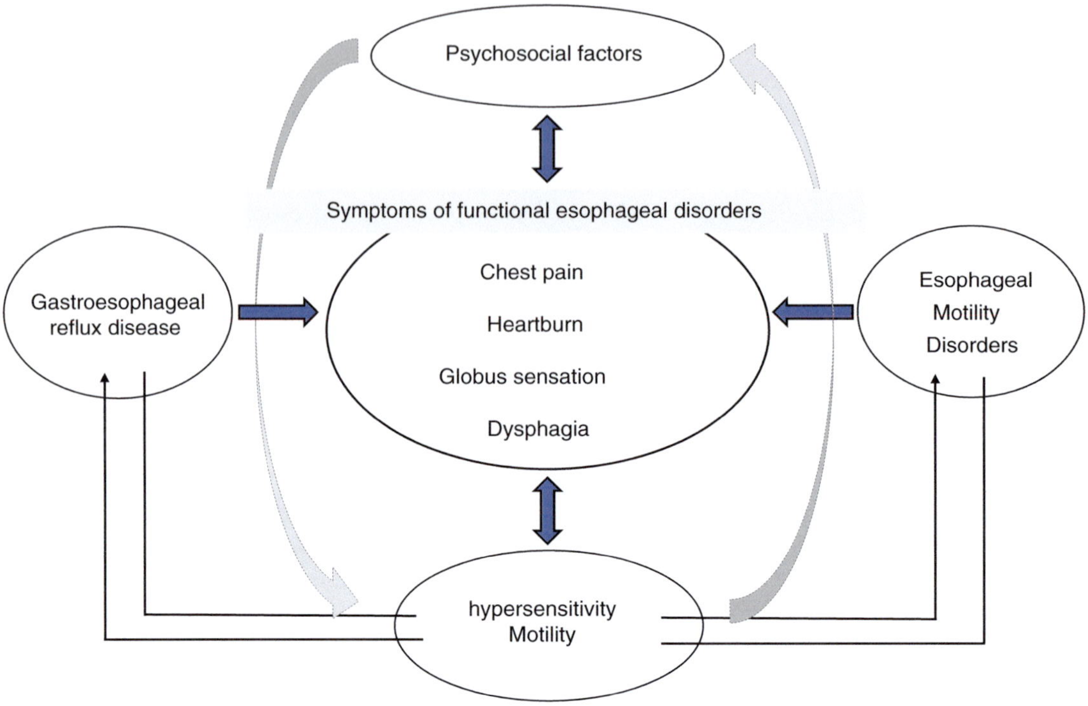

Fig. 10.1 There is an overlap in the pathophysiology of gastroesophageal reflux disease and Esophageal motility disorders, both of which contribute to the symptoms of functional esophageal disorders

NCCP patients suggests that emotional stress such as anxiety may enhance pain experiences.

4 Diagnostic Criteria and Examinations

Since NCCP is a general term for chest pain not originating from the heart, it is necessary to first confirm the absence of organic or functional heart disease through detailed cardiovascular examinations. In daily clinical practice, as shown in Fig. 10.2, if various tests such as stress tests and coronary angiography indicate a poor correlation between chest pain and heart disease, further tests are conducted to identify non-ischemic, non-cardiac chest pain [13]. Common diseases encountered in daily clinical practice that fall under NCCP include GERD, esophageal motility disorders, and anxiety disorders such as panic disorder, and it is important not to overlook these conditions. Additionally, chest pain originating from respiratory diseases, musculoskeletal disorders, and large vascular diseases should be considered, and the initial onset time, occurrence time (postprandial, at rest, during sleep, etc.), duration, relationship with food intake, weight loss, dysphagia, heartburn, and presence of allergic diseases should be confirmed. Although there are no physical symptoms directly linked to NCCP differentiation, warning signs such as dysphagia, odynophagia, recent weight loss, anorexia, and anemia during examination may suggest gastrointestinal malignancy. Since GERD is the most common cause of NCCP, upper gastrointestinal endoscopy is essential.

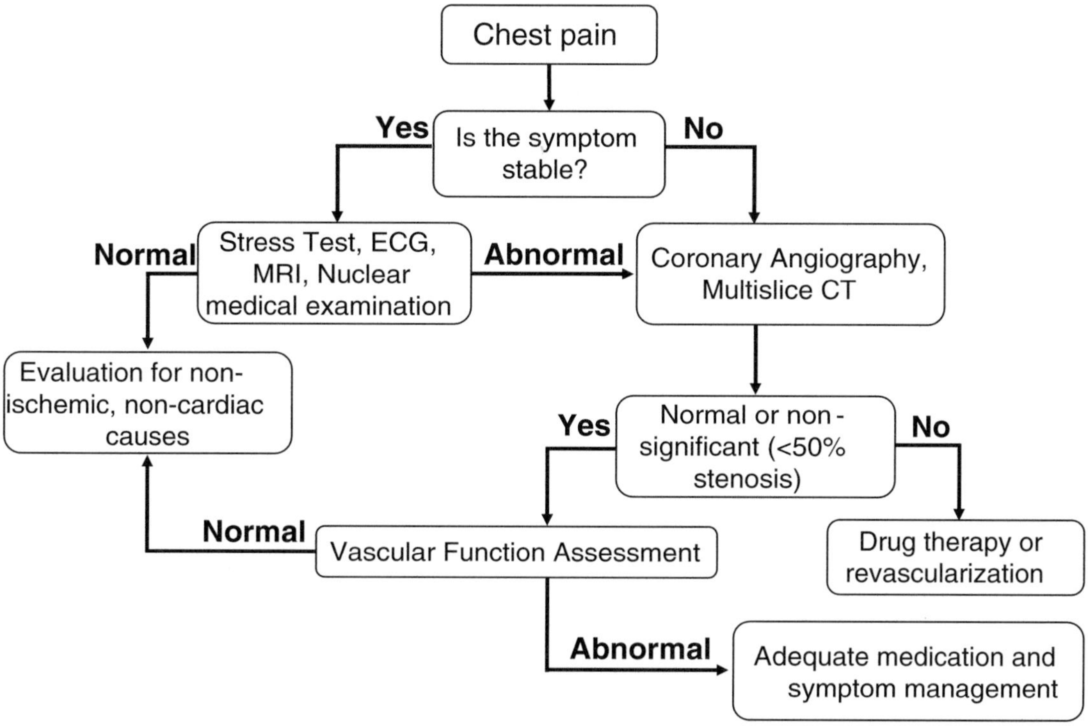

Fig. 10.2 Diagnostic methods for non-cardiac chest pain (NCCP). (Adapted from Reference [1])

Figure 10.3 shows the diagnostic flowchart for NCCP patients [14]. Upper gastrointestinal endoscopy is performed to exclude organic diseases and confirm the presence or absence of mucosal damage. If mucosal damage is present, its treatment is prioritized. If endoscopic mucosal damage is not observed but GERD is suspected as the cause, diagnostic treatment with proton pump inhibitors (PPIs) is recommended. If symptoms improve with PPI administration, GERD-related NCCP can be diagnosed. If PPI is ineffective, 24-hour esophageal impedance-pH monitoring is conducted. Calculating the symptom index, which indicates the correlation between symptoms and reflux, allows understanding of the pathophysiology of non-erosive reflux disease (NERD), reflux hypersensitivity, and functional heartburn. In cases with dysphagia, esophageal motility disorders are suspected, and esophageal manometry is performed. If chest pain occurs at least once a week, and 24-hour esophageal impedance-pH monitoring shows no correlation between symptom onset and reflux, and esophageal manometry excludes esophageal motility disorders, functional chest pain is diagnosed [9].

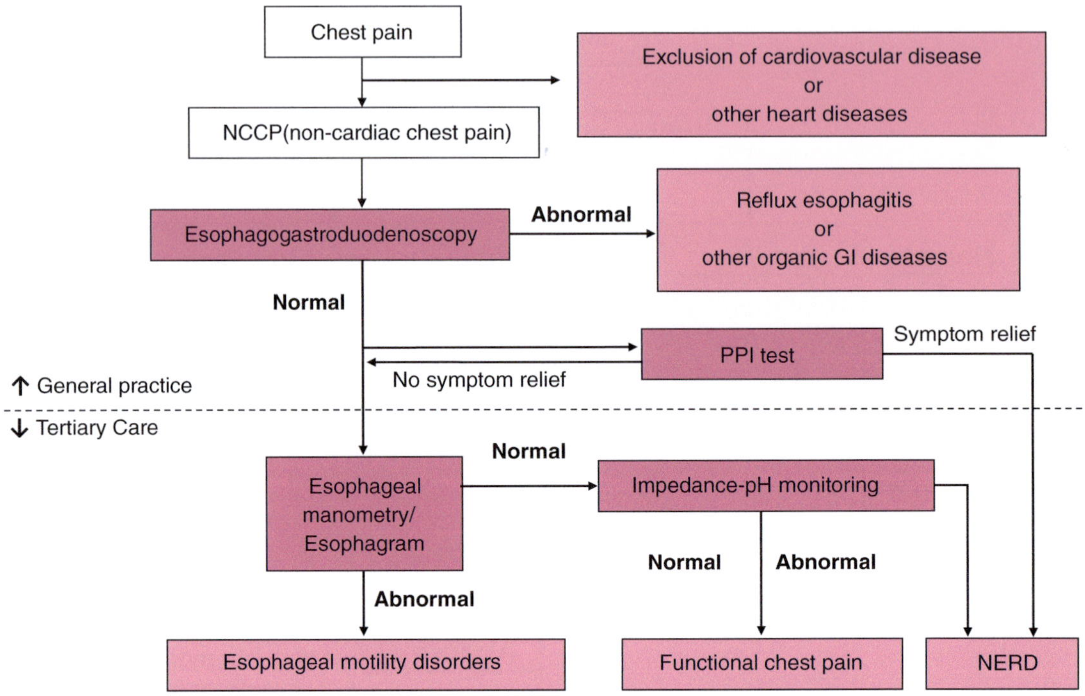

Fig. 10.3 Diagnostic flowchart for NCCP. (Reproduced with permission from Reference [14])

5 Differential Diagnosis and Complications

When examining patients with chest pain, it is crucial to differentiate and exclude serious life-threatening conditions first. Important differential diagnoses include ischemic heart disease, acute aortic dissection, acute pulmonary thromboembolism, tension pneumothorax, spontaneous esophageal rupture, esophageal cancer and other gastrointestinal cancers, and eosinophilic esophagitis. However, while electrocardiograms and blood tests can exclude urgent ischemic heart disease when chest pain persists, differentiation is not always easy when symptoms subside. Typical angina pectoris chest pain occurs during exercise, but GERD can also be induced by exercise. Nitrates and calcium channel blockers, frequently used in the treatment of ischemic heart disease, can lower LES pressure and induce GERD, necessitating caution even in patients diagnosed with ischemic heart disease, as GERD may coexist and act as a compounding factor. Spontaneous esophageal rupture, a condition where the anatomically weak left lower esophageal wall tears due to vomiting, leading to mediastinitis, can be fatal if diagnosis and treatment are delayed. Although rare, it can suddenly occur in healthy individuals. Chest pain is the main symptom, and if severe pain and high inflammatory markers are present without cardiovascular issues, spontaneous esophageal rupture should be suspected, and a chest CT scan should be performed to avoid missing the diagnosis. Esophageal cancer rarely presents with chest pain as an initial symptom. It is asymptomatic in the early stages but can cause dysphagia and chest pain as it progresses. Differentiation is crucial in patients with risk factors for esophageal cancer, such as a history of heavy alcohol consumption and smoking, along with dysphagia. If dysphagia is accompanied by nutritional deficiencies, weight loss, or anemia, immediate endoscopy is necessary to differentiate malignancy. Eosinophilic esophagitis, characterized by numerous eosinophils infiltrating the esophageal epithelium and causing chronic inflammation, leads to esophageal motility and sensory abnormalities, resulting in symptoms such as dysphagia, heartburn, globus sensation, and chest pain, and can cause esophageal strictures. Upper gastrointestinal endoscopy may show characteristic findings such as concentric rings, linear furrows, and white plaques, but these findings may be absent, necessitating proactive esophageal mucosal biopsy if no causative lesions are identified. Eosinophilic esophagitis is associated with various esophageal motility disorders. Jackhammer esophagus, a type of NCCP characterized by severe chest pain and dysphagia due to strong esophageal contractions, may not show significant eosinophil infiltration in the esophageal epithelium but may exhibit eosinophilic infiltration in the muscularis propria, known as eosinophilic esophageal myositis, complicating diagnosis [15]. Mental abnormalities are present in 17–43% of NCCP cases, with 24–70% having panic disorder and 11–22% having depression [2]. These conditions are not explained by clear organic disease causes, involve physical complaints causing distress, and interfere with daily life, classifying them as functional somatic syndromes with high comorbidity of anxiety and depression [16].

6 Treatment

When diagnosing GERD-related NCCP, if upper gastrointestinal endoscopy reveals mucosal damage indicative of reflux esophagitis, excessive gastric acid reflux is likely the cause of chest pain, and treatment with acid suppression therapy such as PPIs or potassium-competitive acid blockers (P-CABs) is warranted. Even in the absence of clear mucosal damage, NERD should be suspected, and the course of chest pain with PPI administration should be observed.

Esophageal motility disorders account for 30% of non-GERD-related NCCP cases and are significant conditions. In clinical practice, patients presenting with angina-like chest pain are often suspected of having angina, and nitrates or calcium channel blockers, effective for chest pain due to esophageal motility disorders, are frequently administered, leading to potential misdiagnosis as angina through therapeutic diagnosis. Even if nitrates or calcium channel blockers are effective, the presence of esophageal motility disorders such as achalasia should be suspected and actively differentiated. Symptoms of functional esophageal disorders, including functional chest pain, are attributed to visceral hypersensitivity, necessitating pharmacotherapy to alter esophageal pain perception and psychological intervention. Tricyclic antidepressants, which have both central nervous system modulation and peripheral visceral analgesic effects, can increase esophageal pain thresholds but require caution due to anticholinergic side effects [2]. Selective serotonin reuptake inhibitors (SSRIs) reduce chest pain in non-GERD-related NCCP regardless of psychological test improvement [17]. Anxiolytics are effective for panic disorder coexisting with NCCP but require caution due to the potential for drug dependence. NCCP patients are known to have high comorbidity with psychiatric disorders such as depression and anxiety. Psychotherapy is useful for NCCP patients with hypochondriasis or panic disorder, and cognitive-behavioral therapy improves quality of life and reduces chest pain in NCCP patients without panic disorder.

7 Prognosis

NCCP has a better prognosis compared to cardiac chest pain. From the perspective of pathological cardiac events, patients with esophageal-origin functional chest pain have a very low incidence of myocardial infarction and cardiac-related mortality, less than 1%, over a 10-year follow-up period once the diagnosis is confirmed [18]. However, compared to typical GERD symptoms, the symptom resolution rate with PPIs is lower, and the time to effect is longer. Emotional stress factors such as anxiety and fear, in addition to decreased pain thresholds, contribute to the condition, often necessitating relatively long-term treatment.

8 Conclusion

In addition to the general diagnosis and treatment of NCCP, this section discussed the involvement of decreased pain thresholds, emotional stress such as anxiety, and psychosocial factors in the pathophysiology. Due to these pathophysiological mechanisms, NCCP is prone to delayed diagnosis and treatment. Therefore, it is essential to conduct detailed medical interviews to understand the pathophysiology, perform appropriate tests, and use suitable medications for each condition. A psychosomatic approach, similar to the treatment of functional somatic syndromes and chronic pain, is also desirable.

Take-Home Message

For NCCP, it is necessary to conduct a comprehensive search considering various diseases from other fields, including chest pain related to esophageal-origin GERD and esophageal motility disorders. To ensure an accurate diagnosis, it is essential to investigate the relationship between esophageal functional abnormalities and chest pain using esophageal pH monitoring and esophageal manometry. However, due to the invasive nature of these tests, they are rarely performed in practice. Therefore, observing changes in chest pain intensity based on body position (standing or supine) and during swallowing, as well as evaluating the improvement of chest pain with acid suppression therapy, is recommended as relatively simple methods.

Competing Interests The author(s) has no competing interests to declare that are relevant to the content of this manuscript.

References

1. Fass R, et al. Noncardiac chest pain: diagnostic evaluation. Dis Esophagus. 2012;25:89–101.
2. Fass R, et al. Noncardiac chest pain. J Clin Gastroenterol. 2008;42(5):636–46.
3. Locke GR, et al. Prevalence and clinical spectrum of gastroesophageal reflux: a population-based study in Olmsted County, Minnesota. Gastroenterology. 1997;112(5):1448–56.
4. Eslick GD, et al. Non-cardiac chest pain: squeezing the life out of the Australian healthcare system? Med J Aust. 2000;173(5):233–4.
5. Ferguson SC, et al. Esophageal manometry in patients with chest pain and normal coronary arteriogram. Am J Gastroenterol. 1981;75:124–7.
6. Vakil N, et al. The Montreal definition and classification of gastroesophageal reflux disease: a global evidence-based consensus. Am J Gastroenterol. 2006;101:1900–20; quiz 1943.
7. Tanimura T. A study on the frequency of gastroesophageal reflux disease in emergency department visits for non-cardiac chest pain. Nippon Shokakibyo Gakkai Zasshi. 2008;105:54–9. (in Japanese).
8. Dekel R, et al. Assessment of oesophageal motor function in patients with dysphagia or chest pain -the Clinical Outcomes Research Initiative experience. Aliment Pharmacol Ther. 2003;18:1083–9.
9. Drossman DA, et al. Rome IV-functional GI disorders: disorders of gut-brain interaction. Gastroenterology. 2016;150:1257–61.
10. Fass R, et al. Non-cardiac chest pain: an update. Neurogastroenterol Motil. 2006;18:408–17.
11. Rao SS, et al. Unexplained chest pain: the hypersensitive, hyperreactive, and poorly compliant esophagus. Ann Intern Med. 1996;124:950–8.
12. Lembo AJ. Visceral hypersensitivity in noncardiac chest pain. Gastroenterol Clin N Am. 2004;33:55–60.
13. Bugiardini R, et al. Angina with "normal" coronary arteries: a changing philosophy. JAMA. 2005;293:477–84.
14. Akiyama J. Clinical symptoms and diagnostic flowchart for non-cardiac chest pain (NCCP). In: Japanese Society of Gastroenterology, ed. Guidelines for the diagnosis and treatment of esophageal motility disorders. Tokyo: Nankodo; 2006. p. 56–8. (in Japanese).
15. Sato H, et al. Proposed criteria to differentiate heterogeneous eosinophilic gastrointestinal disorders of the esophagus, including eosinophilic esophageal myositis. World J Gastroenterol. 2017;23:2414–23.
16. Nagata K. Diagnosis of functional somatic syndromes. Mod Physician. 2006;26:283. (in Japanese)
17. Varia I, et al. Randomized trial of sertraline in patients with unexplained chest pain of noncardiac origin. Am Heart J. 2000;140:367–72.
18. Kemp HG, et al. Seven year survival of patients with normal or near normal coronary arteriograms: a CASS registry study. J Am Coll Cardiol. 1986;7:479–83.

11 Diagnosis and Treatment of DGBI of the Esophagus, Globus, Functional Dysphagia

Tomomi Machida

Abstract

Globus is defined as the sensation of a lump in the throat or a feeling of discomfort. Functional dysphagia is defined as the sensation of food stucking or passing poorly through the esophageal body. A definitive diagnosis requires ruling out organic or functional diseases that induce similar symptoms. Although the pathophysiology and treatment are not fully established, symptoms often improve or resolve without treatment in many patients. Therefore, treatment should focus on explanation of the pathological condition and reassurance. Medication should be limited to short periods due to side effects. Psychosocial factors can significantly influence symptoms and reduce patients' quality of life. Therefore, a comprehensive approach that includes psychosocial aspects is necessary. Holistic medical care is always necessary.

Keywords

Globus · Functional dysphagia · High resolution manometry · pH-impedance study · PPI-resistant globus · Impair bolus transport/ bolus retention · Nonspecific esophageal motility disprders · Esophageal visceral sensory abnormalities · Esophageal distension disorders · Psychosocial factors

T. Machida (✉)
Department of Psychosomatic Medicine, Tohoku Rosai Hospital, Sendai, Japan

1 Globus, Functional Dysphagia

1.1 Globus

1.1.1 Concept

Globus is defined as a sensation of a lump or foreign body in the throat, which is persistent or intermittent and not associated with pain. This symptom is typically recognized along the midline between the thyroid cartilage and the manubrium of sternum notch [1].

1.1.2 Epidemiology

The symptom is frequently observed, with reports indicating that over 46% of individuals who do not seek medical attention experience it [1]. The prevalence is three times higher in women under the age of 50, with more severe cases also being more common, leading to a higher frequency of medical consultations among women. The symptom persists for more than 3 years in 75% of patients and for more than 7 years in 50% of patients [2].

1.1.3 Etiology and Pathophysiology

Potential causes of symptom induction include structural lesions, gastroesophageal reflux dis-

H. Kaneko et al. (eds.), *Disorders of Gut-Brain Interaction*,
https://doi.org/10.1007/978-981-95-6974-8_11

ease (GERD), heterotopic gastric mucosa in the proximal esophagus (ectopic gastric mucosa, inlet patch), and esophageal motility disorders. Notable structural abnormalities such as tumors or severe inflammation are accompanied by alarm signs (e.g., dysphagia, odynophagia, weight loss), making it difficult to classify them as simple globus symptoms. Minor abnormalities in the pharyngolaryngeal region (e.g., cervical webs, hypertrophy of base of tongue) are also considered, but data supporting their etiological role are limited.

GERD is one of the primary etiological factors for symptom induction. Major physiological hypotheses include (i) laryngopharyngeal reflux directly stimulating the oropharynx and inducing mucosal inflammation, (ii) reflex contraction of the upper esophageal sphincter (UES) in response to acid exposure or distension stimuli in the esophagus, and (iii) sensory projection from the esophagus to the neck via hypersensitive afferent vagal pathways. GERD is confirmed in 23–68% of patients with symptoms [3], but the response rate to proton pump inhibitors (PPIs) varies significantly across studies.

Ectopic gastric mucosa is thought to be associated with symptoms through acid secretion from the gastric mucosa, *Helicobacter pylori* infection, and sensory hypersensitivity. There are reports of significant symptom improvement following argon plasma coagulation of inlet patches [4].

Esophageal motility disorders are often identified in patients with PPI-resistant globus. Increased UES pressure is frequently observed, and symptom relief after botulinum toxin injection suggests a correlation between symptoms and UES pressure elevation. High-resolution manometry with esophageal pressure topography (HRM with EPT) evaluations have reported esophageal motility disorders in 47.9% of PPI-resistant globus patients. These include nonspecific motility disorders that impair bolus transport, such as discontinuity of body contractions, reduced peristalsis, and decreased lower esophageal contraction pressure.

Additionally, in globus patients, esophageal stimuli are perceived in the neck, and symptoms can be induced even by low-pressure distension stimuli. Therefore, sensory abnormalities, such as excessive sensory projection from the esophagus to the neck, are also emphasized [3].

Overall, it is suggested that bolus retention in the esophagus due to peristaltic dysfunction causes esophageal distension, which stimulates the vagus nerve, leading to UES pressure elevation and globus symptoms [5].

The relationship between symptoms and psychological stress or mood disorders is inconsistent, and no specific psychological or personality traits have been reported for the symptoms. However, many patients report symptom exacerbation due to strong emotions or significant stress events within 2 months before onset. Therefore, stress and the resulting mood and emotions are considered auxiliary factors in the occurrence and exacerbation of globus symptoms [1].

1.1.4 Diagnostic Criteria and Examination

Diagnosis is based on the Rome IV diagnostic criteria.

Diagnostic Criteria for globus. Criteria must be fulfilled for past 3 months with symptom onset at least 6 months before diagnosis with a frequency of at least once a week. Must include all of the following.

1. Persistent or intermittent, nonpainful, sensation of a lump or foreign body in the throat with no structural lesion identified on physical examination, laryngoscopy, or endoscopy.
   (a) Occurrence of the sensation between meals
   (b) Absence of dysphagia or odynophagia
   (c) Absence of a gastric inlet patch in the proximal esophagus
2. Absence of evidence that gastroesophageal reflux or eosinophilic esophagitis is the cause of the symptom.
3. Absence of major esophageal motor disorders (achalasia/EGJ outflow obstruction, diffuse esophageal spasm, jackhammer esophagus, absent peristalsis).

Currently, there are no biomarkers or "gold standards" for diagnosis. A systematic review of symptoms and medical history is necessary, considering the possibility of other diseases with similar symptoms. If the medical history suggests other diseases or *alarm* signs (e.g., throat pain, odynophagia, dysphagia, hoarseness, weight loss) are confirmed, careful evaluation of the pharyngolaryngeal and esophageal regions via endoscopy is required. Additionally, potential structural abnormalities or lymph node enlargement should always be assessed. For patients with consistent symptoms/history and no *alarm* signs, laryngoscopy under local anesthesia by an otolaryngologist is recommended due to its low invasiveness and high reassurance effect. If organic abnormalities in the oropharynx are excluded, further detailed examinations to exclude GERD, gastric inlet patches, and major esophageal motility disorders should be conducted. However, since all the excluded diseases are benign, an algorithmic approach starting with PPI therapy is considered appropriate (Fig. 11.1) [2]. There are no systematic data on the dosage or duration of PPI administration for globus symptoms, but it is a rapidly effective drug, and evaluation after 4–8 weeks of administration is appropriate. If PPI is ineffective, upper gastrointestinal endoscopy should be considered if not previously performed. The purpose is to evaluate esophageal mucosal lesions, structural abnormalities, and inlet patches, which have recently been highlighted in diagnostic criteria. If no abnormalities are found on upper gastrointestinal endoscopy, esophageal manometry (HRM with EPT) should be considered. If major esophageal motility disorders are excluded by manometry, the patient can be definitively diagnosed with globus [1, 2].

1.1.5 Treatment

Symptoms persist for a long time, but up to 50% of patients experience symptom relief or resolution without treatment. Therefore, the mainstay of treatment is explanation of the pathophysiological condition and reassurance. Although there are reports

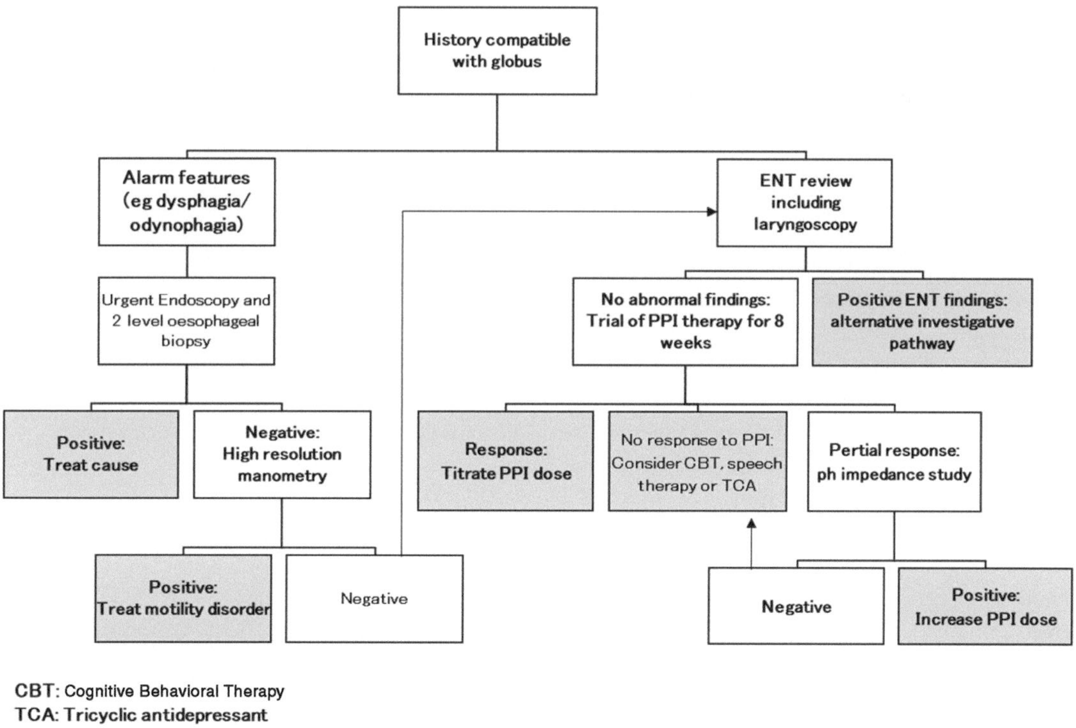

Fig. 11.1 Diagnostic flowchart for globus. (Created from Reference [2])

of the effectiveness of antidepressants, they are not established treatments, and their use should be limited to short periods due to side effects. Recently, behavioral therapy and relaxation therapy have gained attention, with reports of symptom relief through relaxation techniques aimed at reducing pharyngeal tension, such as yawning and water swallowing, by speech therapists. Relaxation methods have been shown to be more effective than reassurance-based interventions [1].

1.2 Functional Dysphagia

1.2.1 Concept

Functional dysphagia is defined as a sensation of food sticking or passing poorly through the esophageal body.

1.2.2 Epidemiology

The exact prevalence is unknown but is considered low. It has been reported that structural abnormalities that could cause symptoms were confirmed in 3/4 of patients complaining of dysphagia through upper gastrointestinal endoscopy [6]. It is presumed that the prevalence decreases further when major esophageal motility disorders are identified through esophageal function tests [7].

1.2.3 Etiology and Pathophysiology

Dysphagia is associated with bolus retention in the esophagus [1]. Major esophageal motility disorders are established diseases, and even if bolus retention is observed, it cannot be considered the cause of functional dysphagia [8]. On the other hand, nonspecific esophageal motility disorders, such as weak contractions or ineffective esophageal motility (discontinuity of body contractions), can induce dysphagia. In GERD patients, bolus transport is impaired due to reduced contraction pressure (below 30–40 mmHg) or discontinuity of contractions (over 3 cm) in the esophageal body [9]. Additionally, the relationship between reduced bolus expulsion force due to motility disorders and increased acid reflux exposure time in the esophagus has been noted. Weak contractions and ineffective esophageal motility are well correlated with symptoms and are considered the cause of intermittent dysphagia in many patients, although not definitively proven.

Sensory abnormalities are also an important etiological factor. Stimulation of the lower esophagus with acid exposure or balloon distension induces dysphagia along with excessive contractions and peristaltic disorders in the esophageal body. In GERD patients, peripheral sensory hypersensitivity due to mucosal inflammation caused by chemical stimuli such as acid induces dysphagia. Additionally, induced sensory hypersensitivity increases sensitivity to balloon distension stimuli, leading to peristaltic disorders. Thus, the relationship between dysphagia and abnormal sensitivity to esophageal distension stimuli is emphasized, but it cannot be concluded that esophageal lumen stimulation directly induces peristaltic disorders. Currently, peristaltic disorders are considered secondary [1].

Overall, as with other esophageal functional disorders, esophageal motility disorders and visceral sensory abnormalities are thought to exist independently and influence each other in functional dysphagia.

Information on the impact of psychological factors on functional dysphagia is limited. However, in patients with both dysphagia and nonspecific esophageal motility disorders, psychological stress, anxiety disorders, depressive disorders, and somatization disorders are frequently observed compared to patients with other etiologies. Acute stress experiments suggest that central factors can induce esophageal motility disorders (increased contraction pressure, continuous *synchronous* contractions) that may affect bolus transport [10].

1.2.4 Diagnostic Criteria and Examination

Diagnosis is based on the Rome IV diagnostic criteria.

Diagnostic criteria for functional dysphagia. Criteria must be fulfilled for the past 3 months with symptom onset at least 6 months before diagnosis with a frequency of at least once a week.

1. Sense of solid and/or liquid foods sticking, lodging, or passing abnormally through the esophagus.
2. Absence of evidence that esophageal mucosal or structural abnormality is the cause of the symptom.
3. Absence of evidence that gastroesophageal reflux or eosinophilic esophagitis is the cause of the symptom.
4. Absence of major esophageal motor disorders (achalasia/EGJ outflow obstruction, diffuse esophageal spasm, jackhammer esophagus, absent peristalsis).

The diagnostic process begins with a careful medical history to evaluate and exclude organic abnormalities of the oral/pharyngeal region (e.g., GERD) and diseases with similar symptoms (e.g., globus, xerostomia, odynophagia).

Exclusion of GERD and eosinophilic esophagitis is crucial for diagnosing functional dysphagia, it is necessary to PPI therapy and performed upper gastrointestinal endoscopy with biopsy (Fig. 11.2) [11]. Recently, the increasing frequency of eosinophilic esophagitis has highlighted the importance of upper gastrointestinal endoscopy, but esophageal barium swallow tests for solid food ingestion are also useful for evaluating minor structural and motility abnormalities and should be used as needed. If structural abnormalities are excluded by these tests, esophageal manometry (HRM with EPT) is performed to exclude major esophageal motility disorders. Additionally, pH monitoring tests should be considered for patients with dysphagia accompanied by heartburn or reflux symptoms. Functional luminal imaging probe (EndoFLIP) is useful for evaluating esophageal distension disorders associated with eosinophilic esophagitis. High-frequency ultrasound endoscopy is also useful for evaluating coordination disorders between the circular and longitudinal muscles, which are associated with excessive esophageal motility. However, the correlation between findings from EndoFLIP or high-frequency ultrasound endoscopy and dysphagia symptoms is weak, and their use is currently limited to research.

In 1/3 to 2/3 of patients with dysphagia without other etiologies, nonspecific esophageal motility disorders (e.g., contraction pattern

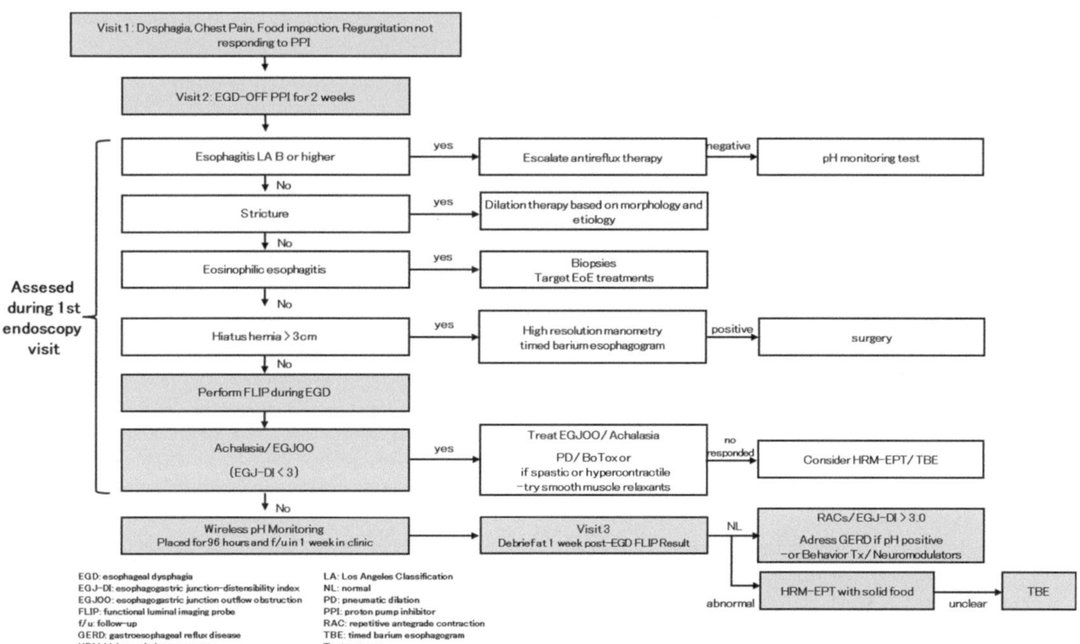

Fig. 11.2 Diagnostic and treatment flowchart for dysphagia. (Created from Reference [11]). When all structural and functional abnormalities are thoroughly examined and excluded, a diagnosis of functional dysphagia can be made

abnormalities, peristaltic disorders, LES pressure elevation) that can impair bolus transport are observed on HRM with EPT, and their association with dysphagia symptoms is confirmed. Although the observed nonspecific esophageal motility disorders are not specific findings for dysphagia patients, they are considered sufficient for diagnosing functional dysphagia [11].

1.2.5 Treatment

Symptoms may improve or resolve over time, so excessive treatment approaches are unnecessary. In mild cases, reassurance and simple non-pharmacological methods (e.g., avoiding foods that trigger symptoms, thorough chewing, washing down food with water) are expected to be effective. In more severe cases, pharmacological trials are useful. Since some dysphagia symptoms are related to acid reflux, a short-term acid suppression trial (PPI for 2–4 weeks) should be considered. Other medications that may be tried include smooth muscle relaxants, anticholinergic agents, anxiolytics/antidepressants. Smooth muscle relaxants are effective when nonspecific esophageal spastic motility disorders are associated with symptoms. Additionally, tricyclic antidepressants are useful for visceral hypersensitivity if other treatments are ineffective. However, the mechanisms of action of these drugs are unclear, and their efficacy is not confirmed, so they should be discontinued promptly if ineffective.

Mechanical interventions may be considered for some patients. In patients with intermittent dysphagia without identifiable etiologies, slight stenosis that are often missed by general tests may be associated with symptoms. Bougie dilation with 50-54F has shown symptom improvement in 68–85% of patients, and similar effects are expected in patients with nonspecific esophageal spastic motility disorders [1].

1.2.6 Prognosis

Globus and functional dysphagia are benign conditions that may improve or resolve spontaneously, but symptoms often persist for years. While psychosocial stress affects symptoms, the symptoms themselves can be stressors, reducing patients' quality of life (QOL). Various psychological therapies (e.g., behavioral therapy, breathing techniques, biofeedback) have been reported to help control symptoms and reduce medical consultation behavior, highlighting the importance of collaborative treatment between physicians and mental health professionals [12].

2 Conclusion

The diagnosis of functional esophageal disorders such as globus and functional dysphagia requires the exclusion of organic/functional diseases that induce similar symptoms. However, few cases lead to a definitive diagnosis after such exclusions. Information on pathophysiology and treatment is also insufficient, but the impact of psychosocial factors on symptoms is significant, and holistic medical care is always required.

Take-Home Message
In the context of globus and functional dysphagia, the gold standard for pathophysiology and treatment has not yet been established. Therefore, it is necessary to adopt a comprehensive approach that includes psychosocial aspects, alongside diagnosis and treatment based on flowcharts, and to consider various factors in patient care.

Competing Interests The author(s) has no competing interests to declare that are relevant to the content of this manuscript.

References

1. Aziz Q, et al. Esophageal disorders. Gastroenterology. 2016;150:1368–79.
2. Harvey PR, et al. Managing a patient with globus pharyngeus. Frontline Gastroenterol. 2018;9:208–12.
3. Noriaki M, et al. Pathophysiology and treatment of patients with globus sensation—from the viewpoint of esophageal motility dysfunction. J Smooth Muscle Res. 2014;50:66–77.
4. Brechmann T, et al. Argon plasma coagulation of gastric inlet patches of the cervical esophagus relieves vocal and respiratory symptoms in selected patients. Dig Dis Sci. 2023;68(5):1936–43.
5. Babaei A, et al. Upper esophageal sphincter during transient lower esophageal sphincter relaxation: effects of reflux content and posture. Am J Physiol Gastrointest Liver Physiol. 2010;298:G601–7.

6. Bill J, et al. Diagnostic yield in the evaluation of dysphagia: experience at a single tertiary care center. Dis Esophagus. 2018;31(6).
7. Kwan AC, et al. Validation of Rome II criteria for functional gastrointestinal disorders by factor analysis of symptoms in Asian patient sample. J Gastroenterol Hepatol. 2003;18:796–802.
8. Pandolfino JE, et al. Distal esophageal spasm in high-resolution esophageal pressure topography: defining clinical phenotypes. Gastroenterology. 2011;141:469–75.
9. Roman S, et al. Weak peristalsis in esophageal pressure topography: classification and association with dysphagia. Am J Gastroenterol. 2011;106:349–56.
10. Galmiche JP, et al. Functional esophageal disorders. Gastroenterology. 2006;130:1459–65.
11. Triggs J, et al. Recent advances in dysphagia management. F1000Res. 2019;8:F1000 Faculty Rev-1527.
12. Megan E, et al. The role of a health psychologist in the management of functional esophageal complaints. Dis Esophagus. 2015;28:428–36.

Diagnosis and Treatment of Motility Disorder of the Esophagus, Non-Erosive Reflux Disease (Including Reflux Hypersensitivity)

12

Noriyuki Kawami and Katsuhiko Iwakiri

Abstract

Non-erosive reflux disease (NERD) is a condition characterized by reflux symptoms such as heartburn and regurgitation without esophageal mucosal break. Some patients with NERD are considered to have the mild type of reflux esophagitis. However, other patients have different pathophysiologies that cannot be explained by the mild type of reflux esophagitis. According to the Rome IV criteria, NERD is classified into the following types. One type is narrowly defined or true NERD in which acid exposure in the esophagus is excessive. Another type is reflux hypersensitivity in which acid exposure in the esophagus is normal but symptoms are related to reflux (mainly weakly acidic reflux) due to esophageal hypersensitivity. The third type of NERD is functional heartburn in which acid exposure in the esophagus is normal and symptoms are unrelated to reflux. Approximately half of the patients with NERD are resistant to proton pump inhibitor (PPI) therapy. In PPI-resistant patients, mosapride, acotiamide, rikkunshito, or alginate are additionally administered (off-label use for NERD). Providing adequate explanations to reassure patients and establish a good patient–physician relationship and considering evaluating pathophysiology at a specialized institution for refractory patients are important. Anti-reflux surgery is an option of treatment for patients with reflux-related symptoms.

Keywords

Gastroesophageal reflux disease (GERD) · Non-erosive reflux disease (NERD) · Reflux esophagitis · Reflux hypersensitivity · Functional heartburn · pH impedance monitoring

1 Non-erosive Reflux Disease (NERD) (Including Reflux Hypersensitivity)

1.1 Concept

Non-erosive reflux disease (NERD) is a condition characterized by reflux symptoms such as heartburn and regurgitation without endoscopic evidence of esophageal mucosal break. Generally, NERD refers to this broad definition. Gastroesophageal reflux disease (GERD) encompasses both reflux esophagitis (with or without symptoms) and NERD (Fig. 12.1) [1]. According to the Rome IV criteria for functional gastrointestinal disorders, NERD is classified into the fol-

N. Kawami (✉) · K. Iwakiri
Department of Gastroenterology, Nippon Medical School, Graduate School of Medicine, Tokyo, Japan
e-mail: s5038@nms.ac.jp

H. Kaneko et al. (eds.), *Disorders of Gut-Brain Interaction*,
https://doi.org/10.1007/978-981-95-6974-8_12

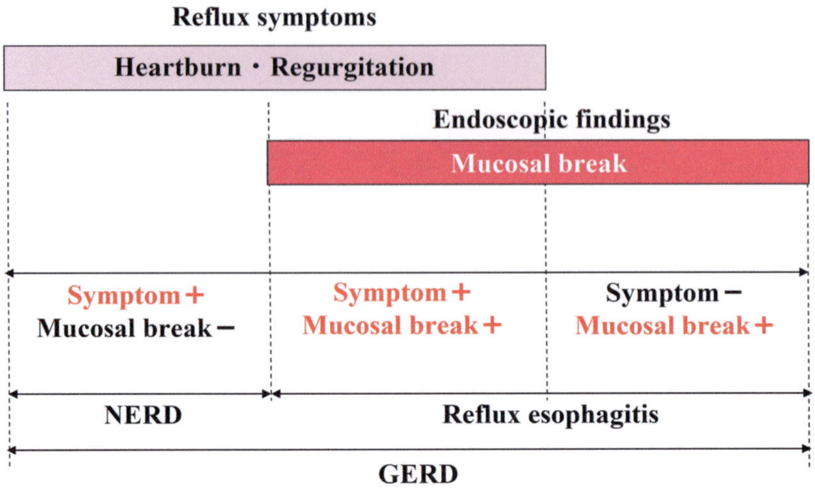

Fig. 12.1 Classification of GERD

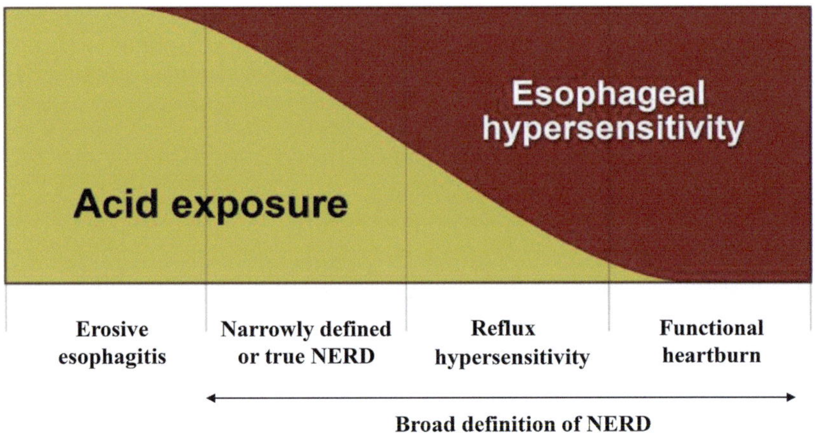

Fig. 12.2 Classification of NERD according to Rome IV criteria for functional gastrointestinal disorders. (Created from Reference [2])

lowing types. One type is narrowly defined or true NERD in which acid exposure in the esophagus is excessive. Another type is reflux hypersensitivity in which acid exposure in the esophagus is normal but symptoms are related to reflux (mainly weakly acidic reflux) due to esophageal hypersensitivity. The third type of NERD is functional heartburn in which acid exposure in the esophagus is normal and symptoms are unrelated to reflux (Fig. 12.2) [2]. In this context, functional heartburn is discussed in detail in Chap. 9. This article provides an overview of the broad definition of NERD.

1.2 Epidemiology

A systematic review of GERD prevalence indicates that the prevalence of reflux esophagitis is 12.0% on average, while the prevalence of GERD symptoms, including NERD, is 17.7% on average, which is higher than the prevalence of reflux esophagitis [3]. This finding is due to the fact that, in Japan, approximately 60% of GERD cases are NERD [4].

Clinical features differ between NERD and reflux esophagitis. Factors associated with reflux esophagitis include hiatal hernia, high BMI, mild gastric mucosal atrophy, and *H. pylori* non-infection. In contrast, NERD is more common in women and younger individuals, with fewer cases of hiatal hernia, lower body weight, severe gastric mucosal atrophy, and higher *H. pylori* infection rates [5]. Some patients with NERD are considered to have the mild type of reflux esophagitis. However, other patients have different pathophysiologies that cannot be explained by the mild type of reflux esophagitis, and clinical manifestations also differ between the two conditions.

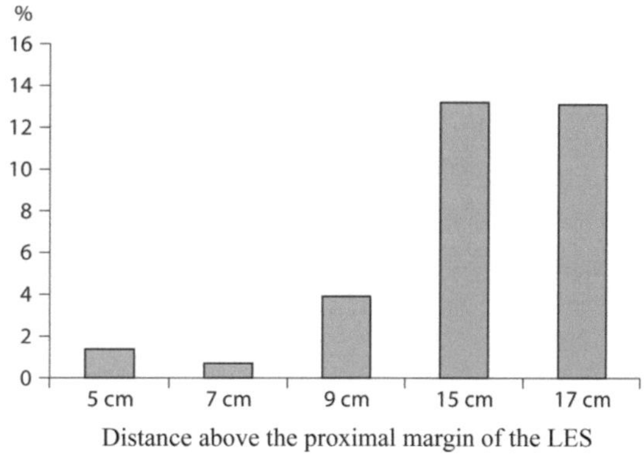

Fig. 12.3 Proportion of symptomatic reflux episodes at each impedance site in PPI double-dose resistant NERD patients [8]

1.3 Etiology and Pathophysiology

1.3.1 Pathophysiology of NERD

Patients with NERD have been pointed out that exhibit esophageal hypersensitivity compared to those with reflux esophagitis. Balloon distension in NERD patients causes symptoms at smaller balloon diameters than in healthy individuals, and acid infusion into the esophagus induces stronger symptoms compared to reflux esophagitis patients. This phenomenon occurs not only with acid but also with saline infusion; therefore, it is thought to be due to esophageal hypersensitivity [6, 7].

However, hypersensitivity alone cannot fully explain symptom occurrence. Several factors, in addition to hypersensitivity, contribute to symptom manifestation. Proximal reflux in the esophagus is more likely to cause symptoms than reflux confined to the distal esophagus. In our previous study, multichannel intraluminal impedance pH (MII-pH) monitoring in PPI-resistant patients with NERD showed that the percentage of symptomatic reflux episodes was 13–14% in the proximal esophagus compared with approximately 1% in the distal esophagus (5 and 7 cm above the lower esophageal sphincter [LES]) (Fig. 12.3) [8]. Additionally, our investigation of esophageal motility in NERD patients revealed that while the occurrence rate of primary peristalsis and amplitude of primary and secondary peristalsis were similar to those in healthy individuals, the occurrence rate of secondary peristalsis was significantly lower in NERD patients compared to healthy individuals (Fig. 12.4) [9]. The reduced occurrence of secondary peristalsis, especially at night when swallowing is infrequent, may facilitate the proximal reflux in the esophagus. Given that proximal reflux is an important factor associated with symptomatic reflux, it has become evident from the perspective of esophageal motility that patients with NERD are more prone to symptomatic reflux.

Saliva secretion is considered important in suppressing excessive acid exposure, along with peristalsis. However, saliva secretion has not been extensively studied. We focused on saliva secretion as a treatment for GERD other than acid suppression and found that saliva secretion was significantly lower in true NERD patients compared to healthy individuals [10]. There are gender differences in saliva secretion, with reduced secretion reported in women. Considering reports that NERD is more prevalent among women, it is possible that reduced salivary secretion may also play a role in its pathophysiology.

1.3.2 Causes of PPI-Resistant NERD

While many cases of reflux esophagitis achieve mucosal healing and symptom improvement with proton pump inhibitors (PPIs) or potassium-competitive acid blockers (P-CABs), about half of NERD cases are resistant to drug therapy [11]. In our investigation of 53 cases of PPI double-dose resistant NERD, we first examined the presence of eosinophilic esophagitis via endoscopy

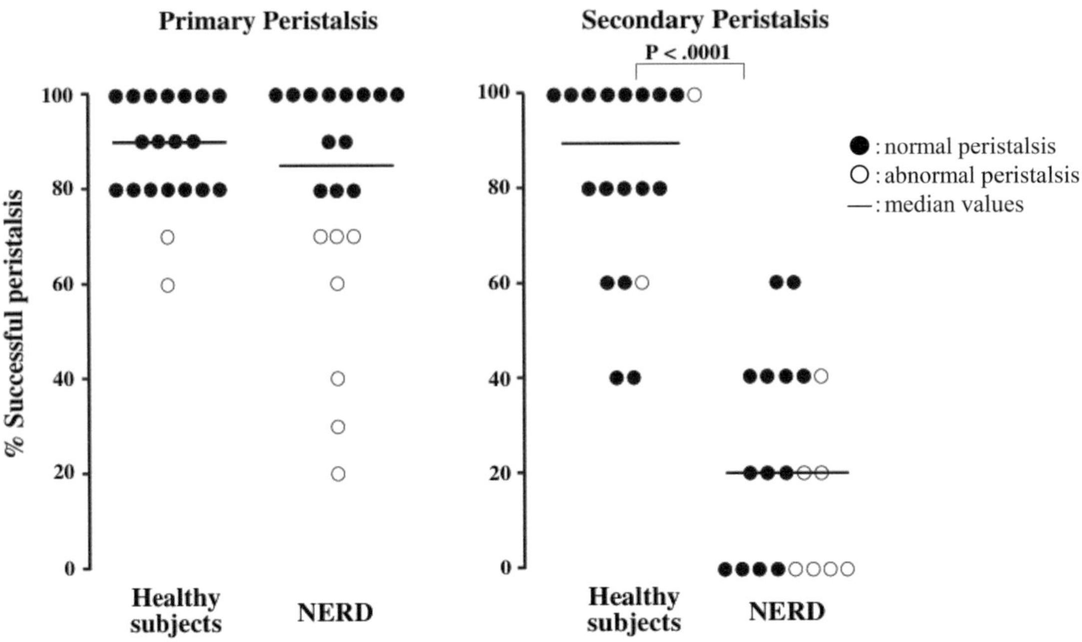

Fig. 12.4 Occurrence rates of primary and secondary peristalsis in healthy individuals and NERD patients [9]

and diagnosed one case with eosinophilic esophagitis. For the remaining 52 cases with unknown diagnoses, esophageal manometry was performed, revealing that four cases had primary esophageal motility disorders. Thus, eosinophilic esophagitis and esophageal motility disorders were identified as causes of symptoms, rather than reflux. Next, MII-pH monitoring was conducted to examine the relationship between symptoms and reflux. We found that in 43.4% of cases, the symptoms were associated with liquid reflux (acid reflux in 9.4% of cases and non-acid reflux in 34% of cases). Additionally, 23 cases (43.4%) had been diagnosed as functional heartburn in which the symptoms were not associated with reflux (Fig. 12.5a) [12]. In patients with symptoms caused by acid reflux, inadequate acid suppression may be the cause. When the causes of vonoprazan 20 mg-resistant NERD (off-label use for NERD) were investigated using the same method, symptoms were associated with liquid reflux in 41.9% of cases. These results were similar to those in a study of PPI-resistant NERD, but there were no symptoms caused by acid reflux, and all symptoms were caused by non-acid reflux (Fig. 12.5b) [13]. Thus, the cause of PPI-resistant NERD was not acid reflux but hypersensitivity to liquid reflux (reflux hypersensitivity).

1.4 Diagnostic Criteria and Examination

1.4.1 Symptom-Based Diagnosis

Typical symptoms of GERD, including NERD, are heartburn and regurgitation. However, extraesophageal symptoms (chronic cough, laryngopharyngeal discomfort, sore throat, and non-cardiac chest pain) may also occur and can sometimes be the only symptoms. Self-administered questionnaires summarizing symptoms suggestive of GERD are useful not only for diagnosis but also for assessing treatment efficacy. Representative questionnaires include the FSSG (F Scale), QUEST, and GERD-Q, with sensitivities and specificities around 70%. Patients with NERD tends to have higher symptom scores compared to patients with reflux esophagitis, but it is difficult to differentiate NERD from reflux esophagitis based on symptoms alone.

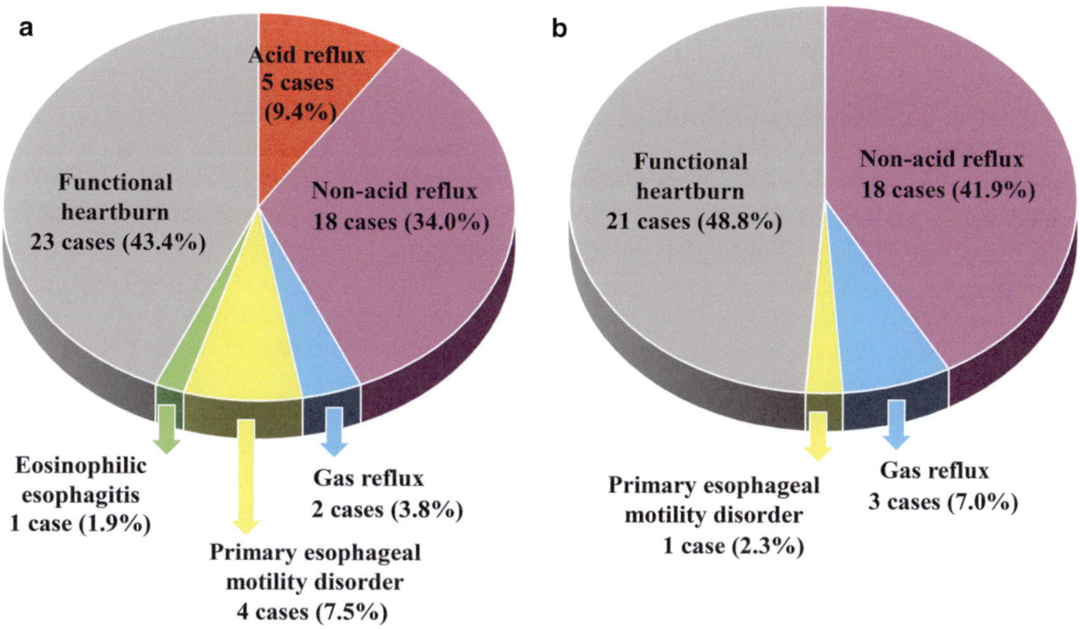

Fig. 12.5 (**a**) Causes of PPI double-dose resistant NERD (53 cases). (Created from Reference [12]). (**b**) Causes of P-CAB resistant NERD (43 cases). (Created from Reference [13])

1.4.2 Esophagogastroduodenoscopy

To diagnose NERD, esophagogastroduodenoscopy is necessary to confirm the absence of esophageal mucosal break. When performing endoscopy, it is recommended to do so before treatment or after discontinuing treatment for at least 2 weeks, as PPI or P-CAB administration can obscure the distinction between NERD and reflux esophagitis or the severity of reflux esophagitis. The Los Angeles classification is used to evaluate esophageal mucosal break, and the absence of Grade A or higher mucosal break indicates NERD. In Japan, the revised Los Angeles classification, which includes Grade M (color change type), is widely used. However, the objective diagnosis and clinical significance of minimal change (Grade M) are insufficiently studied, and Grade M is generally treated as NERD.

1.4.3 MII-pH Monitoring and Esophageal Manometry

In PPI-resistant GERD patients, esophageal pH monitoring in use of PPI is useful for evaluating gastric pH status, esophageal acid exposure time, and the relationship between acid reflux and symptoms. However, some NERD patients, who account for about 60% of GERD cases, experience symptoms due to non-acid reflux (weakly acidic reflux or gas reflux), making it difficult to evaluate reflux with esophageal pH monitoring alone. Therefore, MII-pH monitoring, which can evaluate non-acid liquid reflux and gas reflux, has been increasingly used. MII-pH monitoring allows classification of NERD into true NERD, reflux hypersensitivity, and functional heartburn according to the Rome IV criteria for functional gastrointestinal disorders.

Esophageal manometry evaluates esophageal motility function. Recently, high-resolution manometry, which measures with 36 pressure sensors at 1 cm intervals from the proximal stomach to the pharynx, has been used for detailed evaluation of esophageal motility function. Performing esophageal manometry in patients with GERD, including those with NERD, allows evaluation of transient LES relaxation (TLESR), which is the main mechanism of reflux, hiatal hernia (TLESR), which is the main mechanism of reflux, hiatal hernia, esophagogastric junction (EGJ) barrier function, and clearance ability by esophageal motility.

1.5 Differential Diagnosis and Complications

1.5.1 Primary Esophageal Motility Disorders

In our investigation of the causes of PPI-resistant NERD mentioned above, 4 out of 53 cases (7.5%) were due to primary esophageal motility disorders, with 3 cases diagnosed as jackhammer esophagus (hypercontractile esophagus according to the latest Chicago classification) [12]. Although the main symptoms of the patients with jackhammer esophagus are dysphagia and chest pain, some patients complain chest discomfort, making it difficult to diagnose esophageal motility disorders solely through endoscopy. It is essential to always consider esophageal motility disorders as differential diagnosis for NERD.

1.5.2 Eosinophilic Esophagitis

The prevalence of eosinophilic esophagitis has been increasing in Japan. While dysphagia is often the main symptom, some patients experience heartburn and anterior chest discomfort, leading to a diagnosis of PPI-resistant NERD. Eosinophilic esophagitis typically presents with characteristic endoscopic findings such as furrows, rings, and exudates. Diagnosis is confirmed by esophageal mucosal biopsy showing more than 15 eosinophils per high-power field. Many patients have a history of allergic diseases such as asthma, and it is important to take a medical history.

1.5.3 Supragastric Belching

Belching is one of the symptoms of GERD. There are two types of belching: gastric belching (GB), in which air is expelled from the stomach, and supragastric belching (SGB), in which air is expelled from the esophagus [14]. GB occurs when air that has been swallowed with food and accumulated in the stomach expands the gastric fundus, and reflux into the esophagus occurs via TLESR and is expelled through the mouth. General belching is GB. However, in SGB, the LES does not generally relax, abnormal diaphragmatic contraction causes considerable negative pressure in the esophagus, and relaxation of the upper esophageal sphincter (UES) allows air to flow into the esophagus. The air does not enter the stomach due to the closed EGJ and is expelled directly from the esophagus. GB and SGB cannot be differentiated based on symptoms or physical findings alone; MII-pH monitoring or esophageal manometry is required for differentiation. Cognitive behavioral therapy (abdominal breathing) is effective in suppressing excessive SGB. SGB is considered to be involved in the pathophysiology of some PPI-resistant GERD cases.

1.5.4 Rumination Syndrome

Rumination syndrome (RS) is characterized by repeated regurgitation of food into the mouth and subsequent swallowing without nausea. RS is induced when intragastric pressure increases because of involuntary contraction of the abdominal wall muscles and exceeds the pressure at the EGJ [15]. Some patients diagnosed with PPI-resistant GERD have been reported to have RS. Similar to SGB, cognitive behavioral therapy using abdominal breathing is effective.

1.5.5 Functional Dyspepsia and Irritable Bowel Syndrome

Patients with GERD, including NERD, are prone to comorbid functional gastrointestinal disorders such as functional dyspepsia (FD) and irritable bowel syndrome (IBS). In a study using Rome III criteria, approximately 10% of FD cases were comorbid with GERD, but the frequency increased to 30–40% when the location and duration of symptoms were interpreted broadly [16]. Another study targeting health screening patients found that the frequency of GERD comorbidity in IBS patients was 16%, compared to 6.4% in non-IBS patients, with an odds ratio of 2.81 [17]. It is important to consider comorbid functional gastrointestinal disorders when treating NERD patients.

1.6 Treatment

Since the use of vonoprazan for NERD is not covered by insurance, PPIs are administered for

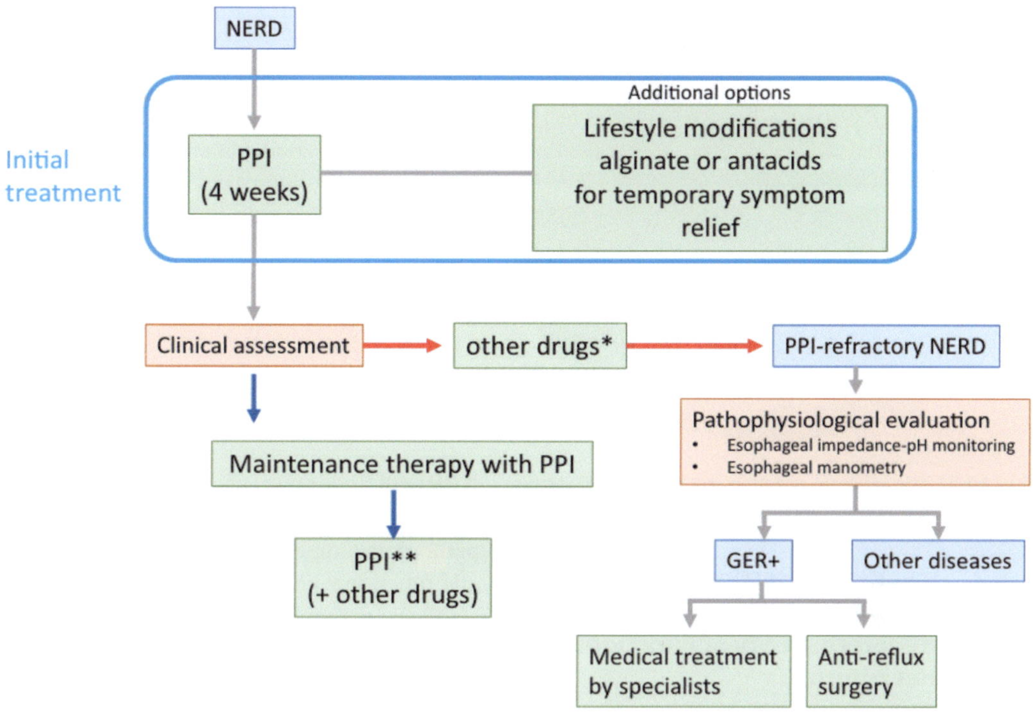

*Prokinetics or Japanese herbal medicine
**Minimal doses of PPI or on-demand therapy may be used

Fig. 12.6 Treatment flowchart for NERD [1]

NERD (Fig. 12.6) [1]. When PPIs are administered for 2–4 weeks, approximately half of the cases show symptom improvement [11]. Many NERD cases responsive to PPIs are considered true NERD, while PPI-resistant NERD cases may involve reflux hypersensitivity or functional heartburn.

1.6.1 Responsive to PPIs (True NERD)

Reflux symptoms in NERD patients vary, with some experiencing daily symptoms and others having symptoms only 2–3 days a week or during specific periods. Patients who experience symptoms immediately after discontinuing medication require continuous administration, while those who do not have symptom recurrence after discontinuation may benefit from on-demand therapy. However, to achieve stable acid suppression with PPIs, continuous administration for at least 3–5 days is necessary. Vonoprazan 20 mg achieves a gastric pH of 4 or higher within approximately 2.5 hours, making it suitable for on-demand therapy (although on-demand therapy with vonoprazan is not covered by insurance). In a study of 30 NERD (true NERD) patients whose symptoms were controlled with PPIs, on-demand therapy with vonoprazan 20 mg (maximum one tablet per day) for 8 weeks showed no difference in satisfaction, F-scale scores, or pre-breakfast gastrin levels compared to the PPI maintenance therapy group. The median number of tablets taken over 8 weeks was 11 (range 3–28), with 30% of patients taking more than 2 tablets per week regularly, 56.6% taking vonoprazan temporarily during symptom periods, and 13.3% taking less than 2 tablets per month. On-demand therapy with vonoprazan 20 mg was effective for NERD patients responsive to PPIs (Fig. 12.7) [18].

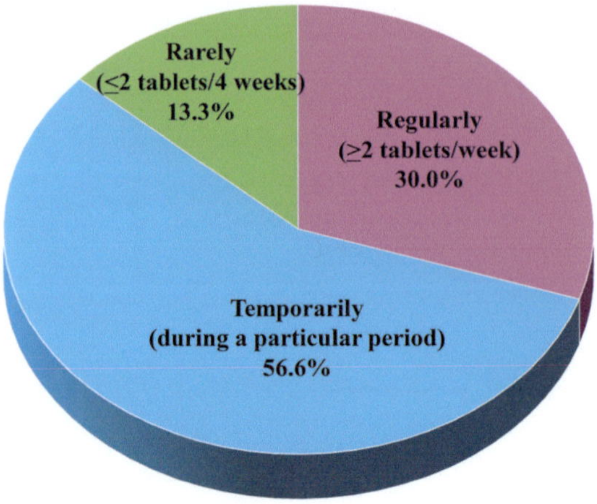

Fig. 12.7 Administration pattern of vonoprazan during the period of on-demand therapy in NERD patients [18]

1.6.2 Insufficient Response or Non-responsive to PPIs (Reflux Hypersensitivity or Functional Heartburn)

For NERD cases with insufficient response to PPIs, the Japanese guidelines recommend additional administration of mosapride, acotiamide, rikkunshito, and alginate (off-label use for NERD) (Fig. 12.6) [1]. The American Gastroenterological Association (AGA) expert review reports the usefulness of antidepressants for treating reflux hypersensitivity and functional heartburn [19]. Tricyclic antidepressants (TCAs) (e.g., imipramine), selective serotonin reuptake inhibitors (SSRIs) such as fluoxetine for reflux hypersensitivity or functional heartburn, and SSRIs such as citalopram for reflux hypersensitivity have shown an improvement in symptoms. However, it is difficult to use these antidepressants in Japan because they are not approved for NERD.

Anti-reflux surgery is also a treatment option for true NERD and reflux hypersensitivity. However, recent international consensus guidelines recommend performing MII-pH monitoring before anti-reflux surgery for reflux hypersensitivity to strictly evaluate the relationship between reflux and symptoms, and surgery should only be performed in cases with clear reflux-related symptoms [20].

PPI-resistant NERD patients with reflux hypersensitivity or functional heartburn are often refractory to treatment. It is important to provide thorough explanations to reassure the patient and to establish a good patient-doctor relationship. Symptoms may worsen due to stress, and sleep disorders can exacerbate hypersensitivity, making it important to assess sleep disturbances. Addressing anxiety and stress can sometimes lead to symptom relief.

2 Conclusion

NERD includes patients with mild type of reflux esophagitis (true NERD) and those with different pathophysiologies such as reflux hypersensitivity and functional heartburn. It is important to understand the pathophysiology of NERD and to treat it appropriately.

Take-Home Message
NERD has different pathophysiologies from reflux esophagitis and can be difficult to treat. It is important to provide adequate explanations to reassure patients and establish a good patient-physician relationship. In patients whose symptoms do not improve, physicians should consider evaluating the pathophysiology at a specialized institution.

Competing Interests The author(s) has no competing interests to declare that are relevant to the content of this manuscript.

References

1. Iwakiri K, et al. Evidence-based clinical practice guidelines for gastroesophageal reflux disease 2021. J Gastroenterol. 2022;57:267–85.
2. Aziz Q, et al. Functional esophageal disorders. Gastroenterology. 2016;150:1368–79.
3. Fujiwara Y. Recent epidemiology of GERD in the Japanese population. Nihon Shokakibyo Gakkai Zasshi. 2017;114:1781–9.
4. Fujiwara Y, et al. Epidemiology and clinical characteristics of GERD in the Japanese population. J Gastroenterol. 2009;44:518–34.

5. Fass R. Erosive esophagitis and nonerosive reflux disease (NERD): comparison of epidemiologic, physiologic, and therapeutic characteristics. J Clin Gastroenterol. 2007;41:131–7.
6. Miwa H, et al. Oesophageal hypersensitivity in Japanese patients with non-erosive gastro-oesophageal reflux diseases. Aliment Pharmacol Ther. 2004;20(Suppl 1):112–7.
7. Nagahara A, et al. Increased esophageal sensitivity to acid and saline in patients with nonerosive gastro-esophageal reflux disease. J Clin Gastroenterol. 2006;40:891–5.
8. Iwakiri K, et al. Characteristics of symptomatic reflux episodes in patients with nonerosive reflux disease who have a positive symptom index on proton pump inhibitor therapy. Digestion. 2010;82:156–61.
9. Iwakiri K, et al. Defective triggering of secondary peristalsis in patients with non-erosive reflux disease. J Gastroenterol Hepatol. 2007;22:2208–11.
10. Koeda M, et al. Saliva secretion is reduced in proton pump inhibitor-responsive non-erosive reflux disease patients. Esophagus. 2021;18:900–7.
11. Miwa H, et al. Efficacy of rabeprazole on heartburn symptom resolution in patients with non-erosive and erosive gastro-oesophageal reflux disease: a multicenter study from Japan. Aliment Pharmacol Ther. 2007;26:69–77.
12. Kawami N, et al. Pathogenesis of double-dose proton pump inhibitor-resistant non-erosive reflux disease, and mechanism of reflux symptoms and gastric acid secretion-suppressive effect in the presence or absence of helicobacter pylori infection. Digestion. 2017;95:140–5.
13. Kawami N, et al. Pathogenesis of potassium-competitive acid blocker-resistant non-erosive reflux disease. Digestion. 2018;98:194–200.
14. Kessing BF, et al. The pathophysiology, diagnosis and treatment of excessive belching symptoms. Am J Gastroenterol. 2014;109:1196–203.
15. Kessing BF, et al. Objective manometric criteria for the rumination syndrome. Am J Gastroenterol. 2014;109:52–9.
16. Ohara S, et al. Survey on the prevalence of GERD and FD based on the Montreal definition and the Rome III criteria among patients presenting with epigastric symptoms in Japan. J Gastroenterol. 2011;46:603–11.
17. Kaji M, et al. Prevalence of overlaps between GERD, FD and IBS and impact on health-related quality of life. J Gastroenterol Hepatol. 2010;25:1151–6.
18. Hoshikawa Y, et al. Efficacy of on-demand therapy using 20-mg vonoprazan for non-erosive reflux disease. Esophagus. 2019;16:201–6.
19. Fass R, et al. AGA clinical practice update on functional heartburn: expert review. Gastroenterology. 2020;158:2286–93.
20. Pauwels A, et al. How to select patients for antireflux surgery? The ICARUS guidelines (international consensus regarding preoperative examinations and clinical characteristics assessment to select adult patients for antireflux surgery). Gut. 2019;68:1928–41.

13 Diagnosis and Treatment of Motility Disorder of the Esophagus, Achalasia

Junichi Akiyama

Abstract

Achalasia is a rare esophageal motility disorder caused by impaired relaxation of the lower esophageal sphincter (LES) and loss of esophageal peristalsis, leading to dysphagia and regurgitation. Though the cause is unknown, autoimmune or infectious factors are suspected. It typically affects adults aged 30–60 and is diagnosed using endoscopy, barium esophagram, and high-resolution manometry (HRM). HRM is the gold standard for diagnosing achalasia, providing pressure measurements throughout the esophagus and enabling classification into three subtypes. Additional testing, like FLIP and timed barium esophagram, may help in inconclusive cases. Treatments aim to reduce LES pressure and improve esophageal emptying. Options include medications, botulinum toxin injections, pneumatic dilation (PD), laparoscopic Heller myotomy (LHM), and per-oral endoscopic myotomy (POEM). While drugs and botulinum toxin offer short-term relief, PD and myotomy provide longer-lasting effects. POEM is especially effective across all subtypes, including Type III, but is associated with higher rates of gastroesophageal reflux compared to LHM. Recent studies suggest POEM may offer superior outcomes, but treatment should be tailored based on achalasia subtype and patient condition. Accurate diagnosis and individualized therapy are key to improving symptoms and long-term outcomes.

Keywords

Achalasia · High resolution manometry · Timed barium esophagram · FLIP pneumatic dilation · Laparoscopic myotomy · Per-oral endoscopic myotomy

J. Akiyama (✉)
Division of Gastroenterology and Hepatology, National Center for Global Health and Medicine, Tokyo, Japan

H. Kaneko et al. (eds.), *Disorders of Gut-Brain Interaction*,
https://doi.org/10.1007/978-981-95-6974-8_13

1 Concept

Achalasia is a primary esophageal motility disorder characterized by impaired relaxation of the lower esophageal sphincter (LES) and disrupted peristalsis in the esophageal body, leading to difficulty in passing food and liquids from the esophagus to the stomach [1]. The etiology is unknown, but infectious or autoimmune causes are suspected. The loss of inhibitory neurons in the esophageal myenteric plexus disrupts the balance between excitatory and inhibitory neural activity, resulting in increased basal LES pressure, loss of LES relaxation, and absence of normal esophageal peristalsis. Certain tumors can cause achalasia as a direct obstruction or a paraneoplastic syndrome (pseudoachalasia).

2 Epidemiology

Achalasia can occur across a wide age range, from children to the elderly, but is most common between the ages of 30 and 60, with no gender preference. The reported incidence ranges from 0.03 to 1.63 per 100,000 persons per year.

3 Symptoms

The main symptom is dysphagia for solids and liquids (70–97%), which progresses slowly over months to years. Other symptoms include regurgitation of undigested food or saliva (75–91%), chest pain (about 50%), heartburn (40–60%), and respiratory symptoms such as coughing due to aspiration (10%). The frequency and severity of symptoms vary depending on the degree of LES dysfunction. The Eckardt score, used to assess symptom severity, is calculated based on the frequency of dysphagia, regurgitation, chest pain, and weight loss, with a total score range of 0–12 points. Higher scores indicate more severe symptoms [2]. Generally, a post-treatment score of 3 or higher indicates treatment failure.

4 Examination and Diagnostic Criteria

Diagnosis of achalasia involves upper gastrointestinal endoscopy (EGD), barium esophagram, and esophageal manometry. Functional lumen imaging probe (FLIP) can be used as an auxiliary diagnostic tool. Figure 13.1 shows the diagnostic algorithm for suspected achalasia [3].

4.1 Upper Gastrointestinal Endoscopy (EGD)

EGD is performed to differentiate organic diseases that can cause dysphagia, such as eosinophilic esophagitis, esophageal webs, and stenosis. Characteristic EGD findings in achalasia include retention of food residues or liquids, dilatation of the esophageal lumen, whitish thickening of the esophageal mucosa (due to inflammation from food residues), and functional narrowing at the esophagogastric junction (concentration of esophageal folds (rosette), wrapping, and inversion into the stomach) [4]. However, early achalasia may not show abnormalities on EGD.

In elderly patients with new-onset dysphagia and rapid weight loss, pseudochalasia due to tumor invasion of the esophagus should be ruled out by CT or endoscopic ultrasound.

4.2 Barium Esophagram

In healthy individuals, ingested barium flows smoothly into the stomach without retention in the esophagus, whereas in achalasia patients, barium outflow into the stomach is delayed, indirectly diagnosing insufficiency of LES relaxation. Radiographic findings in achalasia include a bird-beak appearance at the esophagogastric junction, esophageal dilatation due to passage obstruction, and retention of contrast medium in the esophagus [4]. Timed barium esophagram (TBE), which observes the height of the barium

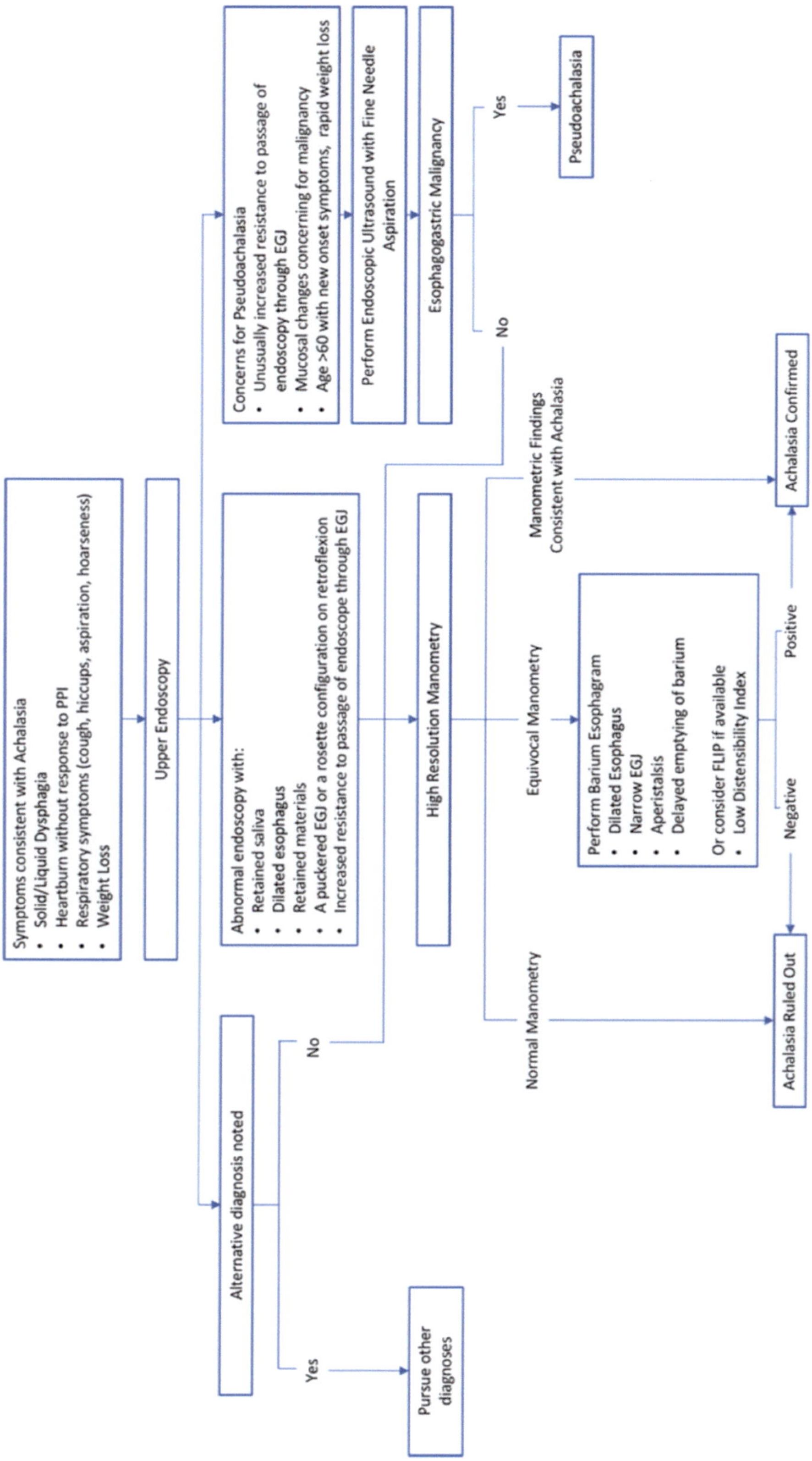

Fig. 13.1 Diagnostic algorithm for achalasia

column in the esophagus at 1, 2, and 5 minutes after ingestion, is helpful in diagnosing achalasia and monitoring post-treatment. Additionally, following TBE, ingesting a 13 mm barium tablet and checking for retention in the esophagus after 5 minutes is another method (Fig. 13.2) [5]. The diagnostic accuracy of achalasia is 85% sensitivity and 86% specificity when barium retention is observed at 2 cm or more after 5 minutes on TBE, and the accuracy increases to 79.5–100% when considering barium tablet retention [5].

Traditionally, achalasia was classified into spindle, flask, and sigmoid types based on barium esophagram. The revised "Guidelines for the Treatment of Esophageal Achalasia (4th Edition)" in 2012 divided achalasia into straight type (St type) including spindle and flask types, and sigmoid type (Sg type), with advanced sigmoid type (aSg type) characterized by strong rightward deviation of the esophagus forming an L-shape [4]. The degree of esophageal dilatation is classified by maximum transverse diameter into Grade I (<3.5 cm), Grade II (≥3.5 cm and <6.0 cm), and Grade III (≥6.0 cm).

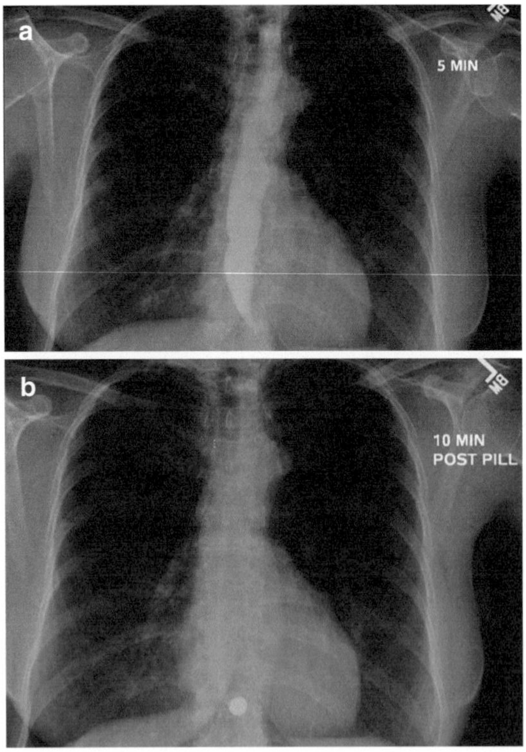

Fig. 13.2 Esophagography [5]. (**a**) TBE image (5 minutes) in a patient with Type II achalasia, showing barium retention in the esophagus. (**b**) Barium tablet retention 5 minutes after ingestion (10 minutes after starting TBE) in the same patient

4.3 Esophageal Manometry

High-resolution esophageal manometry (HRM) is the gold standard for diagnosing achalasia. HRM uses a catheter with 36 pressure sensors spaced 1 cm apart to continuously measure pressure from the upper esophageal sphincter (UES) to the LES. Pressure changes are displayed in color topography, facilitating easy visualization of esophageal motility.

The Chicago classification, proposed for diagnosing esophageal motility disorders using HRM, was updated to the 4th edition in 2021, along with a technical review on achalasia [6, 7]. HRM-specific parameters include integrated relaxation pressure (IRP), distal latency (DL), and distal contractile integral (DCI). IRP indicates the degree of LES relaxation after UES relaxation during swallowing, with values above the normal upper limit indicating deglutitive LES relaxation failure. The normal upper limit of IRP varies depending on the equipment in use. The contractile deceleration point (CDP) is where the propagation speed of the 30 mmHg isobaric contour slows between the esophageal body and the diaphragmatic esophageal enlargement. The time from UES relaxation to CDP is defined as DL and is used to diagnose premature contractions (spastic contractions).

Achalasia is characterized by deglutitive LES relaxation failure, resulting in high IRP values. Based on esophageal body motility patterns, achalasia is classified into three subtypes: Type I achalasia with 100% failed peristalsis, Type II achalasia with 100% failed peristalsis and ≥20% swallows with panesophageal pressurization (PEP), and Type III achalasia with ≥20% swallows with premature/spastic contraction and no evidence of peristalsis (Fig. 13.3, Table 13.1) [6]. The frequency of each subtype is Type II achala-

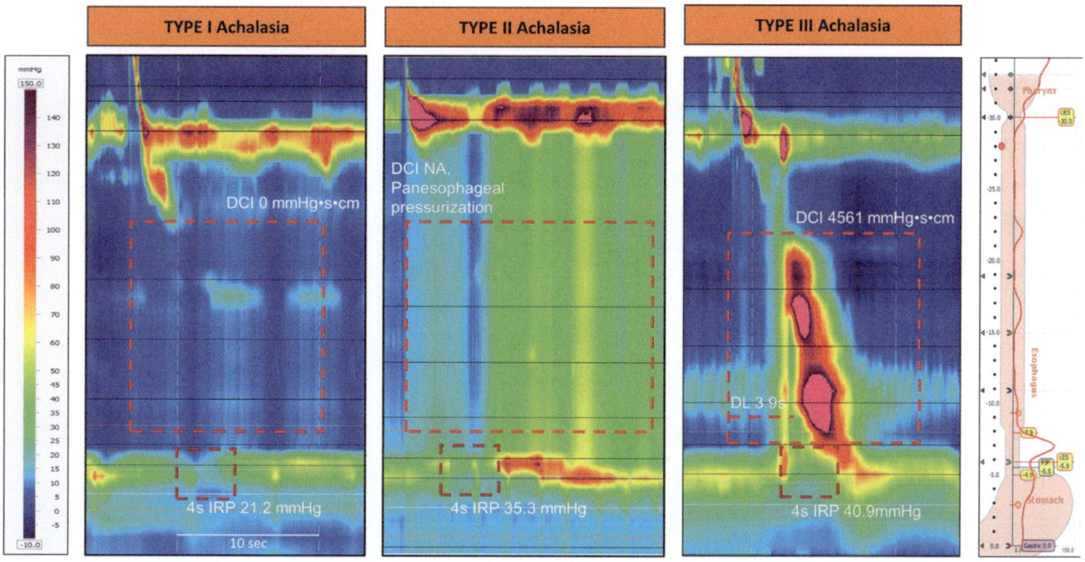

Fig. 13.3 Classification of achalasia by HRM [6]

Table 13.1 Classification of achalasia according to the Chicago Classification (4th Edition) [6]

Disorder	Definition
Type I achalasia	IRP abnormal and 100% failed peristalsis
Type II achalasia	IRP abnormal, 100% failed peristalsis, and ≥20% panesophageal pressurization
Type III achalasia	IRP abnormal and ≥20% premature/ spastic contractions with no normal peristalsis

sia (50–70%), Type I achalasia (20–40%), and Type III achalasia (about 5%).

If HRM does not meet the diagnostic criteria for achalasia, it is considered inconclusive, and supportive testing such as TBE and/or FLIP is required (Fig. 13.4) [7]. This includes cases with high IRP but partial peristaltic waves in the esophageal body (inconclusive achalasia if PEP or premature peristalsis is present, otherwise EGJOO), and cases with 100% failed peristalsis but normal IRP (inconclusive achalasia).

4.4 Functional Lumen Imaging Probe (FLIP)

FLIP is used as an auxiliary diagnostic tool when HRM does not meet the diagnostic criteria for achalasia, resulting in inconclusive achalasia [7]. FLIP uses a catheter with multiple impedance electrodes, and a balloon surrounding the catheter is gradually inflated in the esophagus to measure cross-sectional area and pressure. FLIP evaluates EGJ distensibility and esophageal body contraction patterns. In achalasia, EGJ distensibility is reduced, and diminished or absent contractile response is observed, while normal repetitive antegrade contractions (RAC) are often absent.

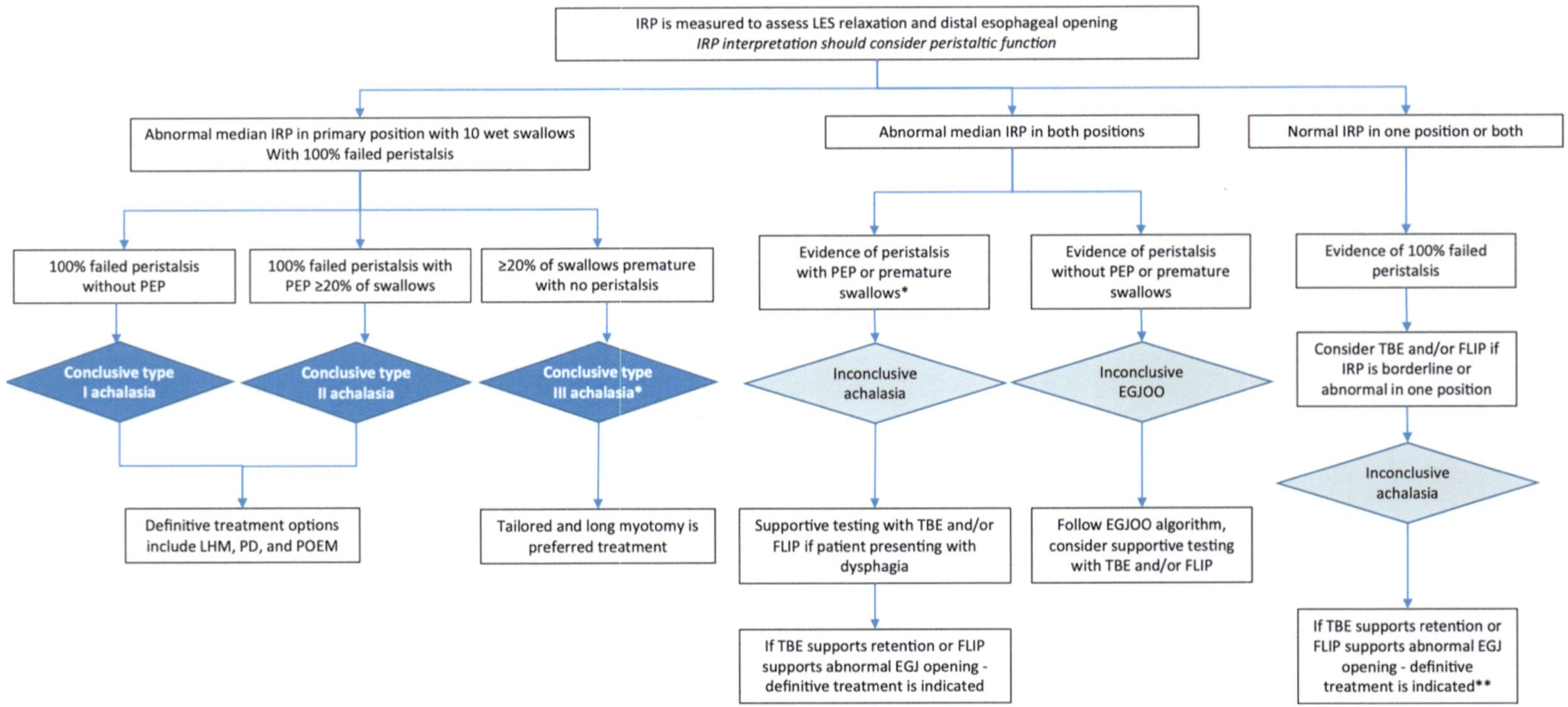

Fig. 13.4 Diagnostic algorithm for achalasia according to the Chicago Classification (4th edition) [7]

5 Treatment

The treatment goals for achalasia are to relieve LES relaxation failure, promote esophageal emptying into the stomach, improve symptoms, and prevent complications such as aspiration and esophageal dilation. Current treatment options include pharmacotherapy, botulinum toxin injection, pneumatic dilation, surgical myotomy, and per-oral endoscopic myotomy (POEM) (Fig. 13.5) [8].

5.1 Pharmacologic Therapy

Pharmacologic therapy for esophageal achalasia includes smooth muscle relaxants such as calcium channel blockers (sublingual nifedipine 10–30 mg before meals) and nitrates (sublingual isosorbide dinitrate 5 mg before meals). However, due to low efficacy, short duration of effect, and side effects such as headache and hypotension, pharmacologic therapy should only be considered in very few select patients with achalasia as a bridge to more effective therapy or in cases where other treatments are not indicated.

5.2 Botulinum Toxin Injection

Botulinum toxin inhibits acetylcholine release from motor nerve endings, leading to a decrease in LES pressure. Endoscopic injection of botulinum toxin (100 U) into the LES muscle layer improves symptoms in approximately 80% of patients initially, but only lasts for several months up to about a year [9]. Due to its short duration of effect, it is generally reserved for patients with a limited life expectancy or who are too sick to undergo endoscopic treatments (dilation or myotomy) or surgical treatments.

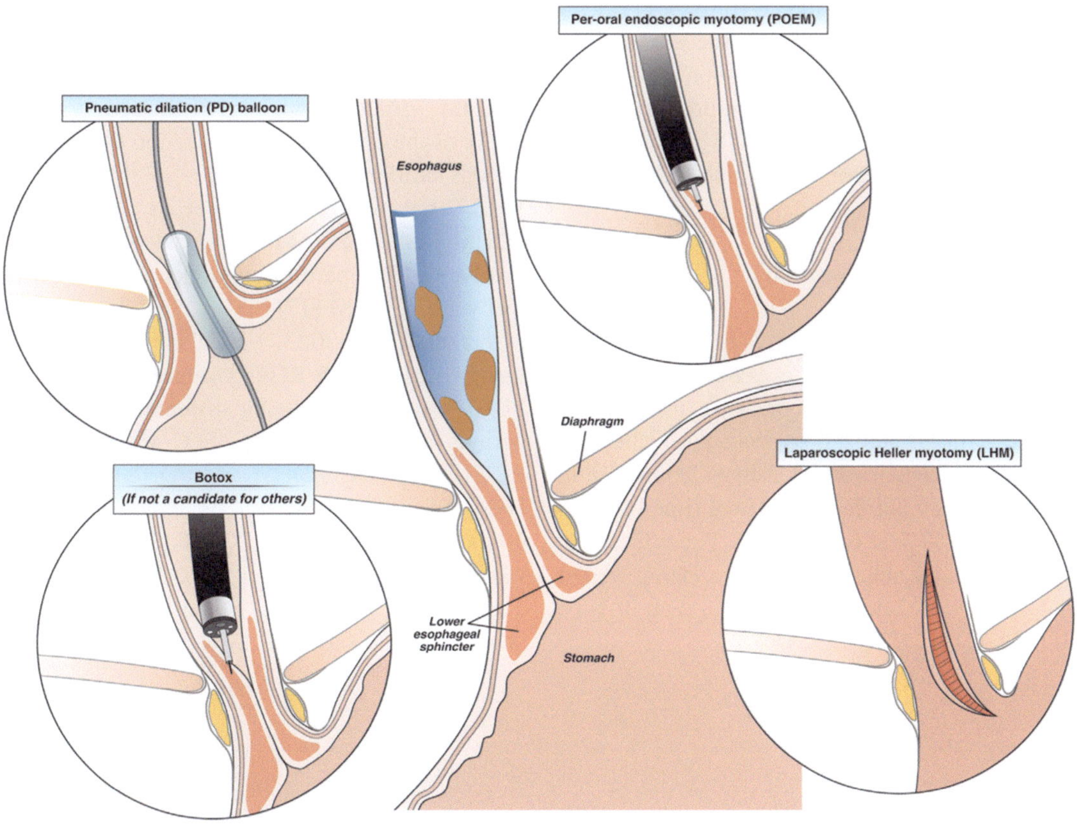

Fig. 13.5 Treatment of achalasia [8]

5.3 Pneumatic Dilation

Endoscopic balloon dilation (pneumatic dilation: PD) involves placing a guidewire using an endoscope and inserting a specialized balloon for achalasia treatment (30, 35, 40 mm) along the guidewire. The balloon is then expanded to disrupt the LES, thereby reducing LES pressure. FLIP can be used to confirm the esophageal lumen diameter during dilation.

Generally, the safety of PD is relatively high, with a perforation risk of about 2% (1% requiring surgery) [10]. The efficacy of a single PD ranges from 66% to 88% at 1 year but declines to 25–29% at 10 years [10]. Therefore, PD may need to be repeated as necessary. In a randomized controlled trial (RCT) comparing PD and laparoscopic Heller myotomy (LHM), the 5-year efficacy was similar (82% vs. 84%), but 25% of cases required multiple PDs due to symptom recurrence [11]. The efficacy of PD varies by achalasia subtype, being higher in Type II (84%) than in Type I (61%) and Type III (31%) [12].

Predictors of PD treatment success include female gender, age >45 years, esophageal diameter >3 cm, Type II achalasia, improved barium clearance on post-treatment TBE, and post-treatment LES pressure <10 mmHg [13].

5.4 Surgical Myotomy

Laparoscopic Heller myotomy (LHM) is a surgical procedure that directly cuts the muscle fibers of the LES to reduce LES pressure, usually performed with an anti-reflux procedure. The success rate of LHM in RCTs ranges from 82% to 90% at 2 years but decreases over time (89% at 6 months to 57% at 6 years) [3]. The efficacy of LHM varies by achalasia subtype, being higher in Type I (81%) and Type II (92%) than in Type III (71%) [12].

5.5 Per-Oral Endoscopic Myotomy (POEM)

POEM is a technique that approaches the muscle layer through the submucosal layer from the esophageal lumen using an oral endoscope and performs myotomy. This method cuts only the inner circular muscle while preserving the outer longitudinal muscle. POEM has high efficacy, with long-term success rates of over 90% at 5–7 years [14]. Because of ability to tailor and lengthen the myotomy, POEM may be especially effective for type III achalasia. POEM exhibited excellent results for all achalasia subtypes: Type I (95%), Type II (97%), and Type III (93%) [12].

However, unlike LHM, POEM does not include an anti-reflux procedure, raising concerns about postoperative GERD. A 2018 meta-analysis found that POEM had higher rates of GERD symptoms (odds ratio 1.69, $p < 0.0001$), reflux esophagitis (odds ratio 9.31, $p < 0.0001$), and acid reflux on pH monitoring (odds ratio 4.30, $p < 0.0001$) compared to LHM [15]. A 2019 RCT reported that the incidence of reflux esophagitis at 2 years was higher in POEM (44%) than in LHM (29%), although the incidence of severe reflux esophagitis (LA classification Grade C or D) was similar [16].

In 2019, a method to prevent GERD after POEM, called POEM+F, was devised, which involves adding partial fundoplication endoscopically after POEM [17].

As of August 2023, 1 RCT comparing LHM and POEM [16], 5 RCTs comparing LHM and PD (with 2 reports being different observation periods of the same trial) [11, 18–22], and 2 RCTs comparing POEM and PD [23, 24] have been reported. These reports indicate that the efficacy of LHM and POEM is both around 90%, while PD is slightly lower at 54–86%. The variability in PD efficacy is attributed to non-standardized protocols, different balloon sizes, and varying tolerance for repeated dilation in case of symptom recurrence.

A meta-analysis examining the efficacy of botulinum toxin injection, PD, LHM, and POEM by achalasia subtype reported that (1) POEM was more effective than LHM in treating Type I and III (Type I: odds ratio 2.97, $p = 0.03$; Type III: odds ratio 3.50, $p = 0.007$); (2) POEM was the most effective for all subtypes (Type I 95%, II 97%, III 93%); (3) PD was slightly less effective than POEM and LHM in Type II, but the difference was not statistically significant; and (4) botulinum toxin injection was less effective for all subtypes [12].

6 Conclusion

The advent of HRM has made the diagnosis of achalasia simple and accurate, establishing HRM as the gold standard. However, TBE and FLIP are useful for cases where the diagnosis is uncertain. In addition to PD, more effective treatments such as LHM and POEM are now available for achalasia. It is crucial to consider the achalasia subtype and select the appropriate treatment for each case.

Take-Home Message

Achalasia is characterized by LES relaxation failure and esophageal body motility disorders. Diagnosis involves EGD, barium esophagram, and HRM, with HRM classifying achalasia into Types I–III. Treatment options include pharmacologic therapy, botulinum toxin injection, endoscopic balloon dilation, surgical myotomy, and POEM, with POEM being the most effective for all subtypes.

Competing Interests The author(s) has no competing interests to declare that are relevant to the content of this manuscript.

References

1. Iwakiri K. Diagnosis and balloon dilation of achalasia. J Jpn Soc Gastroenterol. 2012;109:710–21. (in Japanese).
2. Eckardt AJ, et al. Treatment and surveillance strategies in achalasia: an update. Nat Rev Gastroenterol Hepatol. 2011;8:311–9.
3. Pomenti S, et al. Achalasia: diagnosis, management and surveillance. Gastroenterol Clin N Am. 2021;50:721–36.
4. Guidelines for the treatment of esophageal achalasia, 4th ed. Japanese Society of Esophageal Diseases. Kanehara Publishing; 2012. p. 3–21. (in Japanese).
5. Blonski W, et al. Timed barium swallow: diagnostic role and predictive value in untreated achalasia, esophagogastric junction outflow obstruction, and non-achalasia dysphagia. Am J Gastroenterol. 2018;113(2):196–203.
6. Yadlapati R, et al. Esophageal motility disorders on high-resolution manometry: Chicago classification version 4.0((c)). Neurogastroenterol Motil. 2021;33:e14058.
7. Khan A, et al. Chicago Classification update (version 4.0): technical review on diagnostic criteria for achalasia. Neurogastroenterol Motil. 2021;33:e14182.
8. Patel DA, et al. Motility disorders: current approach to diagnostics and therapeutics. Gastroenterology. 2022;162:1617–34.
9. Pasricha PJ, et al. Intrasphincteric botulinum toxin for the treatment of achalasia. N Engl J Med. 1995;332:774–8.
10. Katzka DA, et al. Review article: an analysis of the efficacy, perforation rates and methods used in pneumatic dilation for achalasia. Aliment Pharmacol Ther. 2011;34:832–9.
11. Moonen A, et al. Long-term results of the European achalasia trial: a multicentre randomised controlled trial comparing pneumatic dilation versus laparoscopic Heller myotomy. Gut. 2016;65:732–9.
12. Andolfi C, et al. Meta-analysis of clinical outcome after treatment for achalasia based on manometric subtypes. Br J Surg. 2019;106:332–41.
13. Patel DA, et al. Idiopathic (primary) achalasia: a review. Orphanet J Rare Dis. 2015;10:89.
14. Modayil RJ, et al. Peroral endoscopic myotomy: 10-year outcomes from a large, single-center U.S. series with high follow-up completion and comprehensive analysis of long-term efficacy, safety, objective GERD, and endoscopic functional luminal assessment. Gastrointest Endosc. 2021;94:930–42.

15. Schlottmann F, et al. Laparoscopic Heller myotomy versus peroral endoscopic myotomy (POEM) for achalasia: a systematic review and meta-analysis. Ann Surg. 2018;267:451–60.
16. Werner YB, et al. Endoscopic or surgical myotomy in patients with idiopathic achalasia. N Engl J Med. 2019;381:2219–29.
17. Inoue H, et al. Peroral endoscopic myotomy and fundoplication: a novel NOTES procedure. Endoscopy. 2019;51:161–4.
18. Persson J, et al. Treatment of achalasia with laparoscopic myotomy or pneumatic dilatation: long-term results of a prospective, randomized study. World J Surg. 2015;39:713–20.
19. Hamdy E, et al. Comparative study between laparoscopic Heller myotomy versus pneumatic dilatation for treatment of early achalasia: a prospective randomized study. J Laparoendosc Adv Surg Tech A. 2015;25:460–4.
20. Borges AA, et al. Pneumatic dilation versus laparoscopic Heller myotomy for the treatment of achalasia: variables related to a good response. Dis Esophagus. 2014;27:18–23.
21. Boeckxstaens GE, et al. Pneumatic dilation versus laparoscopic Heller's myotomy for idiopathic achalasia. N Engl J Med. 2011;364:1807–16.
22. Kostic S, et al. Pneumatic dilatation or laparoscopic cardiomyotomy in the management of newly diagnosed idiopathic achalasia. Results of a randomized controlled trial. World J Surg. 2007;31:470–8.
23. Kuipers T, et al. Peroral endoscopic myotomy versus pneumatic dilation in treatment-naive patients with achalasia: 5-year follow-up of a randomised controlled trial. Lancet Gastroenterol Hepatol. 2022;7:1103–11.
24. Ponds FA, et al. Effect of peroral endoscopic myotomy vs pneumatic dilation on symptom severity and treatment outcomes among treatment-naive patients with achalasia: a randomized clinical trial. JAMA. 2019;322:134–44.

14 Diagnosis and Treatment of Motility Disorder of the Esophagus, Diffuse Esophageal Spasm (Distal Esophageal Spasm)

Tomoyuki Koike and Masahiro Saito

Abstract

Diffuse esophageal spasm (DES), redefined as distal esophageal spasm in the Chicago Classification v4.0, is a rare esophageal motility disorder characterized by premature contractions in the distal esophagus without impaired esophagogastric junction relaxation. Patients typically present with intermittent dysphagia and non-cardiac chest pain, symptoms often difficult to distinguish from angina. Although the etiology remains unclear, dysfunction of nitric oxide–mediated inhibitory pathways have been suggested. High-resolution manometry is central to diagnosis, requiring at least 20% premature contractions with normal integrated relaxation pressure. Imaging may reveal a "corkscrew" esophagus, while endoscopy often yields nonspecific findings. DES must be differentiated from achalasia type III, esophagogastric junction outflow obstruction, and secondary motility disorders. No established treatment exists; management begins with reassurance and proton pump inhibitors, followed by smooth muscle relaxants (nitrates, calcium channel blockers), phosphodiesterase inhibitors, or antidepressants. Endoscopic and surgical options, including balloon dilation, botulinum toxin injection, and peroral endoscopic myotomy (POEM), are considered in refractory cases. DES may progress to achalasia, suggesting a disease spectrum. Advances in manometric criteria and minimally invasive endoscopic therapy are improving diagnostic accuracy and therapeutic outcomes, but further studies are required to clarify long-term prognosis and optimize treatment strategies.

Keywords

Diffuse esophageal spasm (DES) · Distal esophageal spasm (DES) · Non-cardiac chest pain (NCCP) · High-resolution manometry (HRM) · Chicago classification · Esophageal motility disorders · Nitroglycerin · Calcium channel blockers · Anticholinergics · Per-oral endoscopic myotomy (POEM)

T. Koike (✉) · M. Saito
Division of Gastroenterology, Tohoku University Graduate School of Medicine, Sendai, Japan
e-mail: tkoike@rd5.so-net.ne.jp

H. Kaneko et al. (eds.), *Disorders of Gut-Brain Interaction*,
https://doi.org/10.1007/978-981-95-6974-8_14

1 Concept

The primary function of the esophagus is to transport food from the pharynx to the stomach through peristaltic movements. Diffuse esophageal spasm (DES) is a condition characterized by normal peristaltic movements, but occasionally persistent synchronous contractions occur. The main symptoms are dysphagia and intermittent substernal pain, which are causes of non-cardiac chest pain (NCCP). DES, along with achalasia, is one of the esophageal motility disorders. However, various issues, including its definition, have been proposed, and strictly defined cases of DES are rare, with many potentially being overdiagnosed [1]. Recently, with the development and dissemination of high-resolution manometry (HRM), the Chicago classification has clarified the concept of this disease. DES is now diagnosed and classified as "distal esophageal spasm (DES)," which shows abnormalities in esophageal body peristaltic waves without esophagogastric junction (EGJ) relaxation failure (Tables 14.1, Figs. 14.1, and 14.2)

Table 14.1 Diagnostic thresholds and definitions in the Chicago Classification

Assessment	Pressure topography metrics	Definition	Diagnostic threshold	Additional considerations
Relaxation pressure across the esophagogastric junction in response to deglutition	Integrated relaxation pressure (IRP)	Mean of the 4 s of maximal deglutitive relaxation in the 10-s window beginning at UES relaxation, contiguous or non-contiguous, referenced to gastric pressure	Abnormal deglutitive IRP relaxation: Supine median IRP ≥ 15 mmHg (Medtronic) Supine median IRP ≥ 22 mmHg (Laborie/Diversatek) Upright median IRP ≥ 12 mmHg (Medtronic) Upright median IRP ≥ 15 mmHg (Laborie/Diversatek)	IRP > 12 mmHg (Medtronic) on rapid drink challenge (RDC) or IRP > 25 mmHg (Medtronic) on solid test meal supports outflow obstruction
Esophageal peristalsis	Distal Contractile Integral (DCI)—Contractile Vigor	Amplitude × duration × length (mmHg·s·cm) of the distal esophageal contraction exceeding 20 mmHg from the transition zone to the proximal margin of the LES	Normal Contraction: DCI 450 to 8000 mmHg·s·cm Weak Contraction: DCI ≥ 100 and < 450 mmHg·s·cm Failed Peristalsis: DCI < 100 mmHg·s·cm Hypercontractile Swallow: DCI > 8000 mmHg·s·cm Ineffective Swallow: weak contraction or failed peristalsis	Intact contractile response on multiple rapid swallow (MRS): DCI < 100 mmHg·s·cm during MRS and DCI greater than single swallow mean DCI following MRS
	Contractile wavefront integrity	Contiguity of peristalsis in an isobaric contour of 20 mmHg	Ineffective Swallow: Peristaltic break greater than 5 cm in setting of a DCI ≥ 450 mmHg·s·cm	
Latency of deglutitive inhibition	Distal latency (DL)	Interval between UES relaxation and CDP	Premature/Spastic contraction: DL < 4.5 s in setting of a DCI ≥ 450 mmHg·s·cm	
Pressurization	Isobaric Contour		Panesophageal pressurization: isobaric contour of ≥30 mmHg Intrabolus pressurization: isobaric contour of ≥20 mmHg in the supine position (Medtronic)	Panesophageal pressurization >20 mmHg on RDC or solid test meal supports outflow

Created from References [2]

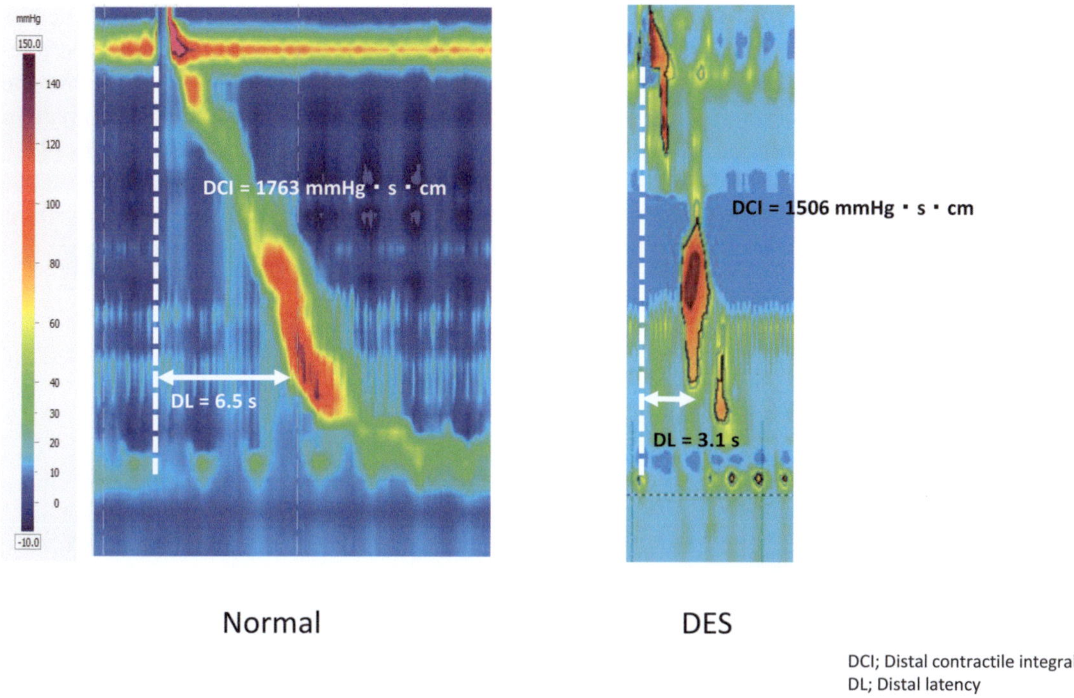

Fig. 14.1 HRM Findings in Normal and DES Cases. Refer to Table 14.1 for abbreviations used in the figure. High-resolution manometry (HRM) displays pressure in color. There are two high-pressure zones: the upper high-pressure zone is the upper esophageal sphincter, and the lower high-pressure zone is the esophagogastric junction. Upon swallowing, peristaltic waves propagate from the upper to the lower esophagus following pharyngeal contraction. The evaluation of EGJ relaxation involves IRP, the assessment of peristaltic wave contraction strength involves DCI, and the time from swallowing to the arrival of the peristaltic wave at the lower esophagus is defined as DL to evaluate primary peristaltic waves

[2, 3]. According to the latest Chicago classification version 4.0, the diagnosis of DES requires esophageal symptoms (dysphagia, NCCP) and at least 20% premature contractions in the presence of normal EGJ relaxation [2].

2 Etiology

While gastroesophageal reflux and stress are considered triggers, the exact cause of DES remains unclear. There are reports suggesting that a coordination disorder involving the nitric oxide (NO) system is significant.

3 Epidemiology

DES is a rare disease, and its exact prevalence is unknown. However, it is reported that the incidence is 0.2 per 100,000 people annually. Kusano et al. reported that among 100 consecutive cases suspected of esophageal motility disorders based on chest pain and dysphagia, 7 cases were diagnosed as DES [4]. Despite the diagnostic challenges, reports from Japan are few. DES can occur at any age but is more common in nervous women aged 40–60, with familial cases also reported. Additionally, 3–5% of cases may progress to typical achalasia.

4 Pathophysiology

Although normal peristaltic waves are usually observed, DES is characterized by persistent and repetitive abnormal contraction movements. Two or more repetitive synchronous contractions with at least 20% of the contractile movements of water swallowing, more than two peaks of repetitive contractions, increased amplitude or height of peristaltic waves, spontaneous contractions, and incomplete relaxation of lower esophageal sphincter (LES) pressure were considered characteristic findings of DES [4, 5]. According to the Chicago classification version 4.0, DES is diagnosed based on HRM results as shown in the flowchart in Figs. 14.2 and 14.3. Specifically, since LES dysfunction is not observed, the integrated relaxation pressure (IRP) is below the upper limit of normal, and the contraction pattern shows at least 20% premature contractions [2].

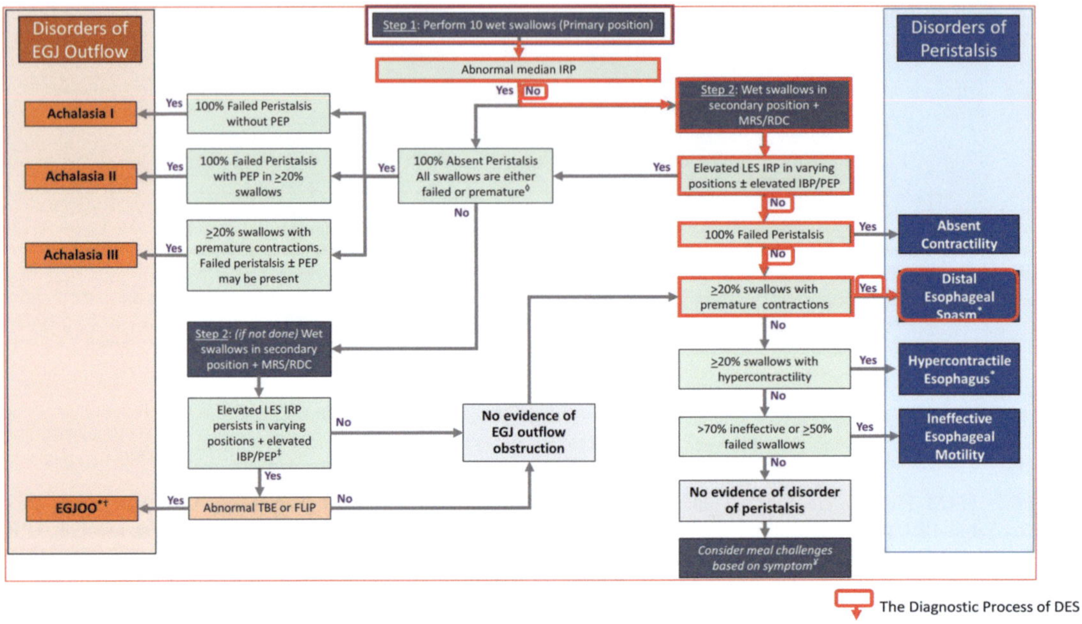

Fig. 14.2 Diagnostic Flowchart of Chicago Classification Version 4.0. (Created from References [2]). This flow diagram represents a conceptual model of a state of the art algorithm that defines the flow process of how the CCv4.0 diagnosis is generated within the constructs of the various phases of the protocol. In this conceptual model, the current protocol allows for some flexibility if the diagnosis is conclusive with 10 swallows in either the primary supine or upright position and allows for a sequenced progression of the protocol to help confirm or rule out the diagnosis. This flow diagram represents the optimal flow process; however exceptions will exist based on the fact that some cutoffs are arbitrary and that the model assumes that a motility expert or a highly qualified motility technician or nurse is performing the protocol and analysis. *Denote manometric patterns of unclear clinical relevance. A clinically relevant conclusive diagnosis requires additional information which may include clinically relevant symptoms and/or supportive testing (as detailed in the document). †Patients with EGJ obstruction and presence of peristaltic swallows would fulfill strict criteria for EGJOO and may have features suggestive of achalasia or other patterns of peristalsis defined by criteria for disorders of peristalsis: EGJOO with spastic features, EGJOO with hypercontractile esophagus, EGJOO with ineffective motility, or EGJOO with no evidence of disordered peristalsis. ‡RDC, solid test swallows, and/or pharmacologic provocation with amyl nitrite or cholecystokinin (if available) can be instituted here to assess for obstruction. ◊Patients previously defined absent contractility based on 10 swallows in the primary position may have achalasia if the IRP is elevated in the alternate position, with the RDC, and/or with MRS. These cases should be considered inconclusive for type I or II achalasia as appropriate and evaluated further with TBE/FLIP. ¥ If no evidence of a disorder of peristalsis or EGJ outflow in a patient with high probability of a missed EGJOO, a solid test meal can be added to rule out an obstructive pattern; if abnormal then possibility of a mechanical obstruction should be readdressed. In a patient with regurgitation or belching postprandial high-resolution impedance monitoring to assess for rumination/belching disorder. IRP integrated relaxation pressure, MRS multiple rapid swallow, RDC rapid drink challenge, LES lower esophageal sphincter, IBP intrabolus pressurization, PEP panesophageal pressurization, EGJ esophagogastric junction, EGJOO EGJ outflow obstruction, TBE timed barium esophagram, FLIP functional lumen imaging probe

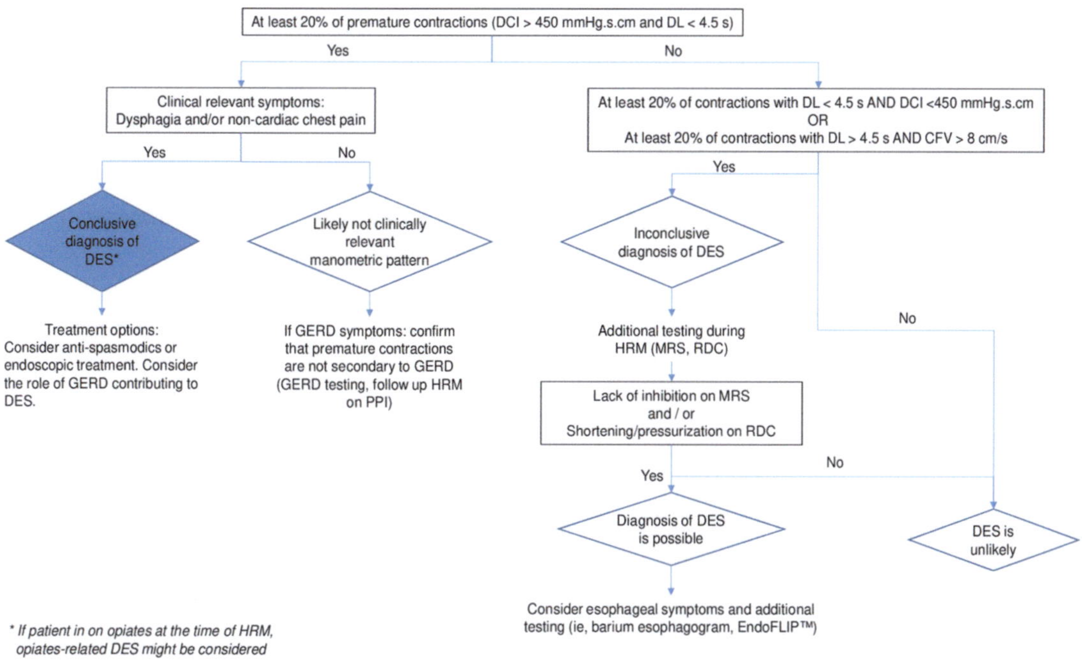

Fig. 14.3 Clinical algorithm for the diagnosis of distal esophageal spasm (DES) according to the version 4.0 of the Chicago Classification. (Created from Reference [3])

5 Pathology

Hypertrophy of the longitudinal muscle and muscularis mucosa of the esophagus is observed on macroscopic examination. Histologically, there is no loss of neurons in the myenteric plexus, but infiltration of inflammatory cells is noted. Additionally, Wallerian degeneration (changes resulting from impaired signal transmission from the distal end of nerve fibers to the peripheral regions) of the vagus nerve esophageal branches has been reported.

6 Symptoms

The main symptoms are dysphagia (approximately 70%) and chest or upper abdominal pain (approximately 80–90%). The pain is severe and radiates to the back, neck, and upper arms. It is often difficult to distinguish from angina, including the response to nitroglycerin, but 50% of cases are related to meals, and nocturnal pain is suggested to be associated with saliva swallowing. Dysphagia and upper abdominal pain are intermittent and non-progressive, occurring with both liquid and solid foods, and are exacerbated by hot or cold substances. These symptoms can lead to reduced food intake and weight loss.

7 Diagnosis

Esophagography shows various findings, but typically a corkscrew (spiral, beaded appearance) is observed. However, DES usually shows normal peristaltic waves, so abnormal findings may not be observed depending on the timing of imaging.

Endoscopy may show several ring-like contractions reflecting continuous synchronous contractions, but the findings may be unclear.

For both esophagography and endoscopy, administration of antispasmodics during the examination may inhibit esophageal motility and cause DES to be missed, so it is necessary to consider performing the examination without antispasmodics if DES is suspected. As mentioned earlier, HRM shows IRP below the upper limit of normal and at least 20% premature contractions (distal latency; DL <4.5 s: DL; the interval from upper esophageal sphincter (UES) relaxation to the contractile deceleration point (CDP)—the point where the propagation velocity of the 30 mmHg isobaric contour slows, observed between the tubular esophagus and the diaphragmatic esophageal ampulla) in swallows [2]. Evaluating IRP is crucial for diagnosing this disease. Missing LES dysfunction can lead to misdiagnosing achalasia as DES.

Cholinesterase inhibitors like edrophonium and pentagastrin and balloon dilation can induce chest pain in patients. Twenty-four-hour pH impedance monitoring is useful for identifying concomitant GERD, with reports indicating that 20–50% of patients have reflux esophagitis.

8 Differential Diagnosis

Esophageal manometry findings similar to DES can be seen in diabetes, alcohol dependence, amyloidosis, systemic sclerosis, and GERD. However, increased peristaltic wave amplitude helps differentiate DES from diabetes, GERD, and alcoholic neuropathy. If IRP is unclear in HRM, differentiating DES from achalasia Type III becomes difficult. Reports suggest that DES can progress to achalasia, indicating that DES and achalasia may be on the same disease spectrum with different severities [3]. Eosinophilic esophagitis is also a differential diagnosis, which can be diagnosed by biopsy from the esophagus.

9 Treatment

There is no established treatment for DES due to its unknown cause. It is important to reassure patients that their chest pain is esophageal rather than cardiac in origin. Explaining this to patients often alleviates symptoms. Pharmacotherapy often starts with proton pump inhibitors (PPIs), because the symptoms of DES are similar to those of GERD, GERD and DES often coexist, esophageal manometry findings in GERD and DES can be similar, and GERD can cause chest pain.

If symptoms do not improve with PPIs, medications that relax esophageal smooth muscle are administered to facilitate the passage of food and alleviate dysphagia and chest pain. These medications often include long-acting nitroglycerin, calcium channel blockers (nifedipine, diltiazem), and anticholinergics [2].

Additionally, sildenafil, which increases nitric oxide (NO) in esophageal smooth muscle, has been tried for achalasia and is expected to be effective for DES as well. Although antidepressants do not affect esophageal motility disorders, they are reported to alleviate subjective symptoms [2]. Furthermore, in Japan, β-agonists, opioid receptor agonists like trimebutine, and Kampo medicine such as Shakuyakukanzoto have been reported to be effective treatments. If pharmacotherapy is ineffective, balloon dilation of the lower esophageal sphincter or botulinum toxin injection is effective. Surgical myotomy was previously performed for refractory cases, but recently, per-oral endoscopic myotomy (POEM) has rapidly gained popularity due to its advantages, such as not leaving scars and its excellent treatment outcomes [6]. POEM has also been reported to be useful for DES, and further accumulation of cases and long-term prognosis studies are expected [7].

Take-Home Message

DES is a disorder characterized by abnormalities in esophageal body peristaltic waves without LES dysfunction, requiring differentiation from achalasia and EGJOO based on IRP < upper limit of normal. The characteristic feature of esophageal body peristaltic waves is at least 20% premature contractions (DL < 4.5 s). Therefore, evaluating IRP is crucial for diagnosing this disease. Missing LES dysfunction can lead to misdiagnosing achalasia Type III as DES.

Competing Interests The author(s) has no competing interests to declare that are relevant to the content of this manuscript.

References

1. Pandolfino JE, et al. American Gastroenterological Association: AGA technical review on the clinical use of esophageal manometry. Gastroenterology. 2005;128:209–24.
2. Yadlapati R, et al. Esophageal motility disorders on high-resolution manometry: Chicago classification version 4.0©. Neurogastroenterol Motil. 2021;33(1):e14058.
3. Roman S, et al. Chicago Classification Update (v4.0): technical review on diagnostic criteria for distal esophageal spasm. Neurogastroenterol Motil. 2021;33(5):e14119.
4. Kusano M, et al. Esophageal motor function in non-achalasia motility disorders. Nihon Shokakibyo Gakkai Zasshi. 2003;100:1095–105. (in Japanese)
5. Spechler SJ, et al. Classification of esophageal motility abnormalities. Gut. 2001;49:145–51.
6. Inoue H, et al. Peroral endoscopic myotomy (POEM) for esophageal achalasia. Endoscopy. 2010;42:265–71.
7. Khashab MA, et al. Peroral endoscopic myotomy is effective and safe in non-achalasia esophageal motility disorders: an international multicenter study. Endosc Int Open. 2018;6(8):E1031–6.

Diagnosis and Treatment of Motility Disorder of the Esophagus, Ineffective Esophageal Motility in Systemic Sclerosis

15

Shigeto Koizumi and Katsunori Iijima

Abstract

Systemic sclerosis is the collagen disease most frequently associated with gastrointestinal lesions. This section primarily discusses esophageal lesions in systemic sclerosis.

Keywords

Esophageal motility disorders · Collagen diseases · Systemic sclerosis (SSc) · Esophageal peristaltic waves · Esophagogastric junction (EGJ) · Lower esophageal sphincter (LES) pressure · Reflux esophagitis

1 Concept

Upon swallowing, primary peristaltic waves propagate from the oral to the anal side of the esophagus, transporting ingested material. The esophagogastric junction (EGJ) presents a high-pressure zone that prevents gastric contents from refluxing into the esophagus. Swallowing temporarily relaxes the EGJ, allowing esophageal contents to enter the stomach. Esophageal motility disorders disrupt this sequence of functions.

Esophageal motility disorders can be classified into primary esophageal motility disorders, where the cause is unknown, and secondary esophageal motility disorders, which occur as a result of underlying diseases. Diseases that can cause secondary esophageal motility disorders include collagen diseases, endocrine/metabolic disorders, neuromuscular diseases, infections, allergic diseases, and malignancies [1]. Table 15.1 lists the main diseases that can cause secondary esophageal motility disorders.

Table 15.1 Major diseases causing secondary esophageal motility disorders

Disease group	Diseases
Collagen diseases	Systemic sclerosis, systemic lupus erythematosus, rheumatoid arthritis, mixed connective tissue disease, Sjögren's syndrome, polyarteritis nodosa
Endocrine/metabolic diseases	Diabetes mellitus, thyroid diseases, amyloidosis
Neuromuscular diseases	Myasthenia gravis, Parkinson's disease
Infections	Trypanosoma cruzi infection, post-polio syndrome
Allergic diseases	Eosinophilic esophagitis
Malignancies	Malignancies causing secondary achalasia

Created from Ref. [1]

S. Koizumi (✉)
Gastroenterology, Koizumi Hospital, Akita, Japan
e-mail: s-hoskoizumi@leaf.ocn.ne.jp

K. Iijima
Gastroenterology, Akita University Graduate School of Medicine, Akita, Japan
e-mail: kiijima@med.akita-u.ac.jp

H. Kaneko et al. (eds.), *Disorders of Gut-Brain Interaction*,
https://doi.org/10.1007/978-981-95-6974-8_15

2 Esophageal Lesions in Collagen Diseases

Major collagen diseases presenting with gastrointestinal lesions include systemic sclerosis (SSc), systemic lupus erythematosus (SLE), rheumatoid arthritis (RA), mixed connective tissue disease (MCTD), Sjögren's syndrome, and polyarteritis nodosa (PN). The main factors causing gastrointestinal lesions due to collagen diseases are (1) abnormal gastrointestinal peristalsis due to increased connective tissue, (2) mucosal damage due to ischemic changes from vasculitis and resulting circulatory failure, and (3) gastrointestinal dilation and decreased peristalsis due to collagen fiber proliferation and muscle tissue atrophy/degeneration [2, 3]. Additionally, secondary factors related to the treatment of collagen diseases, such as non-steroidal anti-inflammatory drugs (NSAIDs) and steroids, also contribute [3].

This section primarily discusses esophageal lesions in systemic sclerosis.

3 Systemic Sclerosis

Systemic sclerosis is a chronic disease characterized by (1) fibrosis due to fibroblast activation, (2) immune abnormalities involving autoantibodies such as anti-topoisomerase I (Scl-70) antibodies and anti-centromere antibodies, and (3) vascular disorders. It affects not only the skin, causing skin sclerosis and Raynaud's phenomenon, but also various organs including the gastrointestinal tract, lungs, kidneys, and heart [4].

In Japan, it is estimated that 20,000–30,000 people are affected, but considering the large number of mild cases, the actual prevalence is likely higher. The disease commonly occurs between the ages of 30 and 50, with a female-to-male ratio of 14:1, and is more common in women than in men. Raynaud's phenomenon is often the initial symptom, followed by skin sclerosis starting from the extremities and spreading centrally. The disease progresses through stages: the edematous stage with predominant dermal edema, the sclerotic stage with increased collagen fiber bundles forming sclerotic plaques, and the atrophic stage with thinning and atrophy of the sclerotic plaques after their expansion [3, 5].

4 Esophageal Lesions in Systemic Sclerosis

Systemic sclerosis is the collagen disease most frequently associated with gastrointestinal lesions, affecting the entire gastrointestinal tract, with the esophagus being the most commonly involved site. It is reported that 50–90% of systemic sclerosis patients have esophageal lesions [6, 7].

4.1 Pathophysiology

Esophageal lesions in systemic sclerosis are caused by increased connective tissue and atrophy of muscle in the esophageal muscularis propria, leading to decreased lower esophageal sphincter (LES) pressure and peristaltic abnormalities (reduced or absent peristaltic waves in the esophageal body) [7, 8]. These esophageal motility disorders cause food passage obstruction, leading to secondary esophageal dilation and reflux esophagitis. Reflux esophagitis is observed in 60% of systemic sclerosis patients [9], and in severe cases with significant reduction in esophageal peristaltic waves and LES function, decreased acid clearance in the esophagus can lead to severe reflux esophagitis. Approximately 40% of systemic sclerosis patients develop esophageal stenosis [9, 10].

4.2 Symptoms

Common symptoms include a sensation of food sticking, dysphagia, heartburn, and hiccups.

4.3 Examination and Diagnosis

1. Esophagography: It shows spindle-shaped dilatation of the esophageal lumen, findings

of gastroesophageal reflux, and delayed passage of contrast due to decreased peristalsis [11]. In addition to dilatation of transverse axis, shortening of longitudinal axis often leads to hiatal hernia. Similar spindle-shaped dilation is observed in achalasia, but achalasia is distinguished by LES dilation disorder.

2. Endoscopy: Reflux esophagitis is commonly observed. Hiatal hernia and esophageal dilation may also be present. If esophageal dilation is observed without EGJ stricture, systemic sclerosis should be considered. Unlike achalasia, systemic sclerosis does not show EGJ passage obstruction. Other findings include Candida esophagitis, often seen in patients taking steroids or acid-suppressing drugs [12]. Histopathological findings primarily show fibrosis deeper than the mucosal surface, making endoscopic biopsy evaluation generally difficult [3]. Long-term cases may develop esophageal stenosis or Barrett's esophagus due to reflux esophagitis, with reports of Barrett's adenocarcinoma, which should be noted [13].
3. Esophageal Manometry: High-resolution manometry (HRM) is used to evaluate esophageal motility. Esophageal motility disorders in systemic sclerosis are characterized by decreased peristaltic wave amplitude in the smooth muscle region. If esophageal motility is reduced but still present, it is classified as ineffective esophageal motility (IEM); if mid-to-lower esophageal motility is completely impaired, it is classified as absent contractility [12].
4. 24-Hour Esophageal pH Monitoring and 24-Hour Esophageal Impedance-pH Monitoring: These tests evaluate gastroesophageal reflux. Systemic sclerosis often coexists with interstitial pneumonia, which is also associated with gastroesophageal reflux. Studies using 24-hour esophageal impedance-pH monitoring in systemic sclerosis patients have shown a significant correlation between the degree of gastroesophageal reflux and the severity of interstitial pneumonia [14].

4.4 Treatment

There is no established treatment for esophageal lesions in systemic sclerosis, and symptomatic treatment is provided for each condition. In addition to patient education on dietary intake, pharmacotherapy with antacids, mucosal protectants, and prokinetics are also administered [6].

For gastroesophageal reflux, treatment is similar to that for typical GERD, with proton pump inhibitors (PPIs) or potassium-competitive acid blockers (P-CABs) being administered [15]. However, reports indicate that even with high-dose PPIs, some systemic sclerosis patients still experience abnormal acid reflux [16]. Alginates may also be co-administered. For esophageal clearance disorders due to decreased peristalsis and LES function, prokinetics such as serotonin 5-HT4 receptor agonists and dopamine antagonists are recommended in addition to acid-suppressing drugs. These medications have been shown to increase esophageal peristaltic pressure and promote esophageal clearance [17–20]. Although there is insufficient evidence for systemic sclerosis, the herbal medicine Rikkunshito has been reported to improve symptoms [21]. Other medications, such as anticholinergics, calcium channel blockers, and β-blockers, may decrease peristaltic motility and LES pressure, so caution is needed when using these drugs [22].

Lifestyle modifications are also important, including avoiding high-fat meals, sweets like chocolate, spicy foods, alcohol, and smoking; consuming low-residue meals in small, frequent portions; avoiding meals before bedtime; staying upright for several hours after meals; and elevating the upper body during sleep [5, 15].

Gastroesophageal reflux can be present even in asymptomatic stages and is associated with worsening pulmonary fibrosis, which directly affects prognosis. Therefore, early testing and treatment intervention for gastroesophageal reflux are suggested [11, 23].

For severe esophageal strictures, balloon dilation or surgical treatment may be considered, but symptoms may worsen, so careful consideration is needed for treatment indications [3].

5 Other Collagen Diseases and Esophageal Motility Disorders

1. Systemic Lupus Erythematosus (SLE): Esophageal motility disorders are observed in about 70% of patients. Generally, the severity of esophageal motility disorders is mild, but severe esophageal motility disorders and esophageal ulcers can occur. The upper esophagus is often affected, while the EGJ is relatively less affected. Patients often receive immunosuppressants like steroids, and Candida esophagitis is frequently observed [1, 3, 12].
2. Rheumatoid Arthritis (RA): Esophageal motility disorders are reported in over 30% of patients. Decreased lower esophageal motility and EGJ barrier function leads to GERD. The upper esophagus is also often affected. RA patients frequently have iron deficiency anemia due to impaired iron utilization, and webs from Plummer-Vinson syndrome may be observed [1, 3, 12].
3. Mixed Connective Tissue Disease (MCTD): Shows esophageal motility disorder patterns similar to systemic sclerosis, but the upper esophageal sphincter is also frequently affected [1, 3, 12].
4. Sjögren's Syndrome: Esophageal motility disorders are observed in over 30% of patients. The upper esophagus is often affected, and the upper esophageal sphincter is also frequently involved [1, 3, 12].

Take-Home Message
This section has provided an overview of esophageal involvement in collagen vascular diseases, with a primary focus on systemic sclerosis. Systemic sclerosis is the collagen disease most commonly associated with gastrointestinal manifestations, affecting the entire gastrointestinal tract, with the esophagus being the most frequently involved organ. When evaluating patients with systemic sclerosis, it is critical to maintain a high index of suspicion for gastrointestinal involvement, particularly esophageal lesions. Thorough history-taking—including inquiry into symptoms, dietary habits, alcohol and tobacco use, and current medications—is essential. Currently, there is no established disease-modifying therapy for systemic sclerosis; therefore, management is primarily symptomatic and tailored to the specific clinical presentation. Careful evaluation and appropriate diagnostic testing are necessary to optimize individualized treatment strategies. I hope this review will be a useful resource in your clinical practice.

Competing Interests The author(s) has no competing interests to declare that are relevant to the content of this manuscript.

References

1. Kuribayashi S, et al. Esophageal motility disorders. In: Gastrointestinal syndrome, Special Issue of Japanese Clinical Syndrome Series No.10. 3rd ed; 2020. p. 36–40. (in Japanese).
2. Umeno J, et al. Gastrointestinal lesions in collagen diseases. Stomach Intest. 2012;47:818. (in Japanese).
3. Funaki Y, et al. Esophageal lesions in collagen diseases. In: Gastrointestinal syndrome, Special Issue of Japanese Clinical Syndrome Series No. 10. 3rd ed; 2020. p. 47–51. (in Japanese).
4. Moriyama T, et al. Systemic sclerosis. In: Yao T, editor. Atlas of stomach and intestine I, upper gastrointestinal tract. 2nd ed. Igaku-Shoin; 2014. p. 44. (in Japanese).
5. Asano Y, et al. Diagnostic criteria, severity classification, and treatment guidelines for systemic sclerosis. J Dermatol. 2016;126:1831–96. (in Japanese).
6. Iijima K. Esophageal lesions associated with systemic diseases. Clin Esophagol. 2015;1:132–4. (in Japanese).
7. Nakamura S, et al. Scleroderma (systemic sclerosis). Stomach Intest. 2003;38:535–41. (in Japanese).
8. Hozumi H, et al. Diseases with esophageal lesions. Clin Gastroenterol. 2008;23:285–91. (in Japanese).
9. Zamost BJ, et al. Esophagitis in scleroderma. Prevalence and risk factors. Gastroenterology. 1987;92:421–8.
10. Rose S, et al. Gastrointestinal manifestations of scleroderma. Gastroenterol Clin N Am. 1998;27:563–94.
11. Ozeki K, et al. Esophageal lesions in systemic sclerosis. In: Kinoshita Y, et al., editors. Gastroenterology for specialists, 3rd ed. Igaku-Shoin; 2021. p. 70–72. (in Japanese).

12. Kuribayashi S, et al. Esophagitis in systemic sclerosis - including other collagen diseases. Gastrointest Endosc. 2019;31:1185–9. (in Japanese).
13. Moriyama T, et al. Esophageal lesions in scleroderma (systemic sclerosis). Gastrointest Endosc. 2014;26:1766–7. (in Japanese).
14. Savarino E, et al. Gastroesophageal reflux and pulmonary fibrosis in scleroderma: a study using pH-impedance monitoring. Am J Respir Crit Care Med. 2009;179:408–13.
15. Japanese Society of Gastroenterology. GERD treatment guidelines 2021. 3rd ed. Nankodo; 2021. (in Japanese).
16. Stern EK, et al. Abnormal esophageal acid exposure on high-dose proton pump inhibitor therapy is common in systemic sclerosis patients. Neurogastroenterol Motil. 2018;30.
17. Cho YK, et al. Effect of mosapride combined with esomeprazole improves esophageal peristaltic function in patients with gastroesophageal reflux disease: a study using high resolution manometry. Dig Dis Sci. 2013;58:1035–41.
18. Agrawal A, et al. Bethanechol improves smooth muscle function in patients with severe ineffective esophageal motility. J Clin Gastroenterol. 2007;41:336–70.
19. Scarpellini E, et al. The effects of itopride on esophageal motility and lower esophageal sphincter function in man. Aliment Pharmacol Ther. 2011;33:99–105.
20. Broad J, et al. Regionally dependent neuromuscular functions of motilin and 5-HT4 receptors in human isolated esophageal body and gastric fundus. Neurogastroenterol Motil. 2014;26:1311–22.
21. Hasegawa M, et al. Experience with rikkunshito for GERD associated with scleroderma. Clin Dermatol. 2011;53:1767–70. (in Japanese).
22. Kirby DF, et al. Evaluation and management of gastrointestinal manifestations in scleroderma. Curr Opin Rheumatol. 2014;26:621–9.
23. Christmann RB, et al. Gastroesophageal reflux incites interstitial lung disease in systemic sclerosis: clinical, radiologic, histopathologic, and treatment evidence. Semin Arthritis Rheum. 2010;40:241–9.

16 Case Discussion, Heartburn

Toshimi Chiba

Abstract

This chapter reports a case of functional heartburn in a female in her 60s. Approximately 6 months ago, her heartburn worsened. Upper gastrointestinal endoscopy confirmed the diagnosis of NERD, and she was treated with potassium-competitive acid blocker (P-CAB) vonoprazan fumarate without symptom improvement, prompting her to seek further evaluation and treatment. High-resolution manometry (HRM) and high-resolution impedance manometry (HRIM) showed no evidence of esophageal motility disorders. After discontinuing potassium-competitive acid blocker (P-CAB), 24-hour esophageal multichannel intraluminal impedance pH (MII-pH) monitoring was performed, and both the symptom index (SI) and symptom-associated probability (SAP) were negative. Since both SI and SAP were negative, the patient was diagnosed with functional heartburn. Due to resistance to acid-suppressing drugs, anxiolytic tandospirone citrate was administered, and its efficacy was confirmed. Psychological factors may also be involved in functional heartburn.

Keywords

Functional heartburn · Non-erosive reflux disease · Reflux hypersensitivity · MII-pH · Symptom index · Symptom association probability · Potassium-competitive acid blocker · Proton pump inhibitor · Tandospirone citrate · Psychological factors · SSRI

1 Introduction

Heartburn and regurgitation are typical symptoms of gastroesophageal reflux disease (GERD). The Montreal classification defines GERD as a disease in which the reflux of stomach contents causes troublesome symptoms or complications [1]. According to the Rome IV criteria, if endoscopy shows no injury to the esophageal mucosa but reflux symptoms are present, esophageal pH or impedance-pH monitoring can be used to classify

T. Chiba (✉)
Division of Internal Medicine, Department of Oral Medicine, Iwate Medical University, Morioka, Japan
e-mail: toschiba@iwate-med.ac.jp

H. Kaneko et al. (eds.), *Disorders of Gut-Brain Interaction*,
https://doi.org/10.1007/978-981-95-6974-8_16

the disease into non-erosive reflux disease (NERD), reflux hypersensitivity, or functional heartburn [2]. In clinical practice, proton pump inhibitors (PPIs) are often used to treat heartburn symptoms, but some cases do not respond to this treatment.

2 Case Presentation (Functional Heartburn)

Patient: 67-year-old female
Chief Complaint: Heartburn
Past History: Hypertension since age 60
Family History: Unremarkable
Allergy History: Unremarkable
Smoking History: None
Alcohol Consumption: Occasional
History of Present illness: The patient had experienced postprandial heartburn for some time without significant impact on daily life. However, approximately 6 months ago, her heartburn worsened. Upper gastrointestinal endoscopy performed at a local clinic showed NERD, and she was treated with potassium-competitive acid blocker (P-CAB) vonoprazan fumarate for 8 weeks without symptom improvement, prompting her to seek further evaluation and treatment.
Physical Examination: Unremarkable

3 Clinical Course

Upper gastrointestinal endoscopy (Fig. 16.1) was performed again, no significant organic lesions were revealed in the esophagus or esophagogastric junction (EGJ), and esophageal biopsy showed no eosinophil infiltration. High-resolution manometry (HRM) (Fig. 16.2) and high-resolution impedance manometry (HRIM) showed no evidence of esophageal motility dis-

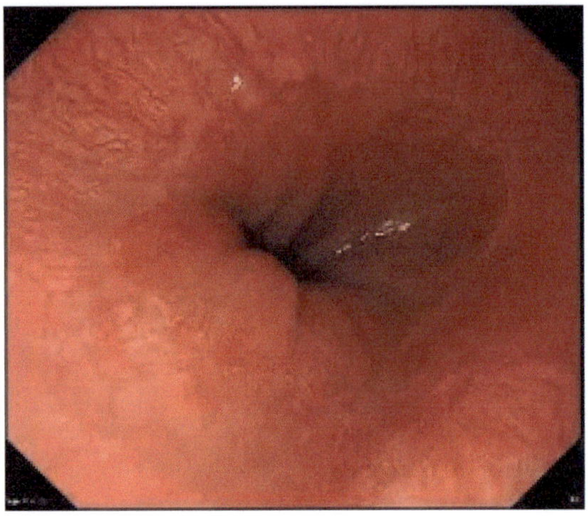

Fig. 16.1 Endoscopic finding of the esophagogastric junction. No findings of erosive reflux esophagitis were observed

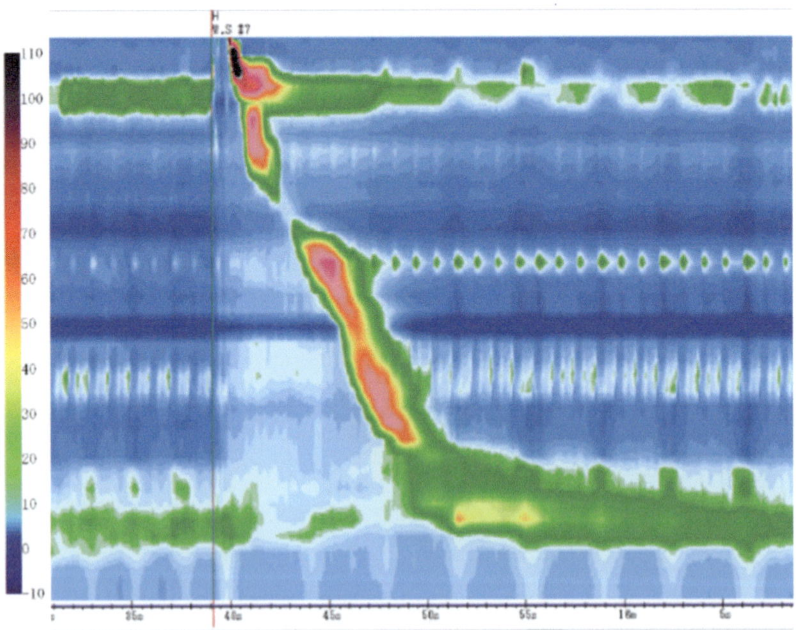

Fig. 16.2 High-resolution esophageal manometry. No findings of esophageal motility disorders, including primary peristaltic waves, were observed

orders, including primary peristaltic waves. After discontinuing P-CAB for 1 week, 24-hour esophageal multichannel intraluminal impedance pH (MII-pH) monitoring was performed, showing a symptom index (SI) of 25% and a symptom association probability (SAP) of 86.5%, both negative. Based on these findings, the patient was diagnosed with functional heartburn. Due to her resistance to acid-suppressing drugs, she was treated with the anxiolytic tandospirone citrate, which proved effective (tandospirone citrate is approved for treating depression, anxiety, agitation, and sleep disorders in psychosomatic conditions).

4 Discussion

PPI-resistant NERD includes functional heartburn and reflux hypersensitivity, and their treatment remains a challenge in GERD management. Differentiation involves evaluating the relationship between reflux and symptoms using SI and SAP (SI is defined as positive if the proportion of symptoms caused by reflux accounts for 50% or more of the total number of symptoms over 24 hours; SAP is calculated based on the results of the MII-pH monitoring to determine the relationship between symptom and reflux, with a positive result if the probability is 95% or higher). Functional heartburn is diagnosed when both SI and SAP are negative, while reflux hypersensitivity is diagnosed when either SI or SAP is positive.

According to the Rome IV criteria, if endoscopic findings of GERD are not observed, it is recommended to discontinue PPI for approximately 1 week and then perform impedance-pH monitoring [2]. Approximately half of NERD patients are PPI-resistant, with functional heartburn accounting for 43.4% and reflux hypersensitivity for 39.6% of these cases [3]. In P-CAB-resistant NERD, functional heartburn accounts for 48.8% and reflux hypersensitivity for 41.9% [4]. Coexistence of heartburn symptoms with functional dyspepsia or irritable bowel syndrome is observed in 30–50% of cases [5, 6], leading to decreased health-related quality of life (HRQOL) [7].

Psychological factors are implicated in functional heartburn, and the efficacy of tricyclic antidepressants and selective serotonin reuptake inhibitors (SSRIs) is considered. In this case, the patient's heartburn worsened without a clear trigger and showed resistance to P-CAB treatment. After explaining the significance and side effects of anxiolytic treatment, tandospirone was administered, resulting in symptom improvement.

Take-Home Message

If upper gastrointestinal endoscopy reveals no significant organic disease and heartburn symptoms do not improve with PPI or P-CAB treatment, and if there is a coexistence of functional dyspepsia or irritable bowel syndrome leading to decreased QOL, consider specialized testing and treatment.

Competing Interests The author(s) has no competing interests to declare that are relevant to the content of this manuscript.

References

1. Vakil N, et al. The montreal definition and classification of gastroesophageal reflux disease: a global evidence-based consensus. Am J Gastroenterol. 2006;101:1900–20.
2. Aziz Q, et al. Esophageal disorders. Gastroenterology. 2016;150:1368–79.
3. Kawami N, et al. Pathogenesis of double-dose proton pump inhibitor-resistant non-erosive reflux disease, and mechanism of reflux symptoms and gastric acid secretion-suppressive effect in the presence or absence of *helicobacter pylori* infection. Digestion. 2017;95:140–5.
4. Kawami N, et al. Pathogenesis of potassium-competitive acid blocker-resistant non-erosive reflux disease. Digestion. 2018;98:194–200.
5. Jones MP, et al. Overlap of heartburn, functional dyspepsia, and irritable bowel syndrome in a population sample: prevalence, temporal stability, and associated comorbidities. Neurogastroenterol Motil. 2022;34:e14349.
6. de Bortoli N, et al. Overlap of functional heartburn and gastroesophageal reflux disease with irritable bowel syndrome. World J Gastroenterol. 2013;19:5787–97.
7. Yao X, et al. The impact of overlapping functional dyspepsia, belching disorders and functional heartburn on anxiety, depression and quality of life of Chinese patients with irritable bowel syndrome. BMC Gastroenterol. 2020;20:209.

Case Discussion, Chest Pain

17

Masahiko Inamori

Abstract

There are many diseases that must be differentiated from chest pain, including so-called "killer diseases" such as myocardial infarction and aortic dissection.

We observed a 58-year-old man who visited our hospital complaining of chest pain. Electrocardiography, chest CT, coronary angiography with acetylcholine provocation testing, and upper gastrointestinal endoscopy showed no abnormalities, and he was diagnosed with non-cardiac chest pain (NCCP) due to GERD. A potassium-competitive acid blocker (P-CAB) was administered, and the frequency of chest pain decreased.

GERD is the most common cause of NCCP, with esophageal motility disorders being less frequent.

Keywords

Chest pain · Heartburn · Non-cardiac chest pain · GERD · Non-erosive reflux disease · Potassium-competitive acid blocker

M. Inamori (✉)
Department of Medical Education, Yokohama City University of School of Medicine, Yokohama, Japan
e-mail: inamorim@yokohama-cu.ac.jp

1 Introduction

When considering diseases that cause chest pain, cardiovascular conditions such as angina pectoris, myocardial infarction, aortic valve stenosis, and aortic dissection are often the first to come to mind. These conditions require urgent treatment and can be fatal; hence they are referred to as "killer diseases" and are taught to medical students and interns. However, the causes of chest pain are not limited to cardiovascular diseases; they also include gastrointestinal disorders, musculoskeletal disorders, pulmonary diseases, herpes zoster, and psychiatric conditions, collectively conceptualized as non-cardiac chest pain (NCCP) [1]. Among NCCP, gastrointestinal disorders are frequently cited, including gastric ulcers, biliary diseases like cholecystitis, acute pancreatitis, and intra-abdominal masses [2]. Many of these are believed to originate from the esophagus [1–3]. This article presents a case managed collaboratively by cardiology and gastroenterology departments.

2 Case Presentation (Chest Pain)

Patient: 58-year-old male.
Chief Complaint: Chest pain.
Past History: Atopic dermatitis since age 10; hypertension managed with medication since

H. Kaneko et al. (eds.), *Disorders of Gut-Brain Interaction*,
https://doi.org/10.1007/978-981-95-6974-8_17

age 36; history of anaphylactic shock at age 40, carries epinephrine auto-injector.

Family History: Father underwent surgery for gastric cancer at age 65.

Allergy History: Allergic to shrimp, crab, mackerel.

Smoking History: Smoked 20 cigarettes/day for 38 years since age 20.

Alcohol Consumption: Occasional drinking.

Occupation: IT technician.

History of Present illness: At age 50, upper gastrointestinal endoscopy during a health checkup revealed mild reflux esophagitis, but it did not significantly impact daily life, so no medication was prescribed, and the condition was monitored. At age 55, the patient experienced chest pain and visited a cardiologist. The chest pain occurred about twice a month, both at rest and during exertion, lasting about 5 minutes and radiating to the neck, raising suspicion of angina. Comprehensive evaluations including 12-lead ECG, stress ECG, Holter ECG, and cardiac ultrasound revealed no abnormalities, and the patient was advised to take nitroglycerin during chest pain episodes. Six months ago, the frequency of chest pain increased twice a week, prompting another visit to the cardiologist. Additional tests including coronary CT were performed, but no abnormalities were found, leading to suspicion of NCCP and referral to our gastroenterology department.

Examination Findings: Height 160 cm, weight 60 kg (unchanged since age 50). Temperature 36.6 °C. Blood pressure 128/78 mmHg, pulse 80/min, regular. Erythema, papules, and crusts observed on the skin. No anemia or jaundice in the conjunctiva. No palpable cervical lymph nodes or thyroid. Clear heart sounds and breath sounds. Flat, soft abdomen without tenderness. No edema in the lower legs.

Urine Findings: Protein (−), glucose (−).

Blood Findings: RBC 4.60 × 10^4/μL, Hb 13.7 g/dL, Ht 41%, WBC 7300/μL (eosinophils 8%), platelets 24.0 × 10^4/μL. Total protein 7.9 g/dL, albumin 4.2 g/dL, total bilirubin 0.9 mg/dL, AST 20 U/L, ALT 22 U/L, LD 220 U/L, ALP 102 U/L, amylase 90 U/L, BUN 22 mg/dL, creatinine 1.2 mg/dL, blood glucose 102 mg/dL, CRP 0.1 mg/dL, IgE 260 IU/mL.

3 Clinical Course

During the medical interview, no clear relationship between chest pain and meals or body position was identified. The patient did not report heartburn, acid regurgitation, a sensation of food sticking, nausea, vomiting, bloating, abdominal pain, abdominal distension, diarrhea, or constipation. He did not feel significant stress at work or home, although his responsibilities had shifted from fieldwork to management with age. Considering esophageal-related NCCP, upper gastrointestinal endoscopy and esophagography were performed, along with cervical-thoracic CT to exclude other organic diseases.

The upper gastrointestinal endoscopy revealed mild cloudiness in the lower esophagus but no significant mucosal damage. No esophageal fluid retention, tortuosity, spiral contractions, esophageal rosette, or pinstripe pattern indicative of esophageal motility disorders were observed [4]. Additionally, no ringed furrows, longitudinal furrows, luminal narrowing, or white plaques indicative of eosinophilic esophagitis were found [5], and biopsy pathology showed no eosinophil infiltration. The stomach and duodenum had no notable findings. Esophagography revealed no significant abnormalities. Cervical-thoracic CT showed no significant lesions, including lung disease, and no esophageal wall thickening.

Based on these findings, the patient was diagnosed with non-erosive reflux disease (NERD) and started on potassium-competitive acid blocker (P-CAB) vonoprazan fumarate. After starting medication, the frequency of chest pain decreased to about once every 2 weeks but persisted. After consulting with the patient and the previous physician, coronary angiography was performed, revealing no significant coronary stenosis, and acetylcholine provocation testing showed no abnormalities. Subsequently, the frequency of chest pain further decreased to about once every 3 months.

4 Discussion

This case presented NCCP without heartburn. The exact cause of chest pain remains unidentified, but clinical course suggests that acid-suppressing medication contributed to symptom improvement, and reassurance from ruling out organic disease through coronary angiography may have also played a role. The patient's history of atopic dermatitis and anaphylactic shock suggests that allergic mechanisms might contribute to symptom onset, although eosinophilic esophagitis has been ruled out.

Further examinations to consider for this patient include esophageal pH-impedance monitoring and esophageal manometry. Traditional pH monitoring primarily evaluates acid reflux, but impedance measurement can assess reflux of liquids and air. SI (symptom index) and SAP (symptom association probability) quantitatively evaluate the relationship between symptom occurrence without reflux. High-resolution esophageal manometry is now mainstream and useful in the diagnosis of esophageal motility disorders such as achalasia and diffuse esophageal spasm [6].

According to Fass et al. [1], the most common cause of NCCP is GERD, with esophageal motility disorders being less frequent. Esophageal hypersensitivity is observed in both conditions, and panic disorder, anxiety disorder, and depression are common comorbidities. Systematic reports on the relationship between allergies and NCCP are limited, warranting further investigation.

Take-Home Message

The causes of chest pain extend beyond cardiovascular diseases, which can be a Killer disease, to include gastrointestinal disorders and other conditions, conceptualized as non-cardiac chest pain (NCCP). GERD is the most common cause of NCCP, with esophageal motility disorders being less frequent.

Competing Interests The author(s) has no competing interests to declare that are relevant to the content of this manuscript.

References

1. Fass R, et al. Noncardiac chest pain: epidemiology, natural course and pathogenesis. J Neurogastroenterol Motil. 2011;17:110–23.
2. Onoda K, et al. Chest pain seen by gastroenterologists (special issue: how to diagnose daily diseases—chest pain). Reg Med. 2014;28:302–7. (in Japanese).
3. Fass R, et al. Noncardiac chest pain. J Clin Gastroenterol. 2008;42:636–46.
4. Kuribayashi S, et al. Endoscopic diagnosis of esophageal motility disorders. Gastroenterol Endosc. 2015;57:2503–12. (in Japanese).
5. Abe Y, et al. Technique explanation: diagnosis of eosinophilic esophagitis. Gastroenterol Endosc. 2014;56:3378–93. (in Japanese).
6. Kuribayashi S, et al. Technique explanation: tips and precautions for esophageal manometry in the diagnosis and treatment of achalasia. Gastroenterol Endosc. 2018;60:1095–106. (in Japanese).

Case Discussion, Dysphagia 18

Shuhei Agawa and Seiji Futagami

Abstract

Dysphagia can be caused by neurological disorders such as stroke, muscular disorders such as dermatomyositis, and esophageal disorders such as esophageal cancer or achalasia. Eosinophilic esophagitis is difficult to distinguish from gastroesophageal reflux disease based on symptoms alone. We present a case in which a patient presented with dysphagia and was diagnosed with eosinophilic esophagitis following endoscopic examination. Eosinophilic esophagitis is definitively diagnosed through biopsy during endoscopy. The use of the EREFS system, a characteristic finding, is useful, and it is important to always consider differential diagnosis while performing endoscopy.

Keywords

Dysphagia · Eosinophilic esophagitis · Endoscopy · EREFS system · Inflammation

1 Introduction

Dysphagia refers to the difficulty in moving food or liquids from the pharynx to the stomach. It can be caused by neurological disorders such as stroke, muscular diseases like dermatomyositis, and esophageal conditions such as esophageal cancer and achalasia. In gastrointestinal diseases, dysphagia is often described as a sensation of food sticking. Functional gastrointestinal disorders frequently associated with dysphagia include gastroesophageal reflux disease (GERD), achalasia, and eosinophilic esophagitis. Diagnosis often involves upper gastrointestinal endoscopy with biopsy, esophagography, and manometry. Treatment varies depending on the condition; for achalasia, it may include pharmacotherapy, surgery, and peroral endoscopic myotomy (POEM), while for eosinophilic esophagitis, treatment often involves proton pump inhibitors (PPIs) and dietary elimination therapy.

2 Case Presentation (Sensation of Food Sticking)

Chief Complaint: Sensation of food sticking

History of Present Illness: The patient occasionally experienced a sensation of food sticking during meals and sought evaluation and treatment.

Past History: Allergic conjunctivitis

Allergies: None

S. Agawa (✉) · S. Futagami
Department of Internal Medicine, Division of Gastroenterology, Nippon Medical School, Tokyo, Japan
e-mail: seiji-f@nms.ac.jp

H. Kaneko et al. (eds.), *Disorders of Gut-Brain Interaction*,
https://doi.org/10.1007/978-981-95-6974-8_18

3 Clinical Course

Blood tests revealed no significant findings. Upper gastrointestinal endoscopy was performed to investigate the cause. Endoscopy revealed longitudinal depressions and ulcers in the esophagus, and biopsies were taken (Figs. 18.1 and 18.2). The biopsy showed severe eosinophil infiltration, with more than 150 eosinophils per high-power field, leading to a diagnosis of eosinophilic esophagitis (EoE). Although the specific foods that exacerbated symptoms were not identified, the patient's symptoms improved with PPI therapy.

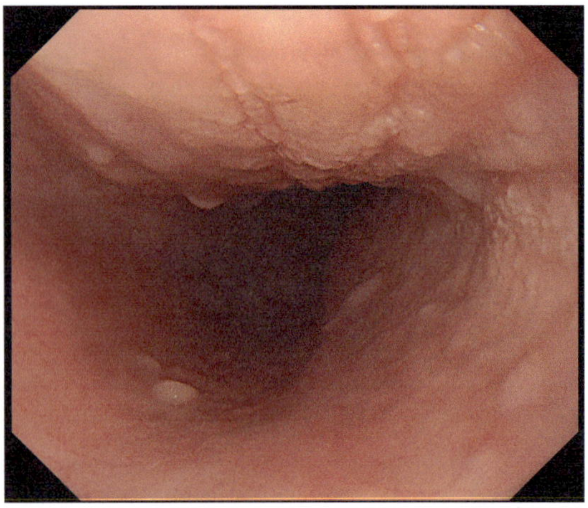

Fig. 18.1 Longitudinal depression (white light)

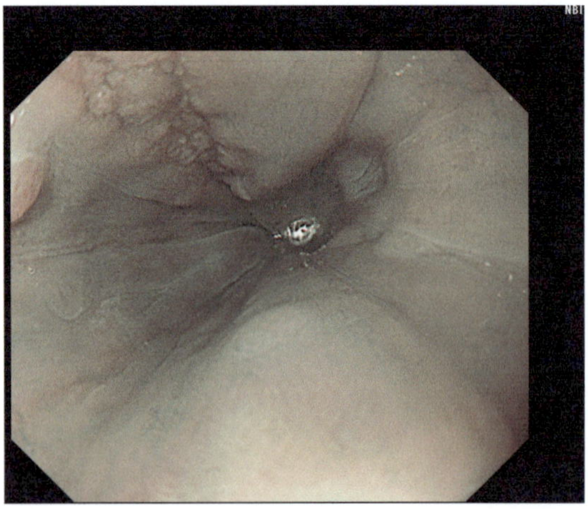

Fig. 18.2 Longitudinal depression (NBI)

4 Discussion

Eosinophilic esophagitis (EoE) is characterized by chronic inflammation predominantly involving eosinophils, localized to the esophagus, leading to fibrosis, esophageal motility disorders, and stricture. Epidemiologically, EoE has a higher prevalence among Caucasian males in Western countries, with reports indicating 20–30 cases per 100,000 people. In Japan, it is relatively more common in young males [1, 2]. Symptoms often include a sensation of food sticking and dysphagia. Unlike *reflux esophagitis*, which has similar symptoms, EoE may not always show characteristic findings on upper gastrointestinal endoscopy. The typical symptom of food sticking arises from esophageal motility disorders caused by chronic inflammation, leading to fibrosis and remodeling of the esophageal wall [3]. Interestingly, symptoms often do not correlate with endoscopic findings or biopsy results.

Characteristic endoscopic findings of EoE include the EREFS system: exudates, rings, edema, furrows, and strictures [4]. Rings and strictures reflect long-term chronic inflammation, while exudates and furrows indicate strong eosinophil infiltration and are useful biopsy sites for diagnosis. However, some cases may not show clear endoscopic findings, making biopsy crucial for diagnosis when EoE is suspected.

PPI therapy is the first-line treatment for EoE. PPIs are thought to maintain the esophageal mucosal barrier function by alleviating mucosal damage from acid reflux, thereby reducing allergen penetration. For PPI-resistant cases, topical steroid therapy is chosen. Although the tissue remission rate is high, the recurrence rate is also high, so maintenance therapy is recommended [5]. For refractory cases, dietary elimination and systemic steroid therapy are considered.

Dysphagia due to functional gastrointestinal disorders cannot always be diagnosed solely based on upper gastrointestinal endoscopy findings. Therefore, when symptoms suggest EoE, biopsy is necessary, and for achalasia, esophageal manometry is required. It is important to always consider these possibilities during diagnosis and treatment.

Take-Home Message

EoE can present with symptoms like food sticking, but diagnosis based on endoscopy alone is difficult, and differentiation from *reflux esophagitis* can be difficult. Additionally, asymptomatic cases identified through biopsies during health checkups do not meet current diagnostic criteria for EoE. Reports indicate that 25–40% of cases are asymptomatic [6]. While active biopsy diagnosis is recommended for symptomatic cases, the management of asymptomatic cases remains a challenge.

Competing Interests The author(s) has no competing interests to declare that are relevant to the content of this manuscript.

References

1. Arias Á, et al. Systematic review with meta-analysis: the incidence and prevalence of eosinophilic oesophagitis in children and adults in population-based studies. Aliment Pharmacol Ther. 2016;43:3–15.
2. Kinoshita Y, et al. Clinical characteristics of Japanese patients with eosinophilic esophagitis and eosinophilic gastroenteritis. J Gastroenterol. 2013;48:333–9.
3. Safroneeva E, et al. Symptoms have modest accuracy in detecting endoscopic and histologic remission in adults with eosinophilic esophagitis. Gastroenterology. 2016;150:581–90.e4.
4. Hirano I, et al. Endoscopic assessment of the oesophageal features of eosinophilic oesophagitis: validation of a novel classification and grading system. Gut. 2013;62:489–95.
5. Philpott H, et al. The role of maintenance therapy in eosinophilic esophagitis: who, why, and how? J Gastroenterol. 2018;53:165–71.
6. Hori K, et al. Do endoscopic features suggesting eosinophilic esophagitis represent histological eosinophilia? Dig Endosc. 2014;26:156–63.

19 Topics, Estimating Esophageal Motility Disorders from Esophagography

Tomoyuki Koike and Masahiro Saito

Abstract

High-resolution manometry (HRM) is the gold standard for diagnosing esophageal motility disorders; however, access to HRM remains limited in clinical practice. In contrast, esophagography is simple, widely available, and useful for evaluating patients with dysphagia or noncardiac chest pain. This chapter presents representative cases of esophageal motility disorders, particularly achalasia and hypercontractile esophagus (jackhammer esophagus), in which characteristic findings can be inferred from esophagography and endoscopy. The role of esophagography in confirming therapeutic efficacy after per-oral endoscopic myotomy (POEM) is also highlighted. For accurate diagnosis and management of esophageal motility disorders, clinicians should integrate HRM with an understanding of esophagographic and endoscopic findings.

Keywords

Esophageal motility disorders · High-resolution manometry (HRM) · Esophagography · Esophageal achalasia · Hypercontractile esophagus (Jackhammer esophagus) · Per-oral endoscopic myotomy (POEM) · Esophagogastric junction outflow obstruction (EGJOO)

1 Introduction

The definitive diagnosis of esophageal motility disorders is achieved through esophageal manometry. Recently, high-resolution manometry (HRM) has been developed as a device for evaluating esophageal motility, enabling detailed diagnosis and understanding of functional esophageal motility disorders (Fig. 19.1) [1]. Furthermore, the Chicago Classification version 4.0 now provides a clear diagnostic flowchart (Fig. 14.2 in Chap. 14) [1]. Although HRM has become widespread in Japan for diagnosing esophageal motility disorders, the number of facilities capable of performing HRM is still limited. On the other hand, because the diagnosis of esophageal motility disorders by esophagography is relatively simple to perform, esophagography is often useful as a reference finding in patients with dysphagia as the primary symptom and intermittent lower sternal pain, known as noncardiac chest pain (NCCP).

T. Koike (✉) · M. Saito
Division of Gastroenterology, Tohoku University Graduate School of Medicine, Sendai, Japan
e-mail: tkoike@rd5.so-net.ne.jp

H. Kaneko et al. (eds.), *Disorders of Gut-Brain Interaction*,
https://doi.org/10.1007/978-981-95-6974-8_19

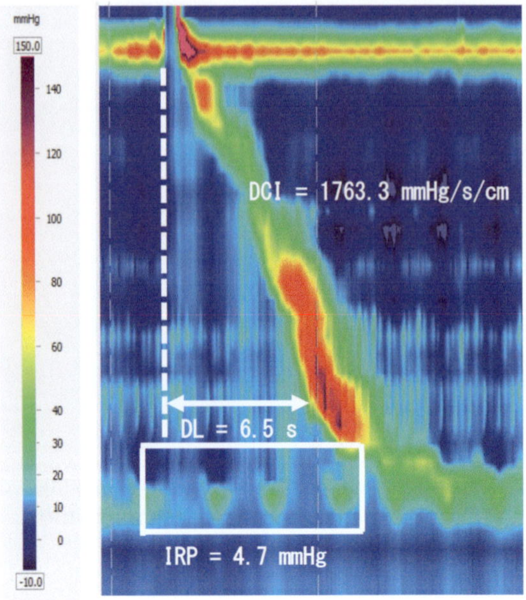

Fig. 19.1 HRM findings of a normal esophagus. HRM displays pressure in color. There are two high-pressure zones: the upper high-pressure zone is the upper esophageal sphincter, and the lower high-pressure zone is the esophagogastric junction. Upon swallowing, a peristaltic wave propagates from the upper to the lower esophagus following pharyngeal contraction. The relaxation of the esophagogastric junction is evaluated using IRP, the contraction strength of the peristaltic wave is assessed using DCI, and the time from swallowing to the arrival of the peristaltic wave at the lower esophagus is defined as DL to evaluate primary peristaltic waves. *Distal Contractile Integral (DCI)*: Amplitude × duration × length (mmHg·s·cm) of the distal esophageal contraction exceeding 20 mmHg from the transition zone to the proximal margin of the LES. *Distal Latency (DL)*: Interval between the upper esophageal sphincter (UES) relaxation and the contractile deceleration point (CDP). *Integrated Relaxation Pressure (IRP)*: Mean of the 4 s of maximal deglutitive relaxation in the 10-s window beginning at UES relaxation, contiguous or non-contiguous, referenced to gastric pressure

This article presents and explains cases where esophageal motility disorders can be inferred from esophagography findings, along with endoscopic findings which are the most frequently performed examinations in Japan.

2 Esophageal Achalasia

Esophageal achalasia is an esophageal motility disorder characterized by impaired relaxation of the lower esophageal sphincter (LES) and peristaltic dysfunction of the esophageal body [1]. In typical cases, achalasia can be suspected relatively easily through both esophagography and endoscopy, as shown in Fig. 19.2. According to the Chicago Classification based on HRM, achalasia is classified into Type I, II, and III (Fig. 14.2 in Chap. 14) [1]. Actual cases are presented in Figs. 19.2 and 19.3.

Recently, per-oral endoscopic myotomy (POEM) has rapidly gained popularity both domestically and internationally as a treatment for esophageal achalasia due to its advantages, such as leaving no scars on the body and its excellent therapeutic outcomes [2]. Post-POEM esophagography reveals that barium, which was previously stagnant and retained, smoothly passes through the esophagogastric junction, indicating improvement in esophageal motility disorders. Thus, esophagography is useful not only for diagnosis but also for confirming therapeutic effects (Figs. 19.3d and 19.4d).

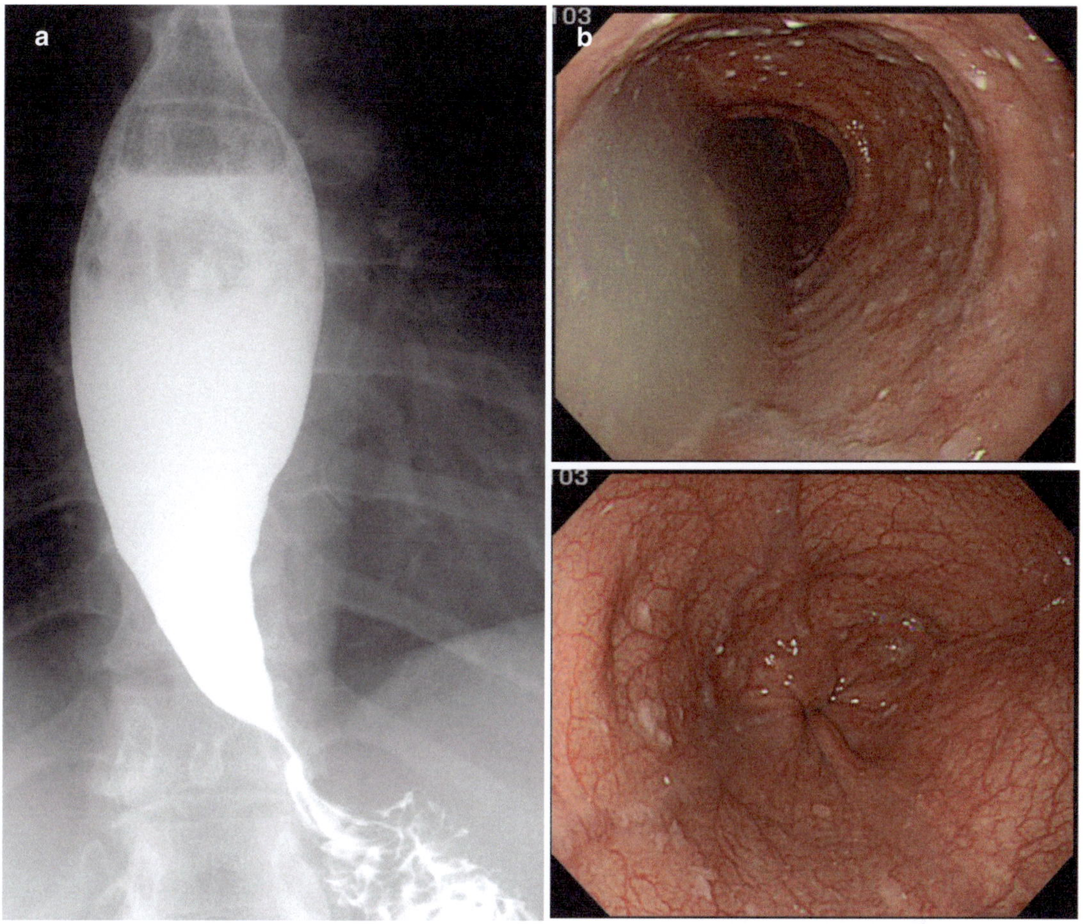

Esophagography Findings

Endoscopic Findings

Fig. 19.2 Esophagography and endoscopic findings of esophageal achalasia. (**a**) Esophagography Findings: Esophageal dilation and barium stasis, mirror formation, and smooth narrowing at the esophagogastric junction (bird's beak appearance at the lower end of the esophagus). (**b**) Endoscopic Findings: Esophageal lumen dilation, stasis of residues, white thickening of the mucosa. The esophagogastric junction is narrowed with circumferential fold concentration (esophageal rosette), but the endoscope passes relatively easily

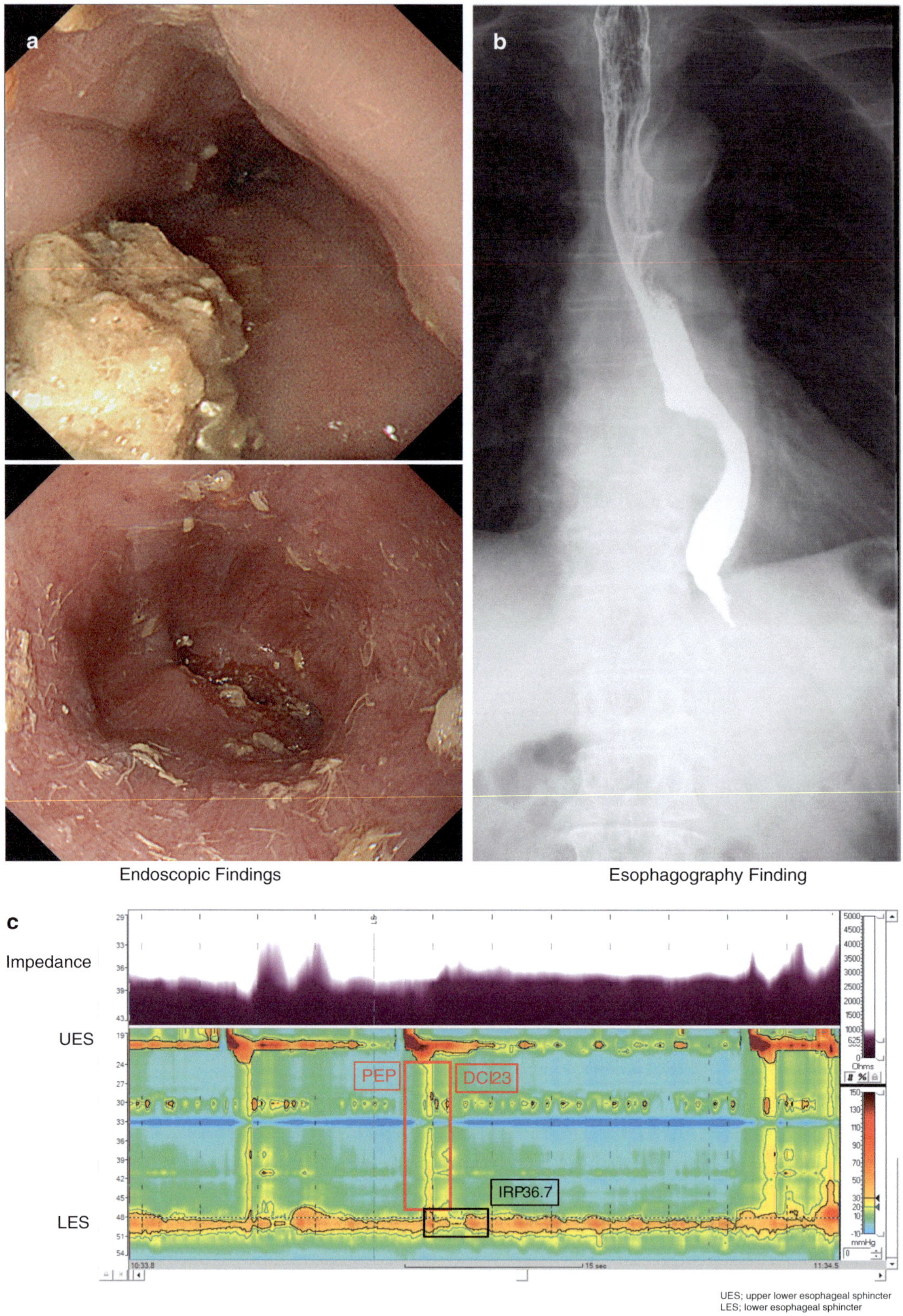
a
b
Endoscopic Findings
Esophagography Finding
c
Impedance
UES
LES
PEP
DCI23
IRP36.7
15 sec
UES; upper lower esophageal sphincter
LES; lower esophageal sphincter

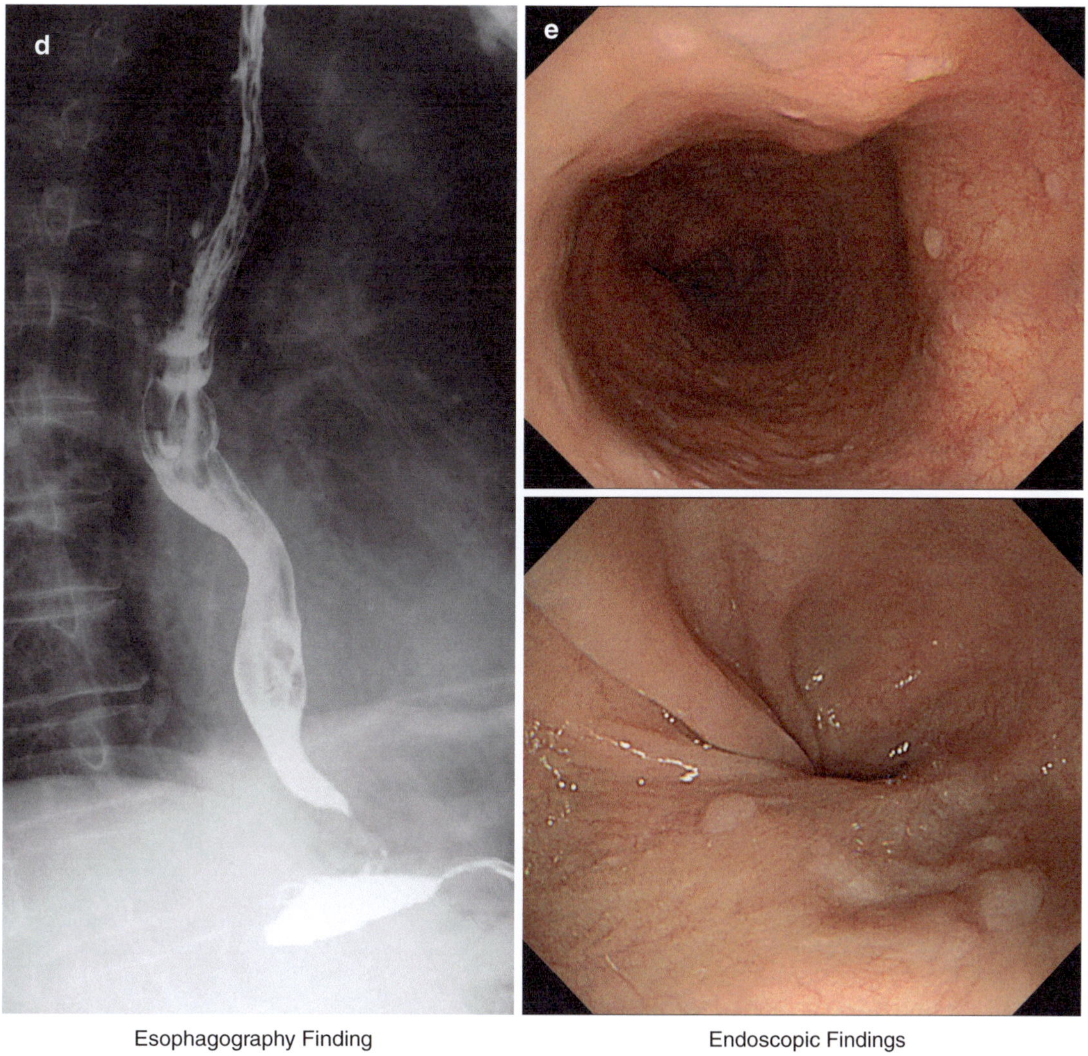

Fig. 19.3 (continued)

Fig. 19.3 (**a**) Endoscopic findings of achalasia type II. A male in his 60s. Endoscopy performed due to dysphagia for one year. Food residues are observed in the esophagus. The esophagogastric junction does not easily dilate with insufflation. (**b**) Esophagography Findings of Achalasia Type II. No esophageal dilation is observed, but barium stasis is noted in the esophagus. (**c**) High-Resolution Esophageal Manometry Impedance (HRIM) Findings of Achalasia Type II. (**d**, **e**) Post-POEM Findings of Achalasia Type II. (**d**) Esophagography Findings: Barium passes smoothly through the esophagogastric junction. (**e**) Endoscopic Findings: No food residues are observed. The scope passes smoothly through the esophagogastric junction

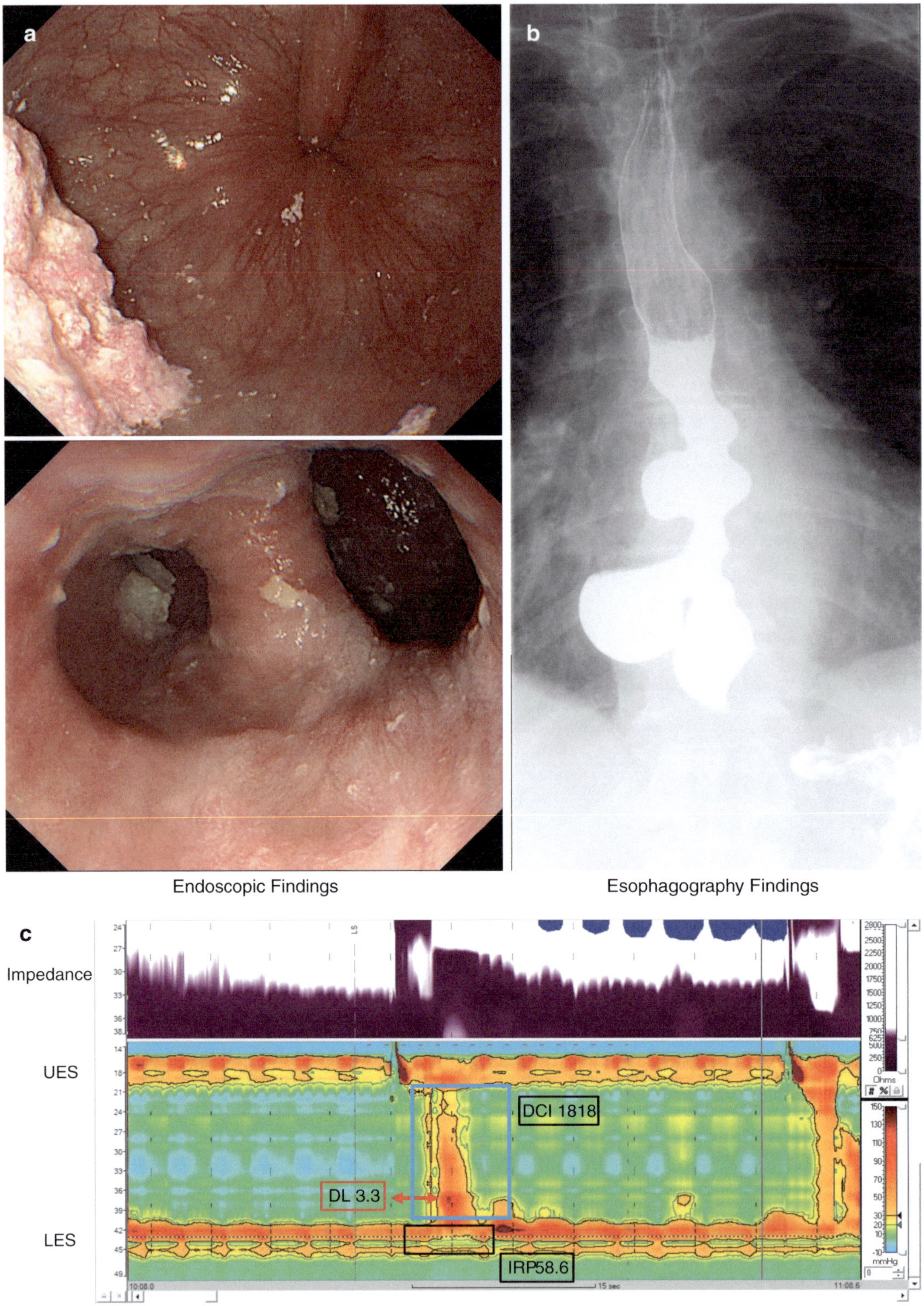

LES (IRP 36.7) failed (DCI<100 mmHg*s*cm) premature (DL<4.5s) 20% premature contractions

UES; upper lower esophageal sphincter
LES; lower esophageal sphincter

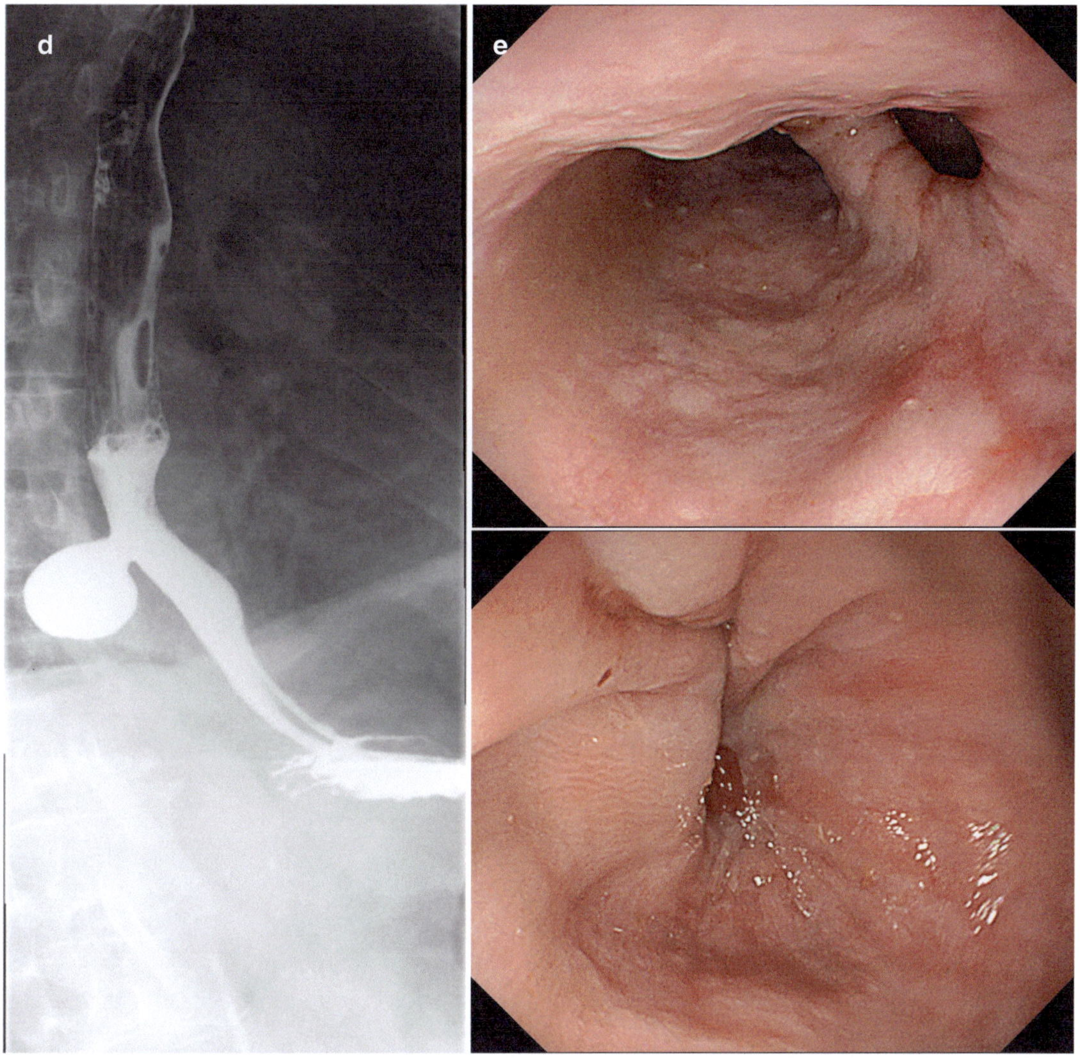

Fig. 19.4 (continued)

Fig. 19.4 (**a**) Endoscopic Findings of Achalasia Type III with Large Diverticulum. A male in his 60s. Endoscopy performed due to dysphagia for five years. Suspected achalasia, symptoms improved with nifedipine, and follow-up was conducted. Food residues are observed in the esophagus. A large esophageal diverticulum is noted. The esophagogastric junction does not easily dilate (esophageal rosette). (**b**) Esophagography Findings of Achalasia Type III with Diverticulum. Barium stasis and abnormal contractions in the esophagus, barium retention in the diverticulum. (**c**) High-Resolution Esophageal Manometry Impedance (HRIM) Findings of Achalasia Type III. (**d**, **e**) Post-POEM Findings of Achalasia Type III with Diverticulum. (**d**) Esophagography Findings: Barium retention in the esophageal diverticulum, but barium passes smoothly. (**e**) Endoscopic Findings: Esophageal diverticulum is noted, but no food residues. The scope passes well through the esophagogastric junction

3 Hypercontractile Esophagus (Jackhammer Esophagus)

Hypercontractile esophagus is a condition characterized by strong contractions of the esophageal body [1]. Cases are presented in Fig. 19.5. Although the diagnosis is made through HRM, abnormal esophageal contractions can also be captured through esophagography in addition to endoscopic findings (Fig. 19.5a, b).

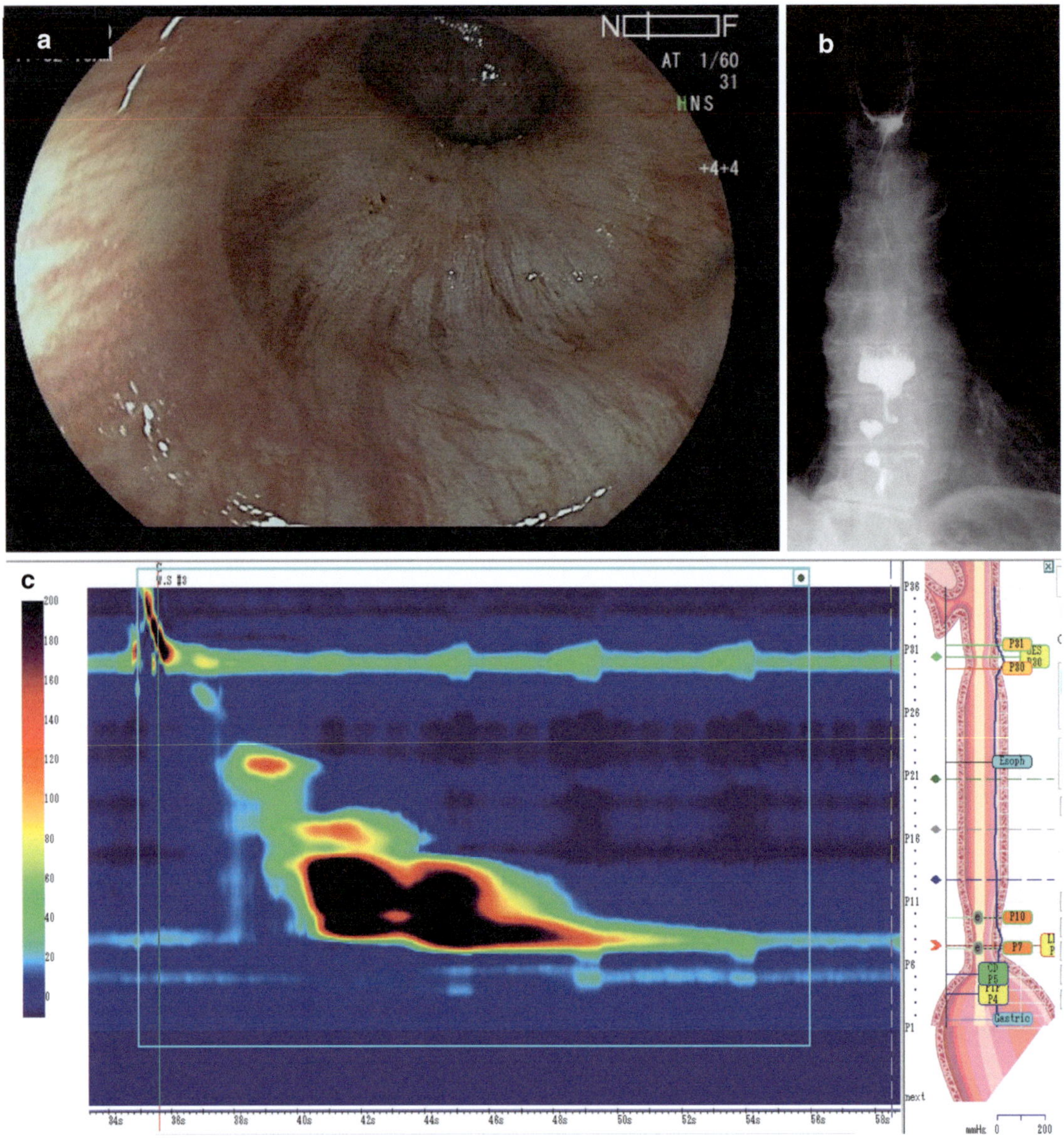

- DCI(Distal contractile integral)12903.3 mmHg/cm/s
- IRP(Integrated relaxation pressure) :19 mmHg

Fig. 19.5 (**a**) Endoscopic Findings of Hypercontractile Esophagus (Jackhammer Esophagus) . A female in her 70s. Dysphagia for several years, unable to drink water, hospitalized. Severe narrowing in the lower esophagus, corkscrew-like appearance on the oral side of the narrowing. (**b**) Esophagography Findings of Hypercontractile Esophagus (Jackhammer Esophagus) . Severe narrowing and beaded appearance in the lower esophagus. Contrast agent stagnates and accumulates at the narrowing. (**c**) High-Resolution Esophageal Manometry (HRM) Findings of Hypercontractile Esophagus (Jackhammer Esophagus). DCI (distal contractile integral): 12903.3 mmHg/s/cm, IRP (integrated relaxation pressure): 19 mmHg

Moreover, the usefulness of esophagography, which can evaluate both esophageal motility and bolus movement, has been reported in the assessment of esophagogastric junction outflow obstruction (EGJOO).

4 Conclusion

Esophageal manometry requires specialized equipment, but esophagography, which has been performed for a long time, is useful for diagnosing esophageal motility disorders and assessing therapeutic effects. It is essential to recognize the importance of esophagography findings in diagnosing esophageal motility disorders. Additionally, esophageal motility disorders can be suspected through endoscopic findings. Care must be taken not to overlook esophageal motility disorders in patients complaining of dysphagia, even if imaging diagnostics do not reveal tumors.

Take-Home Message
High-resolution esophageal manometry (HRM) is a valuable tool for diagnosing esophageal motility disorders; however, access to HRM remains limited to specialized centers. In contrast, esophagography is widely available, making it essential for clinicians to be familiar with the esophagographic features of esophageal motility disorders. In addition, certain endoscopic findings may also raise suspicion for underlying motility abnormalities. Clinicians should maintain a high level of vigilance for esophageal motility disorders in patients presenting with dysphagia, even in the absence of tumor detection on imaging studies.

Competing Interests The author(s) has no competing interests to declare that are relevant to the content of this manuscript.

References

1. Yadlapati R, et al. Esophageal motility disorders on high-resolution manometry: Chicago classification version 4.0©. Neurogastroenterol Motil. 2021;33(1):e14058.
2. Inoue H, et al. Peroral endoscopic myotomy (POEM) for esophageal achalasia. Endoscopy. 2010;42:265–71.

Part IV

Stomach and Duodenum, Basic Edition

Stomach and Duodenum: Anatomy, Physiology of Gastrointestinal Motility, Peptides

20

Kazuhiro Kamada

Abstract

The stomach, located in the upper abdomen from the left hypochondriac to umbilical regions, connects to the esophagus at the cardia and continues through the fundus, body, antrum, and pylorus. The outflow of digested food is regulated by the pyloric sphincter. The stomach has lesser and greater curvatures, with mucosal folds along the greater curvature to aid digestion. It serves as a temporary storage site, initiates protein digestion using gastric acid, kills bacteria, and mixes food through peristalsis before gradually releasing it into the duodenum.

The duodenum is the first 25 cm of the small intestine, C-shaped around the pancreas, and divided into four parts: bulb, descending, horizontal, and ascending. It is retroperitoneal and receives bile and pancreatic juice via the major duodenal papilla, which are essential for digesting proteins, fats, and carbohydrates.

The stomach and duodenum walls share four layers: mucosa (for digestion and absorption), submucosa (containing blood vessels and nerves), muscularis (for contraction), and either serosa or adventitia depending on their location. Hormones play key roles: gastrin from the stomach stimulates gastric acid and enzyme release, while secretin and cholecystokinin (CCK) from the duodenum regulate pancreatic and gallbladder secretions to neutralize acid and aid digestion.

Keywords

Stomach · Duodenum · Anatomy of the digestive tract · Structure of the digestive tract · Gastrointestinal motility · Gastrointestinal peptide

1 Anatomy of the Stomach and Duodenum

1.1 Anatomy of the Stomach and Duodenum (Fig. 20.1)

The stomach is located within the abdominal cavity, extending from the left hypochondrium to the epigastrium and umbilical region. The esophagogastric junction is formed at the site where the esophagus passes through the esophageal hiatus of the diaphragm, leading to the cardia, the entrance of the stomach. The region above the cardia is referred to as the fundus, which is the most dorsal and lowest position when supine. The body of the stomach extends from the cardia to the gastric angle, and the region below the gas-

K. Kamada (✉)
Department of Gastroenterology, Matsushita Memorial Hospital, Moriguchi, Japan
e-mail: k-kamada@koto.kpu-m.ac.jp

H. Kaneko et al. (eds.), *Disorders of Gut-Brain Interaction*,
https://doi.org/10.1007/978-981-95-6974-8_20

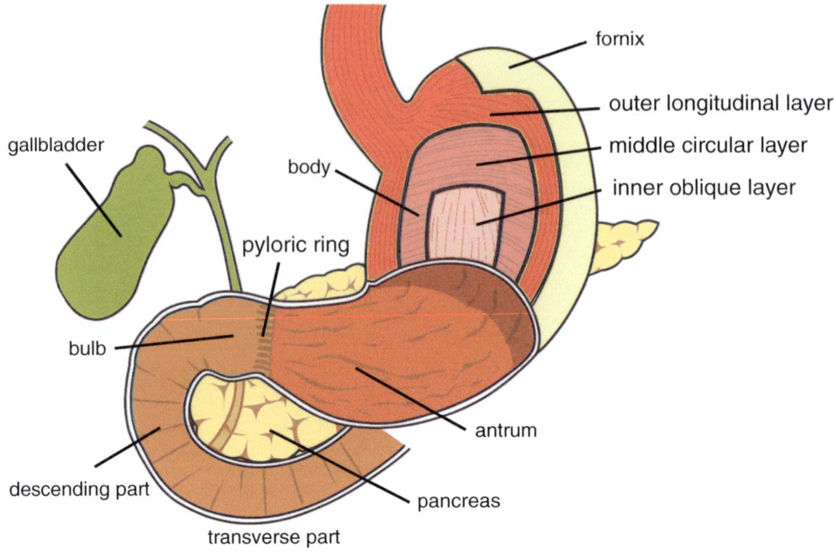

Fig. 20.1 Structure of the stomach and surrounding areas

tric angle is known as the antrum. The anterior wall of the stomach faces the abdomen, while the posterior wall faces the back. The lesser curvature, which is closer to the liver, is shorter, while the greater curvature is longer and curves to the right. The greater curvature of the body of the stomach is lined with longitudinal mucosal folds. The pyloric ring, the exit of the stomach, is surrounded by the pyloric sphincter [1].

The duodenum, continuing from the pylorus of the stomach, is the most proximal part of the small intestine, approximately 25 cm in length. It runs in a C-shape around the head of the pancreas and is fixed to the posterior abdominal wall, lacking a mesentery, thus classified as a retroperitoneal organ, except for the duodenal bulb, which is continuous with the stomach. The duodenum is divided into four parts: the bulb, descending part, horizontal part, and ascending part. The transition points between these parts are known as the superior duodenal flexure, inferior duodenal flexure, and duodenojejunal flexure. The duodenojejunal flexure is anchored to the posterior abdominal wall by the ligament of Treitz, which contains smooth muscle, marking the transition to the jejunum as the small intestine enters the abdominal cavity. The lumen of the duodenum is lined with circular folds, and the descending part contains the major duodenal papilla (*papilla of Vater*), where the common bile duct and pancreatic duct open.

1.2 Structure of the Stomach Wall

The stomach wall consists of four layers: mucosa, submucosa, muscularis, and serosa.

(i) *Mucosa*: The inner surface of the stomach, like other parts of the gastrointestinal tract, is covered by mucosa. The gastric mucosa is composed of simple columnar epithelium made up of surface mucous cells, which secrete mucus to protect the stomach from its potent digestive juice, gastric acid. The mucosa contains deep indentations known as gastric pits (Fig. 20.2). Different glands are present in various regions: cardiac glands around the cardia, fundic glands in the body and fundus, and pyloric glands in the antrum. Cardiac and pyloric glands primarily produce mucus. Fundic glands consist of chief cells that secrete pepsinogen, the precursor of pepsin, mucous neck cells that secrete mucus, and parietal cells that secrete gastric acid and intrinsic factor.

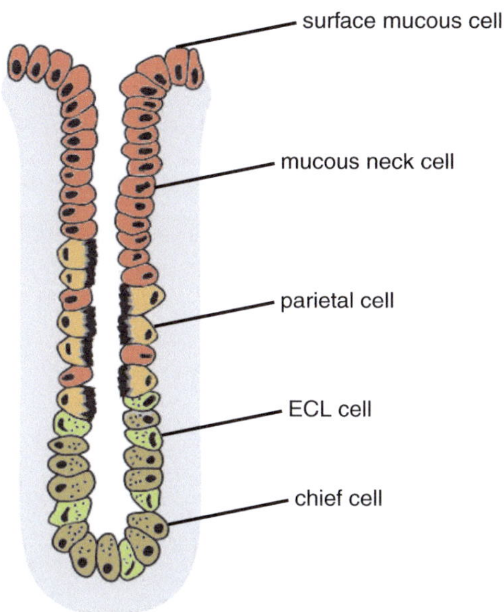

Fig. 20.2 Structure of the stomach wall

Chief cells are located in the deeper parts of the fundic glands, parietal cells are situated above the chief cells, and mucous neck cells are found in the neck of the gland.

Endocrine cells, primarily G cells located in the pyloric glands, secrete gastrin. Gastrin and acetylcholine stimulate enterochromaffin-like (ECL) cells near the parietal cells to release histamine, which binds to histamine (H2) receptors on parietal cells, promoting gastric acid secretion. Additionally, D cells near the G cells in the pyloric glands and the body of the stomach secrete somatostatin, which inhibits the secretion of gastrointestinal hormones such as gastrin, glucagon, and cholecystokinin.

(ii) *Submucosa*: The submucosa is a layer of connective tissue located between the muscularis mucosae and the muscularis propria, supporting the mucosa and maintaining its connection to the muscularis. It contains abundant small blood vessels and lymphatic vessels, along with the Meissner's plexus.

(iii) *Muscularis*: Typically, the muscularis of the gastrointestinal wall consists of two layers: an inner circular layer and an outer longitudinal layer. However, the stomach's muscularis has three layers: an outer longitudinal layer, a middle circular layer, and an inner oblique layer. The outer longitudinal layer continues from the esophagus to the duodenum. Similarly, the middle circular layer extends from the inner circular layer of the esophagus to the duodenum, forming the thickened pyloric sphincter at the pyloric ring. The inner oblique layer is unique to the stomach, surrounding the cardia. Between the longitudinal and circular layers lies the Auerbach's plexus (myenteric plexus) (Fig. 20.1).

(iv) *Serosa*: The outermost layer of the stomach is covered by serosa. The serosa on the anterior and posterior walls of the stomach join at the lesser curvature and greater curvature, forming the lesser omentum and greater omentum, respectively. Blood vessels and nerves supplying the stomach run through the subserosal layer and penetrate the stomach wall.

1.3 Secretion of Gastric Juice

Gastric juice is colorless, transparent, and odorless, with a daily secretion volume of 2–3 L. The main components of gastric juice are gastric acid, pepsin, mucus, and intrinsic factor. Gastric acid is a strong acid with bactericidal properties against bacteria ingested with food. It also converts pepsinogen, secreted by chief cells, into pepsin. Pepsinogen itself is an inactive precursor, but under acidic conditions provided by gastric acid, it becomes active pepsin when the inhibitor and binding peptide are detached. There are two types of pepsinogen: pepsinogen I, primarily found in chief cells of fundic glands, and pepsinogen II, found in mucous cells throughout the gastric mucosa and duodenum [2].

Even during fasting, a small amount of gastric juice is secreted as basal secretion. Gastric juice secretion is regulated by direct stimulation of smooth muscle and mucosa by food bolus and its digestive products, as well as by neural and humoral factors. Stretch receptors in the gastric wall and chemoreceptors in the mucosa transmit stimuli to the medulla via the submucosal plexus, leading to gastric acid secretion through local and neural reflexes. Gastric juice secretion is divided into three phases based on the mechanism of stimulation:

(i) *Cephalic Phase*: Conditioned reflexes such as thinking about food, seeing food, or smelling food, and unconditioned reflexes such as tasting, chewing, and swallowing stimulate the release of acetylcholine from vagal nerve endings, which stimulates gastric gland cells to secrete pepsinogen from chief cells and promote gastric acid secretion from parietal cells. Vagal nerve stimulation also triggers G cells in the pyloric glands to secrete gastrin, which acts on secretory glands via the bloodstream to enhance gastric acid secretion from parietal cells.

(ii) *Gastric Phase*: When food enters the stomach, mechanical stimulation from the stretching of the gastric wall induces gastric acid secretion. This reflex involves both central pathways via the vagal nerve and local pathways via the enteric plexus. The effects include direct stimulation of parietal cells and the release of gastrin into the bloodstream from G cells, promoting gastric acid secretion from parietal cells. When the pH in the stomach rises above 3 due to gastric contents, vagal nerve stimulation triggers the release of gastrin. As digestion progresses and contents are transferred to the duodenum, the pH in the stomach drops again, inhibiting gastrin release and reducing gastric acid secretion through a negative feedback mechanism.

(iii) *Intestinal Phase*: When gastric contents enter the duodenum, gastrin is released from the intestinal mucosa, causing secretion, even in small amounts. Conversely, secretin released from the duodenal mucosa promotes pancreatic juice secretion, neutralizing the acidic gastric contents. Secretin, along with gastric inhibitory peptide (GIP) from K cells in the duodenal wall, cholecystokinin from I cells, and somatostatin from D cells in the pancreas and intestines, inhibits gastrin secretion from G cells in the gastric mucosa and suppresses gastric acid secretion from parietal cells.

Physiologically active substances that act on parietal cells to secrete gastric acid include histamine, gastrin, and acetylcholine. Parietal cells possess histamine H2 receptors that bind histamine from mast cells, gastrin receptors that bind gastrin, and muscarinic M3 receptors that bind acetylcholine [3].

1.4 Structure of the Duodenal Wall

As in the jejunum and ileum, the inner surface of the duodenal lumen has numerous protruding villi. In addition, the surface of the epithelial cells lining the villi have microvilli that form a brush border. The epithelial cells covering the villi have microvilli on their surface, forming a brush border.

Like the stomach, the duodenal wall consists of four layers: mucosa, submucosa, muscularis, and serosa, but there is no mesentery. The submucosal tissue of the duodenum contains branched tubuloalveolar mucous glands called Brunner's glands, which penetrate the muscularis mucosae and open at the base of the intestinal crypts. These glands secrete neutral to alkaline mucus, protecting the duodenal wall by neutralizing the acidic chyme transported from the stomach.

2 Motility of the Stomach and Duodenum

Gastrointestinal motility is regulated by the contraction and relaxation of smooth muscle in the gastrointestinal wall, influenced by neural factors and humoral factors such as gastrointestinal hormones. The gastrointestinal tract contains numerous nerve cells, and its motility is controlled bidirectionally by neural and peptide factors from the gut to the brain and vice versa. Smooth muscle activity is regulated by the autonomic nervous system, comprising the sympathetic and parasympathetic nervous systems. Vagal nerve stimulation, part of the parasympathetic system, enhances gastric motility, tone, and secretion, while sympathetic nerve stimulation inhibits these functions. Additionally, two enteric nerve plexuses exist: the Auerbach's plexus (myenteric plexus) between the longitudinal and circular muscle layers, which regulates muscle function, and the Meissner's plexus (submucosal plexus) in the submucosal tissue, which regulates mucosal function. These plexuses form networks that influence each other [4].

Hormones secreted from the gastrointestinal epithelium are stimulated by digestive products in the gastrointestinal tract and neurostimulatory substances in the blood, leading to secretion from various endocrine cells in the epithelium. These hormones have paracrine effects, acting locally on surrounding cells, and endocrine effects, entering the bloodstream to act on cells in different locations.

2.1 Fasting Contractions

Gastrointestinal motility is classified into two patterns based on pre- and postprandial status. One pattern is fasting contractions, characterized by strong contraction waves observed 6–8 hours after eating. The other pattern is postprandial contractions, consisting of rhythmic contraction waves with weaker contraction strength but occurring regularly after eating. Fasting contractions are marked by interdigestive migrating motor contractions (IMMC), where strong contraction waves propagate regularly towards the anus. After a resting phase of approximately 60–70 minutes, strong contraction waves lasting about 20–25 minutes begin in the stomach and duodenum, propagating towards the anus. Physiologically, IMMC serves to expel food residues and accumulated gastric and intestinal fluids towards the anus, preparing the gastrointestinal tract for the next meal. IMMC is divided into four phases: Phase I is the resting phase (40–60% of one cycle), Phase II is characterized by irregular contractions primarily for mixing (20–30% of one cycle), Phase III is the most distinctive phase with strong contractions lasting 20–25 minutes, propagating towards the anus, and Phase IV is the transition phase with irregular contractions leading back to the resting phase. IMMC is triggered by motilin secreted from endocrine cells in the duodenum and upper jejunum [5].

2.2 Postprandial Contractions

During postprandial contractions, the stomach undergoes receptive relaxation in response to food intake, where the gastric body relaxes to accommodate the incoming food. This physiological response allows the stomach to store a large amount of food and gradually move it towards the anus. As the gastric body is distended by the contents, adaptive relaxation further enhances the relaxation of the gastric body. This reflex, similar to receptive relaxation, is mediated by the inhibition of cholinergic neuron activity and the promotion of non-cholinergic, non-adrenergic inhibitory neuron activity, increasing the stomach's capacity to store food.

Peristaltic contractions in the stomach involve circular contractions originating in the gastric body, propagating through the antrum to the pylorus. These contractions occur at a frequency of 3–4 times per minute in humans, with the peristaltic waves originating from the upper to the middle part of the gastric body, centered around the greater curvature. The peristaltic waves are weak in the gastric body but become stronger as they pass through the angular notch and move from the antrum to the pylorus. The pyloric ring, formed by the thickened circular muscle layer known as the pyloric sphincter, remains contracted. With each peristaltic wave, the gastric contents are propelled towards the pylorus, but most of the contents are pushed back due to the contracted pylorus, resulting in mixing of the contents. Under normal conditions, the pylorus allows the passage of water and liquid components into the duodenum, but solid food remains in the stomach until it is digested to a size of 2–3 mm.

When strong peristaltic waves reach the pylorus, it relaxes slightly, allowing small amounts of chyme to be pushed into the duodenum. As the chyme formation progresses, peristaltic waves become stronger and more frequent, gradually squeezing the food in the gastric body and moving it to the antrum, increasing gastric pressure. When the gastric pressure exceeds the duodenal and pyloric pressures, the pylorus opens, and the contents are gradually sent into the duodenum. This process continues until the stomach is emptied.

Postprandial contractions in the small intestine, including the duodenum, are not uniform continuous peristaltic movements like those in the stomach but change complexly over time. The movements include peristaltic contractions, segmental contractions, and pendular movements. The contents are mixed and stirred by these movements, facilitating digestion and absorption while being transported towards the anus. The speed of movement varies by the region of the gastrointestinal tract, and the patterns of segmental and peristaltic movements are primarily controlled by the enteric nervous system (ENS) within the gastrointestinal wall.

Peristaltic contractions involve coordinated contractions of the circular and longitudinal muscles, moving the contraction ring towards the anus and propelling the gastrointestinal contents expelled from the stomach. Peristaltic contractions are induced by stretch stimuli, where the intestinal wall stretches due to the contents, stimulating the enteric nervous system, primarily the Auerbach's plexus. This stimulation causes sequential contractions of the intestinal wall from the oral side, with the contraction ring moving towards the anus. The speed of peristaltic contractions gradually slows from the duodenum to the terminal ileum [6].

Segmental contractions involve sustained contractions of the circular muscle at regular intervals for several tens of seconds, dividing the intestinal tract into segments. Further contraction of the circular muscle within the segments forms new contraction rings. The circular muscle repeatedly contracts and relaxes in a segmental pattern, pushing the contents on both sides of the contraction ring. When the contraction ring disappears, the contents return to their original position, facilitating mixing with digestive juices.

Pendular movements are caused by periodic contractions and relaxations of the longitudinal muscle layer, resulting in the gastrointestinal tract stretching and contracting along its long axis. This creates a pendulum-like back-and-forth movement of the contents between the oral and anal sides.

3 Upper Gastrointestinal Peptides

Physiologically active substances secreted by nerve cells and gland cells in the gastrointestinal mucosa primarily act in a paracrine manner locally but also enter the bloodstream to act on distant cells. The hormones secreted by the gastrointestinal tract have been studied for their effects on the gastrointestinal tract based on changes in their blood concentrations related to food intake. While their structures and actions are similar, at high concentrations, their effects overlap, but at physiological concentrations, they have distinct actions [7].

3.1 Secretin

Secretin was the first hormone discovered to be secreted by the gastrointestinal tract. Bayliss and Starling, who discovered secretin, named physiologically active substances that are secreted by one organ, transported by the blood, and act on another organ as hormones. Secretin is a peptide hormone consisting of 27 amino acids, secreted by S cells located in the deep glands of the duodenal and upper small intestinal mucosa. The secretion of secretin is induced by the stimulation of the duodenal mucosa by gastric acid and acidic food digested in the stomach flowing into the duodenum from the gastric pylorus.

Secretin promotes the secretion of bicarbonate ions from pancreatic duct cells via cAMP, resulting in the secretion of alkaline pancreatic juice, neutralizing the acidity in the duodenum.

Additionally, secretin inhibits flowing gastric acid into duodenum through the contraction of the gastric pyloric sphincter, enhancement of pancreatic digestive juice secretion by cholecystokinin, and the secretion of somatostatin that inhibits gastrin secretion. This negative feedback mechanism alleviates the acidity in the duodenum, suppressing the secretion of secretin.

3.2 Gastrin

Gastrin is a hormone produced and secreted by G cells located in the mucosa of the gastric pyloric antrum. G cells have a broad base and contain numerous gastrin granules. Gastrin is secreted in response to the presence of proteins in the stomach, an increase in gastric pH, and vagal reflexes. Gastrin binds to gastrin receptors on gastric parietal cells via the bloodstream, promoting gastric acid secretion. It also binds to CCK-B receptors in the duodenum, promoting histamine secretion, which indirectly enhances gastric acid secretion. Additionally, gastrin acts on gastrointestinal mucosa and β-cells in the pancreatic head, promoting the secretion of somatostatin, which inhibits excessive acid secretion. Gastrin also stimulates the secretion of pepsinogen from chief cells, enhances the contraction of the pyloric antrum, induces relaxation of the ileocecal valve, and promotes the growth of the gastric, small intestinal, and colonic mucosa. In autoimmune gastritis, parietal cells are damaged, leading to decreased gastric acid secretion and elevated blood gastrin levels. Gastrin-producing tumors also result in elevated blood gastrin levels due to ectopic gastrin production.

3.3 Cholecystokinin (CCK)

Cholecystokinin (CCK) is secreted by I cells in the upper small intestinal mucosa, with its secretion promoted by the arrival of digestive products in the intestine. CCK stimulates pancreatic enzyme secretion, gallbladder contraction, and relaxation of the sphincter of Oddi, allowing pancreatic juice and bile to flow into the gastrointestinal tract. Initially, cholecystokinin and pancreozymin, a substance promoting pancreatic enzyme secretion, were discovered separately, but they were later found to be the same substance with a sequence of 33 amino acids. CCK exerts its effects by binding to its receptors, which are G protein-coupled receptors classified into CCK-A and CCK-B receptors. Cholecystokinin and gastrin share the same five amino acids at their C-terminus, with CCK-A receptors having a high affinity for CCK and CCK-B receptors having a similar affinity for both CCK and gastrin. Both receptors activate phospholipase C (PLC), producing inositol triphosphate (IP3) and diacylglycerol (DAG). CCK has an appetite-suppressing effect mediated by CCK-A receptors on vagal afferent fibers, transmitting satiety signals to the central nervous system. Other effects include enhancing pancreatic juice secretion, enhancement of the action of secretin to promote contraction of the pyloric sphincter, inhibiting gastric emptying, and increasing motility in the small intestine and colon.

The secretion of CCK is controlled by CCK-releasing peptide in the small intestinal mucosa and monitor peptide produced by the pancreas. When CCK acts, bile and pancreatic juice flow into the duodenum, enhancing the digestion of proteins and fats. These digestive products further promote CCK secretion, creating a positive feedback mechanism. The passage of digestive products through the duodenum, the completion of food breakdown by CCK-releasing peptides and monitor peptides, and the breakdown by excessive protein-degrading enzymes cause the increase in CCK secretion to cease.

3.4 Gastric Inhibitory Polypeptide (GIP)

Gastric inhibitory polypeptide (GIP) is a peptide consisting of 42 amino acids, produced by K cells in the duodenal and jejunal mucosa, and secreted into the bloodstream in response to glucose and fats in the duodenum. Named for its ability to inhibit both gastric juice secretion and gastric motility when administered in large amounts, GIP does not inhibit gastric function at physiological concentrations. Along with GLP-1 (glucagon-like peptide-1), GIP is secreted from the gastrointestinal tract in response to nutrient intake, stimulating pancreatic β-cells and promoting insulin secretion, known as incretin hormones. GIP enhances glucose-dependent insulin secretion and inhibits glucagon secretion, but its effects are diminished in chronic hyperglycemia while GLP-1 is not. GIP also involved in suppressing fat accumulation and obesity. Drugs acting on both GIP and GLP-1 receptors (GIP/GLP-1 receptor agonists) have been clinically applied in diabetes treatment, showing effectiveness in weight reduction in diabetic patients.

3.5 Motilin

Motilin is a polypeptide consisting of 22 amino acids, secreted by enterochromaffin cells and Mo cells in the duodenum and upper jejunum. Its secretion is stimulated by gastric acid and bile acids via muscarinic receptors. Motilin receptors are G protein-coupled receptors located on the enteric nerves and smooth muscles of the stomach and duodenum [8]. Motilin exhibits periodic fluctuations in blood concentration during fasting, with peaks coinciding with the strong contraction phase of interdigestive migrating motor contractions (IMMC). This contraction involves the vagus nerve and 5HT3 receptors. Besides inducing fasting contractions, motilin enhances gastric acid secretion and promotes the secretion of enzymes such as amylase from the pancreas [9]. Erythromycin has been identified as a motilin receptor agonist, and erythromycin derivatives without antibacterial activity were expected to be useful for the treatment of functional gastrointestinal disorders. However, no remarkable effects were obtained, and its clinical application has been limited.

3.6 Ghrelin

Ghrelin is a peptide consisting of 28 amino acid residues, produced by endocrine cells (X/A-like cells) in the gastric body and secreted into the bloodstream. The side chain of the third serine residue is acylated with octanoic acid, an eight-carbon fatty acid, essential for ghrelin's activity. The enzyme required for this acylation (ghrelin O-acyltransferase: GOAT) has also been identified in the stomach. In the bloodstream, ghrelin is deacylated to des-acyl ghrelin. Ghrelin has various physiological effects, including potent growth hormone secretion, appetite stimulation, promotion of gastric juice secretion, enhancement of gastrointestinal motility, vasodilation, and blood pressure reduction, as well as involvement in musculoskeletal, glucose, and lipid metabolism. Conversely, des-acyl ghrelin has antagonistic effects, such as inhibiting feeding behavior and fasting gastric motility. Liver-expressed antimicrobial peptide 2 (LEAP-2) has been identified as an inhibitor of ghrelin, is expressed in the liver and jejunum, binds to the ghrelin receptor GHSR-1a, and inhibiting ghrelin signaling [10]. Due to its diverse effects, ghrelin is expected to have various clinical applications. Ghrelin agonists have shown efficacy in increasing body weight in cancer cachexia patients and are already used as therapeutic agents.

3.7 Somatostatin

Somatostatin, identified as a hormone inhibiting growth hormone secretion from the hypothalamus, exists as somatostatin-14 (SST-14) with 14 amino acids and somatostatin-28 (SST-28) with 28 amino acids. Widely distributed in the body, somatostatin is secreted by gastrointestinal mucosa and D cells in the pancreatic islets, exerting local paracrine effects. Somatostatin inhibits the secretion of gastrin, VIP, GIP, secretin, motilin, and insulin. Its secretion is stimulated by acidic substances in the gastrointestinal lumen, acting as a paracrine manner to inhibit gastrin secretion by gastric juice [11]. Additionally, somatostatin inhibits pancreatic exocrine function, gastric acid secretion, gastrointestinal motility and absorption, and gallbladder contraction. It also reduces visceral blood flow and inhibits cell proliferation, with most of its effects being inhibitory.

Competing Interests The author(s) has no competing interests to declare that are relevant to the content of this manuscript.

References

1. Hiroshi M, et al., editors. Stomach. Nankodo; 1989. (in Japanese).
2. Hall JE. Guyton and hall textbook of medical physiology. 13th ed. Saunders; 2015.
3. Barrett KE, et al. Ganong's review of medical physiology. 25th ed. McGraw-Hill Education/Medical; 2015.
4. Honma K, editor. Standard physiology. 9th ed. Igaku-Shoin; 2019. (in Japanese).
5. Ninomiya I, et al., editors. Standard physiology. 3rd ed. Bunkodo; 2013. (in Japanese).
6. Okada T, editor. Physiology. 2nd ed. Medical View; 2014. (in Japanese).
7. Hongo M. Gastric acid secretion, gastric endocrinology, and gastric motility. Chem Educ. 2017;65:356–7. (in Japanese).
8. Mochiki H, et al. Basics and clinical applications of motilin. Prog Med. 2007;223:545–8. (in Japanese).
9. Mochiki H, et al. Gastrointestinal motility effects of gastrointestinal hormones (Gastrin and Motilin). Gastroenterol Sci. 2022;6:162–5. (in Japanese).
10. Nakazato M, et al. A role for ghrelin in the central regulation of feeding. Nature. 2001;409:194–8.
11. Kaneko H. Somatostatin (Somatostatin-like Peptides). Prog Med. 2007;223:533–8. (in Japanese).

21 Gastroduodenal Motility and Perception Test, Internal Pressure Test and Perception Test, Barostat Method

Tadayuki Oshima

Abstract

The barostat is a specialized device used to measure visceral perceptual thresholds and gastrointestinal (GI) wall distensibility by maintaining constant pressure within a polyethylene balloon positioned in the GI tract. Initially developed for gastric studies, its use has expanded to the small intestine, colon, and rectum. The barostat allows for precise assessment of perceptual thresholds and adaptive relaxation, particularly relevant in disorders of gut-brain interaction (DGBI) such as functional dyspepsia (FD) and irritable bowel syndrome (IBS).

Despite its diagnostic value, the barostat test is invasive, costly, and largely limited to research settings. In FD, it has revealed abnormalities in gastric accommodation and hypersensitivity, contributing to subtype classification and therapeutic evaluation. Pharmacological agents such as Rikkunshito and mosapride have demonstrated beneficial effects in barostat-based assessments. Further research integrating barostat findings with non-invasive imaging modalities—such as SPECT, scintigraphy, and ultrasonography—may enhance the diagnostic utility and clinical applicability of this method. The barostat remains an important tool in advancing our understanding of GI sensory-motor physiology.

Keywords

Adaptive relaxation · Barostat · Disorders of gut-brain interaction · Functional dyspepsia · Gastrointestinal motility · Irritable bowel syndrome · Perceptual threshold · Visceral hypersensitivity

1 Barostat

1.1 What Is a Barostat?

The term "barostat" originates from the Greek words "baro" (pressure) and "stat" (to keep constant). It is an apparatus that controls air flow through tubing connecting the device to a bag placed in the gastrointestinal tract. This device is used to measure (i) the perceptual thresholds and (ii) the distensibility of the gastrointestinal wall. The polyethylene bag is designed to be compliant yet minimally elastic, ensuring that it does not contribute to pressure generation within the system.

T. Oshima (✉)
Department of Gastroenterology, Okazaki City Medical Association, Public Health Center, Okazaki, Japan

Department of Gastroenterology and Metabolism, Nagoya City University Graduate School of Medical Science, Nagoya, Japan

H. Kaneko et al. (eds.), *Disorders of Gut-Brain Interaction*,
https://doi.org/10.1007/978-981-95-6974-8_21

Previously, the volume of air introduced into the bag was used to evaluate perceptual or pain thresholds via gastrointestinal distension. However, since the degree of distension and stimulus intensity can vary among subjects even at the same balloon volume, Malagelada et al. developed a prototype barostat that uses pressure as a more reproducible and quantifiable stimulus [1]. Initially, the barostat was used to measure the distensibility (often expressed as compliance) of the gastric fundus, and later it was applied to other organs such as the small intestine and colon.

The barostat uses a pressure transducer to sense internal pressure and regulates air flow via an automated piston-driven pump.

When set to maintain constant internal pressure in the bag, the device withdraws air during contraction and introduces air during relaxation of the gastrointestinal tract, adjusting the air inflow through computer control to keep the internal pressure constant (Fig. 21.1). The transducer sensing the pressure and the pump controlling the air volume are connected to the device via separate tubes to ensure accurate pressure measurement and control. The pump uses a piston-syringe mechanism to control air volume more precisely.

By changing the internal pressure of the bag over time, the barostat can determine visceral perception and pain thresholds of the target organ based on the subject's symptom reporting. Additionally, by setting the internal pressure of the bag and using the volume of air introduced as an indicator, the distensibility of the gastrointestinal tract can be evaluated. The barostat allows assessment of gastric distensibility, particularly adaptive relaxation of the gastric fundus following a meal. The test can be performed on various parts of the gastrointestinal tract (esophagus, stomach, small intestine, colon, rectum), and balloons of various shapes are used to apply uniform pressure to the walls of each organ, tailored to their anatomical structure (Fig. 21.2).

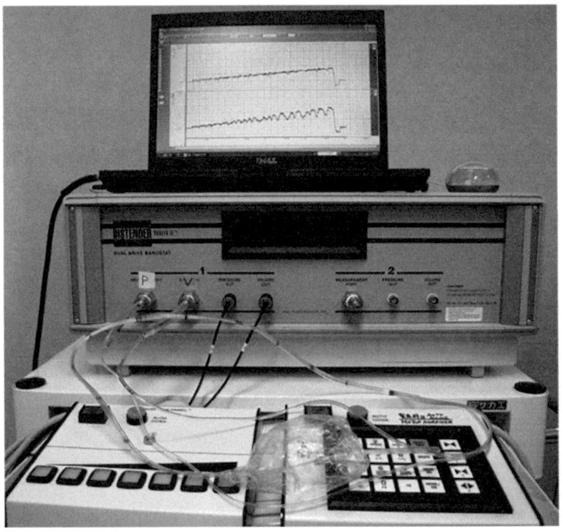

Fig. 21.1 Barostat device

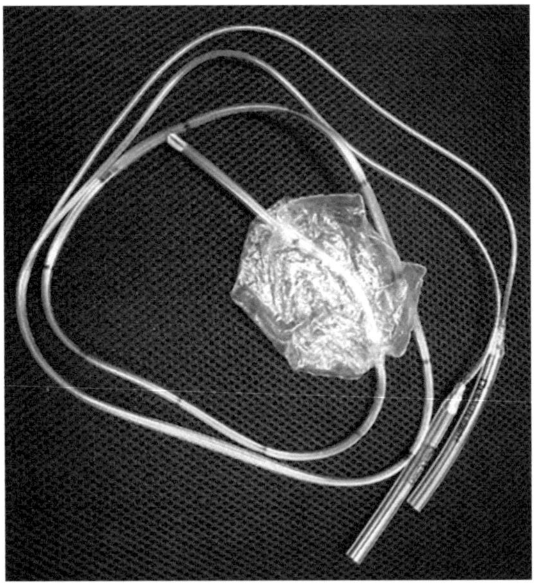

Fig. 21.2 Gastric balloon

1.2 Barostat Test

The barostat test is one of the gastrointestinal function tests that assess (i) visceral perceptual thresholds in response to distension and (ii) the mechanical distensibility of the gastrointestinal wall. Because of the high cost and invasive nature of the device, its use is largely restricted to research settings at specialized facilities, and limited data are available in Japan. Additionally, normal values and standardized measurement methods have not been established, and the test is not covered by public health insurance. Further studies combining the barostat test with non-invasive diagnostics may establish diagnostic criteria for disorders of gut-brain interaction (DGBI). This could make the barostat a more objective and sensitive diagnostic tool.

1.3 Background of the Barostat Test

With increasing interest in DGBI, including functional dyspepsia (FD) and irritable bowel syndrome (IBS), physiological and pathophysiological studies on gastrointestinal motility and perception using the barostat have been conducted in animal models. Although gastrointestinal distension can be easily applied in animal models, evaluating pain is more challenging than in human subjects. Therefore, surrogate indicators such as pulse rate, blood pressure, electrocardiogram, respiratory rate, and electromyographic activity of rectus abdominis muscle contractions have been used to assess pain. In humans, tests began with healthy subjects and were followed by data collection from DGBI patients, which revealed decreased perceptual thresholds and gastric distensibility in gastric barostat tests.

1.4 Relevant Conditions and Diseases

In DGBI such as FD and IBS, one of the underlying pathophysiological mechanisms is visceral hypersensitivity, and this method has been developed as a tool to assess this. Research has primarily focused on the stomach in upper gastrointestinal disorders, with reports on FD. FD patients are known to be susceptible to psychological stress, which is associated with decreased perceptual thresholds. To evaluate this, the barostat test can measure pain thresholds by gradually increasing the intragastric pressure. Additionally, the gastric fundus normally relaxes after a meal to temporarily accommodate ingested food, but this function is impaired in FD, resulting in impaired postprandial adaptive relaxation. This impairment can be detected using the barostat test, which measures adaptive relaxation by maintaining a constant pressure in a balloon placed in the stomach [2].

Further studies are needed to determine whether decreased perceptual thresholds and impaired adaptive relaxation response, as measured by the barostat test, can be used as diagnostic criteria for FD. However, given the heterogeneous nature of FD, these abnormalities may contribute to the subclassification of the disorder.

1.5 Considerations When Performing the Barostat Test

For gastric tests, the tube is inserted either orally or nasally, and for colon and rectal tests, it is inserted anally. Lidocaine-containing jelly or spray, commonly used in endoscopic procedures, should be avoided as it may interfere with measurement accuracy. Moreover, since tube insertion often causes mechanical stimulation, it is advisable to allow a sufficient adaptation period of 10–30 minutes after placement to minimize its influence on the measurements.

1.5.1 Measurement of Perceptual Thresholds

1. The balloon can evaluate perception and pain thresholds by distending the wall of the target gastrointestinal organ.
2. Balloon volume is automatically adjusted to maintain a preset intrabag pressure. As the target pressure is increased (stepwise or as a ramp), the balloon volume and the corresponding pressures at perception and pain thresholds are recorded.
3. Methods of pressure modulation include the stepwise method, which increases pressure stepwise, the ramp method, which gradually

increases pressure at a constant rate; and the phasic method, which applies pressure for a fixed duration, then releases and reapplies it. Each method has advantages and disadvantages, and there is currently no consensus regarding their relative superiority.

1.5.2 Measurement of Distensibility

1. In the stomach, the balloon is placed in the gastric fundus under X-ray fluoroscopy to evaluate the postprandial (adaptive) relaxation response.
2. The barostat bag, connected to the catheter, is usually inserted orally. The catheter is then connected to a barostat device, which controls the internal pressure and volume of the bag.
3. During the measurement, the bag is inflated to apply pressure to the gastrointestinal wall at a level that is not perceived by the subject. Gastrointestinal wall tension is influenced not only by internal pressure but also by intra-abdominal pressure. Therefore, the pressure required to detect abdominal pressure is called the minimal distending pressure (MDP). In the stomach, MDP is approximately 2–8 mmHg and is slightly higher in the duodenum and colon.
4. Air is introduced into the bag to maintain a constant pressure that is 1–2 mmHg above the MDP (referred to as the operating pressure), and changes in balloon volume are measured.
5. Both MDP and the operating pressure should be set below the perceptual threshold so that the subject does not perceive the pressure.
6. Changes in the volume of air introduced into the bag are used to assess variations in gastrointestinal wall tension.

2 Conclusion

The barostat test is not commonly used in clinical practice due to its invasive nature. However, it has demonstrated that some patients with functional dyspepsia exhibit impairments in gastric perception and adaptive relaxation response. Additionally, medications such as Rikkunshito [3] and mosapride have been shown to improve perceptual thresholds and adaptive relaxation responses as assessed by the barostat test.

Future studies should aim to clarify the relationship between these findings and non-invasive tests, such as single photon emission computed tomography (SPECT), scintigraphy, and abdominal ultrasound, to facilitate easier assessment of gastrointestinal motility. The development of pharmacological treatments that improve these abnormalities and relieve symptoms is also desirable.

Take-Home Message

Although the barostat test is invasive, it has demonstrated that some patients with functional dyspepsia exhibit gastric hypersensitivity and impaired adaptive relaxation. Future research should explore how these findings can be integrated with non-invasive tests and guide the development of effective treatments.

Competing Interests The author(s) has no competing interests to declare that are relevant to the content of this manuscript.

References

1. Azpiroz F, et al. Physiological variations in canine gastric tone measured by an electronic barostat. Am J Physiol. 1985;248:G229–37.
2. Tack J, et al. Symptoms associated with hypersensitivity to gastric distention in functional dyspepsia. Gastroenterology. 2001;121:526–35.
3. Miwa H, et al. Impairment of gastric accommodation induced by water-avoidance stress is mediated by 5-HT2B receptors. Neurogastroenterol Motil. 2016;28:765–78.

22 Gastroduodenal Motility and Perception Test, Internal Pressure Test and Perception Test, Drinking Test

Mototsugu Kato

Abstract

The barostat method is the gold standard for evaluating gastrointestinal function, but it is not used as a routine examination because of its high invasiveness. On the other hand, the drinking test is minimally invasive and suitable for routine clinical use. However, various methods of drinking tests have been reported, and there is no standardized method. The drinking test is influenced by visceral hypersensitivity, impaired gastric accommodation, and delayed gastric emptying. FD patients with decreased volume load tolerance have significantly lower drinking volumes and more upper abdominal symptoms with increased drinking volume. A drinking ultrasonography test, which combines the drinking test with external ultrasonography, was developed to evaluate gastric distensibility, gastric emptying, and gastric perception. The drinking ultrasonography test can provide insights into pathophysiological mechanisms to select treatment based on FD pathophysiology.

Keywords

Functional Dyspepsia · Drinking test · Barostat · Gastric hypersensitivity · Impaired gastric accommodation · Delayed gastric emptying · Drinking ultrasonography test

1 Introduction

The pathophysiology of functional dyspepsia (FD) is complex, and not all FD patients exhibit gastrointestinal motility disorders. However, delayed gastric emptying, gastric hypersensitivity, and impaired postprandial gastric accommodation are significant factors [1, 2]. FD is diagnosed based on troublesome abdominal symptoms, and endoscopy is used to exclude organic diseases and diagnose *H. pylori* infection. Although gastrointestinal motility and sensory function tests may be performed in FD, pathophysiological evaluation is not always necessary for FD management. The upper gastrointestinal tract has various physiological functions, and abnormalities in these functions are associated with functional disorders. In FD, adaptive relaxation as a reservoir, acid secretion, contractility, emptying, pyloric function to prevent rapid gastric emptying and duodenal reflux, and gastric visceral perception play important roles.

1.1 Drinking Test

The barostat method is a test for evaluating gastrointestinal function (see Chap. 21). The baro-

M. Kato (✉)
Public Interest Foundation, Gastroenterology, Sapporo, Japan

H. Kaneko et al. (eds.), *Disorders of Gut-Brain Interaction*,
https://doi.org/10.1007/978-981-95-6974-8_22

stat method involves inserting a bag into the stomach and changing the internal pressure to assess compliance. Although it is a standard test, it is highly invasive for routine use [3].

There is no standardized method for the drinking test, and various methods have been reported (Table 22.1). The types of liquids used can be broadly classified into water or nutrient solutions. The loading speed can be classified into intervals of 5 min, 1 min (rapid), or continuous infusion by a pump at 15–30 mL/min (slow). The loading volume can be set to the maximum tolerable volume, a weight-based upper limit, or until certain symptoms appear. Evaluation criteria include total drinking volume, severity of symptoms, and duration of symptoms. Depending on the loading speed and type of liquid, the test is referred to as the rapid water drinking test, rapid nutrient drinking test, slow nutrient drinking test, or satiety drinking test [4].

Table 22.1 Methods of drinking test

Type of liquid	Water	Nutrient	
Loading speed (drinking Interval)	5 min (rapid)	Every minute (rapid) 60–100 mL	Continuous pump infusion (slow) 15–30 mL/min
Loading volume (drinking volume)	Maximum tolerable volume	Upper limit set	Until certain symptoms appear
Evaluation criteria	Total drinking volume	Severity of symptoms	Duration of symptoms

Comparative studies between FD patients and healthy individuals using the drinking test have shown that FD patients have significantly lower drinking volumes in the rapid water drinking test and rapid nutrient drinking test, and significantly lower drinking volumes until symptom onset in the slow nutrient drinking test [5–11] (Fig. 22.1). The drinking test has been proven to have good reproducibility [5, 12]. Additionally, while men tend to have higher drinking volumes than women in the drinking test, multivariate analysis has shown no influence of age, BMI, or gender [13]. In comparisons by the same examiner, the drinking volume is lower in the slow nutrient drinking test than in the rapid water drinking test [13].

The drinking test is influenced by visceral hypersensitivity, impaired gastric accommodation, delayed gastric emptying, and feedback mechanisms to nutrient load, and is considered a

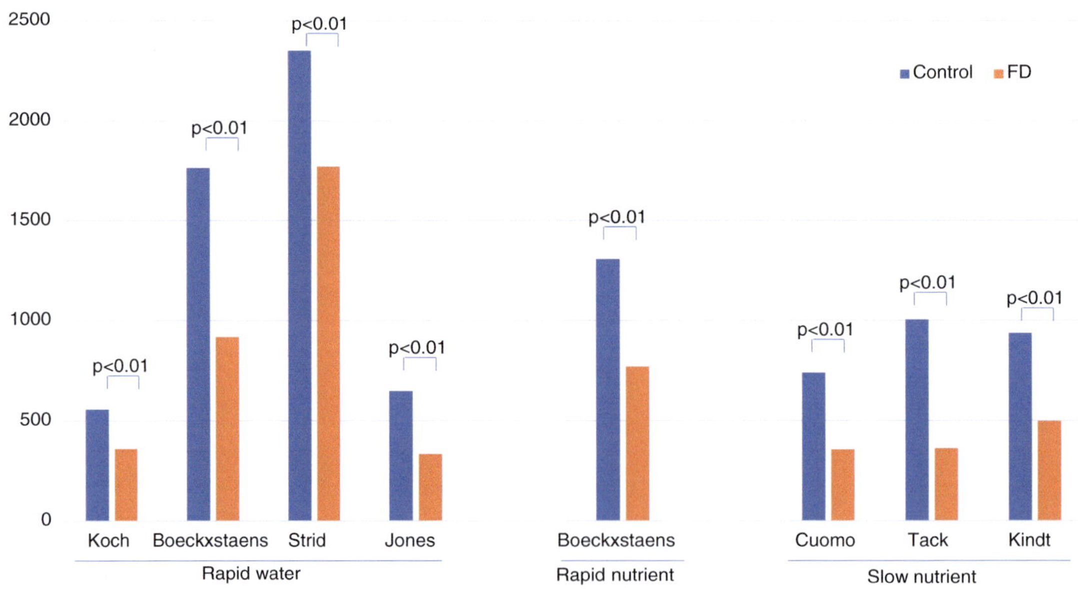

Fig. 22.1 Comparison between healthy individuals and FD patients in the drinking test

comprehensive evaluation of these factors. Comparative studies with the barostat test have reported that many slow nutrient drinking tests reflect the state of gastric accommodation [8, 10, 12]. However, since gastric accommodation takes about 10 min to occur, the rapid drinking test, which is completed within 10 min, is thought to be more influenced by visceral hypersensitivity. Additionally, longer drinking intervals and test durations also involve the influence of gastric emptying capacity.

1.2 Drinking Ultrasonography Test

The authors developed a drinking ultrasonography test that combines the drinking test with external ultrasonography to evaluate gastric distensibility, gastric perception, and gastric emptying [14]. The drinking ultrasonography test is minimally invasive, has a short examination time of approximately 20 min, and can be applied in outpatient settings. Based on the results of the drinking ultrasonography test, subjects can be classified into four categories: abnormal gastric distensibility, abnormal gastric perception, abnormal gastric emptying, and normal.

The method of the drinking ultrasonography test involves fasting for more than 6 h, with the subject in a supine position, using a straw placed at the same height for drinking. The drinking volume is set at 200 mL every 2 min, ending when 800 mL is reached (8 min after the start of the test). If the patient self-determines that drinking is impossible, the test is terminated. Using an ultrasound probe with the spleen as a window, the proximal stomach is observed at its maximum diameter, and the cross-sectional area of the gastric fundus is measured every 2 min of drinking. Simultaneously, abdominal symptoms are evaluated using a visual analog scale (VAS) (0 = no symptoms to 10 = unable to drink due to upper abdominal symptoms). After the end of drinking (or termination), the cross-sectional area of the gastric fundus is measured at 5 min and 10 min post-drinking, with the cross-sectional area of the proximal stomach immediately after drinking set at 100%, and the rate of change in this area measured.

Comparing healthy volunteers with FD patients based on Rome III criteria, the average maximum drinking volume was significantly lower in FD patients (596.2 ± 227.1 mL) compared to healthy individuals (785.0 ± 48.9 mL). Sensory scores indicated hypersensitivity in FD patients at each time point (Fig. 22.2) [15].

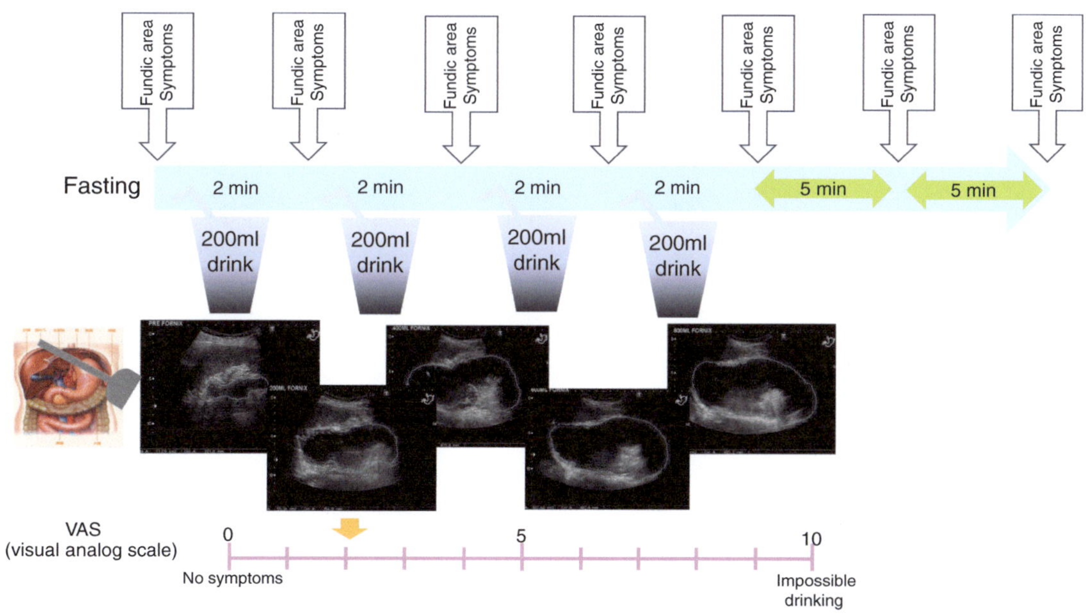

Fig. 22.2 Method of the drinking ultrasonography test

Additionally, FD patients showed a significantly smaller average gastric cross-sectional area at the 800 mL load point (Fig. 22.2). Regarding gastric emptying, in healthy subjects, no cases showed a larger gastric cross-sectional area 10 min after drinking water than immediately after drinking, whereas larger cases were observed in FD patients [14]. Abnormalities are diagnosed when the gastric fundus cross-sectional area and VAS exceed the mean ± SD of healthy individuals, and gastric emptying is abnormal if the emptying rate is <0% at 10 min post-drinking (Fig. 22.3).

In South Korea, a follow-up study using the same method demonstrated significant differences in visceral hypersensitivity and impaired adaptive relaxation between FD patients and healthy individuals, confirming the test's usefulness [16].

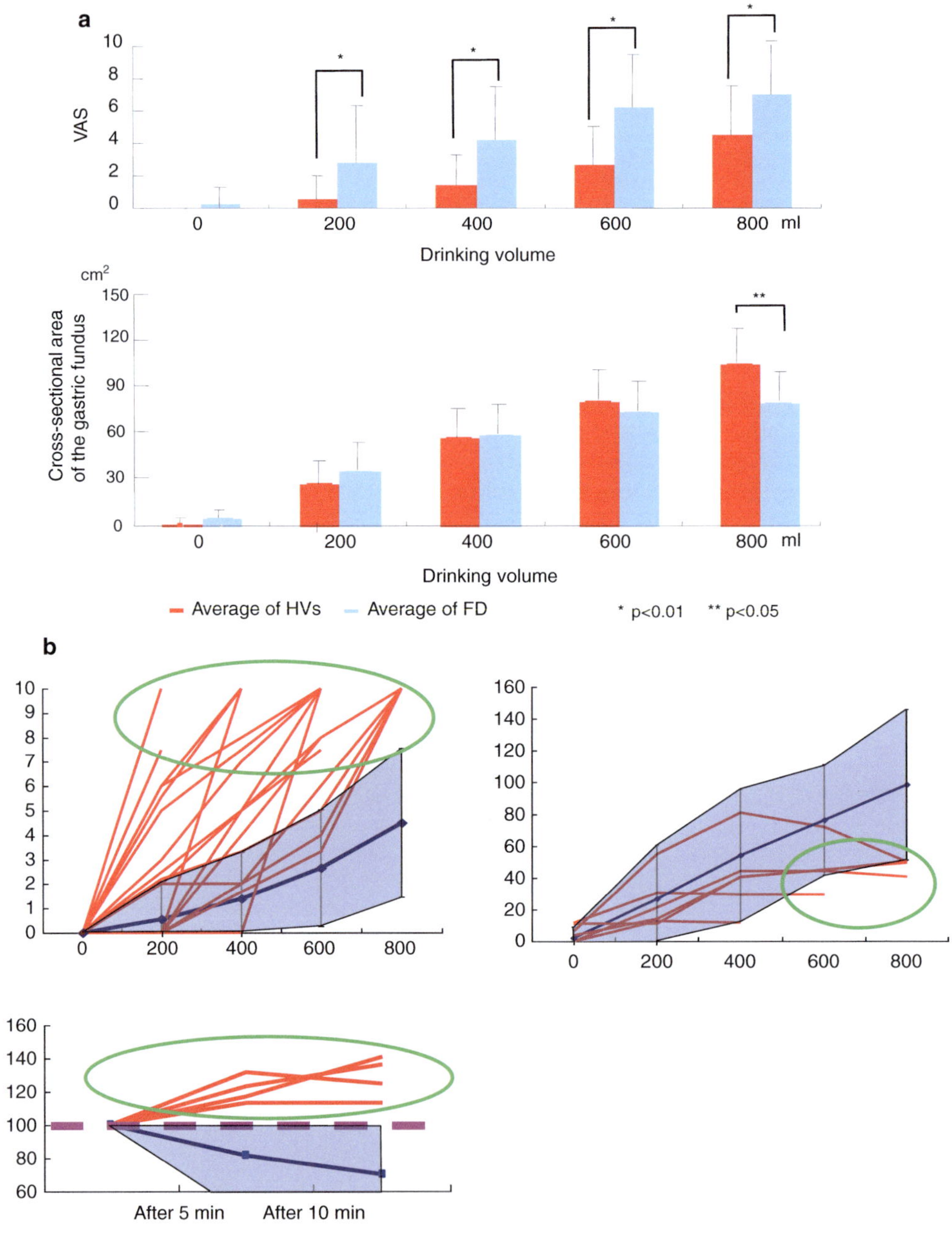

Fig. 22.3 (**a**) Comparison between healthy individuals and FD patients in the drinking ultrasonography test. Top: Perception, Bottom: Distensibility. (**b**) Normal range and abnormal data

2 Conclusion

The drinking test is a simple and minimally invasive test useful for diagnosing FD and should be more widely used in routine clinical practice. Selecting cases where specific drugs or treatments are effective from among FD patients with various underlying pathologies is important, and the drinking ultrasonography test can provide insights into pathophysiological mechanisms. Rome IV presents an algorithm for selecting treatment based on FD pathophysiology, and the future dissemination of the drinking ultrasonography test is anticipated [17].

Take-Home Message

The drinking test utilizes the restricted drinking volume and the appearance of upper abdominal symptoms in FD patients. It is a simple method that can be introduced in any facility. However, since there is no standardized method, it is recommended to refer to reported methods. Empirically, it is advisable to set an upper limit for drinking volume and evaluate the appearance of symptoms.

Competing Interests The author(s) has no competing interests to declare that are relevant to the content of this manuscript.

References

1. Gilja OH, et al. Impaired accommodation of proximal stomach to a meal in functional dyspepsia. Dig Dis Sci. 1996;41:689–96.
2. Kindt S, et al. Impaired gastric accommodation and its role in dyspepsia. Gut. 2006;55(12):1685–91.
3. Nakata K. In: Hongo M, editor. Gastric emptying test, drinking test, visceral perception test, barostat, etc. FD diagnosis Q&A. Nihon Iji Shinposha; 2011. p. 104–11. (in Japanese).
4. Scarpellini E, et al. Nutrient drinking test as biomarker in functional dyspepsia. Am J Gastroenterol. 2021;116:1387–95.
5. Koch KL, et al. Reproducibility of gastric myoelectrical activity and the water load test in patients with dysmotility-like dyspepsia symptoms and in control subjects. J Clin Gastroenterol. 2000;31:125–9.
6. Boeckxstaens GE, et al. Impaired drinking capacity in patients with functional dyspepsia: relationship with proximal stomach function. Gastroenterology. 2001;121:1054–63.
7. Strid H, et al. Impact of sex and psychological factors on the water loading test in functional dyspepsia. Scand J Gastroenterol. 2001;36:725–30.
8. Jones MP, et al. The water load test: observations from healthy controls and patients with functional dyspepsia. Am J Physiol Gastrointest Liver Physiol. 2003;284:G896–904.
9. Cuomo R, et al. Functional dyspepsia symptoms, gastric emptying and satiety provocative test: analysis of relationships. Scand J Gastroenterol. 2001;36:1030–6.
10. Tack J, et al. Assessment of meal-induced gastric accommodation by a satiety drinking test in health and in severe functional dyspepsia. Gut. 2003;52:1271–7.
11. Kindt S, et al. Reproducibility and symptomatic predictors of a slow nutrient drinking test in health and in functional dyspepsia. Neurogastroenterol Motil. 2008;20:320–9.
12. Iida A, et al. Usefulness of a slow nutrient drinking test for evaluating gastric perception and accommodation. Digestion. 2011;84:253–60.
13. Abid S, et al. Satiety drinking tests: effects of caloric content, drinking rate, gender, age, and body mass index. Scand J Gastroenterol. 2009;44:551–6.
14. Kato M, et al. Pathophysiological classification of functional dyspepsia using a novel drinking-ultrasonography test. Digestion. 2010;82:162–6.
15. Hata T, et al. Comparison of gastric motor and sensory functions between functional dyspepsia and healthy subjects using novel drinking-ultrasonography test. Digestion. 2013;87(1):34–9.
16. Kugler T. The usefulness of water-drinking ultrasonography combined test for evaluating patients with functional dyspepsia. Korean J Gastroenterol. 2015;66(2):92–7.
17. Stanghellini V, et al. Gastroduodenal disorders. Gastroenterology. 2016;150:1380–92.

23 Gastroduodenal Motility Test, Gastric Emptying Test, Scintigraphy Test

Toshihiko Tomita

Abstract

Disorders of gastric and duodenal motility are major contributors to upper abdominal symptoms. Impaired adaptive relaxation of the stomach frequently results in early satiety, whereas both delayed and accelerated gastric emptying have been linked to symptom development. A clear understanding of these mechanisms is essential for selecting appropriate treatment, and objective assessments of gastrointestinal motility can provide valuable insights into underlying pathophysiology. However, routine use of such tests is not recommended in daily practice, since specialized equipment is not always available, and functional gastrointestinal disorders are multifactorial, influenced by factors beyond motility alone. Accordingly, current guidelines advocate a selective rather than universal approach to testing. Nevertheless, gastric emptying studies remain clinically useful because they allow detection of impaired accommodation or abnormal emptying patterns. These findings may inform therapeutic choices and support individualized management. Thus, motility tests should be performed selectively, guided by a patient's symptoms and clinical course, rather than applied indiscriminately.

Keywords

Evaluation methods · Motility function · Gastric scintigraphy · Functional dyspepsia

T. Tomita (✉)
Department of Gastroenterology, Faculty of Medicine, Hyogo Medical University, Nishinomiya, Japan
e-mail: tomita@hyo-med.ac.jp

1 Scintigraphy

1.1 Evaluation Methods of Motility Function

Generally, the evaluation methods for gastric and duodenal motility function include intraluminal pressure measurement, sensory testing, gastric adaptive relaxation response, and gastric emptying time measurement (Table 23.1) [1]. Postprandial motility is crucial for gastric motility function, and the adaptive relaxation response of the fundus during meal intake has been previously reported to be associated with dyspeptic symptoms. This adaptive relaxation response is considered a physiological reaction to store food in the fundus postprandially. However, in patients with Functional Dyspepsia (FD), this adaptive relaxation does not occur smoothly, leading to early satiety, and delayed gastric emptying induces bloating [2]. Generally, 20–40% of FD patients exhibit impaired adaptive relaxation, and

H. Kaneko et al. (eds.), *Disorders of Gut-Brain Interaction*,
https://doi.org/10.1007/978-981-95-6974-8_23

10–20% show delayed emptying (Fig. 23.1, Table 23.2) [3, 4].

To date, various methods have been used to evaluate the gastric adaptive relaxation response, including the barostat test, single-photon emission computed tomography (SPECT), magnetic resonance imaging (MRI), external ultrasound, and drinking load tests. The gastric barostat test is known as the gold standard for evaluating the adaptive relaxation response, but due to the need to place a balloon in the stomach, the associated discomfort, invasiveness, and high cost of the equipment, it is not widely used in Japan except in some specialized medical institutions. On the other hand, methods for measuring gastric emptying time include direct methods, such as ultrasound and radioisotope methods that directly image the movement of gastric contents, and indirect methods, such as the acetaminophen method and the 13C breath test, which evaluate gastric emptying time based on the temporal changes of markers absorbed in the small intestine. In particular, gastric scintigraphy is used as the gold standard for measuring emptying time in Western countries.

Table 23.1 Gastric motility function tests

Measurement of gastric emptying time	Acetaminophen Method ^{13}C Breath Test External Ultrasound Examination Radioisotope Method: Scintigraphy is the gold standard modality
Measurement of gastric accommodation	Barostat: Balloon placement in the fundus, measuring the volume of air inflow and balloon pressure over time for evaluation. SPECT MRI External Ultrasound Drinking Load Test

Adapted from Refs. [8, 9]

Table 23.2 Relationship between gastric emptying function and dyspeptic symptoms [3]

Study	*n*	Prevalence (%)	Association
Wegener (1989)	43	30	None
Jian (1989)	28	59	None
Tally (1989)	32	30	None
Waldron (1991)	50	42	None
Klauser (1993)	69	35	None
Scott (1993)	75	28	None
Perri (1998)	304	33	Postprandial bloating, nausea, vomiting
Talley (2001)	551	24	None
Sarnelli (2003)	392	23	Postprandial bloating, nausea, vomiting

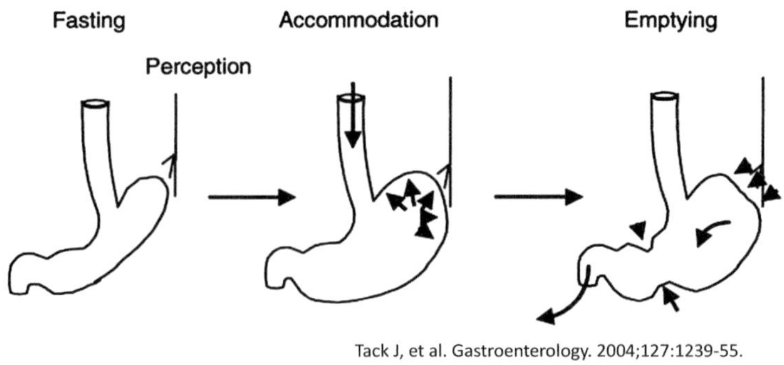

Fig. 23.1 Gastric motility physiology [3]

1.2 Gastric Scintigraphy

Gastric scintigraphy involves the ingestion of a test meal mixed with a radioisotope-labeled compound (99mTc-tin colloid (37 MBq)), followed by imaging with a scintillation camera focused on the epigastric region. The radioactivity in the region of interest (ROI) set in the stomach is measured over time, and gastric emptying time is calculated from the change in radioactivity (e.g., half-emptying time (T half)). Gastric scintigraphy allows direct observation of gastrointestinal movement as images, providing a noninvasive, real-time, and visual method to accurately evaluate gastric motility (Figs. 23.2 and 23.3) [5]. Unlike other methods that can only test liquid meals, gastric scintigraphy can evaluate both liquid and solid meals, allowing for the assessment of gastric motility under physiological conditions. Additionally, it can be

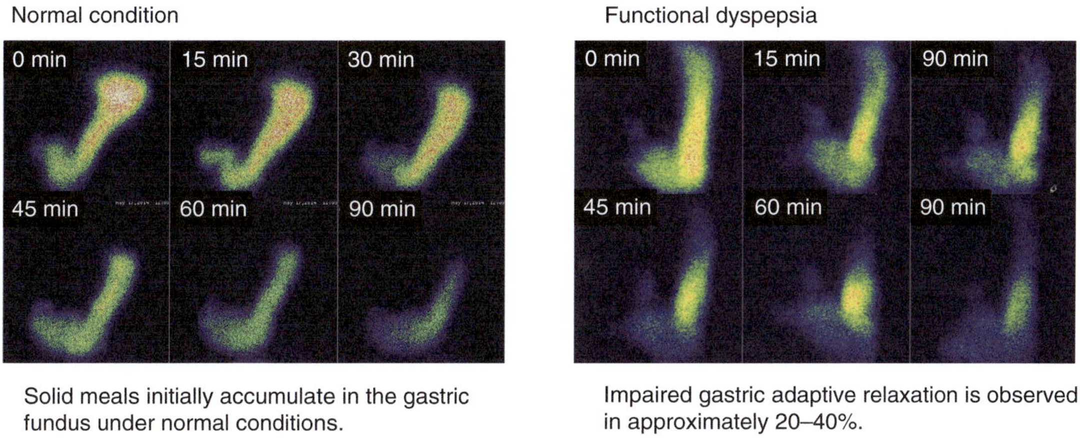

Fig. 23.2 Temporal patterns of gastric motility function in gastric scintigraphy

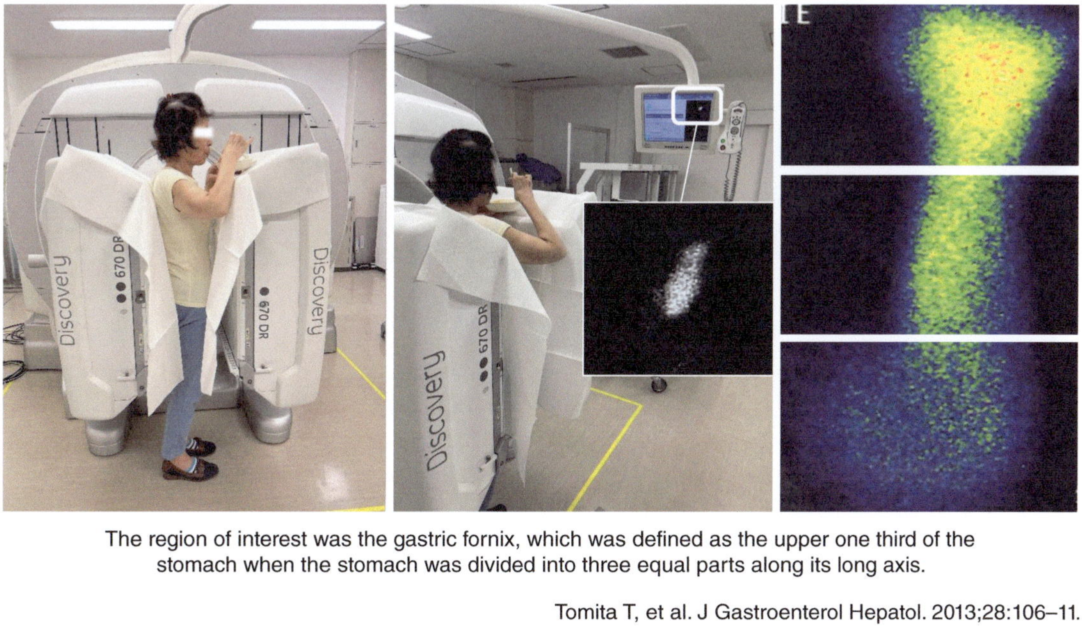

Fig. 23.3 Setting and quantification of regions of interest in gastric scintigraphy [4]

evaluated in different postures, such as sitting or standing. However, since the test involves ingesting a test meal mixed with a radiopharmaceutical, there is radiation exposure. The exposure per test is reported to be 0.2–8 mSv, similar to that of a standard X-ray examination. The need for a gamma camera limits this test to specialized medical institutions.

Traditionally, gastric scintigraphy has been primarily used to measure gastric emptying time. However, we have reported a positive correlation between the results of gastric scintigraphy and the barostat test, an evaluation method for the adaptive relaxation response, by defining the ratio of radioactivity in the fundus to the total gastric radioactivity immediately after ingesting the test meal as gastric storage capacity (Fig. 23.4) [5]. In the future, gastric scintigraphy may be used for comprehensive evaluation of gastric motility, including the adaptive relaxation response, not just for measuring emptying time. In fact, using gastric scintigraphy, we have reported the potential to evaluate the gastric motility of FD patients over time before and after taking acotiamide hydrochloride, suggesting that this test method can be used to evaluate gastric motility in various pathophysiological conditions (Fig. 23.5) [6].

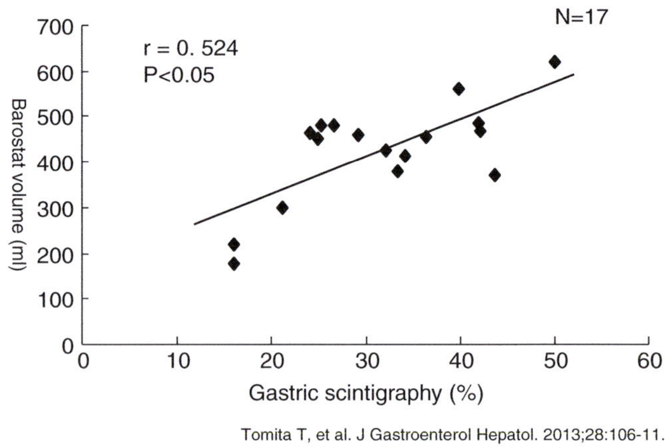

Fig. 23.4 Correlation between scintigraphy and barostat test in evaluating adaptive relaxation response [4]

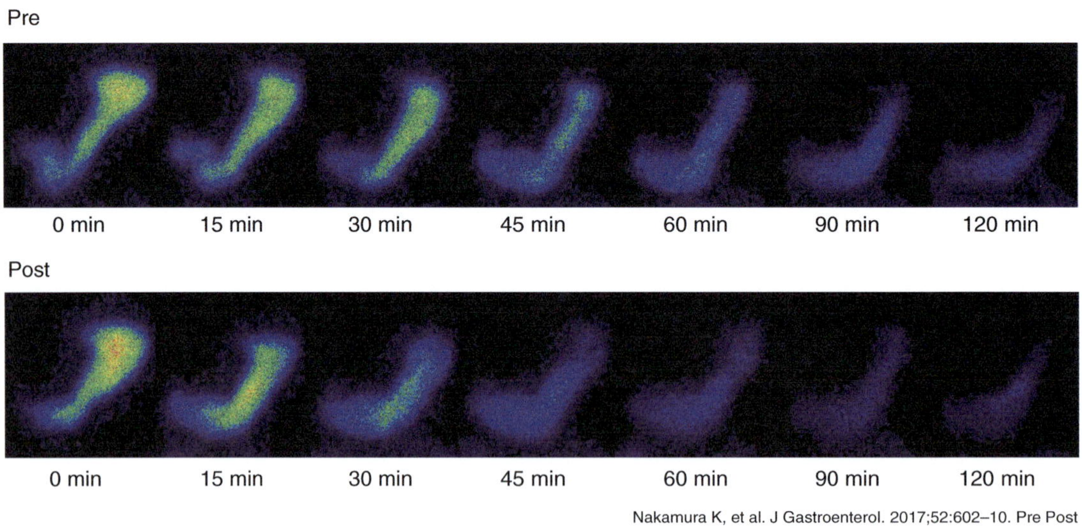

Fig. 23.5 Gastric motility function before and after drug administration

2 Conclusion

Due to issues with testing equipment and the complexity of the pathophysiology of functional gastrointestinal disorders, motility function tests are not recommended for all patients according to guidelines [7]. It is challenging to prove that the direct cause of symptom onset is an abnormality in motility physiology or visceral hypersensitivity with a single test. However, conducting gastrointestinal motility tests can evaluate the presence of impaired adaptive relaxation response or delayed gastric emptying, potentially serving as a basis for selecting appropriate medications.

Take-Home Message
Gastrointestinal motility disorders are one of the factors contributing to the onset of upper abdominal symptoms in functional dyspepsia.

In particular, adaptive relaxation response disorders are associated with early satiety, and it has been recognized that both too rapid and too slow gastric emptying are linked to symptoms. Therefore, evaluating motility function through various tests and understanding the pathophysiology is important for considering optimal treatment strategies.

Competing Interests The author(s) has no competing interests to declare that are relevant to the content of this manuscript.

References

1. Miwa H, et al. Current understanding of pathogenesis of functional dyspepsia. J Gastroenterol Hepatol. 2011;26(Suppl 3):53–60.
2. Tack J, et al. Role of impaired gastric accommodation to a meal in functional dyspepsia. Gastroenterology. 1998;115:1346–52.
3. Tack J, et al. Pathophysiology and treatment of functional dyspepsia. Gastroenterology. 2004;127:1239–55.
4. Asano H, et al. Prevalence of gastric motility disorders in patients with functional dyspepsia. J Neurogastroenterol Motil. 2017;23:392–9.
5. Tomita T, et al. Use of scintigraphy to evaluate gastric accommodation and emptying: comparison with barostat. J Gastroenterol Hepatol. 2013;28:106–11.
6. Nakamura K, et al. Correction to: a double-blind placebo controlled study of acotiamide hydrochloride for efficacy on gastrointestinal motility of patients with functional dyspepsia. J Gastroenterol. 2017;52:602–10.
7. The Japanese Society of Gastroenterology, ed. Clinical practice guidelines for functional gastrointestinal disorders 2021—Functional Dyspepsia (FD), 2nd rev. Nankodo; 2021. (in Japanese).
8. van den Elzen BD, et al. Fundic accommodation assessed by SPECT scanning: comparison with the gastric barostat. Gut. 2003;52:1548–54.
9. Gilja OH, et al. Impaired accommodation of proximal stomach to a meal in functional dyspepsia. Dig Dis Sci. 1996;41:689–96.

24 Gastroduodenal Motility Test, Gastric Emptying Test, ^{13}C-Breath Test

Hidekazu Suzuki

Abstract

The ^{13}C breath test has emerged as a non-invasive, radiation-free method for assessing gastric emptying, offering a practical alternative to traditional scintigraphy. This technique utilizes ^{13}C-labeled compounds—^{13}C-octanoic acid for solids and ^{13}C-acetic acid for liquids—which, after passing through the stomach, are absorbed in the small intestine and metabolized to $^{13}CO_2$, detectable in exhaled breath. While widely implemented, methodological variations have impeded standardization. In Japan, the 44th Smooth Muscle Society Workshop proposed a standardized protocol using ^{13}C-acetic acid for liquid meals. We further addressed the lack of gender-specific reference values by establishing T_{max} cutoffs of 60 min for males and 75 min for females, revealing no sex-based prevalence difference in delayed gastric emptying among functional dyspepsia (FD) patients. Additionally, daily physical activity was found to influence gastric emptying independently. The Cairn ^{13}C-Spirulina Gastric Emptying Breath Test (GEBT), validated against scintigraphy, offers standardized assessment using ^{13}C-labeled Spirulina and gas isotope ratio mass spectrometry. Despite its clinical promise, the ^{13}C breath test lacks national health insurance coverage in Japan and is hindered by procedural variability and logistical demands. Future efforts should focus on broader standardization, procedural simplification, and integration into routine clinical practice through the support of national insurance reimbursement.

Keywords

^{13}C-breath test · Gastric emptying · Gastric accommodation

1 Introduction

Food ingested orally traverses the esophagus and is subsequently stored in the fundus of the stomach, where it is mixed with gastric acid and then emptied into the duodenum. Impairment in any of these processes, or a combination thereof, can result in a variety of symptoms originating from the upper gastrointestinal tract. Conditions such as Parkinson's disease, diabetic or idiopathic gastroparesis, and certain cases of functional dyspepsia (FD) are characterized by reduced gastric motility, particularly delayed gastric emptying. This not only precipitates upper gastrointestinal symptoms but also has secondary effects, such as

H. Suzuki (✉)
Division of Gastroenterology and Hepatology, Department of Internal Medicine, Tokai University School of Medicine, Isehara, Japan
e-mail: hsuzuki@tokai.ac.jp

H. Kaneko et al. (eds.), *Disorders of Gut-Brain Interaction*,
https://doi.org/10.1007/978-981-95-6974-8_24

delayed drug delivery to the duodenum, which in turn delays the onset of medication effects [1]. In such pathophysiological contexts [1, 2], objective evaluation through gastric emptying tests is of paramount importance. Gastric emptying tests can be broadly categorized into direct methods, which observe the test meal reaching the duodenum (e.g., radioisotope (RI) method, ultrasound), and indirect methods, which measure secondary changes in blood or breath after the test meal reaches the duodenum (e.g., acetaminophen method, breath test). Traditionally, the RI method was the gold standard, but due to cost and radiation exposure, alternative tests such as the acetaminophen method and external ultrasound have been developed. Since around 2003, the ^{13}C urea breath test has become widely used for diagnosing *H. pylori* infection and confirming the eradication. Consequently, the measurement of $^{13}CO_2$ using infrared spectrometry has become widespread in domestic medical institutions, leading to the adoption of the ^{13}C breath test for the evaluation of gastric emptying.

1.1 ^{13}C Breath Test

Following the seminal report by Ghoos et al. in 1993 [3], the ^{13}C breath test has gained widespread acceptance in Western countries and has been extensively studied and disseminated by Prof. Koji Nakada at Jikei University in Japan. For solid test meals, ^{13}C-octanoic acid is used, and for liquid test meals, ^{13}C-acetic acid is used as the ^{13}C-labeled compound. These ^{13}C-labeled compounds are not absorbed from the stomach but are rapidly absorbed from the small intestinal mucosa distal to the duodenum after gastric emptying, appearing in the breath via systemic circulation. By examining the temporal changes in the presence ratio of $^{13}CO_2$ in the breath, gastric emptying time (rate) can be measured. The ^{13}C breath test is considered almost equivalent to the quantitative, direct gastric emptying test using radioisotopes (RI) [4]. The ^{13}C method is simple, non-invasive, free from radiation exposure, and does not involve drugs, thus avoiding side effects, making it the most convenient gastric emptying test in clinical practice. However, there was no internationally recognized standard method for its implementation. In 2002, the 44th Japanese Smooth Muscle Society Workshop proposed a standard method using ^{13}C-acetic acid mixed with a liquid meal (200 mL, 200 kcal) [5]. The test involves measuring for 4 h to calculate T_{max} and $T_{1/2}$, or a simplified method measuring for 90 min to evaluate T_{max}.

The test criteria vary depending on the form and calorie content of the test meal, so there is no international standard. In clinical practice, delayed gastric emptying is determined by comparing the effects before and after the test drug intake or with healthy individuals. The results are influenced by the amount, calorie content, composition, and form of the test meal.

1.2 Gender Differences in Gastric Emptying

Despite the widespread use of the ^{13}C-acetic acid breath test for evaluating gastric emptying (particularly liquid emptying), the standard values did not consider gender differences in healthy individuals. Therefore, we recalibrated the standard values of the ^{13}C-acetic acid breath test considering gender differences. Using the gender-adjusted standard values, we clarified the prevalence and clinical characteristics of delayed gastric emptying in FD patients. Specifically, we evaluated gastric emptying in 52 healthy individuals and 126 FD patients using the ^{13}C-acetic acid breath test. The cutoff point for T_{max} for diagnosing delayed gastric emptying was determined based on gender-specific healthy individual data. Additionally, we compared gastroesophageal reflux symptoms, indigestion symptoms, anxiety and depression scores, age, BMI, smoking, and alcohol consumption between the delayed and non-delayed gastric emptying groups. As a result, compared to healthy males, healthy females had delayed gastric emptying (T_{max}, females: males, 53.6±19.3: 42.7±16.9 min, $p = 0.04$), setting the cutoff point for T_{max} at 60 min for males and 75 min for females [6]. With these gender-specific cutoff values, the prevalence of delayed gastric emptying in

FD patients showed no gender difference ($p = 0.68$). Male FD patients with delayed gastric emptying had lower BMI than the non-delayed group. Reflux symptoms were more severe in the delayed gastric emptying group than in the non-delayed group among female patients [6].

1.3 Intensity of Daily Physical Activity and Gastric Emptying

It is believed that the intensity of daily physical activity influences gastrointestinal motility. To investigate the impact on dyspeptic symptoms, we examined the relationship between the intensity of daily physical activity and gastric emptying. Thirty healthy individuals were selected and divided into three groups (low, medium, high) based on the total intensity of physical activity over 1 week. Gastric emptying (liquid emptying) was evaluated using the ^{13}C-acetic acid breath test. Gastroesophageal reflux symptoms, indigestion symptoms, stool form, anxiety and depression scores, and sleep quality scores were also compared. Baseline scores for gastroesophageal reflux symptoms, anxiety, depression, and sleep quality showed no differences among the three groups. Gastric emptying was significantly faster in the low-intensity exercise group compared to the medium-intensity exercise group. Soft stools and alcohol consumption were also associated with daily exercise intensity, but these variables were not confounding factors; daily exercise intensity was independently related to gastric emptying [7].

1.4 Cairn ^{13}C-Spirulina GEBT [8, 9]

Among the gastric emptying tests already used in clinical trials, the Cairn ^{13}C-Spirulina Gastric Emptying Breath Test (GEBT) is non-radioactive, non-invasive, and measures the gastric emptying rate in adults. Spirulina is a genus of algae belonging to the order Oscillatoriales, found in freshwater and brackish environments. The Cairn GEBT, validated against the gold standard gastric scintigraphy method, enables rapid and accurate identification of gastroparesis.

1.5 Procedure of GEBT

After fasting overnight, two pre-meal breath samples are collected. The patient then consumes the ^{13}C GEBT test meal, which consists of 43 mg of ^{13}C-compounds (provided as approximately 100 mg of ^{13}C-Spirulina), six salted crackers, 6 ounces (180 mL) of water, and 27 g of rehydrated, precisely formulated, pasteurized scrambled egg mix (approximately 230 kcal). The scrambled egg meal containing ^{13}C-Spirulina is ground into particles of 1–2 mm in the stomach, allowing passage through the pylorus into the duodenum. In the upper small intestine, the ^{13}C-labeled Spirulina digest (proteins, carbohydrates, fats) is absorbed, metabolized, and excreted as ^{13}C-labeled carbon dioxide ($^{13}CO_2$) in the breath. Breath samples collected in capped glass tubes before and after the test meal are analyzed using gas isotope ratio mass spectrometry (GIRMS) to determine the ratio of $^{13}CO_2$ to $^{12}CO_2$ in each sample. By comparing pre-meal values and measuring the temporal changes in this ratio, the $^{13}CO_2$ excretion rate is calculated, determining the individual's gastric emptying rate. The gastric emptying rate is proportional to the $^{13}CO_2$ excretion rate at any given measurement time t. The results of the Cairn GEBT are reported using the metric "kPCD." At any measurement time t, $kPCD(t) = 1000 \times$ [percentage of the ^{13}C dose (PCD) excreted per minute as $^{13}CO_2$ from the test meal]. Higher kPCD values indicate faster $^{13}CO_2$ excretion rates and faster gastric emptying rates. The test results are displayed as a $^{13}CO_2$ excretion curve, showing the temporal excretion rate (kPCD/min). An increase in the $^{13}CO_2$ excretion rate (kPCD/min) reflects an increase in the gastric emptying rate.

2 Conclusion

Currently, there are no insurance-covered gastric emptying tests in Japan. The ^{13}C breath test for gastric emptying is noteworthy for its non-invasive and simple implementation. However, the test methods vary by each facility, and differences in test meals, measurement points, and reference values make direct comparison of results between facilities challenging. Recently, standardized methods such as GEBT have been adopted, but multiple breath sampling points and prolonged subject restraint time pose challenges for widespread clinical use. Future efforts should focus on further standardizing and simplifying the test methods and achieving insurance coverage.

Take-Home Message

The ^{13}C breath test for gastric emptying primarily uses ^{13}C-octanoic acid for solid test meals and ^{13}C -acetic acid for liquid test meals as labeled compounds. After ingesting the test meal mixed with ^{13}C-labeled compounds, the ^{13}C-labeled compounds are not absorbed from the stomach but are absorbed from the small intestine after gastric emptying, appearing in the breath via systemic circulation. By examining the temporal changes in the presence ratio of $^{13}CO_2$ in the breath, gastric emptying can be measured. The ^{13}C method is simple, non-invasive, non-radioactive, and drug-free, making it highly anticipated in clinical practice. However, it is not yet covered by insurance in Japan, limiting its routine use.

Competing Interests The author(s) has no competing interests to declare that are relevant to the content of this manuscript.

References

1. Arai E, et al. Subthalamic deep brain stimulation can improve gastric emptying in Parkinson's disease. Brain. 2012;135(Pt 5):1478–85.
2. Camilleri M, et al. ACG Clinical Guideline: Gastroparesis. Am. J. Gastroenterol. 117:1197–1220, 2022.
3. Ghoos YF, et al. Measurement of gastric emptying rate of solids by means of a carbon-labeled octanoic acid breath test. Gastroenterology. 1993;104:1640–7.
4. Sanaka M, et al. The Wagner-Nelson method makes the [^{13}C]-breath test comparable to radioscintigraphy in measuring gastric emptying of a solid/liquid mixed meal in humans. Clin Exp Pharmacol Physiol. 2007;34(7):641–4.
5. Nakada K, et al. The report of the workshop entitled "The present and the future in gastric emptying study assessed by ^{13}C breath test -with special reference to the standardization of the method-" at the 44th Annual Meeting of the Japanese Smooth Muscle Society. J Smooth Muscle Res (Jpn Sec.) 2002;6(3):J75–91. (in Japanese).
6. Mori H, et al. Gender difference of gastric emptying in healthy volunteers and patients with functional dyspepsia. Digestion. 2017;95:72–8.
7. Matsuzaki J, et al. Influence of regular exercise on gastric emptying in healthy men: a pilot study. J Clin Biochem Nutr. 2016;59:130–3.
8. DiBaise JK, et al. Effects of low doses of erythromycin on the ^{13}C Spirulina platensis gastric emptying breath test and electrogastrogram: a controlled study in healthy volunteers. Am J Gastroenterol. 2001;96:2041–50.
9. Szarka LA, et al. A stable isotope breath test with a standard meal for abnormal gastric emptying of solids in the clinic and in research. Clin Gastroenterol Hepatol. 2008;6:635–643e1.

25 Gastroduodenal Motility Test, Gastric Emptying Test, Acetaminophen Method

Masashi Matsushima

Abstract

Acetaminophen method is a representative one among the indirect methods for evaluating the gastric motility. Although the method has become rarely used in recent years, understanding its principles, advantages, and disadvantages remains valuable for better understanding of other gastric emptying tests.

Keywords

Acetaminophen · Gastric motility · Paracetamol absorption test · Liquid diet · Gastric emptying

Functional gastrointestinal disorders (FGIDs), particularly functional dyspepsia (FD), necessitate the evaluation of gastric storage capacity, gastric and duodenal visceral perception, and gastric emptying, which are considered critical components of the disorders. The gold standard for assessing gastric emptying is gastric emptying scintigraphy. However, the handling of radioisotopes is cumbersome, involves radiation exposure (albeit minimal), is costly, and requires a gamma camera, making it a challenging and uncommon test in routine practice. Direct methods for evaluating gastric contents include ultrasound and non-radiopaque marker methods. Conversely, indirect methods reflect the absorption of administered substances or metabolites from the duodenum. Among these indirect methods, the acetaminophen method (also known as the paracetamol absorption test) has been utilized for a long time and is primarily employed to relatively easily evaluate liquid gastric emptying [1].

Indirect methods involve the oral administration of drugs that are minimally absorbed in the stomach and rapidly absorbed below the duodenum, with monitoring of blood concentrations to evaluate gastric emptying. Acetaminophen is considered to be rapidly absorbed from the small intestinal mucosa, and although it is somewhat absorbed from the gastric intestinal metaplasia mucosa, the absorption in the stomach is negligible compared to the surface area of the small intestinal mucosa. Even in mild malabsorption syndromes, absorption in the duodenum and small intestinal mucosa is not affected [2]. Acetaminophen absorbed into the bloodstream is conjugated with glucuronic acid in the liver and excreted into bile or sulfated and phosphorylated in the kidneys and excreted in urine. Clinically, acetaminophen is frequently used as an analgesic and antipyretic, and although acute toxicity may occur with high doses exceeding 7.5 g/day in adults, the approximately 1.5 g used in this mea-

M. Matsushima (✉)
Department of Internal Medicine (Gastroenterology), Tokai University School of Medicine, Isehara, Japan
e-mail: mmatsush@tokai.ac.jp

H. Kaneko et al. (eds.), *Disorders of Gut-Brain Interaction*,
https://doi.org/10.1007/978-981-95-6974-8_25

surement method is extremely safe and does not have the gastrointestinal mucosal damaging effects seen with non-steroidal anti-inflammatory drugs (NSAIDs). The basic interpretation of the results is based on the temporal blood plasma acetaminophen concentration after administration. If the peak concentration is high or the peak value is reached early, gastric emptying capacity is considered to be enhanced. Conversely, if the peak concentration is low or the peak value is reached late, gastric emptying capacity is considered to be reduced [3].

Postprandial gastric emptying dynamics differ significantly between solid and liquid meals, the latter being emptied more quickly [2]. In healthy individuals, food intake causes relaxation of the gastric fundus (adaptive relaxation), and the ingested food is temporarily stored in this area. Subsequently, liquid components are sequentially emptied from the stomach, while solid food remains in the gastric fundus until most of the liquid is emptied. Strong peristaltic waves (approximately 3 times per minute) originating from pacemaker cells in the upper body move, mix, and grind the solid food in the body and antrum before it is emptied through the pylorus. Although this measurement method is primarily applied to liquid meals, it can also be applied to semi-solid meals.

The original method was reported by Heading et al. in 1973, and its correlation with the gold standard radioisotope method has been verified [3]. After overnight fasting, 1.5 g of acetaminophen is taken with 50 mL of water, with no liquid intake for 2 hours and no food or smoking for 3 hours, followed by blood sampling over 11 hours. Using the obtained plasma, acetaminophen concentration is measured by gas-liquid chromatography. The results showed that the gastric content half-life by the RI method inversely correlated with the peak of plasma acetaminophen concentration and positively correlated with the peak of plasma acetaminophen concentration time.

In Japan, Harasawa et al. introduced and disseminated this method [4]. Harasawa's method uses a semi-liquid meal (OKUNOS-A) with approximately 1 cal/mL as the test meal, and after ingestion with 1.5 g, or 20 mg/kg body weight of acetaminophen, the 45-minute value, which shows the peak or near-peak plasma acetaminophen concentration in many cases, is adopted. This method does not require frequent blood sampling as in the original method, has a shorter test time, and is relatively easy and convenient, leading to widespread use. Additionally, the dye method using 2,2-diphenyl-1-picrylhydrazyl dye has been introduced alongside the HPLC method for measuring acetaminophen. The 45-minute value later showed a good correlation (R value −0.877) with the gold standard RI method [2, 5] (Table 25.1, Fig. 25.1).

In the late 1990s, simulation analysis based on pharmacokinetic theory was used to examine the validity of adopting the 45-minute value [6]. Harasawa's method of single blood sampling at 45 minutes is ideal for screening due to its simplicity and low cost, but there was debate about whether it was inferior to the accuracy of indicators based on multiple blood samples. Acetaminophen reaching the duodenum at a constant rate from the stomach is rapidly absorbed according to the first-order rate constant (Ka), partially metabolized by the liver's first-pass effect, and the remainder (indicating F bioavailability) reaches the systemic circulation,

Table 25.1 A protocol of the acetaminophen absorption test

1. Test Meal[a], mix 1.5 g of acetaminophen or 20 mg/kg with 200 mL of room temperature liquid and stir well.
2. If performing periodic blood sampling, leave the indwelling needle in place after the initial blood draw before the test begins.
3. Administer the test meal orally in the early morning on an empty stomach (no smoking), in a seated position.
4. Maintain a seated position and abstain from food and drink until the test is completed.
5. Perform heparinized venous blood sampling at 45 min (optionally at 15, 30, and 60 min).
6. Centrifuge at 3000 cpm, store plasma components at −20 °C until measurement.

[a]The test meal used is semi-liquid OKUNOS-A (Horinouchi Canning Co., now Horika Foods Co., Niigata, Japan), with a composition similar to the currently sold thick liquid food "Liquid Food A" by the same company: 1 cal/mL (protein 4.8%, fat 2.3%, carbohydrate 15%).

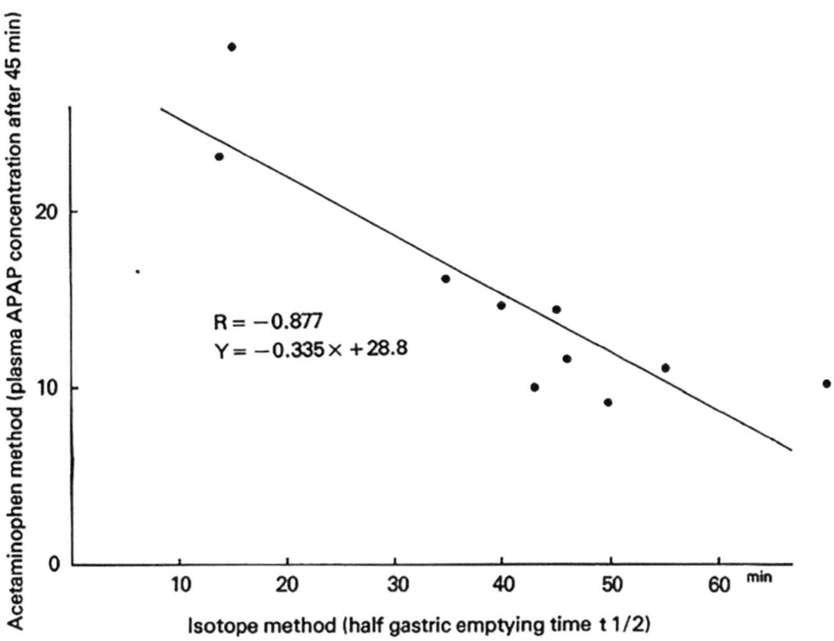

Fig. 25.1 Correlation between the acetaminophen method (45-min value) and the radioisotope method. (Adapted from Reference [5], Figure 1)

distributing to body tissues (Vd) and reaching equilibrium with the systemic circulation, then disappearing from the body according to another first-order rate constant (Kel). The theoretical formula for C45 (acetaminophen 45-minute value) in this model includes Ka, Kel, Vd, and F, and is affected not only by $T_{1/2}$ (half-life) but also by individual differences. When these parameters are varied within a certain range, particularly in cases of gastric emptying enhancement with $T_{1/2}$ less than 0.3 hours, two corresponding $T_{1/2}$ values are theoretically obtained for the C45 value, resulting in unreliable outcomes. On the other hand, in cases of delayed gastric emptying, a certain correlation was recognized despite errors, suggesting that the C45 single blood sampling method is appropriate for screening delayed gastric emptying. Additionally, the validity of other indicators requiring frequent blood sampling, such as C_{max}/AUC (∞), AUC (t)/AUC (2.0), and those requiring only two blood samples, such as C (0.5)/C (0.25) and C (1.0)/C (0.5), has been suggested. The latter two are considered promising due to the practicality of fewer blood samples, but the lack of comparison with the gold standard RI method remains an issue.

Considering the appropriate indicators for this method comprehensively, although there are concerns about its application to cases with extremely enhanced gastric emptying, C45 single blood sampling method would be useful for screening purposes and certain types of analyses in which individual differences can be minimized such as analyzing certain trends between groups and changes before and after interventions.

Take-Home Message

Although the acetaminophen method has become rarely used in recent years, understanding its principles, advantages, and disadvantages remains valuable for better understanding of other gastric emptying tests.

Competing Interests The author(s) has no competing interests to declare that are relevant to the content of this manuscript.

References

1. Inamori M, et al. Measurement methods for gastrointestinal motility. J Jpn Soc Gastroenterol. 2019;116:801–8. (in Japanese).
2. Hasebe T, et al. V. Observation of changes accompanying content movement (1) Acetaminophen. In: Hongo M, editor. Introduction to clinical measurement methods for gastrointestinal motility. Kyowa Kikaku Tsushin; 1996. (in Japanese).
3. Heading RC, et al. The dependence of paracetamol absorption on the rate of gastric emptying. Br J Pharmacol. 1973;47:415–21.
4. Harasawa S, et al. Gastric emptying in normal subjects and patients with peptic ulcer, a study using the acetaminophen method. Gastroenterologia Japonica. 1979;14:1–10.
5. Harasawa S, et al. Gastric emptying in patients with gastric ulcers—effects of oral and intramuscular administration of anticholinergic drug. Tokai J Exp Clin Med. 1982;7:551–9.
6. Sanaka M, et al. Guide for judicious use of the paracetamol absorption technique in a study of gastric emptying rate of liquid. J Gastroenterol. 1998;33:785–91.

Gastroduodenal Motility Test, Gastric Emptying Test, Ultrasonographic Method

26

Hiroaki Kusunoki, Ken Haruma, Noriaki Manabe, Tomoari Kamada, and Jiro Hata

Abstract

Ultrasound is a non-invasive, relatively simple, and repeatable method for examining gastrointestinal motility. We devised a method using consommé soup as a liquid test meal and oyakodon (chicken and egg rice bowl) as a solid test meal to evaluate upper gastrointestinal function using a number of parameters, including proximal gastric distension, gastric emptying, antral motility, and duodenal reflux. This chapter introduces the method and some of the results. Ultrasound has great potential for the future, as it can be used with a variety of test meals and can also evaluate the lower gastrointestinal tract.

Keywords

Ultrasonography (US) · Gastrointestinal motility · Gastric accommodation reflex (GAR) · Motility index (MI) · Duodenogastric reflux (DGR)

1 Ultrasound Method

Extracorporeal ultrasound (US) is a noninvasive, direct method for assessing gastrointestinal contents. Taking advantage of its real-time nature, we have evaluated gastroduodenal motility using a variety of indices, including gastric emptying, antral motility, and duodenogastric reflux (DGR), and have used it in general clinical practice. Any food can be used as a test meal as long as it can be visualized by US immediately after ingestion. However, we use consommé soup as the liquid test meal and Oyakodon (chicken and egg rice bowl) as the solid test meal [1–10, 12, 14]. Consommé soup can be prepared by simply dissolving a standard, commercially available cube-type soup base in 400 ml of hot water. Oyakodon can also be prepared by simply pouring the pre-packaged Oyakodon base, which is available in

H. Kusunoki (✉)
Junpukai Health Maintenance Center Kurashiki, Okayama, Japan

K. Haruma
Department of General Internal Medicine, Kawasaki Medical School General Medical Center, Okayama, Japan
e-mail: kharuma@med.kawasaki-m.ac.jp

N. Manabe
Division of Endoscopy and Ultrasonography, Department of Clinical Laboratory Medicine, Kawasaki Medical School, Okayama, Japan
e-mail: n_manabe@med.kawasaki-m.ac.jp

T. Kamada
Department of Health Care Medicine, Kawasaki Medical School General Medical Center, Okayama, Japan
e-mail: tkamada@med.kawasaki-m.ac.jp

J. Hata
Department of General Medicine, Kawasaki Medical School, Kurashiki, Japan
e-mail: ultrajiro@nifty.com

H. Kaneko et al. (eds.), *Disorders of Gut-Brain Interaction*,
https://doi.org/10.1007/978-981-95-6974-8_26

retort pouches, over packaged rice. Therefore, both test meals can be reproducibly prepared.

The consommé soup we use contains lipids and amino acids, but does not excessively stimulate chemoreceptors. Therefore, it does not induce a gastric inhibitory response (duodenal brake phenomenon) in healthy subjects, and impaired accommodation reflex of the proximal stomach and/or disturbed antral contractions are not observed. However, many patients with functional dyspepsia (FD) exhibit motility dysfunctions that are thought to be the cause of their symptoms (Figs 26.1 and 26.2). Therefore, this test meal can detect various motility differences between FD and healthy subjects (Table 26.1). We currently evaluate gastroduodenal motility using four items: gastric accommodation reflex (GAR) of the proximal stomach, gastric emptying rate (GER), antral contractions (motility index = MI), and duodenogastric reflux (DGR) , or five parameters, including fasting antral area (FAA; assessment of the fasting phase III contractions). We detect some or all of these disfunction in 62.5% of FD patients. However, these results also reflect the fact that, even with multiple parameters, no motility abnormalities are detected in 37.5% of FD patients. It seems difficult to explain the pathophysiology of all FD patients solely through gastrointestinal motility alone (Table 26.2). However, there are many cases in which changes in symptoms correlate with changes in motility dysfunctions. Therefore, gastroduodenal motility testing using US is considered to be extremely beneficial as a clinical approach for FD patients [1–12, 14]. However, because this test method uses a liquid test meal, the movement of contents is caused by a pres-

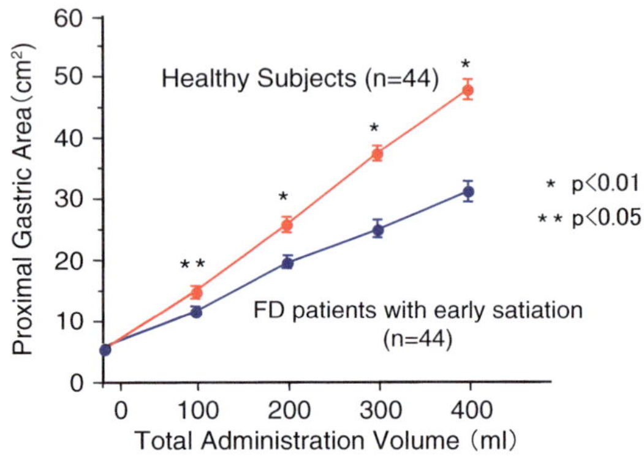

Fig. 26.1 Comparison of changes in the largest cross-sectional area of the proximal stomach after incremental administration of up to 400 ml of water between FD patients who experienced early satiation and healthy subjects: after administration of more than 100 ml water, FD patients showed impaired gastric accommodation reflex in comparison with the healthy subjects

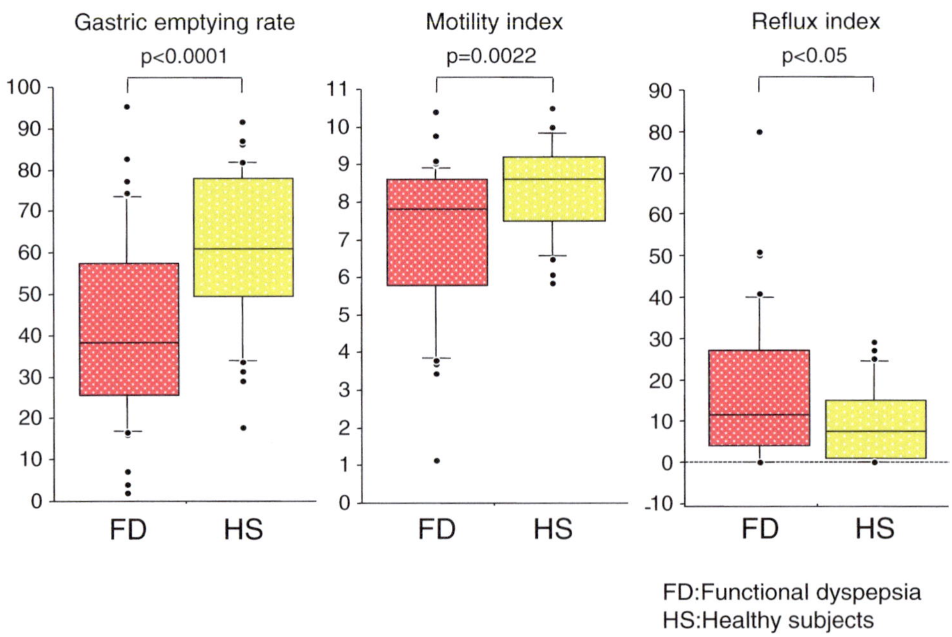

Fig. 26.2 Difference of the gastric motility in FD patients and healthy subjects

sure gradient between the stomach and duodenum. Gastric pressure is affected by factors such as proximal gastric distension, antral motility, and tonic contractions of the stomach wall, while duodenal pressure is affected by factors such as duodenal contraction and tonic contractions of the duodenal wall. Therefore, it is important to understand that evaluation parameters such as GER and DGR are indices that comprehensively evaluate multiple functions. In addition, to evaluate upper gastrointestinal motility, it is desirable to perform functional tests using not only liquid meals but also solid meals. In this chapter, we will present the actual method and results of our ultrasonographic assessment of upper gastrointestinal motility.

Table 26.1 Difference in gastric motility between FD patients and healthy subjects

	HS ($n = 80$)	FD ($n = 80$)
Antral contractions (number of contractions per 3 min)	9.6 ± 0.1	9.3 ± 0.1
Amplitude (area relaxed - area contracted) × 100 / area relaxed (%)	81.7 ± 1.7	65.0 ± 2.5*
Motility index (mean amplitude × antral contractions)	7.9 ± 0.2	6.1 ± 0.3*
Gastric emptying rate (antral cross-sectional area at 1 min after sitting - area at 15 min) × 100 / cross - sectional area at 1 min (%)	63.9 ± 1.7	43.0 ± 2.2*
Duodenogastric reflux (number. of DGR per 5 min × distance of the color signals from the pyloric ring)	1.9 ± 0.2	5.5 ± 3.8*

FD Functional dyspepsia, *HS* Healthy subjects
mean ± SE
*$p < 0.01$:(Mann-Whitney U test)

Table 26.2 Prevalence of motility disorders in patients with FD

Function of fasting gastric motility (Dysfunction of phase III contractions)	26.7%
Liquid meal test	
1. Delayed gastric emptying 2. Decreased motility index (Dysfunction of antral contractions) 3. Increased reflux index (DGR↑)	1. 44.6% 2. 20.8% 3. 24.4%
Solid meal test	
Delayed gastric emptying Antral dysfunction in the early postprandial phase	53.3% 33.3%
Dysfunction of the accommodation reflex	77.3% of FD patients with early satiety

1.1 Fasting Antral Area (FAA)

In the fasting period, we evaluated the antral contraction and confirmed that the stomach was in phase I. Then, we fixed the ultrasound probe on a plane where the abdominal aorta, superior mesenteric artery, and antrum were simultaneously visualized (Fig. 26.3), and measured the cross-sectional area of the antrum. The FAA was encircled on the mucosal side of the antrum with the built-in caliper, and the area calculated automatically. Hausken et al. reported that patients with FD have, on average, a significantly larger antrum area than healthy controls [11]. Our results are entirely consistent with their report (Fig. 26.4). We also reported that healthy subjects have significantly smaller antrum area on average after phase III than before phase III (Fig. 26.5). We therefore have reason to believe that the enlarged FAA in FD might be related to fasting phase III dysfunction.

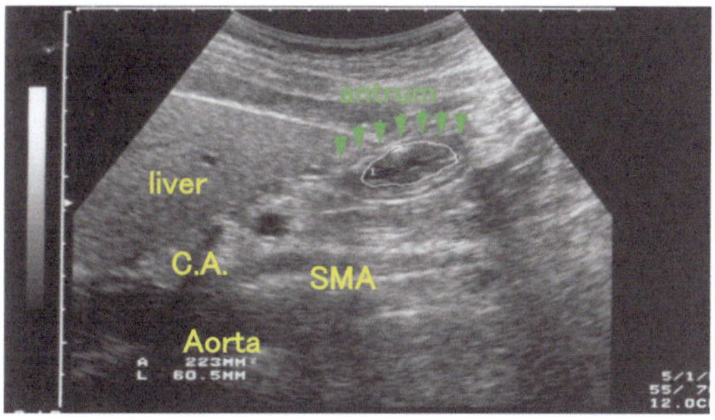

Fig. 26.3 Image of the FAA. An ultrasound probe was positioned vertically to permit simultaneous visualization of the antrum, the superior mesenteric artery, and the abdominal aorta

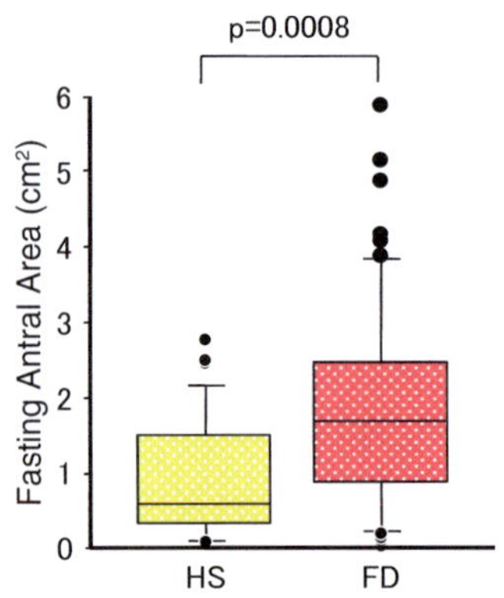

Fig. 26.4 Difference in FAA between healthy subjects and FD patients. FAA of healthy subjects was smaller than that of FD patients

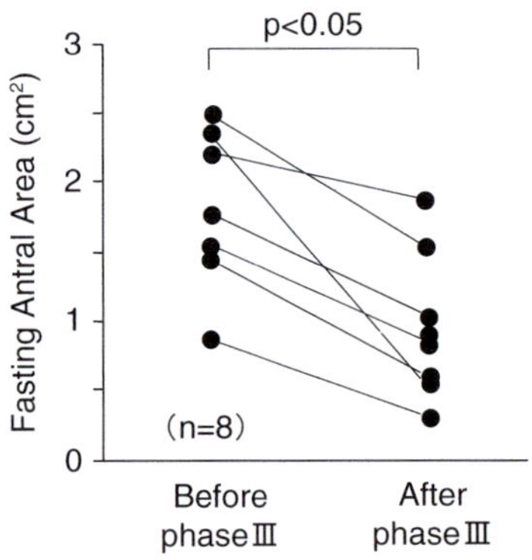

Fig. 26.5 FAA (before phase III vs after phase III). FAA decreased significantly after phase III contractions

1.2 Gastric Motility Test (Liquid Test Meal)

1.2.1 Preparations

1. Ultrasound instrument with Doppler,
2. 1 cube of consommé soup base (Ajinomoto Co., Ltd., Japan),
3. Measuring cup that can measure 400 mL,
4. Paper cup that can measure 100 mL,
5. Flexible straw,
6. Ultrasound image recording paper and image printer

1.2.2 Procedure

- Dissolve one cube of consommé soup base in hot water to prepare a 400 mL liquid test meal (0.38 g protein, 0.25 g fat, 2.3 g sugar per serving, 3.25 kcal /100 mL; Ajinomoto) at 37 °C (Fig. 26.6).
  Ultrasound instruments used included curved array scanners with a 3.75 or 5 MHz transducer (Aplio: Canon Medical Systems, Nasu, Japan).
- Measure the cross-sectional area of the antrum in the fasting state with the patient in a sitting position, using the abdominal aorta and superior mesenteric artery as landmarks (Fig. 26.3).
- Have the subject lie supine on the bed. An ultrasound probe is fixed between the ribs in the left axilla, and the cross-sectional area of the proximal stomach during fasting is measured using the spleen as a window (Fig. 26.7).
- The subject was asked to drink 100 mL of the test meal (total volume 400 mL) four times using a straw while lying supine (Fig. 26.8), and the cross-sectional area of the proximal stomach was measured for each intake. Measurements were taken when the area reached a steady state (1 min after the end of drinking) (Fig. 26.9).
- After approximately 1 min with the subject in a seated position (Fig. 26.10), the ultrasound probe is placed in a position that allows simultaneous visualization of the abdominal aorta and superior mesenteric artery, and the cross-sectional area of the antrum is measured (Fig. 26.11).
- A probe was placed at a position within 3 cm of the pyloric ring where the contraction could be visualized concentrically, and the antral contraction rate and number of contractions were measured over a 3-min period. The product of these values was used as the MI (Motility Index). The contraction rate was calculated from the difference in the cross-sectional area of the antrum at maximum relaxation and maximum contraction (Fig. 26.12).
- The ultrasound probe was fixed in a position that allowed simultaneous visualization of the gastric antrum, pyloric ring, and duodenal bulb, and the movement of contents through the pyloric ring was observed using ultrasound Doppler. The RI (Reflux Index) was calculated by multiplying the distance traveled

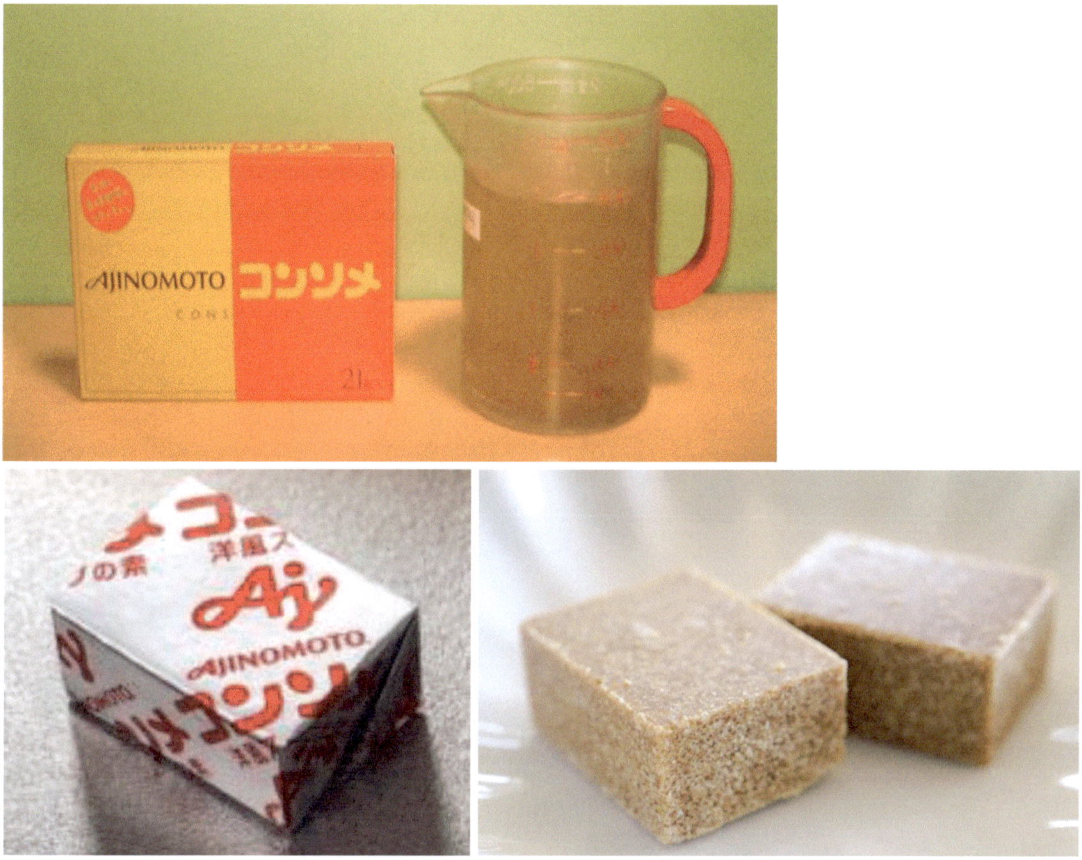

Fig. 26.6 A liquid test meal; 400 mL of consommé soup

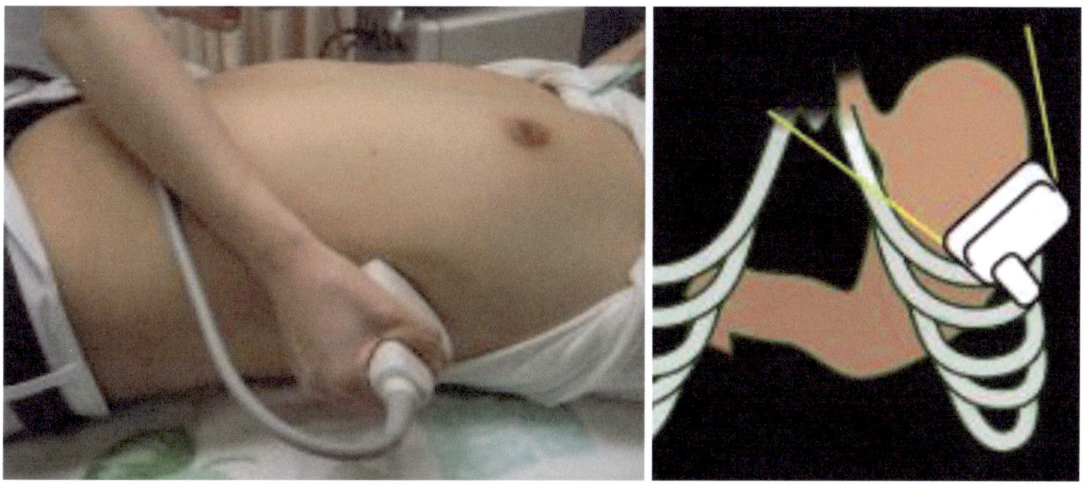

Fig. 26.7 The position of US probe to obtain the cross-sectional area of the proximal stomach. The probe was positioned and maintained in an intercostal space of the left axilla

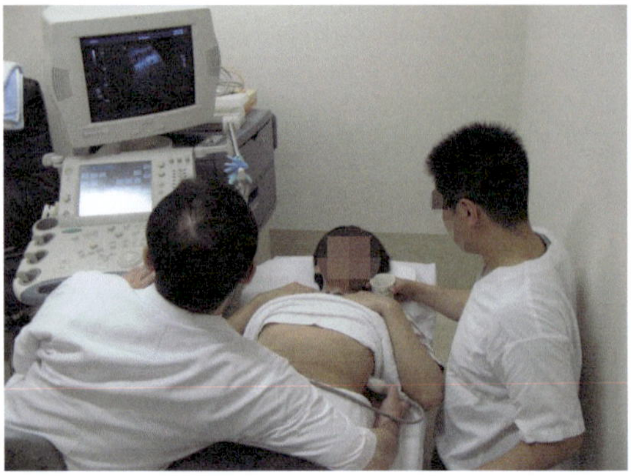

Fig. 26.8 The cross-sectional area of the proximal stomach was measured with the subjects lying on a bed in the supine position

from the pyloric ring by the number of times the reflux signal appeared over a 5-min period (Fig. 26.13).

- After approximately 15 min with the subject in a seated position, the ultrasound probe is again placed in a position where the abdominal aorta and superior mesenteric artery can be visualized simultaneously, and the cross-sectional area of the gastric antrum is measured. This is compared with the value measured approximately 1 min after the subject has been seated, and the excretion rate is calculated from the difference in area (Fig. 26.14).
- Record all images on media.

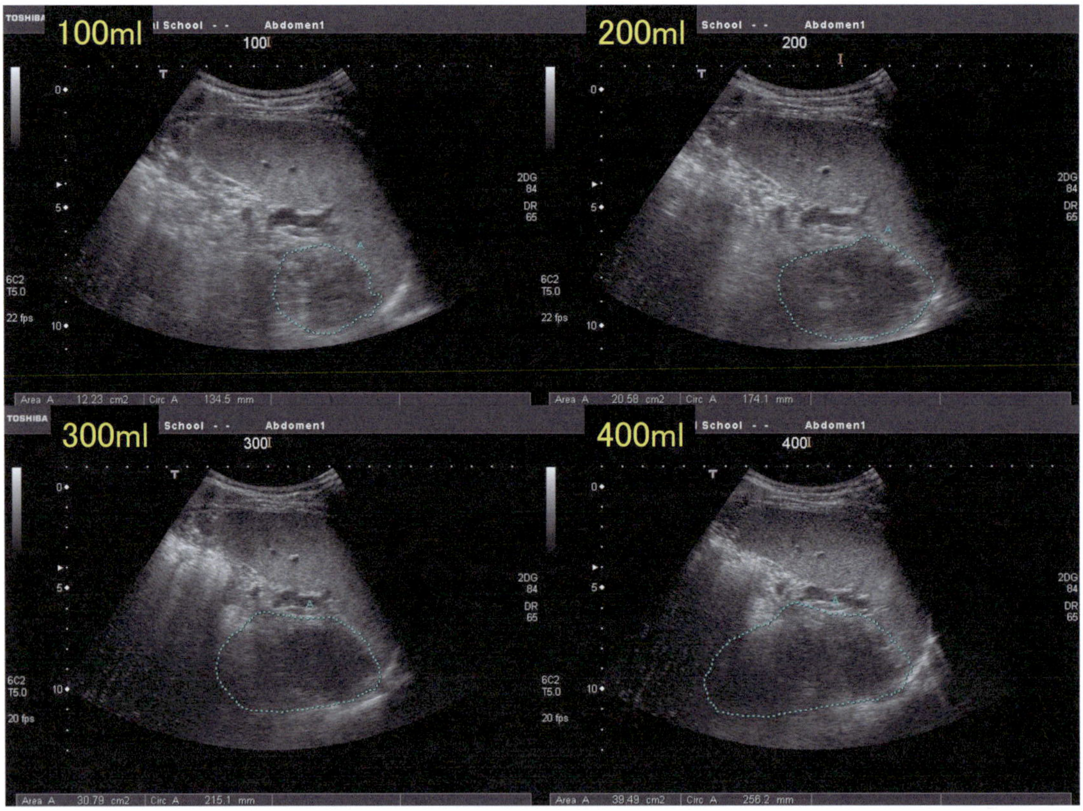

Fig. 26.9 Changes in the US images of the largest cross-sectional area of the proximal stomach after incremental ingestion of up to 400 mL of consommé soup via a straw

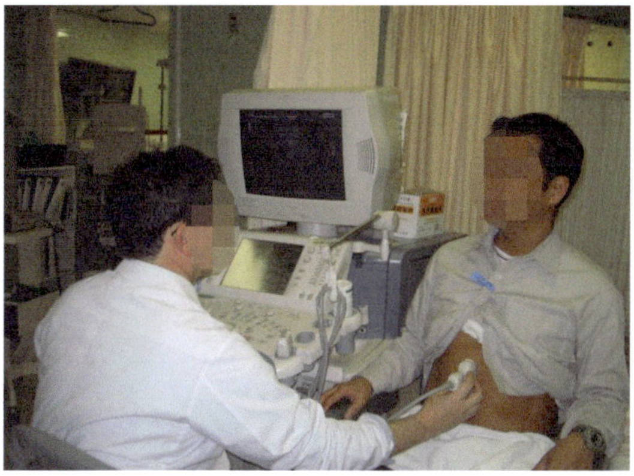

Fig. 26.10 Subjects sat in a chair

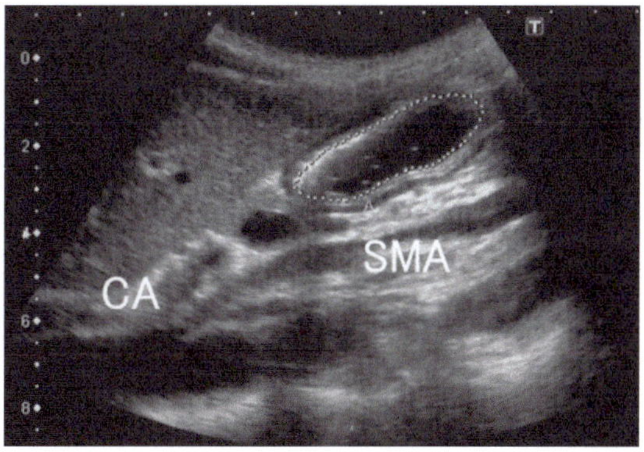

Fig. 26.11 At 1 min after sitting, antral area was measured in the same method

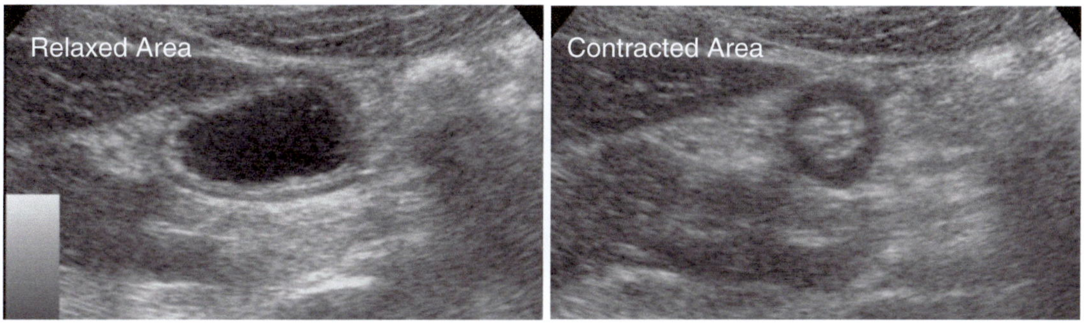

Fig. 26.12 The frequency of antral contractions was defined as the number of contractions per 3 min

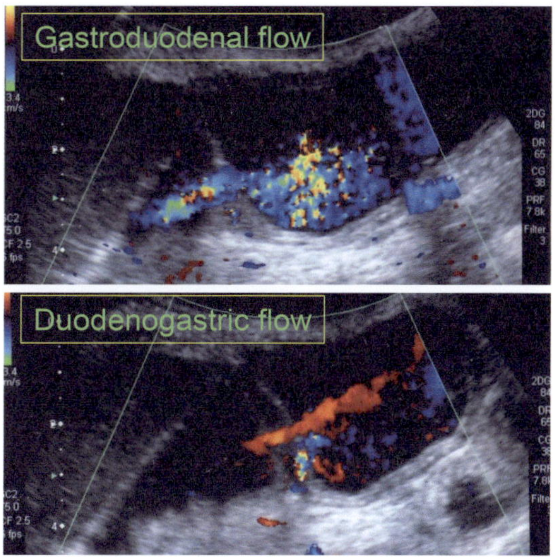

Fig. 26.13 The evaluation of duodenogastric reflux (DGR) with color Doppler ultrasonography

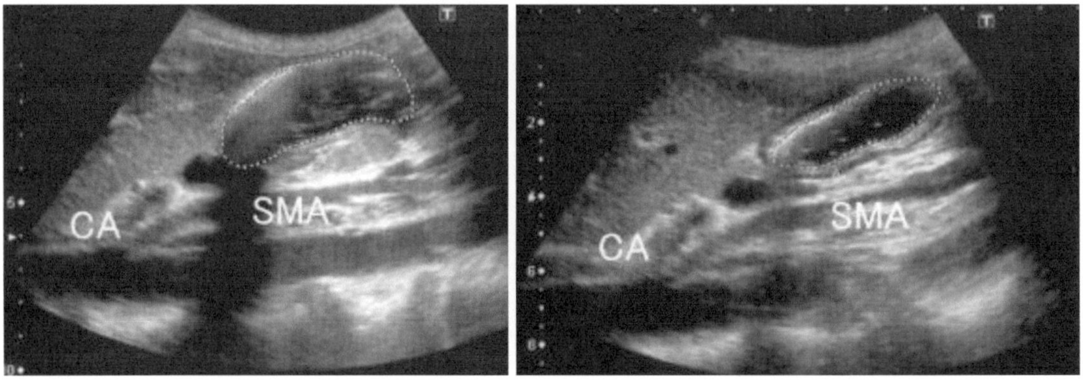

Fig. 26.14 At 15 min after sitting in a chair, the antral area was measured in the same method

1.2.3 Evaluation Items

- Fasting antral Area (FAA)
- Gastric accommodation reflex (GAR) : percent change in proximal gastric cross-sectional area after drinking 100 mL of water for a total of 400 mL.
- Gastric emptying rate (GER): percent change in antral cross-sectional area at 1 min and 15 min after sitting = (A1–A15) × 100/A1 (%)
  Antral cross-sectional area at 1 min after sitting = A1,
  Antral cross-sectional area 15 min after sitting = A15
- Motility index (MI) = contraction rate (%) × number of contractions per 3 min
  Contraction rate (%) = (relaxed area-contracted area) × 100 / relaxed area (%)
- Duodenogastric reflux (DGR) ; Reflux Index (RI) = number of reflux signals (DGR) per 5 min × distance of the color signals from the pyloric ring (cm)

2 Pharmacometrics Using This Method

Although the prevalence of FD is considerable, there are few effective treatments. We underwent pharmacometrics of some medicine. We introduce the results of two pharmacometrics (acotiamide and rikkunshito) from now on.

However, the pathophysiology of FD is heterogeneous; hence some effects on the pathophysiology of FD are needed in the treatment of FD. Therefore, we may have to provide treatment to regulate gastric acid and stress as well as gastrointestinal motility at the same time.

2.1 Acotiamide

Acotiamide, a prokinetic drug, has been available in Japan since 2013. The effect of acotiamide has been established in FD patients, especially in postprandial distress syndrome of FD [8, 12].

In our previous study, the significant difference in the expansion rate in the cross-sectional area of the proximal stomach between the acotiamide group and the placebo group after 400 ml ingestion of a liquid meal (Figs. 26.15 and 26.16). GER significantly accelerated after treatment in the acotiamide group although there was no significant change in the placebo group. However, no significant difference was observed in the MI and RI between the two groups. This observation suggests that acotiamide may be beneficial for FD patients with impaired GAR and delayed gastric emptying [8].

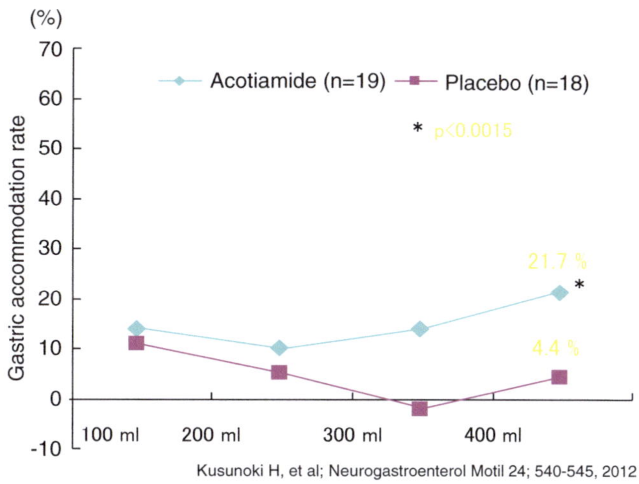

Fig. 26.15 The expansion rate in the cross-sectional area of the proximal stomach between the acotiamide group and the placebo group. There was a significant difference between the two groups after 400 mL ingestion of a liquid test meal

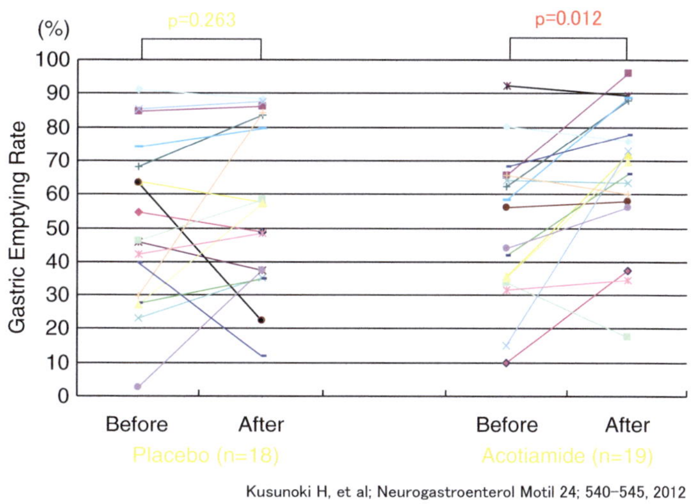

Fig. 26.16 The change in the GER between the acotiamide group and placebo group. GER significantly accelerated after treatment in the acotiamide group, though there was no significant change in the placebo group

2.2 Rikkunshito

A traditional herbal medicine, rikkunshito, has been identified as an effective drug against dyspeptic symptoms (gastric water indigestion = "Inai-teisui") and is widely used for therapy in patients with FD [7, 12, 13]. The percent change in the cross-sectional area of the proximal stomach was significantly greater after treatment with rikkunshito, than that before treatment (Fig. 26.17). Although, the gastric emptying rate and MI increased significantly, there were no significant difference in RI before and after treatment with rikkunshito (Fig. 26.18). This observation suggests that rikkunshito may be beneficial for FD patients with impaired meal-induced GAR and gastric dysmotility [7].

2.3 Gastric Motility Test (Solid Test Meal)

Solid test meal: Using Oyakodon as a solid test meal allows for the evaluation of the time required for complete gastric emptying, the gastric emptying curve, and antral contraction motility.

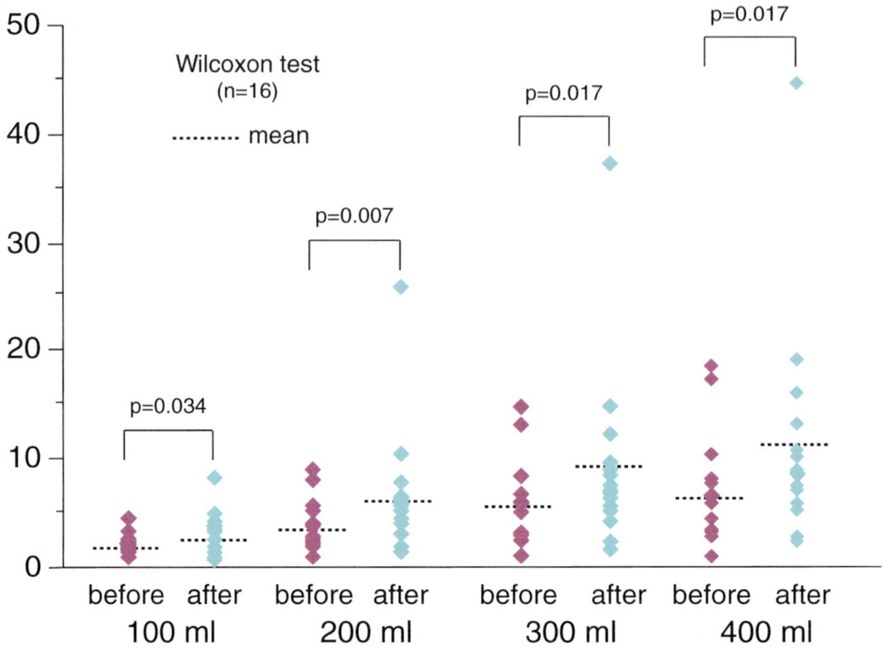

Fig. 26.17 GAR increased significantly after Rikkunshito treatment compared with before treatment

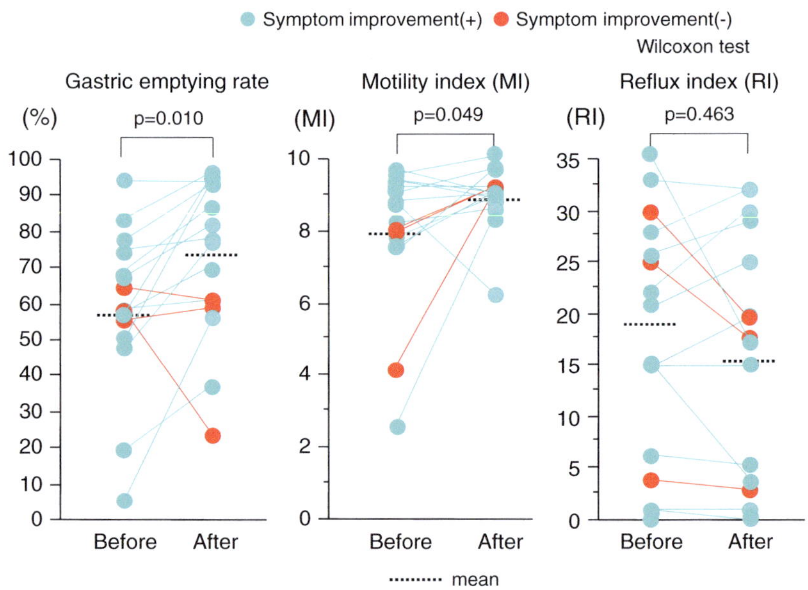

Fig. 26.18 Change in the GER, MI, and RI before and after treatment with Rikkunshito

However, because the distribution of the test meal in the stomach is not as simple as with a liquid meal, measurements of the cross-sectional areas of two locations—the gastric body and antrum—are required to estimate the residual volume of the test meal. The gastric emptying curve is calculated using the value of the antral cross-sectional area + the body cross-sectional area × 3 (Fig. 26.19), which has been confirmed to be nearly identical to the emptying curve obtained with scintigraphy. A drawback is that even with Oyakodon, complete emptying takes approximately 4 h, necessitating even longer observation periods in cases of delayed gastric

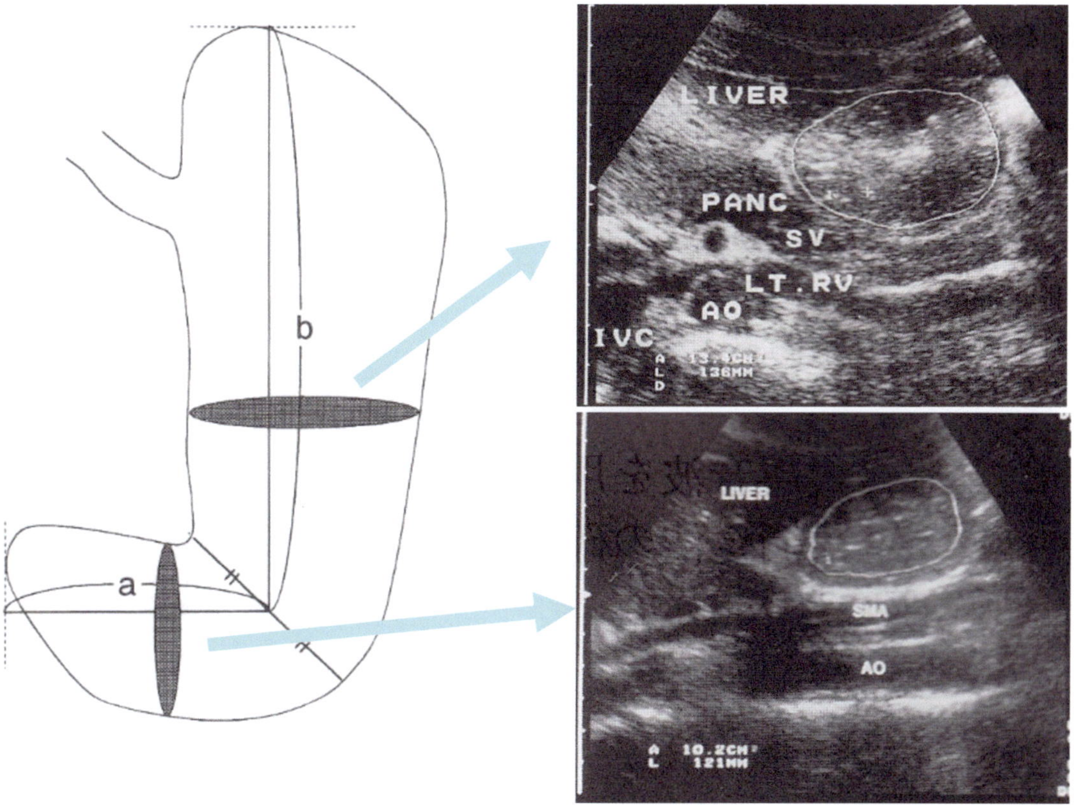

Fig. 26.19 Estimation of residual volume in the stomach after ingestion of a solid test meal (oyakodon). The gastric emptying curve calculated by multiplying the gastric body cross-sectional area by 3 and the antrum cross-sectional area was close to the gastric emptying curve calculated by RI

emptying [3, 14]. However, this method appears to be useful for diagnosing and evaluating the pathology of patients with delayed gastric emptying and gastroparesis, and because it is closer to the actual meal, it can provide more insight than a liquid meal. The gastric emptying kinetics of solid food after pulverization into a porridge are thought to be similar to that of liquid food. However, proximal gastric distension (proximal gastric retention) and antral contractility play a greater role in the process of porridge formation than liquid food, making solid food more useful for assessing these functions. We have reported that gastric emptying after liquid and solid food coincides in approximately 60% of cases (Table 26.3), and we believe that both tests should be performed when assessing gastrointestinal motility. The early antral contraction motility decreased after a solid meal (Fig. 26.20), which is not observed in healthy individuals but only in FD patients, is a phenomenon caused by decreased proximal gastric distension and the resulting abnormal gastric distribution, and is different from the decreased antral contraction mediated by the duodenal brake seen after liquid food administration.

Table 26.3 Incidence of delayed gastric emptying after liquid and solid test meals in FD patients

	Normal gastric emptying (Required)	Delayed gastric emptying (Required)
Normal gastric emptying (solid)	37.5%	21.9%
Delayed gastric emptying (solid)	20.3%	20.3%

Kusunoki et al. [3]

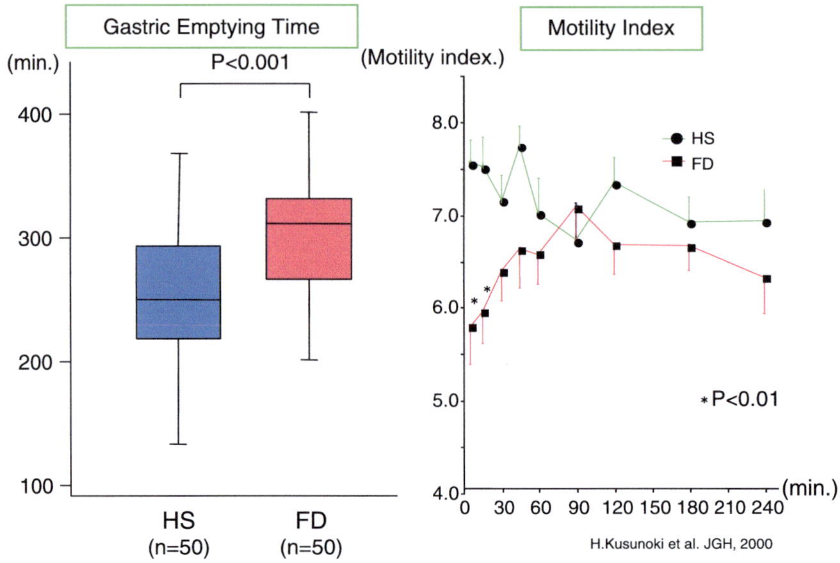

Fig. 26.20 Comparison of gastric emptying time and antral motility between healthy subjects and FD patients. Patients with FD had reduced early postprandial antral motility and delayed final gastric emptying

Competing Interests The author(s) has no competing interests to declare that are relevant to the content of this manuscript.

References

1. Fujimura J, et al. Quantitation of duodenogastric reflux and antral motility by color Doppler ultrasonography. Scand J Gastroenterol. 1994;29:897–902.
2. Okamoto E, et al. Effect of octreotide, a somatostatin analogue, on gastric function evaluated by real-time ultrasonography. Aliment Pharmacol Ther. 1997;11:177–84.
3. Kusunoki H, et al. Real-time ultrasonographic assessment of antroduodenal motility after ingestion of solid and liquid meals by patients with functional dyspepsia. J Gastroenterol Hepatol. 2000;15:1022–7.
4. Haruma K, et al. Real-time assessment of gastroduodenal motility by ultrasonography. Digestion. 2008;77(Suppl 1):48–51.
5. Kusunoki H, et al. Simple and non-invasive assessment of the accommodation reflex of the proximal stomach. J Smooth Muscle Res. 2010;46:249–58.
6. Kusunoki H, et al. Efficacy of mosapride citrate in proximal gastric accommodation and gastrointestinal motility in healthy volunteers. A double-blind placebo-controlled ultrasonographic study. J Gastroenterol. 2010;45:1228–34.
7. Kusunoki H, et al. Efficacy of Rikkunshito, a traditionam Japanese medicine (Kampo), in treating functional dyspepsia. Intern Med. 2010;49:2195–202.
8. Kusunoki H, et al. Therapeutic efficacy of acotiamide in patients with functional dyspepsia based on enhanced postprandial gastric accommodation and emptying: randamized controlled study evaluation by real-time ultrasonography. Neurogastroenterol Motil. 2012;24:540–e251.
9. Hasuo H, et al. Tolerable pain reduces gastric fundal accommodation and gastric motility in healthy subjects: a crossover ultrasonographic study. Biopsychosoc Med. 2017;11:4–10.
10. Yamanaka H. Establishment and clinical application of gastroduodenal motor function test using transabdominal ultrasound. Hiroshima J Med Sci. 1995;43:9–25. (in Japanese)
11. Hausken T, Berstat A. Wide gastric antrum in patients with non-ulcer dyspepsia. Effect of cisapride. Scand J Gastroenterol. 1992;27:427–32.
12. Tominaga K, Kusunoki H, editors. Functional dyspepsia. Springer Nature Singapore Pte Ltd.; 2018. p. 69–90.
13. Tominaga K, et al. Rikkunshito simultaneously improves dyspepsia correlated with anxiety in patients with functional dyspepsia: A randomized clinical trial (the DREAM study). Neurogastroenterol Motil. 2018;30(7):e13319.
14. Tani H. Establishment of gastric motility measurement method after solid meal loading using transabdominal ultrasound. Hiroshima J Med Sci. 1996;44:301–13.

Gastroduodenal Fuction Test, Mucosal Permeability Test

27

Makoto Arai

Abstract

In functional gastrointestinal disorders, it has become clear that duodenal mucosal permeability is related to the pathophysiology of the condition. Ussing chambers have been conventionally used as a standard method for evaluating mucosal permeability. Other methods include the Lactulose/D-Mannitol Test, evaluation of mRNA or protein levels of intercellular junction molecules, and evaluation of intercellular spaces using an electron microscope or a high-magnification endoscope. It has also become possible to measure the impedance and admittance values of the mucosa. Recently, instruments that evaluate admittance values in real time have also been developed. However, the relationship between duodenal mucosal permeability and symptom severity or therapeutic efficacy has not been sufficiently demonstrated. Various gastrointestinal mucosal permeability tests have been developed, and it is important to select the most appropriate testing method in full consideration of the situation (e.g., whether endoscopic examination is possible, whether tissue sampling can be performed, whether real-time evaluation is necessary).

Keywords

Permeability · Leakage · Ussing Chamber · Admittance · Impedance · Intercellular adhesion molecule · Intercellular space · Lactulose/D-Mannitol test

1 Introduction

In normal mucosa, gases, liquids, solutes, and ions permeation through cells or their surroundings. Permeation is also called as "permeability." Increased permeability from the vascular side to the gastrointestinal lumen can be referred to as "leakage." Some reports describe it as "leaky" due to the image of various substances leaking out when the mucosa becomes fragile. The Ussing chamber is considered the gold standard for evaluating mucosal permeability. However, as discussed later, there are issues with this method, and other evaluation methods are also widely used.

M. Arai (✉)
Department of Gastroenterology, Tokyo Women's Medical University Yachiyo Medical Center, Yachiyo, Japan
e-mail: arai.makoto@twmu.ac.jp

H. Kaneko et al. (eds.), *Disorders of Gut-Brain Interaction*,
https://doi.org/10.1007/978-981-95-6974-8_27

1.1 Duodenal Mucosal Permeability Test

1.1.1 Evaluation Using the Ussing Chamber

Devices such as those manufactured by Physiologic Instruments Inc. are used. The Ussing chamber system employs the short-circuit current method to electrophysiologically measure electrolyte transport across epithelial membranes. Theoretically, it is possible to evaluate any membrane. The method for testing using actual human gastrointestinal mucosa is explained (Fig. 27.1) [1]. Tissue is collected using biopsy forceps under endoscopy and sandwiched between a biopsy chamber and slider (aperture area 0.005 cm^2). Hank's balanced salt solution is maintained at a constant temperature (37 °C) in a water bath and oxygenated with O_2/CO_2 (95/5%) while filling the device. After stabilizing the equipment, transepithelial electric resistance (TEER) of the mucosa is measured. Measurements are taken within 10 minutes of biopsy collection, and the average value is obtained using multiple specimens. Another method involves adding fluorescein isothiocyanate (FITC)-dextran 4 high molecular weight (4 kDa) to one chamber and measuring the extent to which it migrates to the other chamber to evaluate permeability. TEER measurement has the advantage of being highly sensitive and capable of measuring rapid reactions in real time, compared to methods that use fluorescent dyes or isotopes. However, it is important to note that the actual electrolytes being transported are unknown, and the measurement is not an evaluation of the steady state since it measures electrolyte transport when a potential difference occurs. It has been reported that TEER is decreased and FITC-dextran permeability is increased in cases of Functional Dyspepsia (FD), and changes before and after proton pump inhibitor administration have also been examined [2, 3].

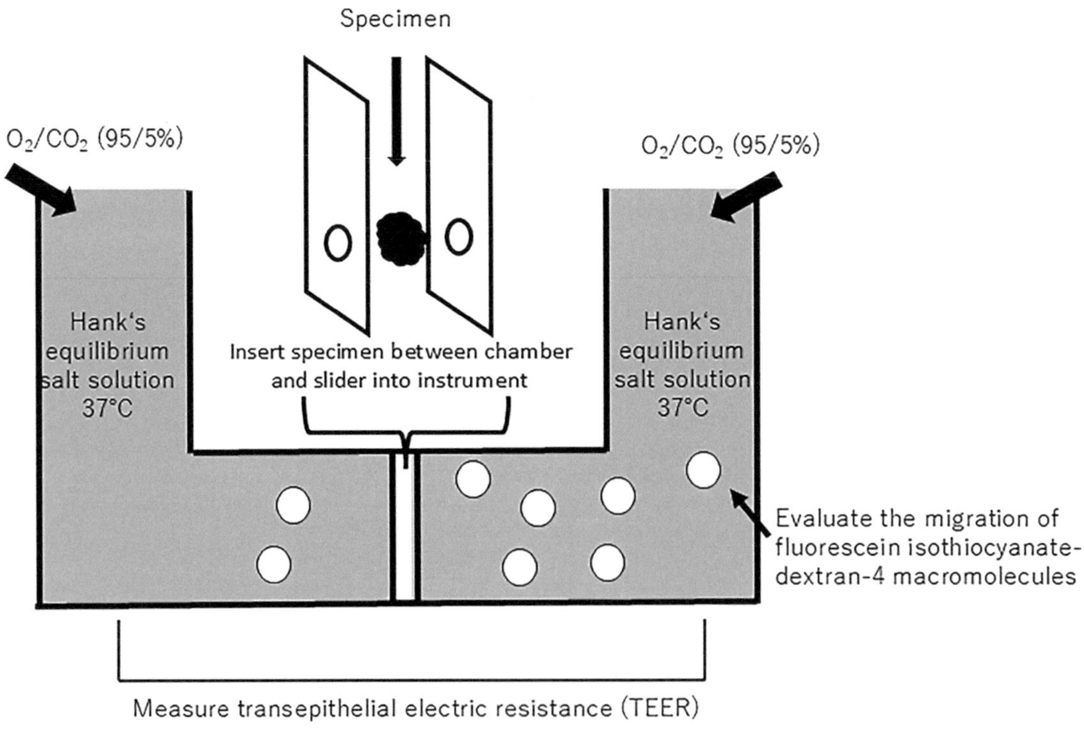

Fig. 27.1 Mucosal permeability test using the Ussing chamber

1.1.2 Lactulose/D-Mannitol Test

The ratio of lactulose to mannitol in urine is measured to evaluate small intestinal mucosal permeability. This test is considered to reflect gastric and duodenal permeability, particularly in the early time period (0–2 or 5 hours). D-mannitol, a smaller molecule, is absorbed via the transcellular uptake, while lactulose, a larger molecule, is absorbed via the paracellular uptake. Under physiological conditions, lactulose is minimally absorbed, but when cell junctions loosen and permeability increases, lactulose absorption increases, raising its concentration in urine and thus increasing the lactulose/mannitol ratio. During the test, after urination, the subject ingests a solution of 5 g lactulose and 2 g mannitol dissolved in 100 mL of water. Urine is collected during the early time period (0–2 or 5 hours) post-ingestion, and the lactulose/mannitol ratio is measured by high-performance liquid chromatography/mass spectrometry (HPLC/MS). A ratio of 0.07 or higher indicates increased permeability [4, 5]. However, it is unclear whether lactulose and mannitol truly have separate absorption pathways, and evaluating the permeability of molecules larger than lactulose (342 Da) is challenging.

1.1.3 mRNA and Protein Expression Analysis of Intercellular Adhesion Molecules

Intercellular adhesion is primarily composed of three major molecular and protein complexes: tight junctions (claudin, occludin, zonula occludens), adherens junctions (E-cadherin, α-, β-catenin), and desmosomes (desmoplakin, desmocollin, desmoglein), which maintain the barrier function of epithelial cells. Tight junction proteins are particularly thought to function primarily in intercellular permeability. The expression levels of tight junction proteins can be evaluated by Western blotting, immunohistochemistry, or quantitative PCR for mRNA expression. Recently, more detailed analyses using next-generation sequencers have become possible. However, it is still unclear whether the expression levels of these proteins directly affect mucosal permeability. Correlations between TEER or FITC-dextran permeability evaluation and the protein expression levels of occludin, E-cadherin, and β-catenin [2], as well as correlations between the mRNA expression levels of zonula occludens and impedancevalues, have been demonstrated [6].

1.1.4 Microscopy and Electron Microscopy

Electron microscopy analysis evaluates the widening of intercellular spaces as increased permeability. These evaluation results are reported to correlate with the results of FITC-dextran migration using the Ussing chamber and tight junction protein expression results [7, 8]. Microscopic observation methods include optical and confocal methods. The optical method, combining CCD and microscopic optics, allows ultra-magnified observation at the cellular and nuclear scale. In February 2018, Olympus released Endocytoscopy (Endocyto®), enabling detailed mucosal surface observation with promising future applications. The confocal method uses a confocal optical system that selectively images only the information at the focal point within living tissue. Mauna Kea Technologies released Confocal Laser Endomicroscopy (Cellvizio®), an endoscope capable of magnified observation at the cellular and nuclear scale. Although not covered by insurance for gastrointestinal use, fluorescein used in ophthalmology rapidly diffuses into the bloodstream and extravascular space after intravenous injection. Observing leakage from capillaries over time allows for the evaluation of gastrointestinal mucosal function. In cases of FD, reports have observed the widening of intercellular spaces and dye leakage [9].

1.1.5 Mucosal Admittance and Impedance

Multichannel intraluminal impedance (MII)-pH monitoring is useful for classifying the pathophysiology of refractory non-erosive reflux disease (NERD), and this device can measure baseline impedance (BI). Impedance indicates the resistance to current flow, with higher values indicating "firm" mucosa. Using this principle, Nakagawa et al. developed high-resolution manometry and impedance (HRM/Z) for the duodenum and small intestine, measuring BI in these areas. BI in the duodenum of FD patients was lower than in healthy individuals [10]. However, real-time measurement results are not obtained, and like esophageal evaluation, long-term device attachment and subsequent analysis are required. The Tissue Conductance Meter (TCM, Japan Ash Co.) can measure mucosal admittance values in real-time under endoscopy (Fig. 27.2). Admittance indicates the ease of current flow and is thought to indicate mucosal fragility. Therefore, admittance values are the inverse of impedance values. The actual measurement is explained. By attaching two applied electrodes to the skin, the low impedance area in the body is controlled to a constant voltage. Under endoscopy, the detection electrode (sensor) is pressed against the target mucosa. The sensor can be inserted and removed through the endoscope forceps channel and can be used with thin endoscopes such as transnasal endoscopes. The measurement time is approximately 0.5 seconds, making it very short. When pressing the sensor against the mucosa, it is necessary to keep the angle and pressure as constant as possible to reduce measurement variability. While some "practice" is required to stably press the sensor tangentially in the esophagus, in the stomach and duodenum, the sensor can be pressed vertically, reducing measurement variability. By contacting the detection electrode with the target mucosal surface, current flows through the mucosa from a constant voltage range to the detection electrode. This detection electrode current is easily affected by mucosa with high BI. The applied voltage is 25 mV, with low frequency (320 Hz) and high frequency (30.7 kHz). In normal mucosa, the intercellular spaces are narrow, and there is little extracellular fluid, so both frequency currents are less affected. In abnormal mucosa, the intercellular spaces are wider, and there is more extracellular fluid. Since extracellular fluid contains electrolytes, low-frequency current is greatly affected by ions and increases, while high-frequency current is less affected. Therefore, by measuring the conductance dependent on low-frequency and high-frequency currents and their differences, mucosal abnormalities are evaluated and quantified as admittance values. Generally, the relationship is current (I) × impedance (Z) = voltage (V), 1/Z = admittance (Y), Y = I/V, and since TCM uses a constant voltage, $Y = 1/Z \propto I$. Admittance values measured using TCM and TEER measured using the Ussing chamber show an inverse correlation, and admittance values are reported to be high in FD cases [1, 6].

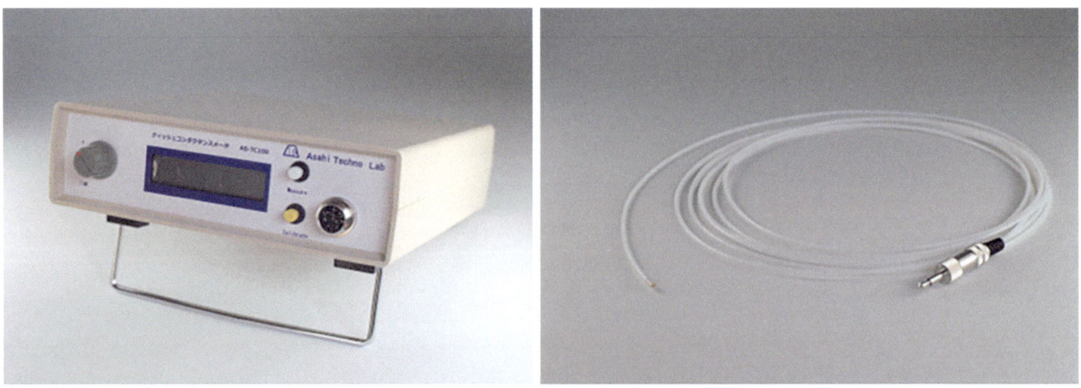

Machine body Detection electrode (sensor)

Fig. 27.2 Tissue conductance meter (main unit and detection electrode). (Provided by Japan Ash Co.)

Table 27.1 Duodenal mucosal permeability test

Evaluation items	Evaluation methods and equipment	Real-time	Endoscopy	Tissue sampling	Functional evaluation
TEER or migration of fluorescein isothiocyanate	Ussing Chamber	Not Possible	Required	Required	Possible
Absorption of lactulose and D-mannitol	Lactulose/D-Mannitol Test	Not Possible	Not needed	Not needed	Possible
Intercellular adhesion molecules, pyroptosis	mRNA and Protein Expression Analysis	Not Possible	Required	Required	Not Possible
Intercellular spaces	Electron microscopy	Not Possible	Required	Required	Not Possible
Intercellular spaces	Endocytoscopy	Possible	Required	Not needed	Not Possible
Leak of fluorescein	Confocal laser endomicroscopy	Possible	Required	Not needed	Possible
Mucosal Admittance	Tissue Conductance Meter	Possible	Required	Not needed	Possible
Mucosal Impedance	High-resolution manometry and impedance	Not Possible	Not needed	Not needed	Possible

TEER transepithelial electric resistance

2 Conclusion

The characteristics of each evaluation method are shown in Table 27.1. There are many reports on the relationship between duodenal mucosal permeability and functional gastrointestinal disorders, but further investigation is needed to determine which test method can serve as an objective indicator related to symptom severity. Currently, there are no test methods covered by Japanese government insurance for evaluating duodenal mucosal permeability. Therefore, at this stage, gastric and duodenal mucosal permeability tests should be conducted as clinical research rather than being directly applied in clinical practice.

Take-Home Message

In functional gastrointestinal disorders, it has become clear that duodenal mucosal permeability is related to the pathophysiology of the condition. However, the relationship between duodenal mucosal permeability and symptom severity or therapeutic efficacy has not been sufficiently demonstrated. Various gastrointestinal mucosal permeability tests have been developed, and it is important to select the most appropriate testing method in full consideration of the situation (e.g., whether endoscopic examination is possible, whether tissue sampling can be performed, whether real-time evaluation is necessary).

Competing Interests The author(s) has no competing interests to declare that are relevant to the content of this manuscript.

References

1. Ishigami H, et al. Endoscopy-guided evaluation of duodenal mucosal permeability in functional dyspepsia. Clin Transl Gastroenterol. 2017;8(4):e83.
2. Vanheel H, et al. Impaired duodenal mucosal integrity and low-grade inflammation in functional dyspepsia. Gut. 2014;63(2):262–71.
3. Wauters L, et al. Proton pump inhibitors reduce duodenal eosinophilia, mast cells, and permeability in patients with functional dyspepsia. Gastroenterology. 2021;160(5):1521–1531.e9.
4. Zhou Q, et al. MicroRNA-29a regulates intestinal membrane permeability in patients with irritable bowel syndrome. Gut. 2010;59(6):775–84.
5. Camilleri M, et al. Understanding measurements of intestinal permeability in healthy humans with urine lactulose and mannitol excretion. Neurogastroenterol Motil. 2010;22(1):e15–26.
6. Komori K, et al. The altered mucosal barrier function in the duodenum plays a role in the pathogenesis of functional dyspepsia. Dig Dis Sci. 2019;64(11):3228–39.
7. Tanaka F, et al. Concentration of glial cell line-derived neurotrophic factor positively correlates with symptoms in functional dyspepsia. Dig Dis Sci. 2016;61(12):3478–85.

8. Narayanan SP, et al. Duodenal mucosal barrier in functional dyspepsia. Clin Gastroenterol Hepatol. 2022;20(5):1019–1028.e3.
9. Nojkov B, et al. Evidence of duodenal epithelial barrier impairment and increased pyroptosis in patients with functional dyspepsia on confocal laser endomicroscopy and "Ex Vivo" mucosa analysis. Am J Gastroenterol. 2020;115(11):1891–901.
10. Nakagawa K, et al. Patients with dyspepsia have impaired mucosal integrity both in the duodenum and jejunum: in vivo assessment of small bowel mucosal integrity using baseline impedance. J Gastroenterol. 2020;55(3):273–80.

Part V

Stomach and Duodenum, Practical Edition

Diagnosis and Treatment of DGBI of the Stomach and Duodenum, Functional Dyspepsia

28

Akihito Nagahara

Abstract

This review explores Functional Dyspepsia (FD), a common disorder classified within FGIDs per Rome IV criteria. It discusses FD's epidemiology, multifactorial etiology—including gut-brain axis, microbiota, and microinflammation—clinical features, diagnostic approaches, and management strategies. Emphasizing lifestyle modification, pharmacotherapy (PPIs, acotiamide, Rikkunshito), and psychosocial support, the article highlights the chronic, recurrent nature of FD and the importance of patient-centered care. Recognizing the complexity of pathophysiology and overlapping subtypes, it underscores the need for thorough evaluation and tailored treatment to improve quality of life.

Keywords

Functional dyspepsia · Concept · Epidemiology · Pathophysiology · Treatment

A. Nagahara (✉)
Department of Gastroenterology, Juntendo University Faculty of Medicine, Tokyo, Japan
e-mail: nagahara@juntendo.ac.jp

1 Concept

Functional Dyspepsia (FD), which is included in functional gastrointestinal disorders (FGIDs), is globally defined and classified by the Rome Committee. The latest version is Rome IV, proposed in 2016. Dyspepsia, derived from Greek, translates directly to "indigestion" and has been used to describe upper abdominal symptoms induced by food intake. The fundamental symptoms of dyspepsia encompass postprandial discomfort and early satiety, with another major symptom being upper abdominal pain or epigastric burning, whether food-related or not. Accompanying symptoms may include flatulence, nausea, and excessive belching [1]. Heartburn may result from impaired adaptive relaxation of the gastric fundus, but as the concept of gastroesophageal reflux disease (GERD) becomes clearer, it is increasingly considered an esophageal symptom [2].

2 Epidemiology

A report by the Rome Committee investigating the global prevalence of FGIDs found that the proportion of individuals with one or more FGIDs was 40.3% in internet surveys and 20.7% in household surveys, with a higher prevalence in women (internet survey odds ratio, 1.7; 95% CI, 1.6–1.7; household survey odds ratio, 1.3; 95%

H. Kaneko et al. (eds.), *Disorders of Gut-Brain Interaction*,
https://doi.org/10.1007/978-981-95-6974-8_28

CI, 1.3–1.4), and was associated with decreased quality of life and frequent medical visits [3]. The prevalence among hospital visitors in Asia surveyed using Rome IV criteria ranged from 3.3% to 20% [4]. In Japan, the prevalence among health check-up recipients was reported to be 11–17%, and among patients visiting hospitals with upper abdominal symptoms, it was 45–54% [2]. Although the prevalence varies significantly depending on the definition and target population, it is undoubtedly a common condition encountered in clinical practice.

3 Etiology and Pathophysiology

The onset of FD, including FGIDs, is thought to be multifactorial, involving lifestyle, genetics, environment, psychosocial factors, gastrointestinal motility disorders, visceral hypersensitivity, and microinflammation of the stomach and duodenum [2]. Thus, individual symptoms do not arise from a single mechanism, making the elucidation of the disease's pathophysiology even more challenging.

Lifestyle factors are known to affect many diseases, and in FD patients, reports indicate decreased physical activity levels, sleep disorders, nausea, and abdominal pain induced by high-fat diets, irregular eating patterns, rapid eating, and nighttime fat consumption. Conversely, tea, fresh fruit, and raw vegetable intake have been reported to negatively correlate with FD [2]. The mechanism of symptom manifestation in FGIDs, including FD, has long been noted to involve the gut-brain axis. There has been debate on whether anxiety and depressive symptoms persist and lead to FD symptoms or whether FD symptoms persist and lead to anxiety and depressive symptoms. Studies on the relationship between psychological distress and FGIDs show that the onset of either condition is 50% each [5], and another prospective study observed significant prior onset of both FGIDs and anxiety/depressive symptoms. These studies have led to the recognition that the gut-brain mechanism in FGIDs is bidirectional.

Furthermore, the relationship between upbringing, genetic factors, and FD has been studied. Maternal separation stress in animal experiments is involved in the onset of FGIDs. In Japan, internet surveys reported a significant correlation between childhood abuse history and dyspepsia patients, with symptom severity [2]. Regarding FD susceptibility genes, several genetic polymorphisms have been reported, but a 2019 meta-analysis did not show involvement of genetic polymorphisms. However, a sub-analysis indicated that G-protein β_3 C825T was associated with increased susceptibility to Epigastric Pain Syndrome (EPS) [6].

Symptom manifestation involves significant roles of gastrointestinal motility and visceral hypersensitivity. In healthy individuals, food intake causes the gastric fundus to expand and temporarily store food through adaptive relaxation, which is impaired in 40–50% of FD patients. Food is expelled into the duodenum by peristalsis, but delayed gastric emptying is observed in 30–60% of FD patients. FD patients have a lower threshold for symptom manifestation in response to balloon distension stimuli inserted into the stomach, with higher pain frequency. Additionally, symptoms are strongly reported with acid or fat infusion into the duodenum. The basal and peak gastric acid secretion levels are similar in both healthy individuals and FD patients, and gastric acid secretion decreases in cases of gastric mucosal atrophy, indicating that symptom manifestation is not due to "excess gastric acid." Evidence has accumulated showing abnormal brain activity in various regions related to visceral hypersensitivity.

Recent research has advanced the understanding of the relationship between FD and microinflammation of the stomach and duodenum. Antigen presentation to T cells by pathogens or food peptides leads to the maturation of naive T cells into TH2 cells, releasing related cytokines (IL-4, IL-5, IL-14), and activating eosinophils, B cells, and mast cells. Additionally, IL-23 secretion from antigen-presenting cells such as dendritic cells, B cells, and macrophages promotes TH17 cell differentiation, and the produced GM-CSF further promotes eosinophil mobilization. The release of inflammatory mediators causes damage to the intestinal barrier and nerves, leading to visceral hypersensitivity and motility disorders, triggering symptoms. Signal transduction cascades result in further cytokine release, potentially causing extraintestinal symptoms such as anxiety and fatigue [5].

Research on gut microbiota in FD has rapidly progressed in recent years. Reports have indicated decreased diversity and increased levels of *Streptococcus, Firmicutes, Rothia, Clostridium, Haemophilus, Actinobacillus, Pseudoclavibacter, Tannerella, and Bifidobacterium, and decreased levels of Prevotella, Veillonella, Actinomyces, Streptococcus,* and *Neisseria*, although results vary among studies. Gut microbiota is strongly influenced by diet, environment, and medications, and differences between fecal and mucosal layer microbiota, as well as interactions among bacterial metabolites such as tryptophan, short-chain fatty acids, and bile salts, present numerous challenges for elucidation. FD can also develop after infectious gastroenteritis. A meta-analysis observed FD onset 6 months after infectious gastroenteritis with an odds ratio of 2.54, 95% CI = 1.76–3.65 [7]. Characteristics include early satiety, weight loss, nausea, and vomiting, with many cases showing impaired adaptive relaxation. Post-infectious FD is thought to involve residual inflammation in the stomach and duodenum.

4 Diagnostic Criteria and Tests

According to Rome IV criteria, FD is defined as having one or more of the following symptoms: "bothersome postprandial fullness," " bothersome early satiation," " bothersome epigastric pain," or " bothersome epigastric burning," with symptoms present for the last 3 months with symptom onset at least 6 months before diagnosis [1]. This is a strict international diagnostic criterion for research purposes. In clinical practice, patient complaints are not limited to these four symptoms, and in Japan, where access to medical facilities is good, patients are likely to visit medical institutions before 6 months. Considering daily clinical practice in Japan, the Japanese guidelines define FD as "a disease presenting chronic epigastric pain or gastric discomfort centered around the epigastrium, despite the absence of organic, systemic, or metabolic diseases causing the symptoms" [2]. The Rome Committee classifies FD into two subtypes based on major symptoms: Postprandial Distress Syndrome (PDS) and Epigastric Pain Syndrome (EPS), with many overlapping cases.

PDS: Characterized by bothersome postprandial fullness and bothersome early satiation occurring at least 3 days per week, with possible postprandial epigastric pain or burning, epigastric bloating, excessive belching, and nausea.

EPS: Characterized by bothersome epigastric pain or bothersome epigastric burning occurring at least 1 day a week, not necessarily postprandial, and may occur during fasting or improve with food intake.

The diagnostic and treatment flowchart is shown in Fig. 28.1. Diagnosis is based on symptom evaluation and exclusion of organic diseases. Comprehensive judgment is made based on symptoms, blood tests, alarm signs, medical history, examination history, and medications, with upper gastrointestinal endoscopy, CT, and abdominal ultrasound performed as needed. If organic diseases are excluded, FD is diagnosed.

Starting treatment without upper gastrointestinal endoscopy raises concerns about missing organic diseases such as gastric cancer. However, in clinical practice, if a patient who underwent endoscopy a few months ago during a health check-up presents with chronic gastric pain or discomfort, treatment is initiated first to quickly alleviate the symptoms, and endoscopy is performed as needed based on the response and subsequent course. Factors such as age, use of antithrombotic drugs or NSAIDs, *H. pylori* positivity, presence of alarm signs, and the interval since the last examination are considered when determining the timing of endoscopy. However, alarm signs alone are not sufficient to accurately diagnose the presence of organic disease and may lead to the risk of missing organic disease. As medical professionals, comprehensive judgment should be made, and immediate testing should be performed if necessary (Fig. 28.2).

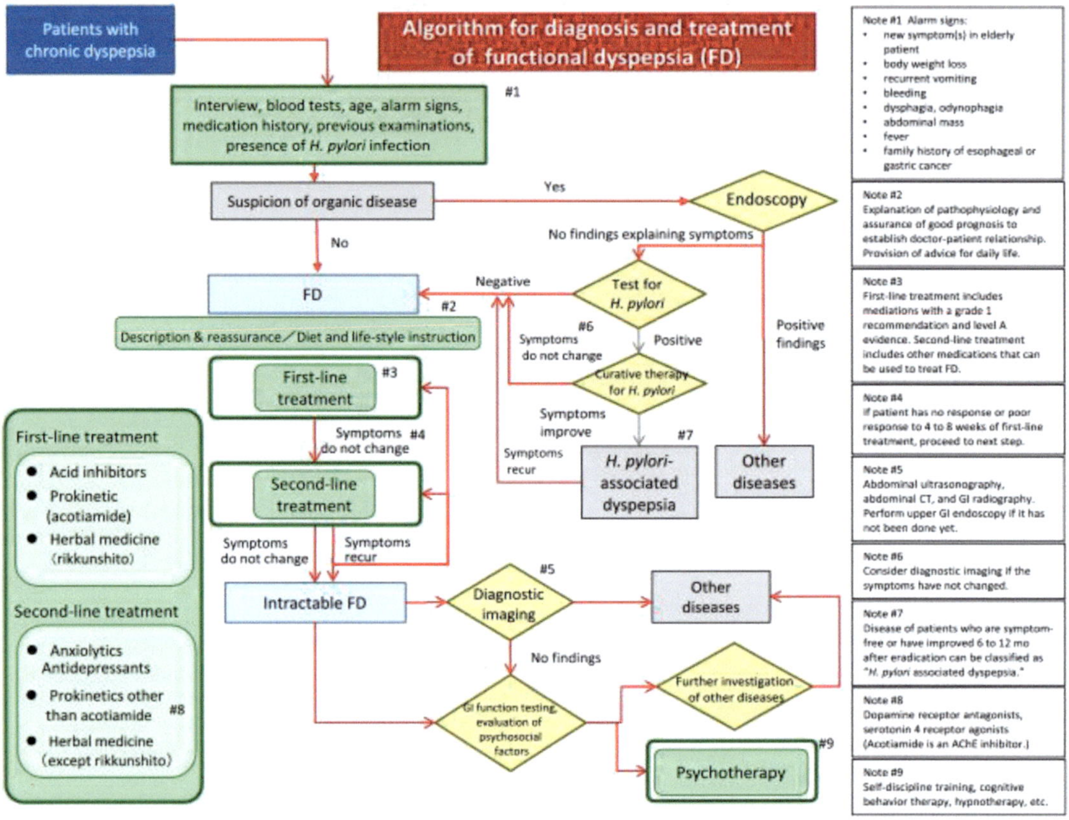

Fig. 28.1 Diagnostic and treatment flowchart for functional dyspepsia (FD)

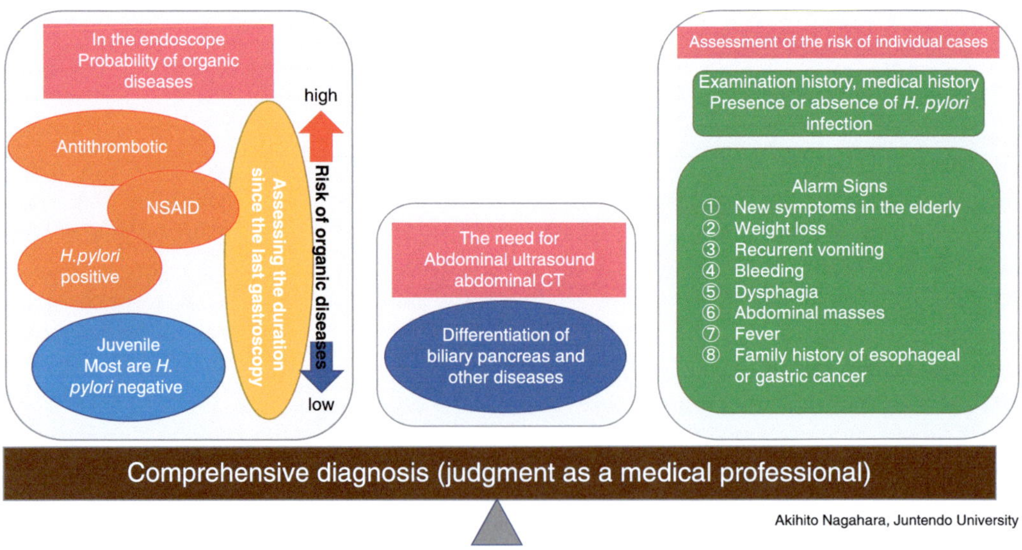

Fig. 28.2 Approach to necessary examinations

5 Differential Diagnosis and Complications

The insurance term "chronic gastritis" encompasses both symptomatic gastritis (symptomatic gastritis) and morphological gastritis (endoscopic gastritis). Most endoscopic gastritis is *H. pylori* gastritis, but the association between *H. pylori* gastritis and symptoms is weak, and many cases are asymptomatic. Additionally, gastric mucosal atrophy, gastric erosion, and histological gastritis are not associated with symptoms. Thus, the single disease name "chronic gastritis" originally confused symptomatic gastritis and morphological gastritis in clinical practice. The advent of FD has finally allowed these to be distinguished.

If symptoms disappear or improve 6 months to 1 year after *H. pylori* eradication therapy, the symptoms are judged to be due to *H. pylori* infection and diagnosed as "*H. pylori*-associated dyspepsia." However, it is painful for symptomatic patients to go without symptom treatment for a year, and in clinical practice, symptom treatment should be initiated alongside eradication.

Comorbidities with FD include irritable bowel syndrome (IBS), gastroesophageal reflux disease (GERD), functional constipation, and anxiety disorders. Additionally, differential diagnosis of biliary and pancreatic diseases, including early chronic pancreatitis, is necessary [2].

6 Treatment

Reports from Japan indicate that SF-8 QOL scores are significantly reduced in FD, GERD, and IBS, and significantly reduced in PDS, EPS, and overlap cases in FD [8]. Thus, the treatment goal is to restore the reduced QOL. FD is a disease defined by symptoms, and since there are no organic lesions or abnormalities in blood biochemical tests, the treatment goal is symptom improvement that satisfies the patient. To achieve this, it is necessary to fully understand the psychosocial background of the patient and build a good patient-physician relationship [2].

Since FD patients often exhibit inappropriate lifestyle habits, proper lifestyle guidance and dietary therapy are fundamental, although evidence in this area is scarce. Recent studies suggest that a diet low in fermentable oligosaccharides, disaccharides, monosaccharides, and polyols (low FODMAP diet) may be effective. Lifestyle guidance and dietary therapy have no disadvantages, and guidelines recommend eating small amounts multiple times instead of large meals, avoiding high-fat foods, providing smoking cessation guidance, and avoiding alcohol and coffee [2].

In pharmacotherapy, the guideline committee's recommendations are divided into strong recommendations and weak recommendations. Strong recommendations include proton pump inhibitors (PPIs), histamine H2 receptor antagonists (H2RAs), acotiamide, and Rikkunshito (Fig. 28.1) [2].

A network meta-analysis of FD treatments indicated that tricyclic antidepressants, H_2RAs, standard/low-dose PPIs, sulpiride/levosulpiride, itopride, and acotiamide were useful, although tricyclic antidepressant trials mostly targeted treatment-resistant patients, and sulpiride/levosulpiride trials were noted for low quality and small sample sizes. A Cochrane review of gastrointestinal motility-improving drugs and acid secretion inhibitors concluded that all were more effective than placebo, but no clear differences were observed between drugs. Based on this evidence, multiple first-line drugs are listed in parallel in the flowchart (Fig. 28.1).

6.1 First-Line Treatment

(i) *Acid Secretion Inhibitors*: PPIs have abundant evidence of efficacy. A multicenter double-blind trial in Japan investigating the effect of rabeprazole on FD found significant improvement in dyspepsia symptom scores (active drug 45.3% vs. placebo 28.2%, $P = 0.027$) and symptom diaries (48.7% vs. 30.0%, $P = 0.016$) with 20 mg of rabeprazole, but no significant difference with high doses (40 mg) [9]. The lack of effect differences between H_2RAs, low-dose PPIs, and standard-dose PPIs highlights the complexity of FD pathophysiology, necessitating patient-specific prescription adjustments based on patient-physician trust. Although H_2RAs have reported efficacy, they pose risks of cognitive decline and delirium in elderly patients [10], and resistance has been reported after several weeks of administration in *H. pylori*-negative cases, requiring careful consideration when prescribing.

Potassium-competitive acid blockers (P-CABs) may be as effective as PPIs [2]. Their strong acid secretion inhibitory effect may be useful in differentiating whether symptoms are acid-related.

(ii) *Acotiamide*: Acotiamide, an acetylcholinesterase inhibitor, demonstrated efficacy in a Japanese clinical trial targeting PDS, with overall improvement rates of 52.2% for acotiamide and 34.8% for placebo after 4 weeks ($p < 0.001$) [11]. It is important to instruct patients to continue taking acotiamide for 4 weeks, as its effect does not disappear immediately after taking a single tablet. A Phase III study in India comparing acotiamide with mosapride reported equivalent efficacy and safety.

(iii) *Rikkunshito*: In a multicenter, double-blind trial, Rikkunshito showed no significant difference in patient improvement rates after 4 weeks (Rikkunshito 14.9%, placebo 11.4%), but significant improvement was observed after 8 weeks (37.7% vs. 22.9%, $p = 0.019$) [12]. This indicates that Rikkunshito is a drug that works gradually over 8 weeks. To maximize its effect, it is important to instruct patients to continue taking it for 8 weeks. Additionally, depressive symptoms also improved. FD is known to frequently co-occur with depression and anxiety disorders, suggesting Rikkunshito may be useful for such patients. A meta-analysis from China comparing Rikkunshito with PPIs and gastrointestinal motility-improving drugs reported a relative risk of 1.21 (95% CI 1.17–1.25, $P < 0.001$) for clinical improvement, improved gastric emptying, and reduced recurrence rates 6 months post-treatment [13].

6.2 Second-Line Treatment

Evaluate symptom changes after prescription, and if the effect is insufficient, prescribe drugs with different mechanisms of action, including second-line drugs.

(i) *Anxiolytics and Antidepressants*: Tricyclic antidepressants have shown efficacy in meta-analyses (risk ratio 0.76, 95% CI: 0.62–0.94), but selective serotonin reuptake inhibitors have not demonstrated efficacy beyond placebo [14]. Tricyclic antidepressants are known for their numerous side effects, requiring careful consideration when prescribing. Sulpiride/levosulpiride, classified as antipsychotics, have antidepressant and gastrointestinal motility-promoting effects. Meta-analysis indicated a risk ratio of 0.50 (95% CI: 0.37–0.67) [15]. Benzodiazepine receptor agonists lack randomized controlled trials for FD and have limited evidence. Additionally, they pose risks of falls in elderly patients and tolerance and dependence with continued use. Tandospirone, a 5-hydroxytryptamine (5HT)1A receptor agonist, has demonstrated efficacy in a Japanese double-blind trial [16].

(ii) *Gastrointestinal Motility-Improving Drugs (Excluding Acotiamide)*: The guidelines list dopamine receptor antagonists (metoclopramide, domperidone, sulpiride, itopride) and serotonin 5-HT_4 receptor agonists (mosapride). Network meta-analysis indicated efficacy over placebo, but no significant difference between metoclopramide and domperidone. Metoclopramide and domperidone pose risks of extrapyramidal symptoms in patients with liver or kidney impairment and elderly patients, and QT prolongation in patients with heart disease, recommending short-term use. Sulpiride poses risks of galactorrhea, Parkinsonism, and dyskinesia, requiring caution, especially in elderly patients. Itopride has fewer side effects but limited evidence [2]. Mosapride demonstrated efficacy for gastric pain and discomfort in a non-blind trial in Japan [17].

This study protocol involved performing upper gastrointestinal endoscopy to exclude GERD, gastric ulcers, and gastric cancer, followed by administration of mosapride or teprenone. In 28% of patients with no abnormalities on endoscopy, symptoms disappeared after being informed of the absence of abnormalities. This highlights the significant impact of healthcare provider interactions on patient symptoms, emphasizing the importance of reassuring patient interactions.

(iii) *Kampo Medicines (Excluding Rikkunshito)*: The guidelines list Hangekobokuto and Kamishoyosan. Hange-koboku-to has been reported to be useful in a small number of cases, and Kamishoyosan has shown significant symptom improvement over motility-improving drugs in a meta-analysis from China (odds ratio, 3.26; 95% CI, 2.24–4.47; $P < 0.001$), and Kamishoyosan plus motility-improving drugs significantly improved symptoms over motility-improving drugs alone (odds ratio, 4.32; 95% CI, 2.64–7.08; $P < 0.001$) [18]. In clinical practice, Anchusan and Hange-shashin-to are empirically prescribed.

(iv) *Combination Therapy*: In clinical practice, combination therapy with acotiamide and acid secretion inhibitors is often seen. However, the efficacy of combination therapy has not been sufficiently studied. A Japanese report evaluating symptom changes with combination therapy of acotiamide and acid secretion inhibitors (famotidine) or placebo using a randomized double-blind method found no significant additive effect of acid secretion inhibitors [19]. On the other hand, a non-randomized, non-blind trial reported improvement in both EPS and PDS symptoms with the combination of PPI and acotiamide. Although the evidence is insufficient, it is worth attempting in clinical practice.

6.3 Other Treatments

Cognitive behavioral therapy, hypnotherapy, autonomic training therapy, and acupuncture have been attempted and reported to be useful, but these treatments are difficult to verify using traditional double-blind trial methods [2]. The current evaluation methods indicate a low level of evidence, but future developments are anticipated. These treatments are challenging for internists, and if upper abdominal symptoms are suspected to be somatic symptoms caused by mental disorders, collaboration between internal medicine and psychiatry/psychosomatic medicine is necessary.

6.4 Subtype-Specific Treatment

FD is divided into PDS and EPS based on the main complaint, but there are many overlapping cases. PDS is characterized by gastric discomfort leading to gastrointestinal motility decline, which suggests the use of gastrointestinal motility-improving drugs. EPS is characterized by gastric pain leading to gastric acid hypersensitivity, which suggests the use of acid secretion inhibitors. While it is easy to understand the treatment approach by estimating the pathology from the main complaint, no significant differences in pathology have been found between PDS and EPS. Both gastrointestinal motility-improving drugs and acid secretion inhibitors are effective for either symptom [9, 11], leading to mixed opinions on drug treatment selection based on the main complaint.

7 Prognosis

Reports indicate a recurrence rate of 20% after 3 months of PPI treatment, with 67% resuming PPI treatment one year after discontinuation [2]. A long-term study of acotiamide in Japan reported a remission rate of 38.0% for patients who discontinued treatment for more than 12 consecutive weeks, and a treatment resumption rate of 54.9% [20], indicating that FD is a disease prone to recurrence. A report examining the survival rate of FGID patients over a maximum of 20 years found no difference in survival rates for dyspepsia [21], and another report indicated that dyspepsia symptoms did not increase mortality rates. Therefore, while FD is prone to recurrence and does not have a favorable prognosis from a quality of life perspective, it does not affect life expectancy.

8 Conclusion

As the circumstances surrounding individuals become increasingly complex year by year, the number of patients with FGIDs is expected to grow. Because FGIDs lack objective, visible markers, appropriate diagnosis and treatment are only possible when physicians have a thorough understanding of the condition. It is essential that not only physicians but all healthcare professionals recognize the nature of these disorders, build trusting relationships with patients, and contribute to bringing relief and hope to those who suffer.

Take-Home Message

Functional dyspepsia (FD) is a symptom-based diagnosis, made after ruling out structural diseases. The Rome IV criteria are globally used, while Japan adopts a more pragmatic clinical definition for real-world practice.

FD has a multifactorial pathophysiology, involving impaired gastric motility, visceral hypersensitivity, psychosocial stress, low-grade inflammation, and alterations in gut microbiota. Brain-gut interactions are now recognized as bidirectional.

Diagnosis is based on symptom evaluation and exclusion of organic disease. Timing of endoscopy is considered depending on alarm features and previous test history. FD is classified into two subtypes: Postprandial Distress Syndrome (PDS) and Epigastric Pain Syndrome (EPS), though overlap is common.

The treatment goal is to improve quality of life (QOL) and patient satisfaction. Lifestyle modification is fundamental, combined with pharmacotherapy. First-line treatments include proton pump inhibitors (PPIs), acotiamide, and Rikkunshito by the guideline.

FD tends to recur but does not affect life expectancy. A trusting physician–patient relationship, grounded in understanding and empathy, is essential for successful management of this invisible but impactful disorder.

Competing Interests The author(s) has no competing interests to declare that are relevant to the content of this manuscript.

References

1. Drossmann DA, et al. Rome IV—functional gastrointestinal disorders: disorders of gut-brain interaction, vol. II. 4th ed. Rome Foundation; 2016.
2. Evidence-based clinical practice guidelines for functional dyspepsia 2021
3. Sperber AD, et al. Worldwide prevalence and burden of functional gastrointestinal disorders, results of Rome Foundation global study. Gastroenterology. 2021;160:99–114.
4. Kamiya T, et al. Questionnaire-based survey on epidemiology of functional gastrointestinal disorders and current status of gastrointestinal motility testing in Asian countries. Digestion. 2020;102:73–89.
5. Black CJ, et al. Functional gastrointestinal disorders: advances in understanding and management. Lancet. 2020;396:1664–7.
6. Du L, et al. Polymorphisms and susceptibility to functional dyspepsia: a systematic review and meta-analysis. Gastroenterol Res Pract. 2019;2019:3420548.
7. Futagami S, et al. Systematic review with meta-analysis: post-infectious functional dyspepsia. Aliment Pharmacol Ther. 2015;41:177–88.
8. Yamawaki H, et al. Impact of sleep disorders, quality of life and gastric emptying in distinct subtypes of functional dyspepsia in Japan. J Neurogastroenterol Motil. 2014;20:104–12.
9. Iwakiri R, et al. Randomised clinical trial: rabeprazole improves symptoms in patients with functional dyspepsia in Japan. Aliment Pharmacol Ther. 2013;38:729–40.
10. Guidelines for safe drug therapy in the elderly 2015. Japanese Geriatrics Society; Japan Agency for Medical Research and Development (in Japanese).
11. Matsueda K, et al. A placebo-controlled trial of acotiamide for meal-related symptoms of functional dyspepsia. Gut. 2012;61:821–8.

12. Tominaga K, et al. Rikkunshito simultaneously improves dyspepsia correlated with anxiety in patients with functional dyspepsia: a randomized clinical trial (the DREAM study). Neurogastroenterol Motil. 2018;30:e13319.
13. Ko SJ, et al. Effects of the herbal medicine Rikkunshito, for functional dyspepsia: a systematic review and meta-analysis. J Gastroenterol Hepatol. 2021;36:64–74.
14. Lu Y, et al. Antidepressants in the treatment of functional dyspepsia: a systematic review and meta-analysis. PLoS One. 2016;11(6):e0157798.
15. Ford AC, et al. Efficacy of psychotropic drugs in functional dyspepsia: systematic review and meta-analysis. Gut. 2017;66:411–20.
16. Miwa H, et al. Efficacy of the 5-HT1A agonist tandospirone citrate in improving symptoms of patients with functional dyspepsia: a randomized controlled trial. Am J Gastroenterol. 2009;104:2779–87.
17. Hongo M, et al. Large-scale randomized clinical study on functional dyspepsia treatment with mosapride or teprenone: Japan Mosapride Mega-Study (JMMS). J Gastroenterol Hepatol. 2012;27:62–8.
18. Qin F, et al. Chinese herbal medicine modified xiaoyao san for functional dyspepsia: meta-analysis of randomized controlled trials. J Gastroenterol Hepatol. 2009;24:1320–5.
19. Hojo M, et al. A randomized, double-blind, pilot study of the effect of famotidine on acotiamide treatment for functional dyspepsia. Digestion. 2017;96:5–12.
20. Matsueda K, et al. A long-term study of acotiamide in patients with functional dyspepsia: results from an open-label phase III trial in Japan on efficacy, safety and pattern of administration. Digestion. 2011;84:261–8.
21. Chang JY, et al. Impact of functional gastrointestinal disorders on survival in the community. Am J Gastroenterol. 2010;105:822–32.

29 Diagnosis and Treatment of DGBI of the Stomach and Duodenum, Belching Disorders

Yasuhiro Fujiwara

Abstract

Belching disorders are bothersome conditions that affect daily quality of life. Belching is divided into gastric belching and supragastric belching according to the location of origin. This chapter reviews the definitions, mechanisms, diagnosis, and treatments of gastric and supragastric belching (GB and SGB).

Keywords

Belching disorders · Gastric belching · Supragastric belching · Esophageal impedance pH monitoring · Cognitive behavioral therapy

1 Concept

Typically, air is swallowed along with food. One of the physiological mechanisms for expelling gas from the body is belching (eructation). Research on belching began with the report by Ingelfinger et al. in 1964, and detailed mechanisms, including transient lower esophageal sphincter relaxation, were reported from the 1970s to the 1990s. With advancements in examination methods, Bredenoord et al. in 2004 used esophageal impedance pH monitoring to investigate belching in detail, revealing two types: gastric belching (GB) expelled from the stomach and supragastric belching (SGB) expelled from the esophagus. Frequent belching can negatively impact quality of life (QOL). The Rome IV criteria list belching disorders as gastroduodenal functional disorders, divided into excessive GB and excessive SGB [1].

2 Epidemiology

The detailed epidemiology of belching disorders is unclear, but an international epidemiological survey of FGIDs involving 33 countries reported a frequency of 1% for belching disorders, lower than other FGIDs. The frequency of belching disorders showed no gender difference and tended to be lower in elderly individuals aged 65 and above, at 0.7% [2]. A survey conducted in Japan found that out of 1998 health check-up recipients, 121 individuals (6.1%) reported frequent belching ("always" or "often"). Frequent belching was associated with heartburn, FD, anxiety/depression, and sleep disturbances [3]. However, epidemiological surveys cannot differentiate between excessive GB and excessive SGB.

Y. Fujiwara (✉)
Osaka Metropolitan University, Osaka, Japan
e-mail: fujiwara@omu.ac.jp

H. Kaneko et al. (eds.), *Disorders of Gut-Brain Interaction*,
https://doi.org/10.1007/978-981-95-6974-8_29

3 Etiology and Pathophysiology

GB is caused by transient lower esophageal sphincter relaxation, the main pathology of GERD. Typically, healthy individuals swallow 6-40 times per meal, ingesting 8–32 mL of air per swallow. Air swallowed accumulates in the proximal stomach, causing transient lower esophageal sphincter relaxation due to gastric fundus distension. Gas in the stomach moves into the esophagus, causing upper esophageal sphincter relaxation and expulsion of gas from the mouth. This phenomenon is highly physiological (Fig. 29.1a). In contrast, SGB does not involve gas expelled from the stomach but occurs due to abnormal diaphragmatic contraction, increasing negative pressure in the esophageal lumen, causing upper esophageal sphincter relaxation and air inflow into the esophagus (inhalation). The lower esophageal sphincter does not relax, so gas in the esophagus is expelled directly from the mouth (Fig. 29.1b). The mechanism of abnormal diaphragmatic contraction in SGB is unclear, but psychological factors or unpleasant somatic sensations are likely involved [4, 5].

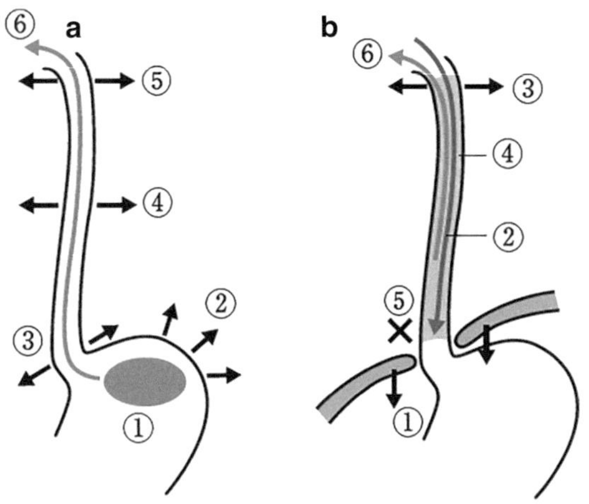

Fig. 29.1 Mechanisms of GB and SGB. (**a**) 1. Air accumulation in the proximal stomach, 2. Gastric fundus distension, 3. Transient lower esophageal sphincter relaxation, 4. Esophageal wall distension, 5. Upper esophageal sphincter relaxation, 6. Gas expulsion. (**b**) 1. Abnormal diaphragmatic contraction, 2. Negative pressure in the esophageal lumen, 3. Upper esophageal sphincter relaxation, 4. Air inflow, 5. No lower esophageal sphincter relaxation, 6. Gas expulsion

4 Diagnostic Criteria and Tests

Both GB and SGB can occur in healthy individuals, but frequent occurrences are considered belching disorders. According to Rome IV diagnostic criteria, bothersome belching (interfering with daily life) from the esophagus or stomach occurring at least four days a week is a mandatory criterion. Symptoms must have been present for six months and persisted for at least three months [1]. Excessive SGB patients may belch up to 20 times per minute, and belching does not occur during conversation, making it possible to suspect during examination. Additionally, belching does not occur when the patient is engrossed in something or during sleep [5]. Although other symptoms are rarely reported, comorbidities such as anxiety disorders, obsessive-compulsive disorder, and bulimia may occur. Frequent belching significantly impairs QOL in many cases [5]. Excessive GB lacks clear clinical features but may be seen in aerophagia associated with mental disorders [1].

Definitive diagnosis requires esophageal impedance pH monitoring [6]. When gas passes through, impedance values rise, and diagnosis is based on the location of the rise and the time it returns to baseline, i.e., changes in impedance values. In GB, impedance values rise retrogradely from the lower esophagus to the upper esophagus and decrease sequentially from the lower esophagus to the upper esophagus (Fig. 29.2a). In SGB, impedance values rise anterogradely from the upper esophagus to the lower esophagus and decrease sequentially from the lower esophagus to the upper esophagus (Fig. 29.2b). In aerophagia, impedance values rise anterogradely from the upper esophagus to the lower esophagus and decrease sequentially from the upper esophagus to the lower esophagus. Thus, esophageal impedance testing can differentiate GB, SGB, and aerophagia [6]. However, automatic analysis software cannot recognize these patterns, requiring manual confirmation of impedance value changes over time, which involves considerable effort. High-resolution esophageal manometry can also differentiate GB and SGB based on upper and lower esophageal sphincter relaxation and belch-

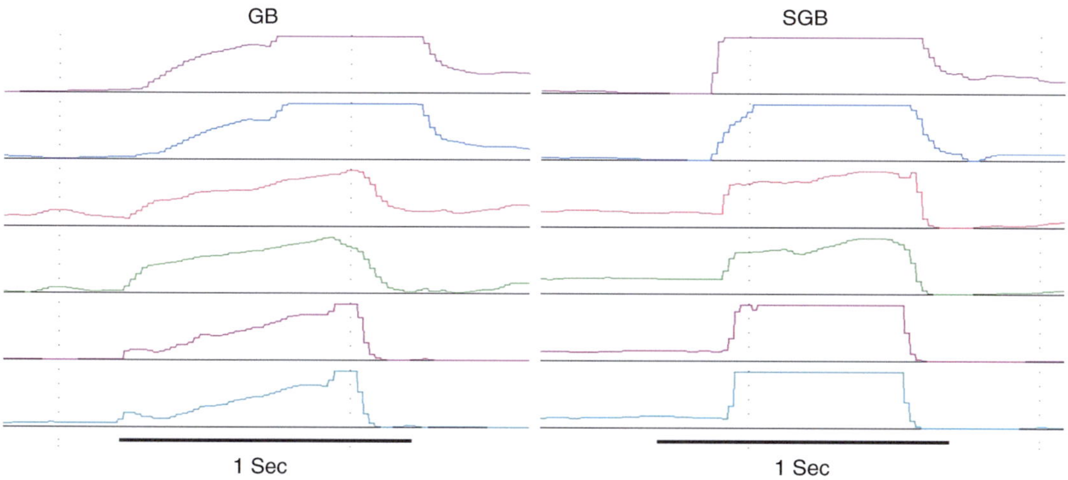

Fig. 29.2 Esophageal impedance findings in GB and SGB

ing during the test. Although Rome IV criteria do not define "excessive" by specific counts, literature suggests that SGB occurring more than 13 times a day is considered excessive [5].

5 Treatment

There are few high-quality clinical trials on the treatment of excessive GB and SGB, and evidence is scarce. Generally, excessive GB is partly due to air swallowing, so lifestyle guidance is important, including (1) eating slowly, (2) reducing swallowing frequency, and (3) avoiding carbonated beverages [1]. There is no effective pharmacotherapy, but $GABA_B$ agonist baclofen, which can reduce the frequency of transient lower esophageal sphincter relaxation, is one treatment option for excessive GB. However, its effect is limited, and many patients find it difficult to continue due to side effects such as headaches [5]. Cognitive behavioral therapy (CBT) has been reported to be effective for excessive SGB [4, 6, 7]. CBT consists of cognitive and behavioral components, including talk therapy and diaphragmatic breathing exercises.

Below are specific examples of diaphragmatic breathing exercises for CBT in excessive SGB [5, 7, 8]. The cognitive component is crucial for improving patient adherence to treatment, including (1) assuring patients that SGB is performed unconsciously and can be stopped with appropriate CBT, (2) explaining the mechanism of SGB (frequent inhalation or swallowing of air into the esophagus, immediately expelled using abdominal muscles, different from normal belching = GB), and (3) identifying premonitory symptoms of SGB (many patients report chest discomfort, but some cannot identify it) and correcting the misconception that these symptoms can be alleviated by SGB. Many excessive SGB patients believe gas originates from within the body, so recognizing this misconception is extremely important. Diaphragmatic breathing as behavioral therapy involves (1) placing both hands on the chest and abdomen, confirming only the abdomen moves up and down during diaphragmatic breathing. The method often involves inhaling for 3 s and exhaling for 3 s, but some literature suggests inhaling for 5–8 s and exhaling for 5–8 s. This exercise prevents the use of abdominal muscles for SGB. (2) Opening the mouth halfway and, if possible, placing the tip of the tongue behind the upper front teeth. This physiologically prevents SGB. (3) Practicing twice a day for 3–5 min and instructing patients to start the exercise when they feel premonitory symptoms. Ideally, patients should be able to live with diaphragmatic breathing throughout the day. CBT treatment involves five sessions at two-week intervals. CBT significantly reduces SGB frequency and improves QOL in excessive SGB patients. Additionally, fewer pre-treatment SGB episodes, lower esophageal hypervigilance scores, and higher CBT proficiency are predictors of sustained CBT effects for 6–12 months [5].

6 Relationship Between SGB and GERD

Regarding SGB, transient lower esophageal sphincter relaxation is reported to be involved in the postprandial pathology of PPI-resistant GERD patients with frequent belching. Although the involvement of SGB in PPI-resistant GERD is lower in Japanese patients compared to British patients, it is reported in approximately 20% of Japanese patients. A prospective comparison of CBT treatment and a control group (no intervention) in PPI-resistant GERD patients with frequent belching showed that CBT improved not only belching frequency but also reflux symptoms, including heartburn, and GERD-related QOL [9]. Additionally, SGB is identified as a phenotype involved in reflux hypersensitivity, a subtype of NERD listed in Rome IV.

Take-Home Message
Belching is a common symptom in GERD and FD patients. Excessive belching (belching disorder) that interferes with daily life is classified into gastric belching and supragastric belching based on the site of occurrence. Differentiation requires esophageal impedance pH monitoring, but if belching does not occur during conversation, supragastric belching should be suspected. Cognitive behavioral therapy is effective for treatment, and referral to a specialized hospital is recommended.

Competing Interests The author(s) has no competing interests to declare that are relevant to the content of this manuscript.

References

1. Stanghellini V, et al. Gastroduodenal disorders. Gastroenterology. 2016;150:1380–92.
2. Sperber AD, et al. Worldwide prevalence and burden of functional gastrointestinal disorders, results of Rome Foundation global study. Gastroenterology. 2021;160:99–114.
3. Fujiwara Y, et al. Heartburn, functional dyspepsia, anxiety/depression, and sleep disturbances are associated with clinically significant belching. J Neurogastroenterol Motil. 2021;27:581–7.
4. Kessing BF, et al. The pathophysiology, diagnosis and treatment of excessive belching symptoms. Am J Gastroenterol. 2014;109:1196–203.
5. Sawada A, et al. Belching in gastroesophageal reflux disease: literature review. J Clin Med. 2020;9:3360.
6. Bredenoord AJ, et al. Aerophagia, gastric, and supragastric belching: a study using intraluminal electrical impedance monitoring. Gut. 2004;53:1561–5.
7. Glasinovic E, et al. Treatment of supragastric belching with cognitive behav-ioral therapy improves quality of life and reduces acid gastroesophageal re-flux. Am J Gastroenterol. 2018;113:539–47.
8. Fujiwara Y, et al. A case of excessive supragastric belching successfully treated with cognitive behavioral therapy. Nihon Shokakibyo Gakkai Zasshi. 2020;117:1081–6. (in Japanese).
9. Ong AM, et al. Diaphragmatic breathing reduces belching and proton pump inhibitor refractory gastroesophageal reflux symptoms. Clin Gastroenterol Hepatol. 2018;16:407–16.

30 Diagnosis and Treatment of DGBI of the Stomach and Duodenum, Nausea and Vomiting Disorders

Haruka Amitani and Akihiro Asakawa

Abstract

Nausea is a subjective symptom characterized by an unpleasant sensation that typically arises in the upper abdomen, anterior chest, or pharynx, creating a desire to vomit. Vomiting is the forceful expulsion of stomach or small intestine contents through the mouth via the esophagus. Diseases causing nausea and vomiting are diverse and not limited to the gastrointestinal system. Chronic nausea and vomiting pose considerable therapeutic hurdles, including difficulties in determining the etiology and effectively managing symptoms. Consequently, following a comprehensive differential diagnosis, it is essential to ascertain if the illness aligns with chronic nausea vomiting syndrome (CNVS), cyclic vomiting syndrome (CVS), or cannabinoid hyperemesis syndrome (CHS). Specifically, CHS was designated as a functional gastrointestinal condition in 2016 and represents a relatively novel disease concept, underscoring the necessity for awareness.

H. Amitani · A. Asakawa (✉)
Department of Psychosomatic Internal Medicine, Kagoshima University Graduate School of Medical and Dental Sciences, Kagoshima, Japan
e-mail: amitani@m3.kufm.kagoshima-u.ac.jp; asakawa@m2.kufm.kagoshima-u.ac.jp

Keywords

Nausea · Vomiting · Chronic nausea vomiting syndrome (CNVS) · Cyclic vomiting syndrome (CVS) · Cannabinoid hyperemesis syndrome (CHS)

1 Concept

Nausea is a subjective symptom characterized by an unpleasant sensation that typically arises in the upper abdomen, anterior chest, or pharynx, creating a desire to vomit. Vomiting is the forceful expulsion of stomach or small intestine contents through the mouth via the esophagus. It is important to distinguish vomiting from regurgitation, which is the expulsion of stomach contents without the involvement of nausea or abdominal muscle contractions.

Nausea and vomiting disorders are classified according to the international diagnostic criteria of Rome IV into three categories: (1) chronic nausea vomiting syndrome (CNVS), (2) cyclic vomiting syndrome (CVS), and (3) cannabinoid hyperemesis syndrome (CHS) [1].

CNVS is characterized by severe nausea and vomiting occurring at least once a week. CVS is distinguished by episodic vomiting that occurs periodically, with at least one week of well-being between episodes [1].

H. Kaneko et al. (eds.), *Disorders of Gut-Brain Interaction*,
https://doi.org/10.1007/978-981-95-6974-8_30

Although the symptoms of CHS are similar to those of CVS, CHS patients are predominantly long-term cannabis users. Cannabis is the most commonly used recreational drug globally, with 2.5% of the world's population (147 million people) using it, and its usage rate continues to increase [2]. According to a 2012 survey by the Ministry of Health, Labour and Welfare, the consumption of medical narcotics for pain relief has been increasing annually in both Western countries and Japan. The United States has the highest consumption, with 1791.5 g of narcotic formulations per million people per day, more than ten times that of Japan. CHS is characterized by severe nausea and vomiting occurring periodically as a result of long-term, heavy use of cannabis or synthetic cannabinoids [2].

CNVS, CVS, and CHS share the common feature of symptoms persisting for more than 6 months.

2 Epidemiology

Chronic unexplained nausea is often associated with gastric or duodenal symptoms [1]. Long-term nausea and vomiting are relatively common symptoms, more frequently observed in women than in men [3]. The prevalence of CNVS in Western countries is 0.8–1.2%, while the prevalence of CVS is 0.7–2% [4]. The prevalence of CHS is currently unknown.

3 Etiology and Pathophysiology

Nausea and vomiting arise from complex pathways converging at the vomiting center in the lateral reticular formation of the medulla. The afferent pathways involved include the oropharynx, gastrointestinal tract, heart, musculoskeletal system, and vestibular system. Signals from these afferent pathways, the chemoreceptor trigger zone (CTZ) at the floor of the fourth ventricle, and the cerebral cortex are transmitted to the nucleus tractus solitarius, stimulating the vomiting center. Key neurotransmitters and hormones involved in this process include histamine, dopamine, norepinephrine, acetylcholine, serotonin, substance P, cortisol, β-endorphin, and vasopressin [5].

Reports on the pathophysiology of CNVS are limited. Gastric dysrhythmias are considered important pathophysiological factors in nausea, vomiting, and gastroparesis, serving as significant peripheral biomarkers [6]. Interstitial cells of Cajal (ICCs), which are fibroblast-like cells located at the enteric nerve ending and myenteric plexus, generate electrical slow waves and act as pacemakers for the gastrointestinal tract. A study comparing full-thickness gastric biopsies from nine CNVS patients with specimens from patients undergoing bariatric surgery and diabetic patients found that CNVS patients had fewer ICCs and signs of structural damage to ICC tissue compared to controls [6]. The reduction in ICCs in CNVS patients was less severe than in diabetic gastroparesis patients. Additionally, abnormalities in the initiation and conduction of slow waves in CNVS patients were similar to those observed in gastroparesis patients. Therefore, it was suggested that CNVS and gastroparesis may represent a continuum of disease in terms of ICC impairment.

The pathophysiology of CVS is not well understood, but CVS shares clinical features with migraines. Acute psychological and physiological stress, sleep deprivation, and menstruation are known to trigger episodic symptoms, followed by periods of relative calm with few symptoms. Migraines are the most prominent comorbidity in CVS, with 24–70% of CVS patients having a family history of migraines [7], suggesting a central nervous system involvement in the pathophysiology of CVS. Additionally, several genetic mutations and mitochondrial DNA polymorphisms have been reported in CVS patients [8].

Regarding CHS, the exact mechanism of action of cannabinoids remains unclear, but the involvement of cannabinoid receptors 1 (CBR1) in the stomach and small intestine, which inhibit gastric emptying and induce nausea and vomiting, has been suggested in the pathophysiology of CHS [9].

4 Differential Diagnosis, Diagnostic Criteria, and Tests

As shown in Table 30.1, diseases causing nausea and vomiting are diverse and not limited to the gastrointestinal system [10]. Acute gastroenteritis, pregnancy, and exogenous toxins are relatively easy to manage if the primary cause is identified. However, chronic nausea and vomiting can pose significant clinical challenges due to the difficulty in identifying the cause and adequately controlling symptoms. Therefore, it is important to differentiate these disorders thoroughly rather than continuing with vague treatments.

The diagnostic criteria for CNVS, CVS, and CHS are shown in Tables 30.2, 30.3, and 30.4, respectively [1]. Diagnostic tests are determined based on clinical symptoms [1]. Biochemical tests can exclude electrolyte and acid-base abnormalities, hypothyroidism, and Addison's disease. Upper gastrointestinal endoscopy, small bowel X-ray, computed tomography (CT), or magnetic resonance imaging (MRI) can evaluate gastric and duodenal diseases and small bowel obstruction. If these test results are normal, gastric emptying evaluation should be considered. In cases of severe symptoms, intraluminal pressure measurements of the stomach and small intestine may be performed to evaluate enteric neuropathy or myopathy [1]. Esophageal pH monitoring should be considered to exclude vomiting as an atypical symptom of GERD. If CHS is suspected but the patient does not disclose cannabis use, drug screening should be considered.

Table 30.1 Differential diagnosis of nausea and vomiting

Central nervous system	Closed head injury, cerebrovascular accident (stroke, hemorrhage), hydrocephalus, intracranial mass lesions, meningitis, encephalitis, abscess, idiopathic intracranial hypertension, migraine, epileptic seizures, vestibular neuritis, Ménière's disease, motion sickness
Gastrointestinal system	Chronic intestinal pseudo-obstruction, gastroparesis, intestinal obstruction, adhesions, esophageal disorders/achalasia, intussusception, malignant tumors, pyloric stenosis, strangulated hernia, volvulus, appendicitis, cholecystitis, cholangitis, hepatitis, inflammatory bowel disease, ischemic bowel disease, pancreatitis, peptic ulcer disease, peritonitis, Functional Dyspepsia (FD), Irritable Bowel Syndrome (IBS)
Infectious diseases	Acute otitis media, pneumonia, bacterial peritonitis, urinary tract infection, pyelonephritis, adenovirus, norovirus, rotavirus
Drugs/toxins	Antiarrhythmic drugs, antibiotics, antiepileptic drugs, chemotherapeutic agents, digoxin, hormonal agents, nonsteroidal anti-inflammatory drugs (NSAIDs), opioids, ethanol, illicit drugs, arsenic, organophosphates/pesticides, ricin, bacterial toxins, foodborne toxins
Metabolic/endocrine system	Thyroid disorders, parathyroid dysfunction, adrenal disorders, diabetic ketoacidosis, pregnancy, paraneoplastic syndrome, uremia
Others	Acute glaucoma, acute myocardial infarction, urolithiasis, pain, anorexia nervosa, bulimia nervosa, anxiety, conversion disorder, depression, psychogenic

Modified from Reference [10]

Table 30.2 Diagnostic criteria for chronic nausea and vomiting syndrome (CNVS)

Diagnosis requires all of the following:
1. Troublesome nausea (i.e., severe enough to affect usual activities) occurring at least one day per week, and/or vomiting occurring at least once per week 2. Exclusion of self-induced vomiting, eating disorders, gastroesophageal reflux, and rumination 3. No evidence of organic, systemic, or metabolic diseases that could explain the symptoms based on routine investigations (including upper endoscopy)
Additionally, the following conditions must be met:
1. Criteria fulfilled for the past three months 2. Symptom onset at least six months before diagnosis

Created from Reference [1]

Table 30.3 Diagnostic criteria for cyclic vomiting syndrome (CVS)

Diagnosis requires all of the following:
1. Typical vomiting episodes with acute onset and duration of less than one week 2. Vomiting occurring at least twice in the past year, and twice in the past six months, with intervals of more than one week between episodes 3. No vomiting between episodes, although other mild symptoms may occur periodically
Additionally, the following conditions must be met:
1. Criteria fulfilled for the past three months 2. Symptom onset at least six months before diagnosis
Supplementary Information: History or family history of migraines

Created from Reference [1]

Table 30.4 Diagnostic criteria for cannabinoid hyperemesis syndrome (CHS)

Diagnosis requires all of the following:
1. Typical vomiting episodes similar in onset, duration, and frequency to those of Cyclic Vomiting Syndrome (CVS) 2. Onset following prolonged excessive use of cannabis 3. Alleviation of vomiting episodes with sustained cessation of cannabis use
Additionally, the following conditions must be met:
1. Criteria fulfilled for the past three months 2. Symptom onset at least six months before diagnosis
Supplementary Information: May be associated with pathological bathing behavior (prolonged hot baths or showers)

Created from Reference [1]

CHS may be overlooked in clinical practice due to a lack of awareness among physicians and patients not disclosing their cannabis use history. Additionally, the clinical presentation of CVS and CHS is similar, leading to frequent misdiagnosis of CHS as CVS.

5 Complications

In addition to migraines, CVS is characterized by autonomic dysfunction symptoms such as complex regional pain syndrome, orthostatic intolerance, parasympathetic reactive disorders to deep breathing, and sympathetic skin response abnormalities [1].

6 Treatment

Research on the treatment of CNVS is limited, but currently available antiemetic agents include histamine H_1 receptor antagonists, muscarinic M1 receptor antagonists, dopamine D_2 receptor antagonists, serotonin 5-HT_3 receptor antagonists, and neurokinin NK_1 receptor antagonists [1]. Serotonin 5-HT_3 receptor antagonists are more effective in controlling vomiting than nausea. For patients with presumed functional causes of nausea and vomiting, tricyclic antidepressants, gastric electrical stimulation, and cognitive-behavioral therapy have been reported to be effective [1].

Mirtazapine, a noradrenergic and serotonergic antidepressant, is frequently used to treat patients with nausea and has recently been shown to be effective in patients with indigestion accompanied by weight loss, making it a promising candidate for the treatment of CNVS [1].

The treatment of CVS is divided into (1) lifestyle modifications, (2) abortive therapy (intervention at the onset of prodromal symptoms to stop vomiting episodes), (3) rescue therapy (during vomiting episodes), and (4) prophylactic therapy (daily preventive treatment) [11]. The main goals are to reduce the frequency and severity of vomiting episodes and improve function and quality of life (QOL).

Lifestyle modifications are important for managing CVS, aiming to avoid specific triggers between vomiting episodes. Abortive therapy should be initiated as early as possible during the prodromal phase. Common interventions include anti-migraine triptans for patients with migraine-like features. If abortive therapy fails and vomiting episodes begin, rescue therapy involves replenishing fluids, electrolytes, and energy while using antiemetics, analgesics, and sedatives to alleviate nausea, vomiting, and pain. Prophylactic therapy is recommended for patients with frequent vomiting episodes (more than once a month) or severe, prolonged vomiting. The first-line prophylactic medication is amitriptyline, which is also used for migraine prevention.

Second-line options include anticonvulsants such as topiramate, zonisamide, and levetiracetam.

The treatment of CHS involves symptomatic therapy with intravenous fluids and antiemetics during the acute phase, with the ultimate goal of discontinuing cannabis use, which is the most effective way to alleviate symptoms [12]. Other treatments include benzodiazepines and tricyclic antidepressants, although there is no clear evidence of their effectiveness. Topical capsaicin application or haloperidol administration are currently the only treatments with confirmed efficacy in randomized controlled trials (RCTs).

7 Conclusion

Nausea and vomiting disorders have fewer research reports compared to functional dyspepsia (FD) and irritable bowel syndrome (IBS), and further research is needed to elucidate their pathophysiology and establish appropriate treatment strategies. It is estimated that the diagnosis of CVS or CHS takes approximately 1–2 years, leading to economic issues due to prolonged testing and medical expenses [2]. CHS was classified as a functional gastrointestinal disorders (FGIDs/DGBI) in 2016. Therefore, it is necessary to provide sufficient information to healthcare providers regarding these relatively new disorders, including CHS.

Take-Home Message
Chronic nausea and vomiting require thorough differential diagnosis to determine whether they fall under CNVS, CVS, or CHS. Particularly for CHS, given the increasing number of cannabis-related arrests in Japan, the incidence of CHS may rise in the future. Therefore, it is crucial to consider CHS when evaluating patients with chronic nausea and vomiting.

Competing Interests The author(s) has no competing interests to declare that are relevant to the content of this manuscript.

References

1. Stanghellini V, et al. Gastroduodenal disorders. Gastroenterology. 2016;150:1380–92.
2. Lapoint J, et al. Cannabinoid hyperemesis syndrome: public health implications and a novel model treatment guideline. Western J of Emerg Med. 2018;19:380.
3. Pasricha PJ, et al. Characteristics of patients with chronic unexplained nausea and vomiting and normal gastric emptying. Clin Gastroenterol Hepatol. 2011;9:567–576.e564.
4. Aziz I, et al. Epidemiology, clinical characteristics, and associations for Rome IV functional nausea and vomiting disorders in adults. Clin Gastroenterol Hepatol. 2019;17:878–86.
5. Andrews PL, et al. Nausea and the quest for the perfect anti-emetic. Europ J Pharmacol. 2014;722:108–21.
6. Törnblom H, et al. Chronic nausea and vomiting: insights into underlying mechanisms. Neurogastroenterol Motil. 2016;28:613–9.
7. Levinthal DJ. The cyclic vomiting syndrome threshold: a framework for understanding pathogenesis and predicting successful treatments. Clin Trans Gastroenterol. 2016;7:e198.
8. Zaki EA, et al. Two common mitochondrial DNA polymorphisms are highly associated with migraine headache and cyclic vomiting syndrome. Cephalalgia. 2009;29:719–28.
9. Galli AJ, et al. Cannabinoid hyperemesis syndrome. Curr Drug Abuse Rev. 2011;4:241–9.
10. Scorza K, et al. Evaluation of nausea and vomiting. Am Family Phys. 2007;76:76–84.
11. Kovacic K, et al. Cyclic vomiting syndrome: a narrative review and guide to management. Headache. 2021;61:231–43.
12. Sandhu G, et al. Prevalence of cannabinoid hyperemesis syndrome and its financial burden on the health care industry, vol. 34. Proceedings (Baylor University. Medical Center); 2021. p. 654–7.

31 Diagnosis and Treatment of DGBI of the Stomach and Duodenum, Rumination Syndrome

Kazunari Tominaga

Abstract

Rumination syndrome is included in the field of functional disorders, but not malignant diseases in gastroenterology. However, unfortunately, recognition of rumination syndrome may not be prevalent. In addition, its pathophysiology remains unclear, and its therapeutic strategy is not established. From the above situation, despite being a benign disease, it markedly impairs patients' quality of life and social functioning. Therefore, according to the diagnostic criteria, differential and definitive diagnosis of rumination syndrome from other similar diseases, such as gastroesophageal reflux disease, belching disorders, and nausea and vomiting disorders, is very important for appropriate treatment, such as cognitive-behavioral therapy. Indeed, stress is involved in the pathophysiology of rumination syndrome. However, daily stress cannot be avoided in general populations, especially for patients with this disease. Therefore, building doctor–patient relationships must be crucial for alleviating patients' stressful, poor condition and improving their condition.

Keywords

Regurgitation · Brain–gut interaction · Functional disorder · Quality of life · Cognitive behavioral therapy

1 Concept

Rumination refers to the act of bringing previously swallowed food back to the mouth to re-chew and re-taste it. Commonly used in the context of ruminant animals, such as cows, sheep, and goats, the defining characteristic of ruminants is their possession of four stomachs (the rumen, reticulum, omasum, and abomasum). The abomasum corresponds to the human stomach, with the other three stomachs preceding it. Unlike monogastric animals, which have only one stomach, ruminants have a significantly different digestive function. In humans, rumination has no physiological significance and is considered pathological, known as rumination syndrome.

In rumination syndrome, small amounts of food are involuntarily (without nausea or vomiting) regurgitated from the stomach to the esophagus and mouth within minutes after eating, re-chewed, and usually re-swallowed. Depending on the situation, the regurgitated food may be swallowed again or expelled. Patients do not report nausea or abdominal pain, and the sensation is often described as similar to belching [1].

K. Tominaga (✉)
Department of Gastroenterology, Osaka Gyomeikan Hospital, Osaka, Japan

H. Kaneko et al. (eds.), *Disorders of Gut-Brain Interaction*,
https://doi.org/10.1007/978-981-95-6974-8_31

2 Epidemiology

Rumination syndrome is commonly observed in infants and in certain populations, such as patients with intellectual disabilities or bulimia. However, it can also occur in the general adult population. There are no definitive reports on the incidence and prevalence of rumination syndrome in adults. Recently, a global epidemiological survey involving 54,127 adults from 26 countries was reported (Fig. 31.1) [2]. In this survey, rumination syndrome was observed in

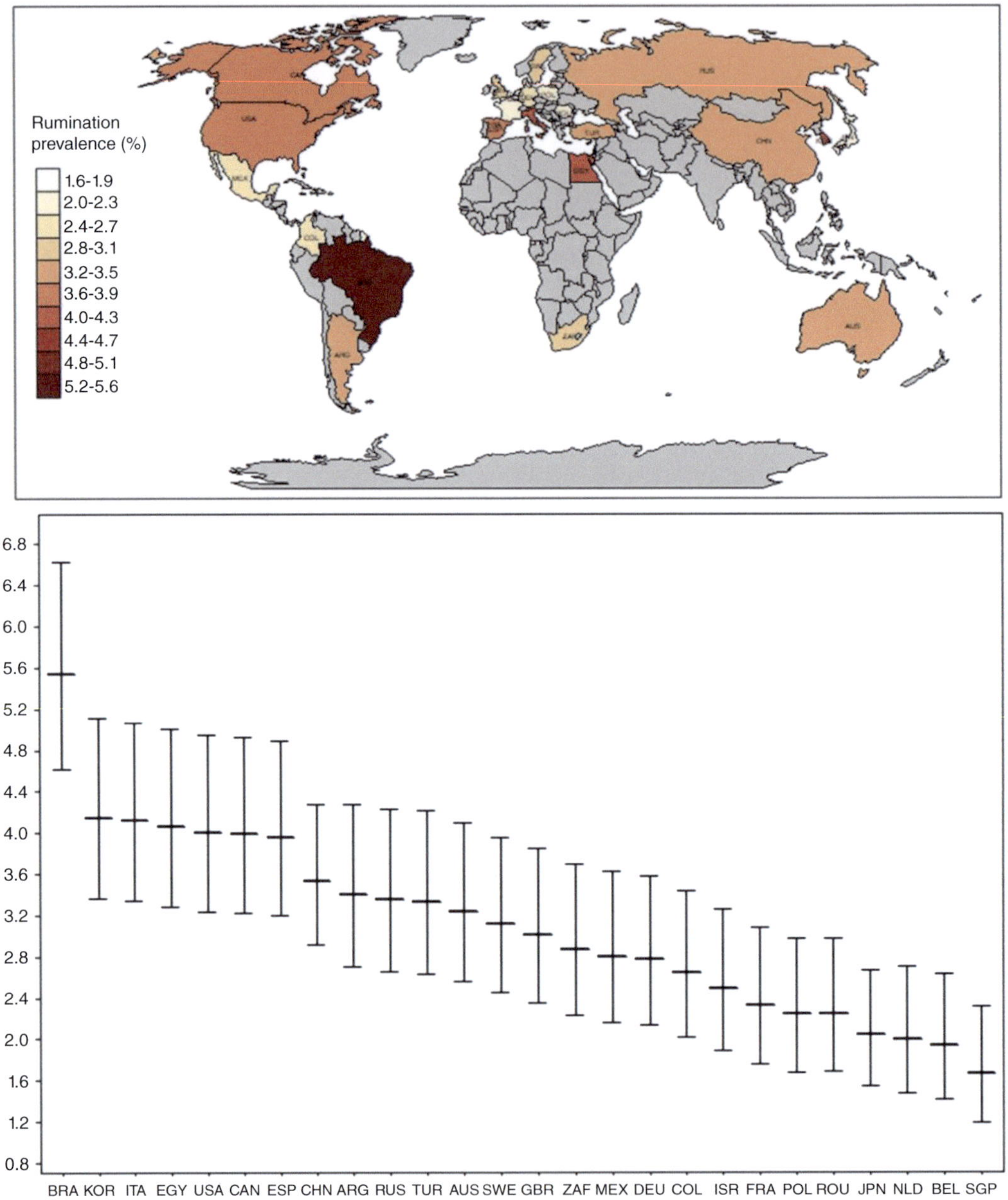

Fig. 31.1 Prevalence of rumination syndrome in general adults in 26 countries [2]. A survey of 54,127 general adults (including 27,549 men, 51%) from 26 countries found that rumination syndrome was present in 3.1% of participants. The average age of those diagnosed was 44.5 ± 15.6 years. The highest prevalence was observed in individuals aged 30–60 years. By country, Brazil had the highest prevalence at 5.5%, while Japan had a relatively low prevalence of approximately 2.0%

3.1% (95% confidence interval: 3.0–3.3%, $n = 1681$) of participants, a higher value compared to previous regional surveys. The highest prevalence was in Brazil (5.5%), and the lowest was in Singapore (1.7%), with Japan at approximately 2.0%. This large-scale survey using the Rome IV diagnostic criteria is the first of its kind, providing reliable data. It is also noted that rumination syndrome may be underdiagnosed, suggesting a higher actual prevalence.

3 Etiology and Pathophysiology

In ruminant animals, rumination is triggered by reverse peristalsis of the esophagus, but there are no reports of reverse peristalsis in humans [3]. Patients with achalasia or Zenker's diverticulum may experience regurgitation of undigested food without nausea, but the pathophysiology of rumination syndrome without esophageal obstruction is largely unknown. Recent studies using 24-hour multichannel intraluminal impedance-pH monitoring (MII/pH) have shown that non-acid reflux (pH > 4) is predominant during regurgitation, and despite frequent reflux episodes, there is no mucosal damage, distinguishing it from gastroesophageal reflux disease (GERD) [4]. Rumination syndrome is also more common in young women [4]. However, the origin of the reflux, the involvement of the acid pocket, and the extent of clearance by swallowing remain unclear.

Given its prevalence in patients with intellectual disabilities and bulimia, rumination syndrome may be a phenotype of eating disorders, possibly resulting from learned maladaptive behaviors. This involves relaxing the lower esophageal sphincter and rhythmically contracting and relaxing the diaphragm to increase intra-abdominal (gastric) pressure, pushing gastric contents into the esophagus and pharynx. Consequently, symptoms such as nausea, pain, and dysphagia do not occur. In stressed patients, rumination itself is not a major concern, but regurgitation and expulsion of food can occasionally lead to weight loss. In infants and young children, environmental factors such as neglect, stressful living conditions, and parent–child relationship issues may contribute to the onset of rumination syndrome.

4 Diagnostic Criteria and Tests

The Rome criteria are the primary diagnostic criteria for functional gastrointestinal disorders like rumination syndrome. The Japanese translation of the Rome III diagnostic criteria describes rumination syndrome as follows [5]:

Both of the following must be present:

- Persistent or recurrent regurgitation of recently ingested food into the mouth, which is then re-chewed, re-swallowed, or expelled.
- Regurgitation is not preceded by retching or vomiting.
- Criteria fulfilled for the last 3 months with symptom onset at least 6 months before diagnosis.

Supplementary Criteria:

- Nausea does not precede regurgitation.
- Regurgitation ceases when the regurgitated material is acidic.
- Regurgitated material may contain pleasant-tasting food.
- Clinical evaluation, sometimes including endoscopy, esophageal motility testing, or both, is necessary.

The Rome IV criteria, published in 2016 [6], are similar. Diagnosis is usually made by inspection, and endoscopy or upper gastrointestinal radiography is required to exclude mechanical obstructions or Zenker's diverticulum. Esophageal manometry and tests to evaluate gastric emptying and antral-duodenal motility may also be performed. Gastric manometry often shows simultaneous pressure increases in the stomach and duodenum during regurgitation, reflecting increased intra-abdominal pressure. However, manometry is not essential for diagnosis [7].

Psychosocial history may reveal underlying psychological stress. The DSM-5 defines the diagnostic criteria for rumination syndrome as follows [8]:

A. Repeated regurgitation of food over a period of at least 1 month, with regurgitated food being re-chewed, re-swallowed, or expelled.
B. The repeated regurgitation is not attributable to an associated gastrointestinal or other medical condition (e.g., GERD and pyloric stenosis).
C. The eating disorder does not occur exclusively during the course of anorexia nervosa, bulimia nervosa, binge-eating disorder, or avoidant/restrictive food intake disorder.
D. If the symptoms occur in the context of another mental disorder (e.g., intellectual disability and other neurodevelopmental disorders), they are sufficiently severe to warrant clinical attention.

These criteria are used for clinical diagnosis but differ slightly from the perspective of gastroenterology.

5 Differential Diagnosis and Comorbidities

In adults, it is important to differentiate rumination syndrome from proton pump inhibitor-resistant GERD. However, distinguishing between persistent postprandial rumination in treatment-resistant GERD and rumination syndrome is challenging, as approximately 20% of patients with treatment-resistant GERD exhibit frequent, persistent postprandial reflux [9]. Therefore, differentiating these conditions based on symptom questionnaires is difficult, and high-resolution manometry may be necessary to evaluate esophageal motility. Recent reports suggest that using a rumination score based on 24-hour MII/pH monitoring (number of non-acid reflux episodes per hour and symptom index) can diagnose rumination syndrome with 91.7% sensitivity and 78.6% specificity, making it useful for differential diagnosis [4].

In infants, differential diagnoses include gastroparesis, pyloric stenosis, hiatal hernia, and Sandifer syndrome, which can be excluded through appropriate physical examination and clinical tests. Additionally, in anorexia nervosa and bulimia nervosa, regurgitation of food due to concerns about weight gain requires differentiation.

6 Treatment

The basic treatment strategies for GERD and rumination syndrome differ significantly. While acid suppression therapy is central to GERD treatment due to the role of the acid pocket in acid reflux, there are no established medications for rumination syndrome, and treatment guidelines are not well-defined. Behavioral therapy, particularly cognitive-behavioral therapy (CBT), has been shown to be effective in alleviating symptoms.

Diaphragmatic breathing (DiaB) involves using the diaphragm instead of the chest muscles for breathing, primarily moving the abdomen during respiration. It is a common treatment for rumination syndrome and can reduce the number of rumination episodes. Another type of breathing, known as slow deep breathing (SlowDB), primarily involves chest breathing and is used to treat increased esophageal pain, potentially benefiting rumination syndrome as well. Both DiaB and SlowDB may improve rumination by altering gastric neural control. Motivated patients with rumination syndrome often respond well to these behavioral therapies (e.g., relaxation, biofeedback, and DiaB). Baclofen may be helpful, but long-term safety and efficacy data are limited.

When rumination syndrome is associated with intellectual disabilities or developmental disorders, treating these conditions can improve symptoms. Treatments for developmental disorders include pharmacotherapy, psychotherapy, and transcranial magnetic stimulation (TMS).

TMS involves applying a special coil to the head to deliver magnetic stimulation to the brain, improving the balance of neural networks and restoring normal activity. TMS is widely used in Western countries, including the United States, but is only available at a few medical institutions in Japan. Compared to pharmacotherapy, TMS has fewer side effects, shorter treatment duration, and can improve developmental disorders.

7 Prognosis

Rumination syndrome is not a life-threatening condition and can occur at any age, including infancy, childhood, adolescence, and adulthood. In infants, it may resolve spontaneously, but there is a risk of severe nutritional deficiencies. Symptoms may be temporary or persist until treated. In adults with intellectual disabilities or other neurodevelopmental disorders, regurgitation and rumination behaviors may serve functions such as self-soothing or self-stimulation. Persistent regurgitation can lead to malnutrition, adversely affecting development and learning abilities. Some individuals may intentionally reduce food intake due to the social undesirability of regurgitation, leading to weight loss and poor health. Overall, rumination syndrome can significantly reduce quality of life (QOL) and impact social life (Fig. 31.2).

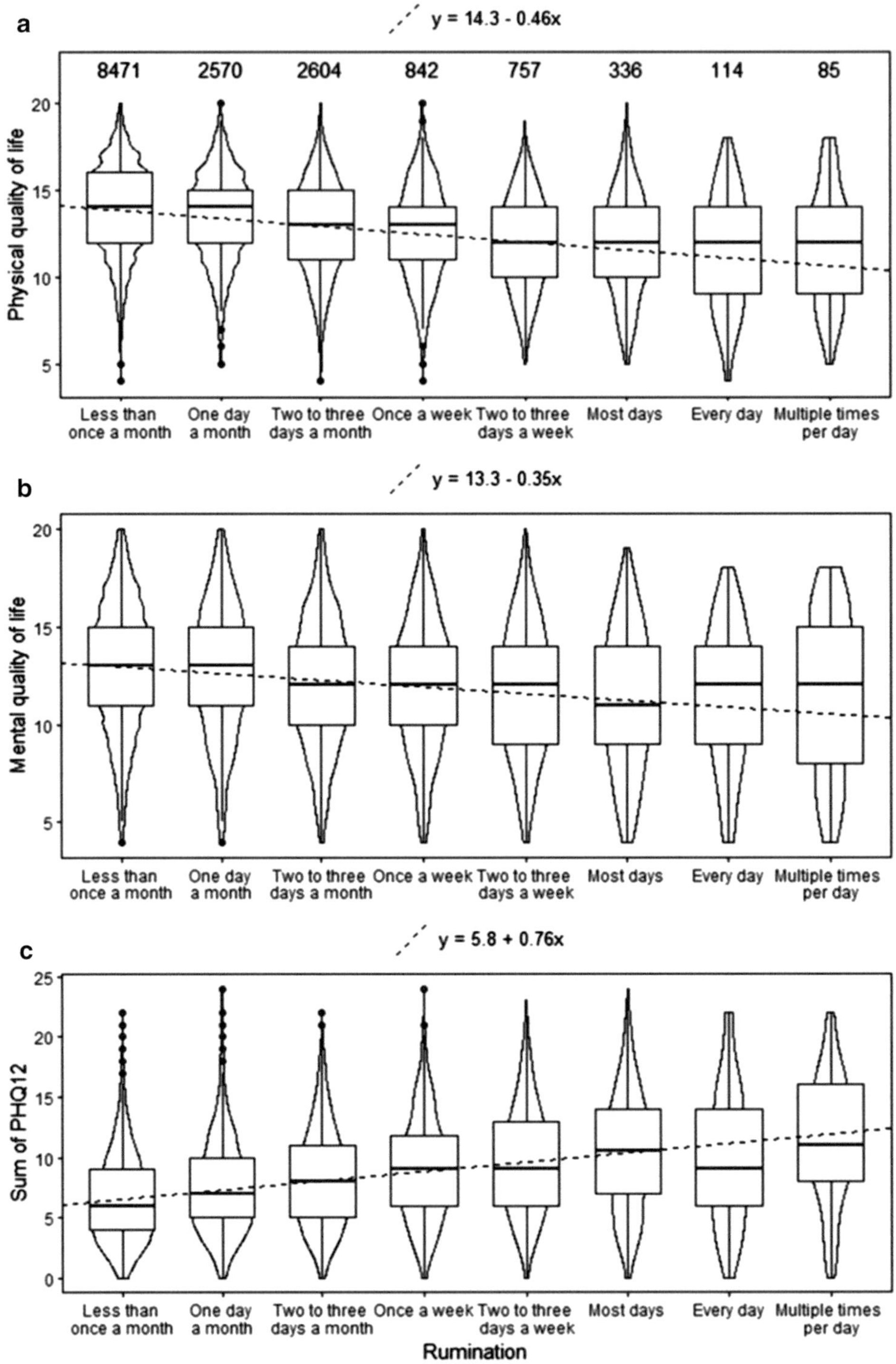

Fig. 31.2 Relationship of rumination frequency with physical/mental QOL and non-gastrointestinal physical symptoms [2]Among individuals diagnosed with rumination syndrome, the correlation between rumination frequency (ranging from less than once a month to multiple times a day in eight stages) and QOL was evaluated using PROMIS Global Health 10 and Patient Health Questionnaire-12 (PHQ-15, excluding three items related to gastrointestinal symptoms). Results showed a negative correlation between rumination frequency and both physical and mental QOL scores. Conversely, rumination frequency positively correlated with the severity of non-gastrointestinal physical symptoms

8 Conclusion

In the Rome IV criteria for gastroduodenal disorders, rumination syndrome is listed as B4, following functional dyspepsia (B1), belching disorders (B2), and nausea and vomiting disorders (B3). The frequency and recognition of rumination syndrome may be low, resulting in an unclear pathophysiology and a lack of established treatments. However, considering the significant reduction in QOL and the impact on social life, addressing this condition is an urgent issue.

Take-Home Message
Rumination differs from common belching and nausea. Key diagnostic criteria include "persistent or recurrent regurgitation of ingested food into the mouth, which is then expelled, re-chewed, or re-swallowed," "regurgitation not preceded by retching or vomiting," "regurgitation ceases when the regurgitated material is acidic," and "regurgitated material may contain pleasant-tasting food." Understanding these situations is crucial for differential diagnosis. While stress may be involved, it is important to explain that rumination syndrome is not life-threatening and to manage it primarily with CBT.

Competing Interests The author has no competing interests to declare that are relevant to the content of this chapter.

References

1. O'Brien MD, et al. The rumination syndrome: clinical features rather than manometric diagnosis. Gastroenterology. 1995;108:1024–9.
2. Josefsson A, et al. Global prevalence and impact of rumination syndrome. Gastroenterology. 2022;162(3):731–42.
3. Sugawa T, et al. A case of rumination syndrome in an adult without intellectual disability. Jpn J Gastroenterol. 2006;103:631–5. (in Japanese)
4. Nakagawa K, et al. Persistent postprandial regurgitation vs rumination in patients with refractory gastroesophageal reflux disease symptoms: identification of a distinct rumination pattern using ambulatory impedance-pH monitoring. Am J Gastroenterol. 2019;114(8):1248–55.
5. Fukudo S, et al. Rome III Japanese version. Kyowa Kikaku. 2008. (in Japanese).
6. Stanghellini V, et al. Gastroduodenal disorders. Gastroenterology. 2016;150(6):1380–92.
7. Malcolm A, et al. Rumination syndrome. Mayo Clin Proc. 1997;72:646–52.
8. Takahashi S, et al. DSM-5 classification and diagnosis of mental disorders. Igaku-Shoin. 2014. (in Japanese).
9. Yadlapati R, et al. Postprandial high-resolution impedance manometry identifies mechanisms of nonresponse to proton pump inhibitors. Clin Gastroenterol Hepatol. 2018;16:211–218.e1.

Diagnosis and Treatment of Motility Disorder, Gastroparesis

32

Hiroto Miwa

Abstract

Gastroparesis (GP) is a disease defined by delayed gastric emptying and dyspeptic symptoms, and it can be associated with the presence of various complications, such as diabetes mellitus, postoperative stomach, and Parkinson's disease. Because GP is basically defined by delayed gastric emptying, measuring gastric emptying is mandatory for diagnosis. However, gastric emptying tests with a solid meal are not commonly performed in many countries besides North America. As a result, the term GP is primarily used in North America and is seldom employed in other regions, including Asian countries.

Patients with GP have symptoms such as early satiety, postprandial fullness, nausea, vomiting, and abdominal pain. We should be careful to differentiate between idiopathic GP and functional dyspepsia (FD) that present chronic dyspeptic symptoms without organic, systemic, or metabolic diseases. However, these two conditions have different features of symptoms. GP often presents with nausea and vomiting, whereas FD rarely includes these symptoms, particularly vomiting. Such symptoms are thought to reflect a relatively strong delay of gastric emptying. Although chronic nausea and vomiting are still rare in Japan, the potential increase in GP patients should be considered due to rising diabetes and Parkinson's disease cases.

Keywords

Functional dyspepsia · Gastric emptying test · Diabetes mellitus · Vomiting

1 Concept

Gastroparesis (GP) is a disorder characterized by delayed gastric emptying in the absence of mechanical obstruction, resulting in symptoms such as early satiety, postprandial fullness, nausea, vomiting, belching, indigestion, and abdominal pain [1]. GP is basically defined by delayed gastric emptying. Therefore, measuring gastric

My expertise: DGBI, *H. pylori* infection, diagnosis, and treatment of GI cancer.

H. Miwa (✉)
Kawanishi City Medical Center, Kawanishi, Hyogo, Japan
e-mail: miwahgi@hyo-med.ac.jp

H. Kaneko et al. (eds.), *Disorders of Gut-Brain Interaction*,
https://doi.org/10.1007/978-981-95-6974-8_32

emptying is required for diagnosis. Typically, gastric scintigraphy and gastric emptying breath tests using solid meals are employed for this evaluation. However, in Japan, gastric scintigraphy is performed in only a few facilities, and gastric emptying breath tests are rarely conducted. Recently, wireless motility capsules and magnetic resonance imaging have also been available for gastric emptying assessment, but these methods are limited to specific facilities. Furthermore, gastric emptying tests in Japan have predominantly used liquid or semi-liquid meals. Although the method using these test meals is simple and practical, there is a matter for discussion about how well the results of the gastric emptying test using liquid meals other than solids reflect actual gastric emptying, and therefore, the reliability of the results has often been questioned. Consequently, the diagnosis of GP has rarely been used in Japan.

However, the limited use of this diagnosis is not unique to Japan. Globally, the term GP is primarily used in North America and is seldom employed in other regions. We conducted a survey on the awareness of this disorder among Asian countries, revealing that nearly 80% of physicians had never or rarely used this diagnosis [2]. Conversely, in North America, the term is frequently used, and there is increasing global interest in functional GI disorders. In fact, there is a growing focus on this disorder at international conferences, driven by the rising number of diabetic patients. Therefore, it is essential for us to acquire accurate knowledge and understanding of this disorder.

2 Epidemiology

GP is defined by delayed gastric emptying without mechanical obstruction and is commonly associated with diabetes. Reports from the United States indicate that the risk of developing GP over a 10-year period is 5.2% for type 1 diabetes patients and 1.0% for type 2 diabetes patients [3]. Idiopathic GP, with unknown causes, is also prevalent alongside diabetic GP. Other causes include postoperative stomach conditions, systemic diseases such as Parkinson's disease and renal failure, drug-induced, and post-viral or bacterial infections. It is estimated that there are over five million patients with GP in the United States, although not all undergo gastric emptying tests. Sometimes, the diagnosis is made based on the presence of food residue during endoscopy. Additionally, GP is often diagnosed based solely on symptoms such as postprandial fullness, nausea, and vomiting [3]. In fact, only 10% of suspected GP patients undergo gastric emptying tests, making the precise prevalence of GP unclear. As mentioned earlier, the term GP is rarely used in Asian countries, including Japan [2], and there are no reports on the actual status of GP. Therefore, it is uncertain whether the term is not used because there are few GP patients in Japan or because the term is not widely recognized.

3 Differential Diagnosis

We should be careful to differentiate between GP and functional dyspepsia (FD) . FD is defined by symptoms in the absence of organic, systemic, or metabolic diseases that could explain the chronic dyspeptic symptoms [4]. GP is a disease defined by delayed gastric emptying and symptoms. The two concepts of disease are fundamentally different. FD must be idiopathic, excluding potential causes such as organic, systemic, or metabolic diseases, whereas GP can be diagnosed even in the presence of various complications if delayed gastric emptying is observed without mechanical obstruction (Fig. 32.1) [4, 5]. It is for this reason that GP is often associated with diabetes. This is the most important difference between the FD and the GP.

On the other hand, when delayed gastric emptying is observed without complications, it is difficult to differentiate between idiopathic GP and FD. Many FD patients exhibit GP-like symptoms without delayed gastric emptying, and the correlation between the degree of gastric emptying abnormality and symptoms is often weak, complicating the discussion. However, it is known that, considering the severity of symptoms, there is a relatively good correlation between gastric emp-

Functional dyspepsia (FD)

Functional dyspepsia (FD) is defined as a condition chronically presenting symptoms centered in the upper abdomen, such as epigastric pain or discomfort, in the absence of any organic, systemic, or metabolic disease that is likely to explain the symptoms. (5)

Rome IV criteria of functional dyspepsia (4)

- At least one of the following four symptoms is present
  - Postprandial distress syndrome (PDS)
    1. Bothersome postprandial fullness
    2. Bothersome early satiety
  - Epigastric pain syndrome (EPS)
    3. Bothersome epigastric pain
    4. Bothersome epigastric burning
- No evidence of organic, systemic, or metabolic disease that is likely to explain the symptoms on routine investigations (including at upper endoscopy)
- Criteria fulfilled for the last 3 months with symptom onset at least 6 months before diagnosis.
- Symptoms must occur at least 3 days a week for PDS, and at least 1 day a week for EPS

Gastroparesis (GP)

Gastroparesis is a disorder characterized by delayed gastric emptying of solid food in the absence of a mechanical obstruction of the stomach, resulting in the cardinal symptoms of early satiety, postprandial fullness, nausea, vomiting, belching and bloating. (1)

Fig. 32.1 Definitions of FD and GP*FD*: A disorder characterized by chronic upper abdominal symptoms, such as epigastric pain and indigestion, in the absence of organic, systemic, or metabolic diseases that could explain these symptoms (Japanese Society of Gastroenterology Clinical Practice Guidelines [5] *GP*: A syndrome characterized by delayed gastric emptying without mechanical obstruction, presenting with symptoms such as early satiety, postprandial fullness, nausea, vomiting, indigestion, and abdominal pain [1]

tying abnormalities and gastrointestinal symptoms. Stanghellini et al. [6] performed scintigraphy on 343 FD patients and found delayed gastric emptying in 33.5%, with a significant correlation between delayed emptying and severe symptoms such as vomiting and postprandial fullness. Thus, delayed gastric emptying itself, as inferred from its mechanism, induces postprandial fullness and vomiting symptoms, but, on the other hand, it may not explain the occurrence of various upper abdominal symptoms, including abdominal pain and early satiety.

4 Pathogenesis and Pathophysiology

There are differences in the characteristic symptoms of GP and FD. GP often presents with nausea and vomiting [7], whereas FD rarely includes these symptoms, particularly vomiting. The reason for the rarity of vomiting in FD is unclear, but it may be because severe gastric emptying disorders are less common in the absence of complications such as diabetes or postoperative stomach conditions. Additionally, the pathophysiology of GP and FD appears to differ. GP is primarily a disorder of delayed gastric emptying, whereas FD involves various factors such as delayed gastric emptying, accelerated gastric emptying, impaired adaptive relaxation response, and visceral hypersensitivity. In clinical practice, psychological factors and stress-induced visceral hypersensitivity also play a role in developing symptoms, even in GP patients. Therefore, the term GP, which attempts to explain patient symptoms solely based on delayed gastric emptying, must be considered precarious.

5 Treatment

Both GP and FD with delayed gastric emptying generally involve pharmacological treatment aimed at improving gastrointestinal motility. However, for relatively severe GP patients, surgical interventions, electrical stimulation, botulinum toxin injections, and gastric-peroral endoscopic myotomy are sometimes performed to improve delayed gastric emptying. Although some FD patients exhibit delayed gastric emptying, few qualify for these treatments. Thus, there are some differences in the treatment approaches for GP and FD.

6 Relationship Between GP and FD

Generally, GP and FD are considered to significantly overlap (Fig. 32.2). FD patients with delayed gastric emptying are regarded as having idiopathic GP without complications. The extent of this overlap is a critical issue. According to somewhat dated data from the United States, among 146 GP patients, 36% had idiopathic GP, 29% had diabetes, 13% had postoperative stomach conditions, and 7.5% had Parkinson's disease [8]. Thus, one-third of GP cases overlap with FD. Conversely, FD patients with delayed gastric emptying are also considered to have idiopathic GP. It is estimated that 10–30% of FD patients exhibit delayed gastric emptying, suggesting a theoretical overlap of 10–30%. However, the prevalence rates of GP (approximately 0.03%) [9] and FD (5–20%) [10] differ by more than 100-fold, making it unrealistic to claim that 10–30% of FD cases are idiopathic GP. In reality, FD rarely involves vomiting, and this discrepancy in prevalence rates may be due to variations in diagnostic criteria for delayed gastric emptying. Nevertheless, with the increasing number of diabetic patients, GP may become more prevalent in Japan, necessitating its consideration in the differential diagnosis of patients with dyspeptic symptoms.

Take-Home Message
Generally, the correlation between delayed gastric emptying and symptoms is considered weak. However, for relatively severe symptoms, there is a correlation between delayed gastric emptying and symptoms such as nausea, vomiting, and postprandial fullness. Although chronic nausea and vomiting are rare in Japan, the potential increase in GP patients due to rising diabetes and Parkinson's disease cases should be considered. GP should be considered in the differential diagnosis for patients presenting with nausea, vomiting, and postprandial fullness.

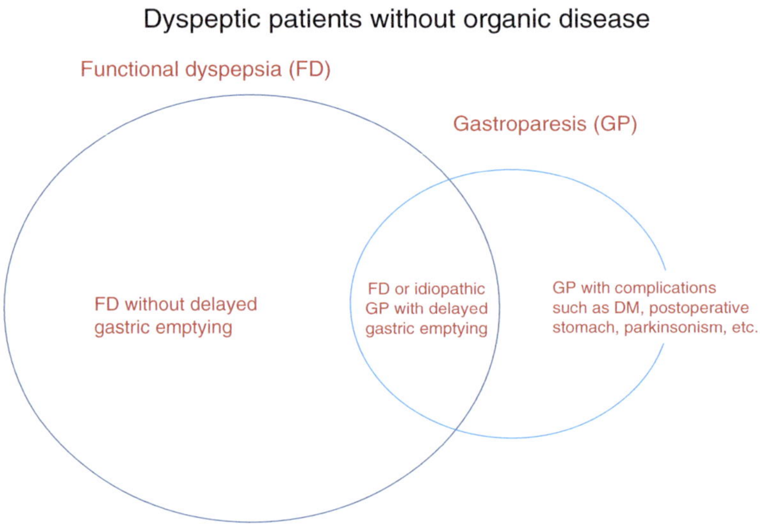

Fig. 32.2 Relationship between FD and GPPatients with upper abdominal symptoms in the absence of organic diseases

Competing Interests The author has no competing interests to declare that are relevant to the content of this chapter.

References

1. Camilleri M, et al. Gastroparesis. Nat Rev Dis Primers. 2018;4:41–60.
2. Oshima T, et al. Knowledge, attitude, and practice survey of gastroparesis in Asia by Asian neurogastroenterology and motility association. J Neurogastroenterol Motil. 2021;27:46–54.
3. Choung RS, et al. Risk of gastroparesis in subjects with type 1 and 2 diabetes in the general population. Am J Gastroenterol. 2012;107:82–8.
4. Stanghellini V, et al. Gastroduodenal disorders. Gastroenterology. 2016;150:1380–92.
5. Miwa H, et al. Evidence-based clinical practice guidelines for functional dyspepsia 2021. J Gastroenterol. 2022;57:47–61.
6. Stanghellini V, et al. Risk indicators of delayed gastric emptying of solids in patients with functional dyspepsia. Gastroenterology. 1996;110:1036–42.
7. Cherian D, et al. Nausea and vomiting in diabetic and idiopathic gastroparesis. Neurogastroenterol Motil. 2012;24:217–22.
8. Soykan I, et al. Demography, clinical characteristics, psychological and abuse profiles, treatment, and long-term follow-up of patients with gastroparesis. Dig Dis Sci. 1998;43:2398–404.
9. Jung HK, et al. The incidence, prevalence, and outcomes of patients with gastroparesis in Olmsted County, Minnesota, from 1996 to 2006. Gastroenterology. 2009;136:1225–33.
10. Oshima T, et al. Epidemiology of functional gastrointestinal disorders in Japan and in the World. J Neurogastroenterol Motil. 2015;21:320–9.

Case Discussion, Postprandial Fullness

33

Fumio Tanaka

Abstract

"Postprandial fullness" is one of the symptoms of dyspepsia and is primarily associated with food intake. Therefore, the Rome IV criteria, which are the diagnostic criteria for functional dyspepsia (FD), identify "bothersome postprandial fullness" as one of the characteristic symptoms of the postprandial distress syndrome subtype of FD. In the management of patients with chronic postprandial fullness, it is important to carefully differentiate possible underlying diseases. Consider the differential diagnosis of systemic diseases such as collagen diseases, endocrine disorders, metabolic diseases, drug-induced causes, and organic gastrointestinal diseases. FD can only be diagnosed after these diseases have been ruled out. The pathophysiology of postprandial fullness involves multiple factors, and the mechanisms by which symptoms arise are complex. For example, delayed gastric emptying and impaired gastric accommodation are considered representative mechanisms. The first-line treatments for FD are acotiamide, gastric acid-secretion inhibitors (proton pump inhibitors and histamine H2 receptor antagonists), and Rikkunshito (a Kampo medicine). Acotiamide is a prokinetic agent and improves gastric emptying and gastric accommodation through acetylcholinesterase inhibition.

Keywords

Postprandial fullness · Postprandial distress syndrome · Delayed gastric emptying · Impaired gastric accommodation · Psychological factors · Acotiamide · Gastric acid-secretion inhibitors · Rikkunshito

"Postprandial fullness" is one of the symptoms of dyspepsia and is primarily associated with food intake. Therefore, the Rome IV criteria, which are the diagnostic criteria for functional dyspepsia (FD), identify "bothersome postprandial fullness" as one of the characteristic symptoms of the postprandial distress syndrome (PDS) subtype of FD [1]. Postprandial fullness can occur in healthy individuals, and it is difficult to establish clear criteria for pathological postprandial fullness. However, the Rome IV criteria include a note that defines it as "severe enough to impact on usual activities."

F. Tanaka (✉)
Department of Gastroenterology, Osaka Metropolitan University Graduate School of Medicine, Osaka, Japan
e-mail: tanaka.f@omu.ac.jp

H. Kaneko et al. (eds.), *Disorders of Gut-Brain Interaction*,
https://doi.org/10.1007/978-981-95-6974-8_33

1 Case Presentation (FD)

Case: 46-year-old female
Chief Complaint: Severe postprandial fullness
Past History: *Helicobacter pylori* eradication at age 28 years
Family History: No notable findings
Allergy History: Pollinosis
Smoking History: None
Alcohol Consumption: Occasional drinking
Regular Medications: None
Current Medical History: The patient has been aware of having a weak stomach since childhood. Two years ago, she experienced severe postprandial fullness and epigastric pain and visited a local physician. Esophagogastroduodenoscopy (EGD) revealed no abnormalities, and treatment with acid secretion inhibitors led to rapid improvement. One year ago, she was promoted at work and given significant responsibilities. However, 3 months ago, severe postprandial fullness recurred. She monitored her condition, but postprandial fullness persisted about 5 days a week, leading to increased anxiety. Consequently, she sought further evaluation and treatment.
Physical Examination: The abdomen was flat and soft, with no surgical scars. Bowel sounds were normal. Mild tenderness was noted in the epigastric region without muscular defense or rebound tenderness. No tenderness was observed in other areas.

2 Clinical Course

Blood tests were conducted to exclude systemic diseases that could cause postprandial fullness, but no abnormalities were found. EGD, abdominal contrast-enhanced CT, and abdominal ultrasound were performed to investigate organic diseases. EGD showed no abnormalities in the esophagus or duodenum, but atrophic gastritis was observed in the stomach. Biopsies from the gastric and duodenal mucosa showed no eosinophilic infiltration of 20 or more cells per high-power field. Both abdominal contrast-enhanced CT and abdominal ultrasound showed no abnormalities, and no stenosis or mass lesions were observed in the gastrointestinal tract. Based on these findings, FD was diagnosed. According to the severe postprandial fullness, the patient was diagnosed with PDS, a subtype of FD. Treatment with the Kampo medicine Rikkunshito at 7.5 g/day was administered orally. After 8 weeks of treatment, the postprandial fullness improved, and the accompanying anxiety also decreased.

3 Discussion

The definition of FD in the Japanese clinical practice guidelines is as follows: FD is defined as "a condition chronically presenting symptoms centered in the upper abdomen, such as epigastric pain or discomfort, in the absence of any organic, systemic, or metabolic disease that is likely to explain the symptoms" [2]. Therefore, to diagnose FD, it is required to first exclude other diseases through history taking and various tests. A diagnostic flowchart for FD starting with postprandial fullness is shown (Fig. 33.1).

Since the publication of the revised second edition of the Japanese clinical practice guidelines in 2021, EGD is not essential for the diagnosis of FD. Instead, the necessity of endoscopy is determined based on the case. For example, if alarm signs (warning signs) are positive, suggesting organic abnormalities, endoscopy is proactively performed. Alarm signs include the appearance of new symptoms in the elderly, weight loss, recurrent vomiting, bleeding, dysphagia, abdominal mass, fever, and a family history of esophageal or gastric cancer.

In this case, EGD was performed due to the history of *Helicobacter pylori* eradication, a history of allergies such as pollinosis, and the persistence of symptoms for 3 months without improvement, and it is necessary to exclude organic diseases. A history of *H. pylori* infection always indicates the possibility of gastric cancer, and a history of allergies suggests the possibility of non-eosinophilic esophagitis (EoE) eosinophilic gastrointestinal diseases (EGIDs). Non-EoE EGIDs is a chronic allergic disease

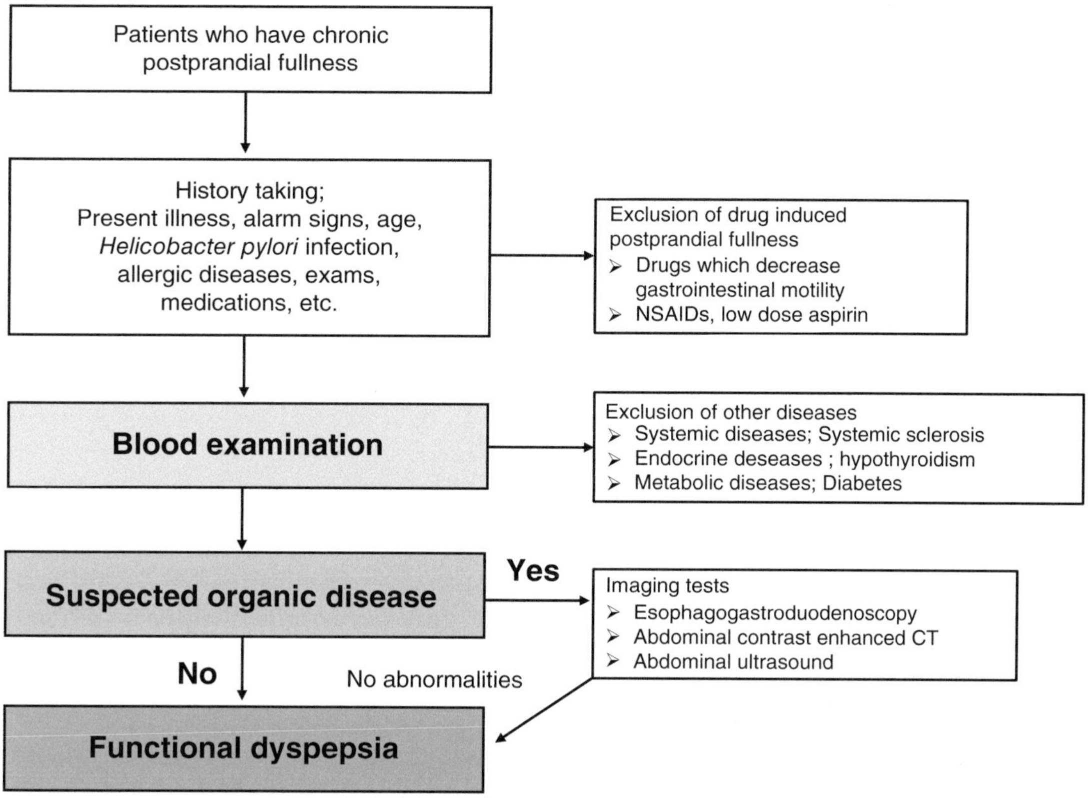

Fig. 33.1 Diagnostic flowchart for FD starting with postprandial fullness

characterized by significant eosinophilic infiltration of 20 or more cells per high-power field in the stomach and duodenum. Even if the endoscopic findings of the stomach and duodenum are normal, biopsy is important to identify eosinophilic infiltration. In this case, no organic abnormalities such as gastric cancer or non-EoE EGIDs were observed on EGD.

H. pylori can also cause dyspeptic symptoms, but in this case, more than a year had passed since eradication, and dyspeptic symptoms persisted; it was determined to be true FD rather than *H. pylori*-associated dyspepsia. In addition to EGD, it is desirable to perform abdominal contrast-enhanced CT and abdominal ultrasound to confirm the absence of organic diseases. For example, if there is advanced cancer or extrinsic compression causing stenosis beyond the stomach, subileus may occur, leading to symptoms such as postprandial fullness, abdominal bloating, vomiting, and abdominal pain due to intestinal dilation and content retention proximal to the stenosis.

FD often coexists with other functional gastrointestinal disorders, and PDS is reported to have a comorbidity risk with irritable bowel syndrome (IBS), particularly constipation-predominant IBS [3]. Therefore, it is important to consider that some cases of postprandial fullness may be associated with constipation.

The pathophysiology of postprandial fullness involves multiple factors, and the mechanisms by which symptoms arise are complex. For example, delayed gastric emptying and impaired gastric accommodation are considered representative mechanisms. Gastric accommodation is a physiological response that allows the proximal stomach to relax and accommodate food when it enters the stomach. Impaired gastric emptying or gastric accommodation can cause pressure on the gastric wall from the gastric contents, stimulating mechanoreceptors distributed in intrinsic primary afferent sensory nerve terminals in the mucosa and muscle layers, potentially leading to postprandial fullness. However, specific nociceptors for postprandial fullness have not yet been identified, and the details remain unclear.

Methods for evaluating gastric emptying include gastric emptying scintigraphy, breath tests, and abdominal ultrasound, but none are covered by Japanese insurance, and currently, these tests are conducted for research purposes in limited facilities, making it difficult to perform them in general clinical settings. Since postprandial fullness can occur due to decreased gastric motility, it is also necessary to exclude secondary systemic and metabolic diseases that can cause decreased gastrointestinal motility. Examples include collagen diseases such as systemic sclerosis, endocrine diseases such as hypothyroidism and hyperparathyroidism, and metabolic diseases such as diabetes. To differentiate these, it is important to conduct blood tests and inquire about the presence of accompanying symptoms outside the gastrointestinal tract, such as joint pain and rashes.

Additionally, it is necessary to ask for a history of medications that can decrease gastrointestinal motility. Examples include anticholinergic drugs such as antidepressants, narcotic analgesics, calcium channel blockers, diuretics, metal ion-containing drugs such as iron and calcium preparations, and L-dopa. The use of drugs that can cause injury to the gastrointestinal mucosa, such as Nonsteroidal anti-inflammatory drugs (NSAIDs) and low-dose aspirin, should also be considered.

FD can only be diagnosed if other diseases and drug-induced factors causing postprandial fullness have been definitely ruled out. Conversely, it is crucial to avoid diagnosing FD without differentiating these conditions. The diagnostic criteria for FD include both Japanese-specific criteria and the Rome IV criteria (Fig 33.2). This case meets both the Japanese and Rome IV criteria for FD. The Japanese criteria are characterized by the absence of a specific disease duration and the absence of consideration of symptom frequency because they allow a broad diagnosis of FD. In contrast, the Rome IV criteria are more stringent and are used for research purposes. Clinically, FD should be diagnosed and treated if the Japanese criteria are in place, even if the Rome IV criteria are not.

Psychological factors such as anxiety and depression may be present in the background of FD patients. In this case, the recurrence of postprandial fullness was triggered by a promotion at work, but in clinical practice, there is not always a triggering episode, and patients may not be aware of it. Although a promotion at work may seem like a positive event socially, it can be a stressful and challenging episode for the individual, depending on their perception. Therefore, it is extremely important to consider the psychological factors and social background of the patient in FD management.

➢ The definition of functional dyspepsia (FD) in the Japanese clinical practice guidelines

'a condition chronically presenting symptoms centered in the upper abdomen, such as epigastric pain or discomfort, in the absence of any organic, systemic, or metabolic disease that is likely to explain the symptoms'

➢ Rome IV diagnostic criteria for FD*

1. One or more of the following**;
(a) Bothersome postprandial fullness
(b) Bothersome early satiation
(c) Bothersome epigastric pain
(d) Bothersome epigastric burning

And

2. No evidence of structural disease (including at upper endoscopy) that is likely to explain the symptoms

* Criteria fulfilled for the last 3 months with symptom onset at least 6 months prior to diagnosis
** For postprandial distress syndrome; Must include (a) and/or (b) at least 3 days a week
** For epigastric pain syndrome; Must include (c) and/or (d) at least 1 day a week

Fig. 33.2 Diagnostic criteria for FD

4 Treatment of FD

The first-line treatments for FD are as follows:

1. Acotiamide
2. Gastric acid-secretion inhibitors (proton pump inhibitors and histamine H2 receptor antagonists)
3. Rikkunshito (a Kampo medicine)

Acotiamide belongs to the category of a prokinetic agent and improves gastric emptying and gastric accommodation through acetylcholinesterase inhibition. Acotiamide has been shown to be effective only for symptoms associated with PDS, such as postprandial fullness and early satiety, and is considered less effective for epigastric pain [4].

The efficacy of proton pump inhibitors has been demonstrated in meta-analyses, with symptom resolution or minimal symptoms observed in 31.1% of the proton pump inhibitor group compared to 25.8% of the placebo group, with a risk ratio of 0.88 (95% confidence interval 0.82–0.94) [5]. However, proton pump inhibitors are not covered by Japanese insurance for FD. Histamine H_2 receptor antagonists have also been shown to be effective in meta-analyses, with similar efficacy to proton pump inhibitors [5]. Potassium-competitive acid blockers have not yet undergone placebo-controlled randomized trials, and their efficacy is currently unclear.

Rikkunshito became a first-line treatment in the revised second edition of the Japanese clinical practice guidelines. Placebo-controlled randomized trials, such as the DREAM study conducted in Japan, have established evidence for its efficacy. Rikkunshito improves gastric emptying and gastric accommodation and enhances the secretion of ghrelin, an appetite-stimulating hormone. In the DREAM study, the response rate to Rikkunshito at 7.5 g/day for 8 weeks was 78.7%, significantly higher than the 63.2% in the placebo group [6]. Symptom-specific efficacy analysis showed particularly high efficacy for symptoms associated with PDS, such as postprandial fullness. Additionally, Rikkunshito has been shown to have an anxiolytic effect, with the degree of anxiety improvement correlating with the improvement in abdominal symptoms.

Take-Home Message
In the management of patients with chronic postprandial fullness, it is important to carefully differentiate possible underlying diseases. Consider the differential diagnosis of systemic diseases such as collagen diseases, endocrine disorders, metabolic diseases, drug-induced causes, and organic gastrointestinal diseases. The differentiation of non-EoE EGIDs has become increasingly important in recent years. FD can only be diagnosed after these diseases have been ruled out.

Competing Interests The author has no competing interests to declare that are relevant to the content of this chapter.

References

1. Stanghellini V, et al. Gastroduodenal disorders. Gastroenterology. 2016;150:1380–92.
2. Miwa H, et al. Evidence-based clinical practice guidelines for functional dyspepsia 2021. J Gastroenterol. 2022;57:47–61.
3. Choi YJ, et al. Overlap between irritable bowel syndrome and functional dyspepsia including subtype analyses. J Gastroenterol Hepatol. 2017;32:1553–61.
4. Xiao G, et al. Efficacy and safety of acotiamide for the treatment of functional dyspepsia: systematic review and meta-analysis. Sci World J. 2014;2014:541950.
5. Pinto-Sanchez MI, et al. Proton pump inhibitors for functional dyspepsia. Cochrane Database Syst Rev. 2017;11:CD011194.
6. Tominaga K, et al. Rikkunshito simultaneously improves dyspepsia correlated with anxiety in patients with functional dyspepsia: A randomized clinical trial (the DREAM study). Neurogastroenterol Motil. 2018;30:e13319.

34 Case Discussion, Epigastric Pain

Hiroshi Mihara

Abstract

Epigastric pain is a hallmark symptom of functional dyspepsia (FD), often challenging to manage when resistant to standard treatments. We present the case of a 46-year-old woman with persistent epigastric pain meeting Rome IV criteria for FD, unresponsive to *Helicobacter pylori* eradication, proton pump inhibitor, and a herbal medicine, Rikkunshito. The patient's symptoms were exacerbated by psychosocial stressors, including a traumatic family history of gastric cancer and unresolved emotional distress. A narrative-based, psychosomatic approach was introduced, integrating elements of cognitive behavioral therapy and whole person care. The physician guided the patient to observe her thoughts, bodily sensations, and emotional responses, fostering self-awareness and emotional regulation. Over 6 months, her symptoms improved, and she was discharged. This case illustrates that treatment-resistant FD may require interventions beyond pharmacological therapy, addressing the patient's cognition and emotion. A strong physician–patient relationship and attentiveness to psychosocial context are vital. Whole person care, involving both problem-solving and narrative modes, can help physicians maintain therapeutic presence under clinical stress. This approach enhances patient-centered care and supports symptom management, even when complete resolution is not possible.

Keywords

Functional dyspepsia (FD) · Epigastric pain syndrome · Treatment-resistant dyspepsia · Rome IV criteria · *Helicobacter pylori* eradication · Cognitive behavioral therapy (CBT) · Psychosomatic medicine · Physician–patient relationship · Somatic symptom disorder · Whole person care

1 Introduction

Epigastric pain is known as a major symptom of functional dyspepsia (FD), and appropriate management for treatment-resistant cases is discussed.

2 Case Presentation

Case: 46-year-old female
Chief Complaint: Epigastric pain
Medical History: Appendectomy at age 15 years

H. Mihara (✉)
Department of Educational Development, Center for Medical Education and Department of General Medicine, Faculty of Medicine, Sapporo Medical University, Sapporo, Japan

H. Kaneko et al. (eds.), *Disorders of Gut-Brain Interaction*,
https://doi.org/10.1007/978-981-95-6974-8_34

Family History: Grandmother and father had gastric cancer

Allergy History and Preferences: None

Background of the Attending Physician: Previously specialized in organ medicine at a core hospital, transferred to a 200-bed general hospital a year ago, and now responsible for general internal medicine outpatient care twice a week.

3 Clinical Course

The patient had been experiencing epigastric pain for the past year and had undergone an upper gastrointestinal endoscopy and received standard medication from a local physician, but symptoms did not improve, leading to a referral. At the time of consultation, the patient met the Rome IV criteria for FD. Physical examination revealed no notable findings, and *Helicobacter pylori* positivity was confirmed. The attending physician informed the patient that the likelihood of a life-threatening condition was low and recommended *H. pylori* eradication therapy. Successful eradication was confirmed 2 months later. However, symptoms persisted, ruling out *H. pylori*-related dyspepsia, and PPI and a herbal medicine, Rikkunshito, were ineffective, leading to a diagnosis of treatment-resistant FD. The attending physician considered whether to try tandospirone citrate, and the following interaction occurred:

Patient: I can't help but worry about my stomach.

Physician: I understand. Please tell me more.

Patient: Yes. I'm approaching the age when my strict father died of gastric cancer, and I can't help but worry that I might get gastric cancer too.

Physician: I see.

Patient: The previous doctor always seemed rushed during consultations, and I didn't feel comfortable talking. But I was so worried about gastric cancer that I finally consulted him, and he got angry, saying, "Don't you trust the endoscopy results?" That's why I decided to come here.

Physician: I understand. Can you tell me more about when your stomach hurts?

Patient: My mother-in-law was a scary person, and whenever I remember her, my stomach hurts. Then I can't help but worry that I might get gastric cancer. But taking medication helps a bit.

Physician: Do you live with your mother-in-law?

Patient: No, she passed away two years ago, and my husband has been living alone for work for the past year.

Physician: Thank you for sharing. It seems that memories of your mother-in-law and anxiety about your father's gastric cancer are affecting your abdominal pain. Next time you feel abdominal pain or anxiety, try to take a deep breath and focus on your breathing. Observe your thoughts, the nature of the pain, and your feelings of anxiety. If possible, keep a diary and show it to me next time.

Patient: I understand. I'll try.

Subsequent Course: Gradually, the patient began to have leftover medication, and six months later, she was discharged with a good prognosis.

4 Discussion

According to the Rome IV criteria, this case is considered treatment-resistant FD (epigastric pain syndrome) [1]. The patient perceived her epigastric pain as severe due to negative emotions triggered by past memories and anxiety related to her father's history of gastric cancer, significantly impacting her daily life. This meets the criteria for somatic symptom disorder in the *Diagnostic and Statistical Manual of Mental Disorders, Fifth Edition* (published by the American Psychiatric Association in 2013). The clinical practice guidelines for FD recommend additional tests and psychosomatic treatment for treatment-resistant FD [2], and the guidelines for psychosomatic medicine emphasize respecting the patient's reasons for consultation and interpretation when selecting treatment methods [3].

Given that the primary cause of this case appears to be anxiety based on past trauma and the father's history of gastric cancer, explanation and cognitive behavioral therapy (CBT) are considered appropriate. The new generation of CBT focuses more on changing responses to cognitive distortions rather than correcting them. The attending physician continued medication treatment while providing training for the patient to observe her thoughts (cognition), the nature of her abdominal pain (sensation), and feelings of anxiety (emotion) as they occur, aiming to help the patient improve her symptoms or eliminate the need for consultation even if symptoms persist.

CBT for FD is considered effective [4, 5], and recent studies have shown the efficacy of the new generation of CBT (Fig. 34.1) [6]. Additionally, internet-based CBT for functional abdominal pain in children has been shown to be cost-effective and effective in randomized controlled trial (RCT) [7]. The clinical practice guidelines for FD propose an algorithm that starts with "explanation and reassurance" and then implements psychosomatic treatment for treatment-resistant FD. However, it is known that the placebo effect obtained during "explanation and reassurance" decreases over time, so it is desirable to consider the patient's cognition and emotions regarding symptoms as much as possible during medication treatment.

Building and maintaining a good patient–physician relationship while thoroughly listening to the psychosocial background is recommended by both the Rome IV and FD clinical practice guidelines [1, 2]. A good patient–physician relationship improves patient satisfaction, treatment adherence, and treatment outcomes. Studies on IBS patients have reported that a good patient–physician relationship reduces the number of necessary follow-up visits [8]. On the other hand, as in the previous physician's case, when the attending physician cannot address the patient's thoughts (cognition) or anxiety (emotion), it can lead to "traumatic experiences" for the patient. This is because the attending physician, faced with a patient suffering from unresponsive symptoms, may experience mental stress and adopt a critical attitude instead of maintaining a harmonious demeanor. How can the attending physician maintain a harmonious attitude while continuously focusing on the patient's symptoms, thoughts (cognition), and anxiety (emotion) during outpatient care for treatment-resistant cases?

The Japanese Society of Internal Medicine Specialist Committee Whole Person Care Working Group proposes two modes for outpatient care: the "problem-solving mode," which focuses on identifying and resolving issues related to the patient's illness, and the "narrative mode," which considers and addresses the patient's suffering from the perspective of its meaning. They advocate for switching between these two modes as needed during outpatient care (Fig. 34.2) [9].

The Whole Person Care program developed at McGill University in Canada, which aims to train healthcare providers to face distressed

Fig. 34.1 Improvement in quality of life after CBT in FD: RCT results

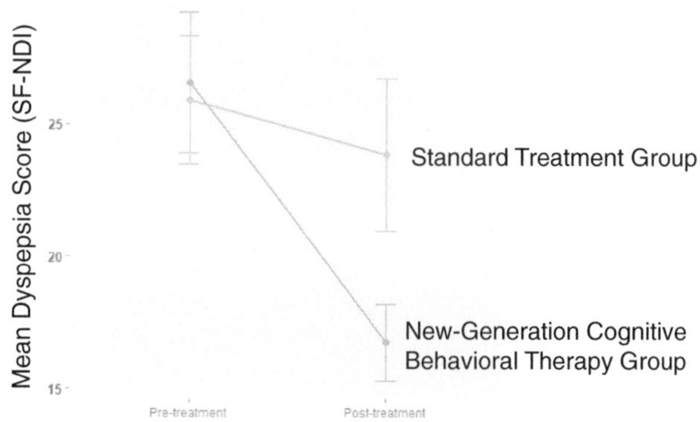

Adapted and reproduced from Reference 6

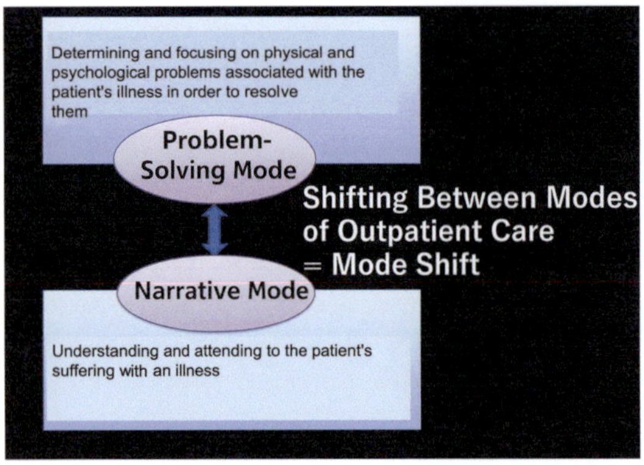

Adapted and reproduced from Reference 9

Fig. 34.2 Shifting between modes of outpatient care: problem-solving mode and narrative mode

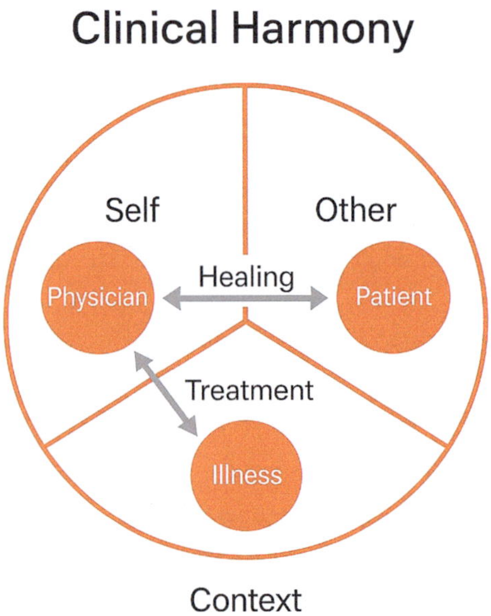

Adapted and reproduced from Reference 10

Fig. 34.3 A harmonious clinical relationship

patients, suggests that healthcare providers, even under high-stress conditions, may adopt critical attitudes. It proposes that healthcare providers have a role not only in diagnosis and treatment but also in supporting patients to face their illness, grow as individuals despite their illness, and accept changes when recovery is not possible (Fig. 34.3) [10]. To continuously face the patient's distress, healthcare providers must also observe their own thoughts (cognition), sensations such as breathing, and feelings of anxiety (emotion) to maintain a harmonious attitude. To deal with the patient's distress, a method 'STOP' has been suggested of immediately adjusting the mind by temporarily stopping thoughts (Stop), taking a deep breath and focusing on the breath (Take a breath), paying attention to physical sensations, thoughts, and emotions (Observe), and then resuming (Proceed) [10].

5 Finally

We examined appropriate responses to patients with treatment-resistant epigastric pain from the perspectives of drug therapy and the mental activities (cognition, sensation, and emotion) of patients and outpatient physicians.

After providing explanation and reassurance, and while administering pharmacological treatment, outpatient physicians should consciously regulate their own emotions, keeping in mind the possibility of treatment-resistant cases. They should help patients to develop the ability to observe and accept their symptoms as they occur, including their thoughts (cognition), the nature of the abdominal pain (sensations), and feelings such as anxiety (emotions).

Take-Home Message

- Epigastric pain is a major symptom of FD and is often persistent and unresponsive to medication.
- This treatment-resistant condition can cause mental stress for both the patient and the attending physician.
- The physician's negative emotions or critical attitudes under stress may lead to "traumatic experiences" for the patient.
- To help the patient stay grounded in the present moment, the attending physician must also cultivate their own awareness to remain present during care.

Competing Interests The author has no competing interests to declare that are relevant to the content of this chapter.

References

1. Mearin F, et al. Bowel disorders. Gastroenterology. 2016;150(6):1393–1407.e5.
2. Miwa H, et al. Evidence-based clinical practice guidelines for functional dyspepsia 2021. J Gastroenterol. 2022;57(2):47–61. Epub 2022 Jan 21.
3. Fukunaga M, et al. Functional dyspepsia (FD). In: Komaki M, et al., editors. Psychosomatic medicine—diagnosis and treatment guidelines 2006. Kyowa Kikaku; 2006. p. 42–62. (in Japanese).
4. Orive M, et al. A randomized controlled trial of a 10-week group psychotherapeutic treatment added to standard medical treatment in patients with functional dyspepsia. J Psychosom Res. 2015;78(6):563–8.
5. Haug TT, et al. Psychotherapy in functional dyspepsia. J Psychosom Res. 1994;38(7):735–44.
6. Teh KKJ, et al. Mindfulness-based cognitive therapy in functional dyspepsia: a pilot randomized trial. J Gastroenterol Hepatol. 2021;36(8):2058–66.
7. Lalouni M, et al. Clinical and cost effectiveness of online cognitive behavioral therapy in children with functional abdominal pain disorders. Clin Gastroenterol Hepatol. 2019;17(11):2236–2244.e11.
8. Owens DM, et al. The irritable bowel syndrome: long-term prognosis and the physician-patient interaction. Ann Intern Med. 1995;122(2):107–12.
9. Tsuchiya S, Imanaga T, Kawaguchi A, et al. Seminar report: whole person care workshop—what is whole person care for a physician in practice? J Jpn Soc Intern Med. 2020;109(6):1155–61. (in Japanese)
10. Hutchinson TA, editor. Whole person care: a new paradigm for the 21st century. New York: Springer; 2011.

35 Case Discussion, Nausea, Vomiting

Mariko Hojo

Abstract

The classification of nausea and vomiting disorders has changed over time, but their pathophysiology and effective treatments remain unclear. Diagnosis relies on excluding organic diseases, and symptomatic management is central.

Keywords

Nausea · Vomiting · Cannabis · Chronic nausea and vomiting syndrome · Cyclic vomiting syndrome · Cannabinoid hyperemesis syndrome

1 Introduction

Nausea is a subjective symptom characterized by an unpleasant sensation of wanting to vomit, occurring in the epigastric, precordial, and pharyngeal regions. Vomiting refers to the forceful expulsion of gastric or intestinal contents through the mouth due to contractions of the rectus abdominis and thoracic wall muscles.

According to the Rome IV criteria, nausea and vomiting disorders are classified into chronic nausea and vomiting syndrome, characterized by distressing nausea or vomiting occurring at least once a week; cyclic vomiting syndrome, characterized by acute episodes of vomiting lasting less than one week and recurring periodically; and cannabinoid hyperemesis syndrome, characterized by vomiting similar to cyclic vomiting syndrome but associated with continuous use of cannabinoids and improvement upon cessation [1].

To diagnose nausea and vomiting disorders, it is necessary to exclude gastrointestinal diseases such as ileus, infectious enteritis, gastrointestinal motility disorders including gastroparesis and pseudo-obstruction; central nervous system diseases such as increased intracranial pressure and cerebrovascular disorders; otolaryngological diseases such as Meniere's syndrome; cardiovascular diseases such as congestive heart failure; endocrine and metabolic diseases such as diabetic coma and uremia; psychogenic diseases such as anorexia nervosa and depression; and drug-induced nausea and vomiting.

Treatment options include antihistamine H_1 receptor antagonists, muscarinic M_1 receptor antagonists, dopamine D_2 receptor antagonists, and serotonin 5-HT_3 receptor antagonists. For chronic nausea and vomiting syndrome, tricyclic antidepressants have been reported to be effective [2]. For cyclic vomiting syndrome, migraine treatments such as triptans may be effective [3]. For cannabinoid hyperemesis syndrome, cessa-

M. Hojo (✉)
Department of Gastroenterology, Juntendo University Faculty of Medicine, Tokyo, Japan
e-mail: mhojo@juntendo.ac.jp

H. Kaneko et al. (eds.), *Disorders of Gut-Brain Interaction*,
https://doi.org/10.1007/978-981-95-6974-8_35

tion of cannabis use is prioritized over antiemetic treatment.

2 Case Presentation (Chronic Nausea and Vomiting Syndrome)

Case: 40-year-old female
Chief Complaint: Nausea
Medical History: None notable
Family History: None notable
Allergy History: None notable
Smoking History: None
Alcohol Consumption: Occasional drinking
Occupational History: Employed at a securities company (trader)
Current Medical History: Nausea symptoms have been present for about 4 years, occurring almost daily. Nausea is present upon waking but does not interfere with waking. There is no loss of appetite, and the severity of symptoms does not change with meals. Vomiting occurs occasionally but not daily, with a frequency of about three times a week at times and once a week at other times. The triggers for vomiting are unclear, but there is a tendency for vomiting to increase after eating out. Upper gastrointestinal contrast examinations during routine check-ups revealed no abnormalities. Since the symptoms did not interfere with daily life, they were left untreated, but due to persistent symptoms, the patient requested further examinations and treatment.
Physical Examination: The abdomen was flat and soft, with normal bowel sounds. There was no tenderness in the abdomen, and neurological examination revealed no abnormalities.

3 Clinical Course

The patient presented with nausea and vomiting without symptoms, such as heartburn or abdominal pain, and no warning signs, such as bleeding, weight loss, or fever. Bowel movements were daily with normal stool consistency. There was no dizziness or history of migraines. There were no signs suggestive of anorexia nervosa or depressive mood. There was no intake of drugs or supplements that could cause nausea. Urine tests, blood tests, and serum biochemical tests revealed no abnormalities, excluding electrolyte imbalances such as hypercalcemia, thyroid diseases, adrenal diseases, and diabetes. Upper and lower gastrointestinal endoscopy, abdominal ultrasound, and abdominal CT scans revealed no abnormalities, excluding gastrointestinal diseases. Head CT also revealed no abnormalities. Based on these findings, the patient was diagnosed with chronic nausea and vomiting syndrome and was instructed to take metoclopramide, which has dopamine D_2 receptor antagonist and serotonin 5-HT_3 receptor antagonist effects, as needed for distressing nausea. During the course of treatment, acotiamide, a cholinesterase inhibitor, was also prescribed for functional dyspepsia presenting with chronic epigastric symptoms without organic disease. After several years of follow-up, nausea disappeared, and occasional vomiting did not interfere with daily life. The reason for symptom improvement is unclear, but the patient was working as a trader at a securities company during the period of severe symptoms, which may have contributed to the stress.

4 Discussion

In the Rome II criteria, functional vomiting was classified as one of the functional gastroduodenal disorders along with functional dyspepsia, with nausea being a symptom of dysmotility-like dyspepsia [4]. However, in the Rome III criteria, nausea was classified as a nausea and vomiting disorder, forming a category within functional gastroduodenal disorders [5]. Nausea and vomiting disorders were further subclassified into chronic idiopathic nausea, which typically does not involve vomiting; functional vomiting, which requires vomiting; and cyclic vomiting syndrome, which has a consistent onset and duration of vomiting and no symptoms when vomiting is absent. In the Rome IV criteria, the subcategories were revised to chronic nausea and vomiting syndrome, cyclic vomiting syndrome, and cannabinoid hyperemesis syndrome [1]. Chronic nausea and vomiting syndrome recognizes the presence of either nausea or vomiting alone. The diagnostic criteria for cyclic vomiting syndrome were partially revised to include a characteristic of having at least 1 week without vomiting between episodes and recognizing the presence of symptoms other than vomiting during vomiting-free periods. Cannabinoid hyperemesis was excluded in Rome III but reclassified as cannabinoid hyperemesis syndrome in Rome IV. Nausea and vomiting disorders have undergone changes in classification and diagnostic criteria with each revision of the Rome criteria based on new literature, and their pathophysiology remains unclear. Nausea and vomiting can occur due to delayed gastric emptying, but symptoms can also occur with normal gastric emptying. Cyclic vomiting syndrome often shows accelerated gastric emptying during vomiting-free periods and delayed gastric emptying during vomiting episodes [6]. Psychological factors such as anxiety disorders or other psychiatric disorders are reported to be present in 20% of cases [7], with 84% of adult cyclic vomiting syndrome patients having anxiety disorders and 78% having mild to moderate depression [8]. Migraines are known to be associated with cyclic vomiting syndrome in children, and reports indicate that 24–70% of adult cyclic vomiting syndrome patients have comorbid migraines or a family history of migraines [6]. Mitochondrial dysfunction has also been implicated in cyclic vomiting syndrome in children [9].

Treatment options include antiemetics, prokinetic agents, tricyclic antidepressants, and triptan medications, but their efficacy is often insufficient. Reports suggest that gastric electrical stimulation [10] and psychotherapy [11] may be effective, but their utility has not been proven.

Nausea and vomiting disorders continue to undergo changes in classification and definition, and their pathophysiology remains unclear. Therefore, effective treatment methods are still unclear. Future research is needed.

Take-Home Message

- Diagnosis requires careful exclusion of organic diseases, central nervous system disorders, otolaryngological diseases, endocrine and cardiovascular diseases, electrolyte imbalances, and drug-induced nausea and vomiting.
- The classification and definition of nausea and vomiting disorders are still evolving, making consistent diagnosis difficult.
- The underlying pathophysiological mechanisms remain unclear, limiting the development of effective treatments.
- In clinical practice, dopamine D_2 receptor antagonists and serotonin 5-HT_3 receptor antagonists are commonly used despite limited evidence-based treatment options.

Competing Interests The author has no competing interests to declare that are relevant to the content of this chapter.

References

1. Stanghellini V, et al. Gastroduodenal disorders. Gastroenterology. 2016;150:1380–92.
2. Patel A, et al. Sensory neuromodulators in functional nausea and vomiting: predictors of response. Postgrad Med J. 2013;89(1049):131–6.
3. Hikita T, et al. Sumatriptan as a treatment for cyclic vomiting syndrome: a clinical trial. Cephalalgia. 2011;31(4):504–7.
4. Talley NJ, et al. Functional gastroduodenal disorders. Gut. 1999;45(Suppl 2):II37–42.
5. Tack J, et al. Functional gastroduodenal disorders. Gastroenterology. 2006;130:1466–79.
6. Abell TL, et al. Cyclic vomiting syndrome in adults. Neurogastroenterol Motil. 2008;20(4):269–84.
7. Prakash C, Clouse RE. Cyclic vomiting syndrome in adults: clinical features and response to tricyclic antidepressants. Am J Gastroenterol. 1999;94(10):2855–60.

8. Namin F, et al. Clinical, psychiatric and manometric profile of cyclic vomiting syndrome in adults and response to tricyclic therapy. Neurogastroenterol Motil. 2007;19(3):196–202.
9. Boles RG, et al. Am J Med Genet A. 2003;120A(4):474–82.
10. Reddymasu SC, et al. Efficacy of gastric electrical stimulation in improving functional vomiting in patients with normal gastric emptying. Dig Dis Sci. 2010;55:983–7.
11. Stravynski A. Behavioral treatment of psychogenic vomiting in the context of social phobia. J Nerv Ment Dis. 1983;171(7):448–51.

Topics, Genetic Polymorphism and Functional Dyspepsia

36

Akiko Shiotani

Abstract

This review focused on genetic polymorphisms that may be associated with susceptibility to functional dyspepsia (FD), based primarily on studies conducted in Japanese populations. G-proteins β3 (*GNβ3*) polymorphisms have been most frequently reported to be associated with FD. The higher frequency of *s/l* and *l/l SCL6A4* genotypes in women patients with epigastric pain syndrome and the *l/l* genotype in postprandial distress syndrome patients was reported. The primiR325 s5981521 T homozygotes leading to reduced post-transcriptional regulation of *SCL6A4* are possibly associated with FD. *TRPV1*G315C, *SCN10A* 2884G, 3275C, and 3218CC are also possible candidate single-nucleotide polymorphisms (SNPs). Genetic polymorphisms associated with FD vary in frequency among different ethnicities and countries, and no consensus has been reached regarding the association between these polymorphisms and the disease. In addition, the associations between *GHRL* and *COX-1* SNPs and subtypes of FD were reported. However, genetic polymorphisms associated with FD vary in frequency among different ethnicities and countries, and no consensus has been reached regarding the association. Recent genome-wide association studies (GWAS) have reported genetic correlations and overlaps between gastrointestinal and psychiatric disorders, highlighting the role of the brain–gut axis.

Further GWAS may lead to applications in personalized medicine.

Keywords

Single-nucleotide polymorphisms · G-protein β3 · Serotonin · *SCL6A4* · microRNA-325 · TRPV1 · *SCN10A*

1 Introduction

Functional gastrointestinal (GI) disorders include representative diseases such as irritable bowel syndrome (IBS) and functional dyspepsia (FD). FD is categorized into postprandial distress syndrome (PDS), characterized by postprandial upper abdominal discomfort, and epigastric pain syndrome (EPS), characterized by epigastric pain. The causes of FD involve multiple factors, including gastric and duodenal motility abnormalities, visceral hypersensitivity, psychosocial factors, genetic factors, environmental (child-rearing) influences, and microinflammation of the GI tract. In PDS, delayed gastric emptying and impaired adaptive relaxation of the stomach

A. Shiotani (✉)
Department of Gastroenterology and Hepatology, Kawasaki Medical School, Kurashiki, Japan
e-mail: shiotani@med.kawasaki-m.ac.jp

H. Kaneko et al. (eds.), *Disorders of Gut-Brain Interaction*,
https://doi.org/10.1007/978-981-95-6974-8_36

post-ingestion are thought to contribute to early satiation.

Genetic polymorphisms refer to variations in the DNA sequence among individuals, including single-nucleotide polymorphisms (SNPs), in which a single nucleotide in the DNA sequence differs, and microsatellite polymorphisms, in which the number of repeats in a repetitive sequence varies. The frequency of these polymorphisms varies among ethnicities and countries, and their association with diseases often yields inconsistent results. In this review, we focus on genetic polymorphisms that may be associated with susceptibility to FD, based primarily on studies conducted in Japanese populations.

2 G-Protein β3 (*GNβ3*)

G-proteins, abbreviated from guanine nucleotide-binding proteins, are intracellular signaling molecules involved in the cellular signal transduction of many membrane-bound receptors. Membrane receptor-associated heterotrimeric G-proteins consist of α, β, and γ subunits, and the β subunit is encoded by the *GNβ3* 45 gene. *GNβ3* is downstream of neurotransmitters such as dopamine, serotonin, and acetylcholine, acting on smooth muscle to influence GI motility. And it is also involved in visceral hypersensitivity via the central nervous system (CNS), such as the spinal cord and cerebrum. The *GNβ3* 825C>T (rs5443) SNP does not involve amino acid substitution, but T allele carriers exhibit enhanced G-protein function, while mL homozygous individuals have impaired signal transduction due to functional decline, which affects the CNS and GI functions.

Genetic polymorphisms of GNβ3 have been investigated and are most frequently reported among the numerous genetic polymorphisms associated with FD. Holtmann et al. first reported the involvement of specific genetic polymorphisms in FD disease susceptibility, identifying the *GNβ3* 825mL allele as a significant risk factor for dyspeptic symptoms. Subsequent studies in Western populations have reported inconsistent results. Some studies have demonstrated an association between the mL/TT allele and dyspeptic symptoms unrelated to meals, while other studies have reported an association between the T allele and FD [1].

In Japanese studies, Tahara et al. examined *GNβ3* rs5443 in 89 FD patients and 94 controls and demonstrated that the TT allele significantly contributed to the occurrence of dyspeptic symptoms in *Helicobacter pylori (H. pylori)*-negative individuals (16.7% vs. 40.5%, mL vs. TT, odds ratio 5.10, 95% CI = 1.21–21) [2]. Oshima et al. reported similar findings, with the TT allele showing a significant association with EPS-like symptoms (odds ratio 2.00, 95% CI = 1.07–3.76) but not PDS-like symptoms (odds ratio 0.68, 95% CI = 0.31–1.51) when adjusted for gender and age. However, the prevalence of *H. pylori* infection is unknown in this study [3]. Shimpuku et al. [4] evaluated gastric motility using the ^{13}C-acetate breath test, finding no significant association with FD overall, while mL homozygotes were associated with delayed gastric emptying. There is a previous study including 74 patients with FD and 64 control subjects; those with a gastric emptying time (Tmax) >60 min were classified as the prolonged Tmax group. Among the PDS patients, excluding gastroesophageal reflux symptoms, the proportion of individuals with the prolonged Tmax was significantly higher in the patient with the 825mL homozygous genotype compared to the T allele carriers (66.7% vs. 25.9%, odds ratio 5.71, 95% confidence interval = 1.12–2.92, $p = 0.045$) [4].

A meta-analysis of 13 case-control studies found no significant association between *GNβ3* 825T allele and FD overall, but a significant association with EPS (odds ratio 1.34, 95% CI = 1.10–1.63, $P = 0.003$) and a trend to association with PDS (odds ratio 1.19, 95% CI = 0.99–1.43, $P = 0.07$). Subgroup analyses in Asian and Western populations also showed no significant associations [5]. Korean studies have denied the association between FGID and *GNβ3*, suggesting phenotypic differences influenced by diet and living environment, with no established consensus.

3 Serotonin (5-HT)-Related Genes

Serotonin (5-HT) is a neurotransmitter synthesized primarily in enterochromaffin cells (EC cells) of the GI tract and acts as a factor regulating the brain–gut connection in the central and peripheral nervous systems. It is involved in various physiological functions such as appetite, sleep, sexual desire, and mood. It also plays a significant role in GI motility and secretion. Synthesized from tryptophan, 5-HT is released from the nerve terminal into the synaptic cleft, where it activates receptors on target cells, and it is taken up into cells by serotonin transporter (SERT). The concentration of 5-HT in the synaptic cleft is increased when uptake is weak due to the *SCL6A4* gene, which encodes SERT. In the *l/l* genotype, the reuptake of 5-HT is strong, and 5-HT levels in the synaptic cleft are reduced [6]. Diarrhea-predominant IBS shows higher frequencies of *l/s* or *s/s* genotypes compared to healthy individuals. However, the *l/l* genotype frequency is less than 6% in Japanese and Korean populations but over 20% in Western populations, indicating ethnic differences and inconsistent associations with IBS. IBS patients frequently exhibit anxiety disorders. A previous Japanese study reported that significantly stronger anxiety was observed in female IBS patients with the *l/l* genotype compared to those with the *s/s* genotype. Conversely, higher anxiety was observed in male patients with *s/s* genotype individuals. The *s/s* genotype is resistant to antidepressants and susceptible to emotional disorders due to environmental stress from childhood [6]. The association of *SCL6A4* with FD is mostly negative, as meta-analyses have denied significant correlations [5]. Japanese studies have reported significantly higher frequencies of *s/l* and *l/l* genotypes in female EPS patients; it is speculated that the *l/l* genotype may be more sensitive to serotonin depletion in women. Other studies matching gender and age report significant associations between *l/l* genotype and PDS (odds ratio 2.32, 95% CI = 1.23–4.37) [1].

MicroRNA-325 (miR325) exhibits strong affinity for the 3′-UTR of *SLC6A4* and contains SNPs, rs5938804 and rs5981521, which are in complete linkage with the coding region of miR325 in the pri-miR325 region. Arisawa et al. [7] reported strong associations between pri-miR325 s5981521 T homozygotes and FD in *H. pylori*-negative patients (odds ratio 8.37, 95% CI = 1.78–39.5). Furthermore, in the wild-type or 3′-UTR mutant form of the *SCL6A4* promoter, the involvement of a SNP in pri-miR325 may lead to reduced post-transcriptional regulation of *SCL6A4*, suggesting a potential association between FD and enhanced SERT function. Five subunit genes (A–E) of 5-HT3 receptors *(HTR3A)* have been identified. Few studies investigate the association between serotonergic function genes and FD. A study in a Caucasian population, including 592 dyspepsia patients, found higher frequencies of *HTR3A* c.-42C>T (C178T, rs1062613) T allele in severe dyspepsia patients (odds ratio 1.50, 95% CI = 1.06–2.20). This association was stronger in women (odds ratio 2.05, 95% CI = 1.25–3.39) and *SCL6A4 l/l* genotype (odds ratio 2.00, 95% CI = 1.01–3.94), with the strongest association in *l/l* genotype in women (odds ratio 3.50, 95% CI = 1.37–8.90) [8]. Associations with *5-HT1A*, *5-HT2A*, and *5-HT2C* have been investigated but remain unclear in FD. Japanese studies on 5-HT2A receptor T102C (rs6313) have reported a low association between this genetic polymorphism and susceptibility to dyspepsia symptoms [1].

4 Transient Receptor Potential Vanilloid 1 (TRPV1)

Noxious stimuli inducing pain are categorized into thermal, chemical, and mechanical stimuli. TRPV1 is a nociceptor receptor expressed in sensory neurons of the GI tract and abundant in the stomach. It is expressed across all layers, including mucosal, smooth muscle, and neural layers, sensing external noxious stimuli and activating mucosal defense mechanisms. Acid is a ligand for TRPV1, with acid hypersensitivity implicated in FD pathogenesis. Chili peppers are believed to have pharmacological effects such as stimulating appetite, promoting digestion, and enhancing the secretion of saliva and gastric juice. However, capsaicin, the main active component of chili peppers, is a TRPV1 agonist that suppresses gastric acid secretion. TRPV1 activation in sensory nerve endings transmits pain signals to the CNS, in the stomach, releasing calcitonin gene-related peptide, nitric oxide (NO), and substance P, promoting healing through vasodilation and increased permeability. Activation of TRPV1 has various effects, including promotion of mucus secretion, blood flow, epithelial cell proliferation, and motility in the colon. The role of TRPV1 expressed in the sensory nerves of the digestive tract is thought to be similar to that in the stomach, such as mucosal protection and wound healing.

The C allele of the *TRPV1* gene's G315C SNP increases TRPV1 protein expression and enhances responsiveness to capsaicin. Tahara et al. [9] examined 98 asymptomatic individuals and 109 FD patients to investigate the *TRPV1*G315C SNP and found a significant inverse correlation between the mL allele and FD (mL vs. others, odds ratio 0.40, 95% CI = 0.38–0.829). In a subgroup analysis, they also reported that mL allele carriers had a lower risk in the EPS group (odds ratio 0.25, 95% CI = 0.09–0.73), the PDS group (odds ratio 0.27, 95% CI = 0.07–0.96), and the *H. pylori*-positive FD group (odds ratio 0.28, 95% CI = 0.10–0.79). Additionally, in a study of 20 randomly selected healthy individuals, they evaluated the occurrence and severity of upper GI symptoms after drinking cold carbonated water and found that C homozygotes had significantly lower severity of digestive tract symptoms and less heaviness in the stomach. This suggests that TRPV1 hyperfunction is thought to be involved in inhibiting FD and may play a greater role in maintaining gastric homeostasis by increasing mucosal blood flow and adaptive relaxation responses rather than transmitting pain signals to the CNS.

5 SCN10A

Voltage-dependent sodium channels are involved in the excitation and transmission of nerve cells and are deeply associated with pain neural transmission. Nine types of voltage-dependent sodium channels (Nav1.1–Nav1.9) have been reported, with Nav1.7, Nav1.3, and Nav1.8 subtypes frequently associated with neuropathic pain. Visceral sensory impulses from the GI tract to the CNS are transmitted via unmyelinated C fibers. The tetrodotoxin resistance (TTX-r) sodium channel Nav1.8 has been identified on C-fibers and plays an important role in the transmission of visceral pain. *SCN10A* is the gene encoding Nav1.8, consisting of 27 exons, three genetic polymorphisms (2884A>G [rs57326399], 3218T>C [rs6795970], and 3275T>C [rs12632942]) with amino acid substitutions in exons 16, 17, and 18. Among these, 3218T>C is a gain-of-function mutation. Genome-wide association studies (GWAS) have reported its involvement in paroxysmal supraventricular tachycardia. Additionally, rs57326399 and rs12632942 are in strong linkage disequilibrium, while 3218T>C is in weak linkage disequilibrium with them. Since the minor alleles are loss-of-function, the haplotype carrying the 2884G, 3218T, and 3275C alleles is presumed to result in a loss of function of Nav1.8.

Arisawa et al. [10] examined these three *SCN10A* SNPs in 297 FD patients and 345 asymptomatic controls and reported a significant association with reduced FD risk. The rs6795970 C homozygote was most significantly associated (odds ratio 0.589, 95% CI = 0.402–0.864, p = 0.0067), and rs57326399 and rs12632942 were also significantly associated with FD, including both EPS and PDS. The haplotype with 2884G, 3275C, and 3218mL alleles was associated with lower FD risk (odds ratio 0.618, 95% CI = 0.448–0.853; p = 0.0034), with a notable association in *H. pylori*-negative subjects (odds ratio 0.463, 95% CI = 0.279–0.9768, p = 0.0029). The *SCN10A* loss-of-function haplotype is particularly associated with the suppression of FD in *H. pylori*-negative individuals.

Similar to TRPV1 and pri-miR325, *SCN10A* genetic polymorphisms are equally involved in both EPS and PDS, suggesting that increased sensitivity to peripheral stimuli is important in the pathogenesis of FD, regardless of subtype [7].

6 Others

Ghrelin is a growth hormone-releasing peptide that also promotes gastric acid secretion and gastric motility. Generally, blood levels of ghrelin increase during fasting and decrease after eating. Fasting ghrelin levels in PDS patients are significantly lower than in healthy individuals, and the postprandial decrease in healthy individuals is not observed in PDS patients. Futagami et al. [11] examined three SNPs in the ghrelin gene (*GHRL* Arg51Gln 346G>A [rs34911341], Leu72Met 408C>A [rs696217], and Gln90Leu 3412T>A [rs4684677]) and preproghrelin 3056T>C (rs2075356) in 23 *H. pylori*-negative EPS patients and 51 PDS patients. They reported that plasma acylated ghrelin levels were significantly lower in FD patients with the preproghrelin rs2075356 T homozygote and were significantly associated with hunger. Additionally, in a study evaluating gastric motility in 74 FD patients and 64 healthy controls, FD patients with the *GHRL* rs4684677 T homozygote had significantly higher depression scores. Although no association of the genetic polymorphisms with peak time in the 13C-acetate breath test was found, FD patients with the *GHRL* rs696217 A homozygote had significantly higher AUC values at 10 and 15 min, indicating an association with early postprandial gastric emptying in FD patients [12].

Cyclooxygenase (COX) is an enzyme crucial for converting arachidonic acid to prostaglandins (PG). COX-1 is distributed throughout the body and has a protective effect on the GI mucosa. Recent studies in Japanese populations have confirmed an association between NSAID-induced ulcers and the *COX-1* T-1676C (rs1340344) SNP, with the T allele being a significant risk factor for NSAID-induced ulcers. Although few studies have investigated the association between *COX-1* genotypes and dyspepsia, the *COX-1* gene promoter rs1340344 has been reported to be significantly associated with EPS in women T allele carriers, although no association was found with FD overall. However, a subsequent study in larger Japanese FD patient cohorts did not find this association [1].

Take-Home Message
Genetic polymorphisms associated with FD vary in frequency among different ethnicities and countries, and no consensus has been reached regarding the association. Recent studies using GWAS with publicly available data sources have reported genetic correlations and overlaps between GI and psychiatric disorders, highlighting the role of the brain–gut axis. Although FD was not included in these studies, it is conceivable that multiple genetic polymorphisms related to the brain–gut axis are involved in FD. Further GWAS research may lead to applications in personalized medicine.

Competing Interests The author has no competing interests to declare that are relevant to the content of this chapter.

References

1. Oshima T, et al. Genetic factors for functional dyspepsia. J Gastroenterol Hepatol. 2011;26(Suppl 3):83–7.
2. Tahara T, et al. Homozygous 825T allele of the GNB3 protein influences the susceptibility of Japanese to dyspepsia. Dig Dis Sci. 2008;53:642–6.
3. Oshima T, et al. The G-protein beta3 subunit 825 TT genotype is associated with epigastric pain syndrome-like dyspepsia. BMC Med Genet. 2010;11:13.
4. Shimpuku M, et al. G-protein β3 subunit 825CC genotype is associated with postprandial distress syndrome with impaired gastric emptying and with the feeling of hunger in Japanese. Neurogastroenterol Motil. 2011;23:1073–80.
5. Du L, et al. Gene Polymorphisms and Susceptibility to Functional Dyspepsia: A Systematic Review and Meta-Analysis. Gene Gastroenterol Res Pract. 2019;2019:3420548.
6. Karg K, et al. The serotonin transporter promoter variant (5-HTTLPR), stress, and depression meta-analysis revisited: evidence of genetic moderation. Arch Gen Psychiatry. 2011 68(5):444–54
7. Arisawa T, et al. Genetic polymorphism of pri-microRNA 325, targeting SLC6A4 3'-UTR, is closely associated with the risk of functional dyspepsia in Japan. J Gastroenterol. 2012 47:1091–8.
8. Mujakovic S, et al. Serotonin receptor 3A polymorphism c.-42C > T is associated with severe dyspepsia. BMC Med Genet. 2011;12:140.
9. Tahara T, et al. Homozygous TRPV1 315C influences the susceptibility to functional dyspepsia. J Clin Gastroenterol. 2010;44:e1–7.

10. Arisawa T, et al. Genetic polymorphisms of SCN10A are associated with functional dyspepsia in Japanese subjects. J Gastroenterol. 2013;48:73–80.
11. Futagami M, et al. The preproghrelin 3056 TT genotype is associated with the feeling of hunger and low acylated ghrelin levels in Japanese patients with Helicobacter pylori-negative functional dyspepsia. Internal Medicine. 2013;52:1155–63.
12. Yamawaki H, et al. Leu72Met408 Polymorphism of the Ghrelin Gene Is Associated With Early Phase of Gastric Emptying in the Patients With Functional Dyspepsia in Japan. J Neurogastroenterol Motil. 2015;21:93–102.

37 Topics, Microinflammation of the Duodenum and Functional Dyspepsia

Shuhei Agawa and Seiji Futagami

Abstract

Functional dyspepsia (FD) is a type of functional gastrointestinal disorder. It is characterized by motility disorders of the stomach and duodenum, such as adaptive relaxation disorder and impaired gastric emptying, with microinflammation of the duodenum known to be a contributing factor. Duodenal microinflammation can be triggered by various causes, including exposure to gastric acid, stress, and the intestinal microbiota. Recent reports have also suggested that early chronic pancreatitis may overlap with refractory FD, and the involvement of the duodenal trypsin receptor, protease-activated receptor-2 (PAR2), is also suspected. Further investigation into the pathophysiology of the condition is warranted.

Keywords

Functional dyspepsia (FD) · Subtle inflammation in the duodenum · Pancreatic enzyme abnormalities · Early chronic pancreatitis · Eosinophil · Protease-activated receptor-2 (PAR2)

S. Agawa · S. Futagami (✉)
Department of Internal Medicine, Division of Gastroenterology, Nippon Medical School, Tokyo, Japan
e-mail: seiji-f@nms.ac.jp

1 Introduction

Functional dyspepsia (FD) is a type of functional gastrointestinal disorders (FGIDs) that does not show abnormalities in blood tests, upper and lower gastrointestinal endoscopy, or abdominal CT scans. FGIDs include FD, characterized by upper abdominal bloating and stomach pain, and irritable bowel syndrome (IBS), which involves severe abdominal pain and discomfort associated with constipation or diarrhea. These conditions often overlap, and the number of patients has been increasing in today's stress-filled society, leading to a growing demand for medical care. The pathophysiology of FD has been increasingly understood, with gastric and duodenal motility disorders being identified in FD patients. One known factor is the presence of subtle inflammation in the duodenum. This section will discuss the relationship between subtle inflammation in the duodenum and the symptoms of FD.

2 The Relationship Between the Stomach and Duodenum in FD

FD is divided into two subgroups based on symptoms: postprandial distress syndrome (PDS), which causes early satiation, and epigastric pain syndrome (EPS), which presents with epigastric

H. Kaneko et al. (eds.), *Disorders of Gut-Brain Interaction*,
https://doi.org/10.1007/978-981-95-6974-8_37

pain. The pathophysiology of these subgroups is known to be related to impaired gastric accommodation and abnormal gastric emptying. Normally, when food is ingested and passes through the esophagus, the fundus of the stomach relaxes to store the food for about 15 min, preventing the rapid influx of high-calorie food into the duodenum. This mechanism, known as gastric accommodation, prevents a rapid rise in blood glucose levels. In FD patients, impaired gastric accommodation leads to inadequate expansion, resulting in early satiation, a symptom of PDS. Additionally, gastric emptying, which involves the rate at which food moves from the stomach to the duodenum, is related to the speed of food inflow into the duodenum. Rapid food inflow, combined with duodenal hypersensitivity, leads to postprandial EPS observed in the EPS group. Thus, in FD, impaired gastric accommodation, abnormal gastric emptying, and subtle inflammation in the duodenum are intricately related, leading to symptom manifestation.

Why does this pathophysiology occur? Many theories have been proposed to explain this pathophysiology. One such theory involves feedback from gastrointestinal hormones such as secretin and cholecystokinin (CCK). The duodenum neutralizes acidic gastric contents through alkaline secretion from Brunner's glands. By adjusting the pH of food and transporting it to the jejunum and ileum, the duodenum controls food transport and nutrient absorption. Therefore, various neuroendocrine cells in the duodenum produce hormones that deeply influence the regulation of gastric emptying by sensing sugars and fatty acids in food. When food enters the duodenum, I cells, K cells, and L cells in the duodenal and distal small intestinal mucosa produce CCK, gastric inhibitory polypeptide, glucagon-like peptide-1 (GLP-1), and peptide YY (PYY), which inhibit gastric emptying. GLP-1, in particular, is known to inhibit gastric emptying by suppressing ghrelin [1, 2].

As previously mentioned, FD patients have impaired gastric accommodation and regulation of gastric emptying. Therefore, rapid inflow of food into the duodenum occurs, leading to postprandial increases in blood glucose and GLP-1, which suppress ghrelin and further inhibit gastric emptying, resulting in reduced inflow of gastric contents into the duodenum [3]. We also focused on gastric emptying immediately after meals in FD patients and reported that the proportion of gastric contents flowing from the stomach to the duodenum at 5 and 15 min post-meal, indicated by area under the curve (AUC)5 and AUC15, was significantly higher compared to healthy individuals [4]. Thus, FD patients experience excessive early postprandial inflow of gastric contents into the duodenum, followed by delayed gastric emptying, leading to seemingly contradictory phenomena. Differences in the movement of food from the stomach to the duodenum compared to healthy individuals may contribute to symptoms and create differences in the duodenal environment.

3 Microinflammation in the Duodenum

The importance of the duodenum in FD symptoms has been previously mentioned. Recently, duodenal mucosal barrier dysfunction and microinflammation have been implicated in symptom manifestation. The duodenal mucosal barrier function is closely interrelated and consists of tight junctions such as occludin, claudin, and zonula occludens protein-1 (ZO-1), adherens junctions including α-catenin, β-catenin, and E-cadherin, and desmosomes like desmoglein-2 (DSG2). These multiple barrier functions protect the duodenum from various aggressive factors, including gastric acid.

In 2014, Vanheel et al. focused on this aspect and reported increased duodenal mucosal permeability due to decreased occludin expression in FD patients [5]. Subsequently, Komori et al. reported decreases in occludin, ZO-1, β-catenin, E-cadherin, and DSG2 [6]. From a visual perspective, Tanaka et al. used electron microscopy to report increased intercellular spaces in the duodenal mucosa of FD patients [7]. Additionally, from a symptom perspective, acid exposure has been reported to cause epigastric pain and a feeling of fullness, suggesting a relationship with pH. FD patients have been noted to have lower duodenal pH during the day [8, 9], and although the detailed mechanism is unknown, it is thought to be related to FD symptoms, linking to the previously mentioned increased mucosal permeability.

In FD patients, differences in the duodenal environment and mucosal barrier function compared to healthy individuals are thought to cause hypersensitivity and impaired gastric emptying. The presence of duodenal mucosal barrier dysfunction in FD patients has been discussed, but why do these changes occur? One cause seems to be subtle inflammation of the duodenal mucosa. One factor of subtle inflammation is acid exposure. As previously mentioned, the duodenum neutralizes acidic gastric contents and is prone to acid exposure. Barrier function impairment due to acid exposure is known in the esophagus, where mucosal barrier dysfunction and hypersensitivity occur in patients with reflux esophagitis [10]. FD patients have been noted to have lower duodenal pH during the day, suggesting that similar conditions may occur in the duodenum due to increased acid exposure. Additionally, the duodenum is exposed to various digestive juices such as pancreatic juice and bile, and their effects cannot be denied. The second factor is psychological stress, which is described in the Rome IV criteria as the brain–gut axis concept. When stress is perceived, corticotropin-releasing hormone is released from the hypothalamus, increasing colonic mucosal permeability and causing symptoms [11]. This aligns with the clinical symptoms of FD, where psychological factors are related to the condition, and the increase in FGIDs in modern society. The third factor is the influence of gut microbiota. Gut microbiota is involved in maintaining mucosal condition through metabolic products, and differences in gut microbiota composition between FD patients and healthy individuals have been reported [12]. This suggests a possible link to the unique mucosal barrier dysfunction in FD. Finally, microinflammation itself is a factor. Increased eosinophil counts in the duodenal mucosa of FD patients have been reported, and the presence of mast cell infiltration suggests the eosinophil-mast cell axis, with potential effects on the nervous system [13]. Thus, various factors intricately interact in the duodenum, creating the pathophysiology of FD (Fig. 37.1).

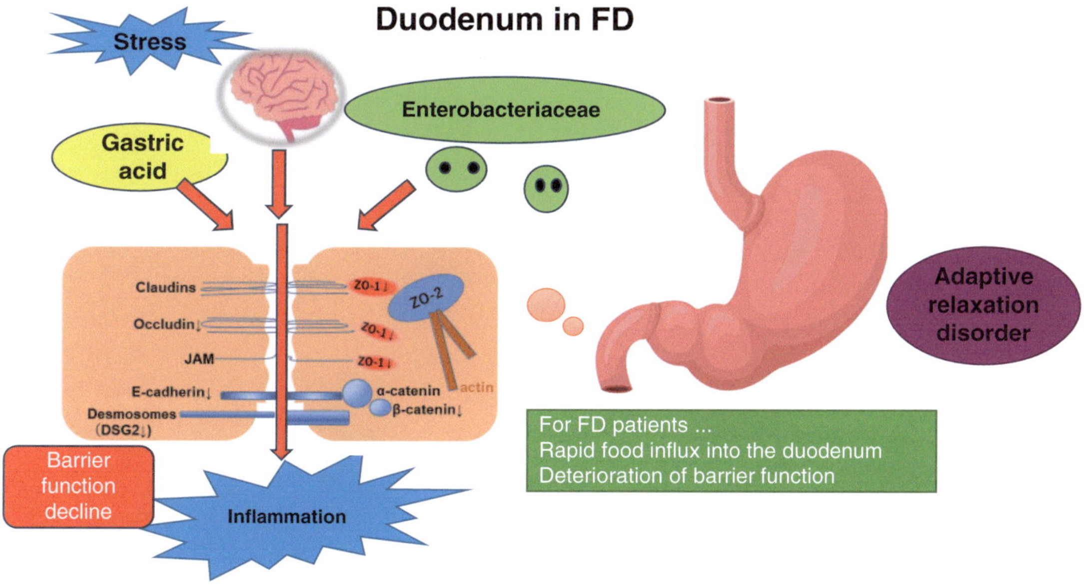

Fig. 37.1 Duodenum in FD (Adapted from Shuhei Agawa et al., Clinical Gastroenterology, 2021, Vol. 36, No. 5). ZO-1 zonula occludens-1, ZO-2 zonula occludens-2, JAM junctional adhesion molecule, DSG2 desmoglein-2

4 Treatment and Association with Pancreatic Diseases

The treatment of FD generally begins with lifestyle modifications such as improving sleep and diet, followed by pharmacotherapy. Pharmacotherapy is divided into first-line and second-line treatments. Historically, acid secretion inhibitors and prokinetics have been used as first-line treatments. The “Evidence-based clinical practice guidelines for functional dyspepsia 2021,” revised in 2021, introduced changes, adding the herbal medicine Rikkunshito as a first-line treatment and limiting gastrointestinal motility enhancers to acotiamide [14]. Consequently, first-line treatments now include proton pump inhibitors, potassium-competitive acid blockers, prokinetic (acotiamide), and herbal medicines (Rikkunshito), either as monotherapy or in combination.

If first-line treatments are insufficient, second-line treatments include other gastrointestinal motility enhancers (mosapride, trimebutine, and metoclopramide), other herbal medicines (Hangeshashinto and Kamishoyosan), and antidepressants (tricyclic antidepressants like imipramine, and anxiolytics like tandospirone). However, in clinical practice, many refractory FD patients with poor symptom improvement from these pharmacotherapies have been reported to have pancreatic enzyme abnormalities, including early chronic pancreatitis [15]. These pancreatic enzyme abnormalities include amylase, lipase, trypsin, elastase-1, and PLA2. Trypsin shows high sensitivity and is a crucial value for evaluation. Interestingly, the symptoms of early chronic pancreatitis include postprandial epigastric pain, which, like FD, does not show clear abnormalities in routine blood tests or abdominal CT scans. Therefore, the guidelines recommend excluding early chronic pancreatitis.

Early chronic pancreatitis is considered a precursor to chronic pancreatitis. Chronic pancreatitis is a fibrotic syndrome caused by persistent subtle inflammation due to factors such as genetics and alcohol consumption, and it is considered a high-risk group for pancreatic cancer. Early diagnosis and treatment of early chronic pancreatitis aim to reduce the risk of pancreatic cancer. Early chronic pancreatitis has symptoms and examination findings very similar to FD. The diagnostic criteria for early chronic pancreatitis, as described in the 2019 Clinical Diagnostic Criteria for Chronic Pancreatitis, are as follows: ① recurrent upper abdominal or back pain, ② abnormal pancreatic enzyme levels in blood or urine, ③ exocrine pancreatic insufficiency, ④ a history of sustained alcohol consumption of more than 60 g/day (pure ethanol equivalent) or pancreatitis-related genetic abnormalities, and ⑤ a history of acute pancreatitis, with at least three of these criteria and imaging findings of early chronic pancreatitis. Imaging findings of early chronic pancreatitis are evaluated using ultrasonic endoscopes and include four criteria: ① hyperechoic foci or strands, ② lobularity, ③ hyperechoic main pancreatic duct margin, and ④ dilated side branches [16]. Based on these diagnostic criteria, it is easy to imagine that active measurement of pancreatic enzymes and endoscopic ultrasound examination, if necessary, are recommended for differentiating FD from early chronic pancreatitis. The importance of differentiating these two conditions lies in the differences in treatment methods. According to Yamawaki et al., the combination therapy of rabeprazole, pancrelipase, and camostat mesilate for early chronic pancreatitis significantly improved epigastric pain compared to FD treatment with rabeprazole and acotiamide. Conversely, continuing conventional FD treatment in early chronic pancreatitis patients tended to worsen epigastric pain [17]. These points highlight the importance of considering pancreatic diseases in the differential diagnosis of refractory FD patients.

5 Pancreatic Enzyme Abnormalities and Microinflammation in the Duodenum

The association between FD and pancreatic diseases requires differentiation due to similar symptoms and examination findings. When considering the symptom manifestation of FD and pancreatic diseases, microinflammation in the duodenum is a likely factor. As previously mentioned, subtle inflammation in the duodenum is observed in FD patients, and similar findings are obtained in patients with pancreatic enzyme abnormalities. The authors focused on trypsin, which shows high sensitivity among pancreatic enzyme abnormalities, and examined the expression of its receptor, PAR2, in the duodenal mucosa. The results showed a correlation between blood trypsin levels and duodenal fluid trypsin levels, as well as an association with eosinophil counts in the duodenal mucosa. Immunostaining also showed significantly higher PAR2 expression in patients with pancreatic enzyme abnormalities (Fig. 37.2). There are many reports on the association between pancreatic enzyme abnormalities and duodenal inflammation, and recent studies have examined the relationship between gut microbiota, pancreatitis, and the risk of pancreatic cancer.

Considering these points, the pathophysiology of FD, traditionally thought to involve the relationship between the stomach and duodenum, including gastric emptying disorders, may be more complex, involving a multi-organ network centered on the duodenum and including the pancreas, in addition to the brain–gut axis. Many aspects remain unclear, and further research is needed to elucidate the pathophysiology.

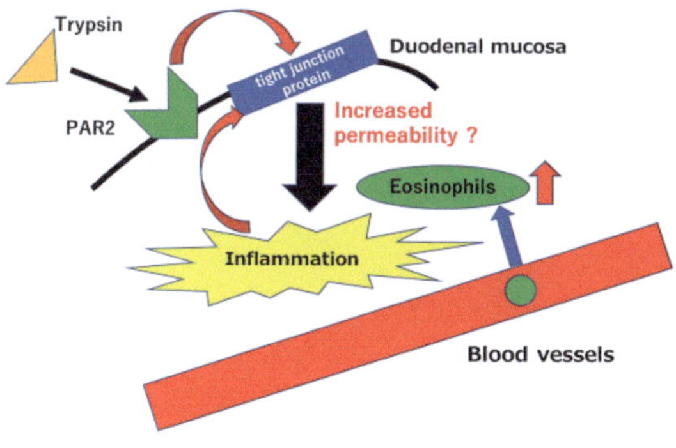

Fig. 37.2 Subtle inflammation in the duodenum mediated by trypsin and PAR2

Take-Home message
Microinflammation in the duodenum is related to the pathophysiology of FD. As previously mentioned, there are several factors contributing to inflammation, and recent reports suggest the involvement of the pancreas, making it important to include early chronic pancreatitis in the differential diagnosis. Given the similarity in symptoms between FD and early chronic pancreatitis, it is recommended to actively measure pancreatic enzymes in refractory FD patients.

Competing Interests The author has no competing interests to declare that are relevant to the content of this chapter.

References

1. Pilichiewicz AN, et al. Load-dependent effects of duodenal lipid on antropyloroduodenal motility, plasma CCK and PYY, and energy intake in healthy men. Am J Physiol Regul Integr Comp Physiol. 2007;293:R2170–8.
2. Ryan AT, et al. Effects of intraduodenal lipid and protein on gut motility and hormone release, glycemia, appetite, and energy intake in lean men. Am J Clin Nutr. 2013;98:300–11.
3. Khoo J, et al. Gastrointestinal hormonal dysfunction in gastroparesis and functional dyspepsia. Neurogastroenterol Motil. 2010;22:1270–8.
4. Yamawaki H, et al. Leu72Met408 polymorphism of the ghrelin gene is associated with early phase of gastric emptying in the patients with functional dyspepsia in Japan. J Neurogastroenterol Motil. 2015;21:93–102.
5. Vanheel H, et al. Impaired duodenal mucosal integrity and low-grade inflammation in functional dyspepsia. Gut. 2014;63:262–71.
6. Komori K, et al. The altered mucosal barrier function in the duodenum plays a role in the pathogenesis of functional dyspepsia. Dig Dis Sci. 2019;64:3228–39.
7. Tanaka F, et al. Concentration of glial cell line-derived neurotrophic factor positively correlates with symptoms in functional dyspepsia. Dig Dis Sci. 2016;61:3478–85.
8. Lee KJ, et al. A pilot on duodenal acid exposure and its relationship to symptoms in functional dyspepsia with prominent nausea. Am J Gastroenterol. 2004;99:1765–73.

9. Bratten J, et al. Prolonged recording of duodenal acid exposure in patients with functional dyspepsia and controls using a radiotelemetry pH monitoring system. J Clin Gastroenterol. 2009;43:527–33.
10. Miwa H, et al. Oesophageal hypersensitivity in Japanese patients with non-erosive gastro-oesophageal reflux diseases. Aliment Pharmacol Ther Suppl. 2004;1:112–7.
11. Wallon C, et al. Corticotropin-releasing hormone (CRH) regulates macromolecular permeability via mast cells in normal human colonic biopsies in vitro. Gut. 2008;57:50–8.
12. Zhong L, et al. Dyspepsia and the microbiome: time to focus on the small intestine. Gut. 2017;66:1168–9.
13. Jung HK, et al. Role of the duodenum in the pathogenesis of functional dyspepsia: a paradigm shift. J Neurogastroenterol Motil. 2018;24:345–54.
14. Miwa H. Evidence-based clinical practice guidelines for functional dyspepsia 2021. J Gastroenterol. 2022;57:47–61.
15. Hashimoto S, et al. Epigastric pain syndrome accompanying pancreatic enzyme abnormalities was overlapped with early chronic pancreatitis using endosonography. J Clin Biochem Nutr. 2017;61:140–5.
16. Japanese Pancreas Society, Committee for Research on Pancreatitis, Subcommittee on Chronic Pancreatitis. Clinical diagnostic criteria for chronic pancreatitis 2019. Pancreas. 2019;34:279. (in Japanese).
17. Yamawaki H, et al. Camostat mesilate, pancrelipase, and rabeprazole combination therapy improves epigastric pain in early chronic pancreatitis and functional dyspepsia with pancreatic enzyme abnormalities. Digestion. 2019;99:283–92.

Part VI

Small Bowel and Colon, Basic Edition

Small Bowel and Colon: Anatomy, Physiology of Gastrointestinal Motility, Peptides

38

Masatomo Ishioh

Abstract

This chapter summarizes the anatomy of the small bowel and colon and the control of gastrointestinal motility. The small intestine comprises mucosa, submucosa, muscularis, and serosa; the myenteric (Auerbach) and submucosal (Meissner) plexuses, with interstitial cells of Cajal, coordinate circular and longitudinal muscle. In the colon, thickened longitudinal bands (teniae coli) form haustra. Motility patterns include peristalsis, segmentation for mixing, and the migrating motor complex (MMC; phases I–IV), which originates in the stomach, traverses the small intestine every 90–120 minutes during fasting, and is replaced postprandially. Colonic function features haustrations, peristalsis, and meal-induced mass peristalsis that drives defecation via rectal distension and sacral–pudendal reflexes. Autonomic inputs modulate but do not generate these rhythms.

Enteroendocrine peptides provide state-dependent control: motilin initiates gastric MMC phase III; ghrelin stimulates appetite and MMC; somatostatin suppresses gastric activity yet can trigger small-intestinal phase III; 5-hydroxytryptamine accelerates MMC propagation. After feeding, cholecystokinin (CCK) (via vagal/CCK1 pathways), glucose-dependent insulinotropic polypeptide, glucagon-like peptide-1, and peptide YY slow upper gastrointestinal transit, coordinate pyloric function, and promote absorption. Stress pathways further tune motility: corticotropin-releasing factor (CRF or corticotropin-releasing hormone) acting on CRF-R2 inhibits gastric activity, whereas CRF-R1 enhances colonic motility. Together, enteric circuits, autonomic inputs, and peptides integrate the feeding state with propulsion and continence.

Keywords

Enteric nervous system · Myenteric plexus · Interstitial cells of Cajal · Migrating motor complex · Peristalsis · Motilin · Corticotropin-releasing factor

1 Anatomy of the Small Bowel and Colon

The small intestine is the longest segment of the gastrointestinal tract, measuring approximately 6–7 m in length, with a diameter that narrows as it progresses distally. The initial portion of the small intestine is the duodenum, a C-shaped structure located superior to the umbilicus. It is

M. Ishioh (✉)
Department of General Medicine, Asahikawa Medical University, Asahikawa, Japan
e-mail: masatomo-ishioht@asahikawa-med.ac.jp

H. Kaneko et al. (eds.), *Disorders of Gut-Brain Interaction*,
https://doi.org/10.1007/978-981-95-6974-8_38

retroperitoneal except for the region connected to the liver via the hepatoduodenal ligament, part of the lesser omentum, and adjacent to the pancreatic head. The jejunum follows, primarily situated in the left upper quadrant, characterized by its thicker walls and prominent circular folds (plicae circulares) running transversely. The ileum, the final segment, is located mainly in the right lower quadrant, with thinner walls and less conspicuous circular folds compared to the jejunum. The ileocecal valve at the terminal ileum regulates the passage of contents into the large intestine (Fig. 38.1). The small intestine's wall comprises four layers: mucosa, submucosa, muscularis, and serosa. The muscularis layer consists of an inner circular muscle layer and an outer longitudinal muscle layer, with the myenteric plexus (Auerbach's plexus) situated between them (Fig. 38.2). The plexus, composed of unmyelinated nerve fibers and nerve cells, includes postganglionic sympathetic fibers, preganglionic and postganglionic parasympathetic fibers, and visceral sensory fibers. Interstitial cells of Cajal exist around the myenteric plexus, which regulate peristalsis in conjunction with the myenteric plexus. Additionally, the submucosal plexus (Meissner's plexus) lies between the submucosa and the circular muscle layer, forming a network with the myenteric plexus and including intercalated neurons, and contributing to the enteric nervous system (ENS) [1]. The composition of nerve fibers in the submucosal plexus is similar to myenteric plexus, although the size of the submucosal plexus is smaller than myenteric plexus, which is involved in the motility of the muscularis mucosae and glandular secretion.

The large intestine extends from the terminal ileum to the anus, measuring approximately 1.5 m in length. It is composed of the appendix, cecum, colon, rectum, and anal canal. The colon is further divided into the ascending colon, right colic flexure (hepatic flexure), transverse colon, left colic flexure (splenic flexure), descending colon, and sigmoid colon. The cecum, with the appendix, begins in the right iliac fossa, ascending as the ascending colon to the right colic flexure beneath the liver, crossing the abdomen as the transverse colon, bending downward at the left colic flexure beneath the spleen, and descending as the descending colon to the left iliac fossa. The sigmoid colon enters the upper part of the pelvis, continuing as the rectum along the posterior pelvic wall, terminating as the anal canal (Fig. 38.1). The histology of the large intestine follows the

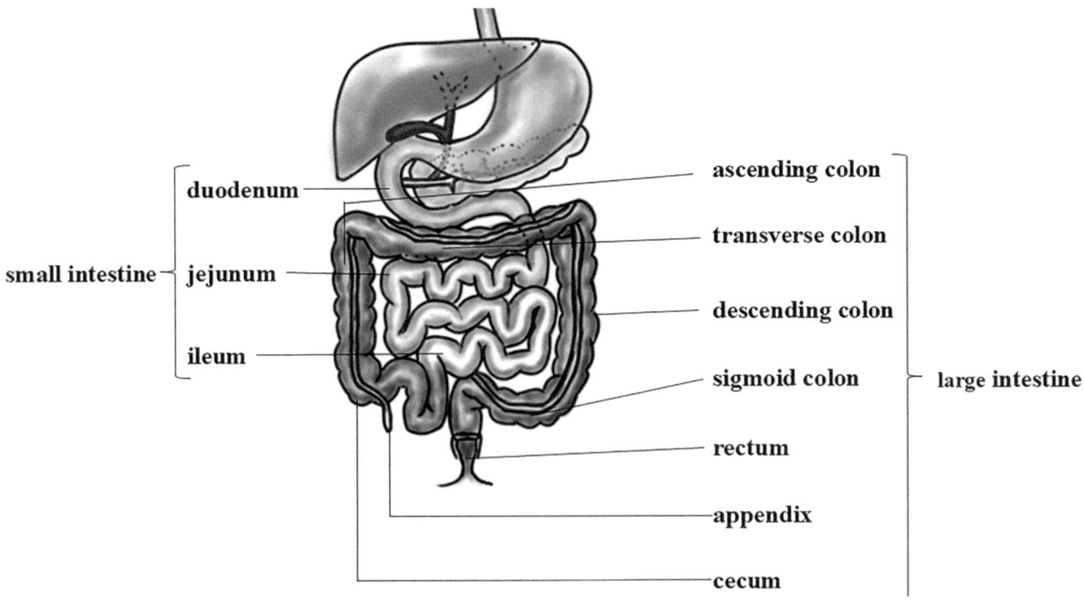

Fig. 38.1 Overall structure of the gastrointestinal tract

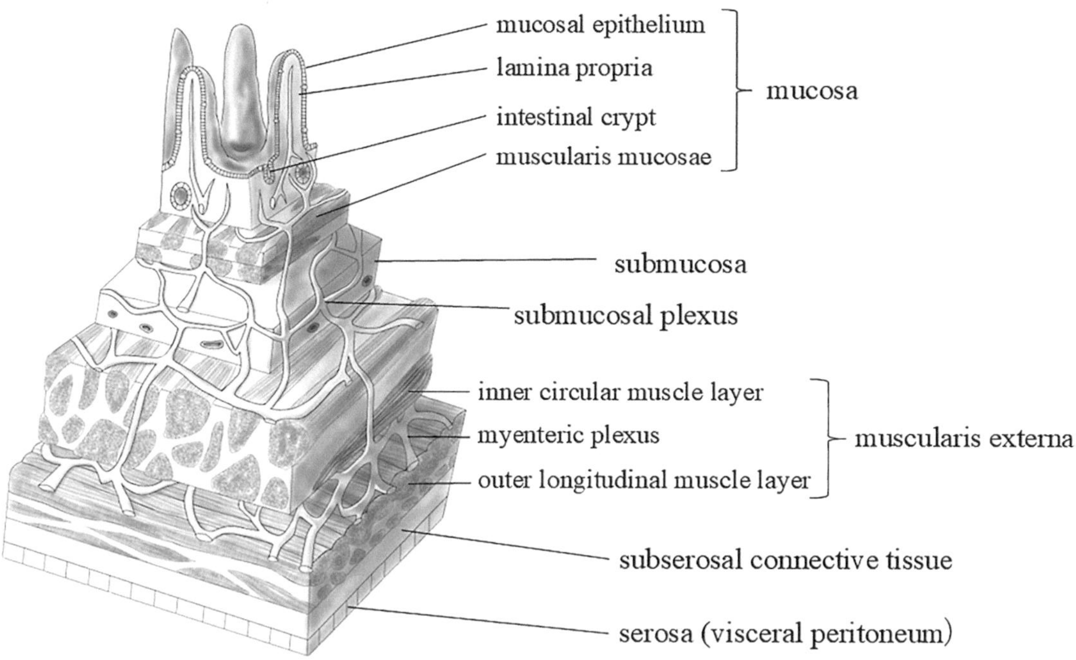

Fig. 38.2 Tissue structure of the gastrointestinal tract (small intestine)

basic gastrointestinal tract structure, with the outer longitudinal muscle layer thickened in parts to form the teniae coli. These teniae coli, comprising the free, omental, and mesocolic teniae, are present along the colon's length, with thinner longitudinal muscle between them. Contractions of the teniae coli create haustra, or sacculations, in the colon wall.

2 Physiology of Gastrointestinal Motility

Gastrointestinal motility is primarily regulated by the intrinsic ENS and extrinsic autonomic nervous system. The ENS, as previously described, consists mainly of the submucosal and myenteric plexuses, which maintain gastrointestinal motility in the absence of neural damage. The autonomic nervous system, mainly the vagus nerve (parasympathetic nervous system) and sympathetic nervous system, controls gastrointestinal motility, but the autonomic nervous system regulates the intensity of gastrointestinal motility without affecting its occurrence.

One type of gastrointestinal motility is peristalsis, which involves coordinated contractions of the circular and longitudinal muscles to propel luminal contents anally. This process is triggered by luminal distension, activating the ENS, which induces contraction of the intestinal wall 2–3 cm orally from the distended segment, with the contraction ring moving anally. Stretch stimuli activate ENS, and cholinergic neurons traveling toward the oral side contract the smooth muscles of the oral side of the contents via substance P and acetylcholine. Simultaneously, ENS activates cholinergic neurons that run toward the anal side, causing the smooth muscles on the anal side to relax via nitric oxide (NO) and vasoactive intestinal peptide (VIP) [2].

In the small intestine, segmenting movements suitable for digestive and absorptive functions are observed. Segmenting movements are similar to peristaltic movements; however, they do not propel the contents of the digestive tract toward the anus. Segmental structures are formed by the contraction of circular muscles at various points. After one contraction ends, the two areas that contracted immediately before the contraction form a new segmental structure. This movement mixes intestinal contents with digestive enzymes, increases contact with the mucous membrane to facilitate nutrient absorption, and makes absorption easier.

These contractions occur more frequently in the duodenum than in the jejunum or ileum, and rhythmic contractions continue until nutrients from the digested contents are absorbed. These rhythmic contractions are caused by interstitial cells of Cajal, which exhibit spontaneous rhythmic fluctuations in membrane potential between −65 and −45 mV. Acetylcholine increases the frequency of spike potentials, while adrenaline decreases it.

During fasting, the small intestine exhibits the migrating motor complex (MMC), a cyclic motility pattern with a 90–120-minute cycle, comprising four phases: phase I (quiescence), phase II (irregular contractions), phase III (intense contractions), and phase IV (rapid decline of contractions). This pattern originates in the stomach and propagates to the distal ileum [3]. The MMC clears residual luminal contents and prevents bacterial overgrowth in the small intestine, known as the housekeeping effect [4]. The MMC is regulated by gastrointestinal peptides and the vagus nerve, with vagotomy abolishing gastric MMC but minimally affecting small intestinal MMC. Feeding interrupts the MMC, transitioning to a postprandial motility pattern influenced by meal composition and fiber content.

The large intestine stores fecal residues, absorbing most remaining water and electrolytes, with motility patterns similar to the small intestine. The phenomenon of segmenting movements in the colon, known as "haustrations," primarily occurs in the cecum and ascending colon. This increases the opportunity for intestinal contents to come into contact with the mucous membrane, promoting nutrient absorption and facilitating the absorption process.

Additionally, peristalsis and mass-peristalsis of the colon are observed for the purpose of transport. Mass-peristalsis occurs several times a day, primarily after meals. These movements are influenced by the expansion of the stomach and duodenum and are known as the gastrocolic reflex. Peristalsis and mass-peristalsis push feces into the rectum, and when the rectum expands, this triggers the defecation reflex through the excitation of pelvic nerves. Even when feces reach the rectum, the external anal sphincter temporarily contracts to prevent immediate defecation. However, as the rectum continues to stretch, the external anal sphincter begins to relax via the pudendal nerve. Additionally, increased intra-abdominal pressure caused by straining or other actions further promotes defecation.

3 Peptides

Gastrointestinal motility is regulated by the ENS, the autonomic nervous system, and bioactive substances such as gastrointestinal peptides. Peptides involved in motility regulation include motilin, ghrelin, somatostatin, 5-hydroxytryptamine (5-HT), cholecystokinin (CCK), glucose-dependent insulinotropic polypeptide (GIP), glucagon-like peptide-1 (GLP-1), and peptide YY (PYY), produced by enteroendocrine cells, which constitute approximately 1% of the intestinal epithelium. Motilin, ghrelin, somatostatin, and 5-HT primarily regulate fasting motility, particularly the MMC, while CCK, GIP, GLP-1, and PYY regulate postprandial motility.

Motilin, a 22-amino acid peptide produced in the duodenum, jejunum, and ENS, fluctuates in plasma concentration during fasting, peaking during the gastric MMC phase III. Studies have shown motilin's important role in initiating gastric MMC phase III [5]. In dogs, anti-motilin serum administration abolishes MMC phase III in the stomach and duodenum but not in the jejunum and ileum. Duodenectomy significantly reduces plasma motilin levels and suppresses gastric MMC phase III, which is restored by motilin administration. Motilin is regulated by various factors, such as pancreatic polypeptide (PP), which decreases plasma motilin levels after the administration of PP intravenously. The blood concentration of PP rises immediately after eating, causing a switch to MMC derived from the duodenum. Motilin is controlled by PP when switching to the postprandial gastrointestinal motility pattern [6]. It has also been reported that duodenal pH affects the activity of motilin. Persistent decrease in duodenal pH prevents the induction of gastric MMC phase III even when plasma motilin concentrations reach their peak. On the other hand, an increase in duodenal pH induces gastric MMC phase III at an early stage, even before motilin concentrations reach their peak. The duodenal pH affects the sensitivity of motilin receptors [7].

Ghrelin, identified as a ligand for the growth hormone secretagogue receptor, shares 21% homology with motilin but does not act on motilin receptors. Produced mainly in the stomach, ghrelin is activated by acylation at the third serine residue by ghrelin *O*-acyltransferase. Ghrelin has been shown to stimulate appetite and, like motilin, induce gastric MMC in various species. Since this effect does not increase plasma motilin levels, it has been suggested that ghrelin may regulate MMC independently of motilin. However, the underlying mechanism has yet to be fully clarified [5].

Somatostatin is produced by neuroendocrine cells in the hypothalamic periventricular nucleus, where it inhibits growth hormone secretion. Additionally, it is produced by endocrine cells in the gastrointestinal tract and interneurons in the ENS, where it suppresses the release of gastrointestinal hormones such as gastrin, CCK, secretin, motilin, VIP, and GIP, as well as pancreatic hormones such as insulin and glucagon. Plasma somatostatin levels peak during duodenal MMC phase III contractions, suggesting its involvement in this phase. Indeed, somatostatin administration inhibits the plasma levels of motilin and PP, suppressing gastric motility while stimulating small intestinal MMC phase III contractions. Similar effects are observed with the administration of the somatostatin receptor agonist octreotide [8].

5-HT is present in the gastrointestinal tract, platelets, and central nervous system and is produced by enterochromaffin cells in the gastrointestinal tract. Studies in humans and dogs have shown that intravenous administration of 5-HT increases the frequency and propagation speed of MMC phase III contractions, while luminal administration does not affect gastrointestinal motility. This indicates that plasma 5-HT levels influence the frequency and propagation speed of MMC phase III contractions [9]. This mechanism may explain the prokinetic effects of 5-HT reuptake inhibitors such as paroxetine and citalopram on small intestinal motility. The subtype of 5-HT receptors involved in gastrointestinal motility varies among species, but in humans, 5-HT enhances gastrointestinal motility via 5-HT3 receptors. Conversely, the 5-HT3 receptor antagonist ondansetron suppresses gastrointestinal motility by inhibiting the increase in plasma motilin levels.

CCK is secreted by I cells in the duodenum and jejunum, promoting gallbladder contraction, relaxation of the sphincter of Oddi, and pancreatic enzyme secretion. Its secretion is stimulated by the entry of gastric contents into the duodenum, leading to pyloric contraction and delayed gastric emptying. Intravenous administration of CCK-8, the most active subtype of CCK, induces pyloric contraction and inhibits upper gastrointestinal motility by promoting the secretion of PYY at physiological blood concentrations, which also suppresses ghrelin-induced appetite stimulation. This effect is mediated by CCK1 receptors, as evidenced by the disappearance of these effects upon administration of the CCK1 receptor antagonist dexloxiglumide. Furthermore, the inhibitory effect on feeding of CCK administration intravenously is abolished by vagotomy, suggesting that the vagus nerve is involved in the gastrointestinal motility inhibition induced by CCK [10]. It is hypothesized that CCK secreted from the intestine acts on CCK receptors produced in the vagal ganglia, stimulating the vagus nerve and transmitting signals to the nucleus tractus solitarius and hypothalamic feeding centers, thereby regulating gastrointestinal motility [11].

GIP is secreted by K cells in the duodenum and jejunum. Experimental studies in dogs have shown that intravenous administration of GIP suppresses motilin-induced spike potentials in the stomach and duodenum, reducing MMC phase III activity. This suggests that GIP is involved in transitioning gastrointestinal motility patterns from fasting to postprandial states. In humans, intravenous administration of GIP does not inhibit gastric emptying [11], but this does not simulate the paracrine effects of postprandial GIP or its first-pass effect through the liver; further analysis is required.

GLP-1 is primarily secreted by L cells in the ileum and colon. Along with PYY, GLP-1 inhibits ileal motility when the distal intestine is exposed to unabsorbed nutrients [12]. Additionally, GLP-1 has been reported to inhibit antral contractions and induce pyloric contraction, thereby delaying gastric emptying. The GLP-1 agonist exenatide improves diarrhea symptoms in patients with short bowel syndrome, while the GLP-1-specific antagonist exendin (9–39) promotes gastric emptying in healthy individuals, suggesting that GLP-1 inhibits gastrointestinal motility in both the stomach and small intestine. Exendin, used in the treatment of type 2 diabetes, often causes diarrhea as a side effect due to stimulation of colonic motility, whereas it does not affect small intestinal motility.

PYY is primarily secreted by L cells in the ileum and colon. PYY exists mainly as PYY1-36 and its degradation product PYY3-36 by dipeptidyl peptidase-4, with the latter being the predominant form. PYY has been confirmed to inhibit upper gastrointestinal motility, as studies using PYY knockout mice have shown enhanced upper gastrointestinal motility. Additionally, PYY, along with neuropeptide Y (NPY), inhibits fluid and electrolyte secretion in the mucosal epithelium via NPY1 and NPY2 receptors, slowing colonic transit [12, 13].

Gastrointestinal motility is also influenced by stress hormones such as corticotropin-releasing factor (CRF, or corticotropin-releasing hormone), which is secreted by various organs, including the brain and gastrointestinal tract, and acts on two receptors, CRF-R1 and CRF-R2 [14]. CRF generally inhibits gastric motility via CRF-R2 and stimulates colonic motility via CRF-R1. Our research suggests that the balance of signaling between CRF-R1 and CRF-R2 determines gastrointestinal motility [14].

Competing Interests The author has no competing interests to declare that are relevant to the content of this chapter.

References

1. Walsh KT, et al. The enteric nervous system for epithelial researchers: basic anatomy, techniques, and interactions with the epithelium. Cell Mol Gastroenterol Hepatol. 2019;8:369–78.
2. Spencer NJ, et al. Enteric nervous system: sensory transduction, neural circuits and gastrointestinal motility. Nat Rev Gastroenterol Hepatol. 2020;17:338–51.
3. Code CF, et al. The interdigestive myoelectric complex of the stomach and small bowel of dogs. J Physiol. 1975;246:289–309.
4. Malagelada C, et al. Small bowel motility. Curr Gastroenterol Rep. 2017;19:26.
5. Deloose E, et al. Motilin: from gastric motility stimulation to hunger signalling. Nat Rev Endocrinol. 2019;15:238–50.
6. Janssens J, et al. Pancreatic polypeptide is not involved in the regulation of the migrating motor complex in man. Regul Pept. 1982;3:41–9.
7. Woodtli W, et al. Duodenal pH governs interdigestive motility in humans. Am J Physiol. 1995;268:G146–52.
8. Barkan AL, et al. Ghrelin secretion in humans is sexually dimorphic, suppressed by somatostatin, and not affected by the ambient growth hormone levels. J Clin Endocrinol Metab. 2003;88:2180–4.
9. Hansen MB, et al. Effect of serotonin on small intestinal contractility in healthy volunteers. Physiol Res. 2008;57:63–71.
10. Viard E, et al. Systemic cholecystokinin amplifies vago-vagal reflex responses recorded in vagal motor neurones. J Physiol. 2012;590:631–46.
11. Asmar M, et al. On the role of glucose-dependent insulintropic polypeptide in postprandial metabolism in humans. Am J Physiol Endocrinol Metab. 2010;298:E614–21.
12. Camilleri M. Integrated upper gastrointestinal response to food intake. Gastroenterology. 2006;131:640–58.
13. Tough IR, et al. Endogenous peptide YY and neuropeptide Y inhibit colonic ion transport, contractility and transit differentially via Y_1 and Y_2 receptors. Br J Pharmacol. 2011;164:471–84.
14. Nozu T, et al. A balance theory of peripheral corticotropin-releasing factor receptor type 1 and type 2 signaling to induce colonic contractions and visceral hyperalgesia in rats. Endocrinology. 2014;155:4655–64.

Small Bowel and Colonic Motility Test, Small Bowel and Colonic Motility

39

Takatsugu Machida

Abstract

The small and large intestines possess inherent motility due to the coordinated actions of interstitial cells of Cajal, the myenteric plexus, and smooth muscle. Normal small intestinal motility exhibits distinct patterns during fasting and postprandial periods. Fasting motility consists of phase I (quiescence), phase II (sporadic irregular contractions), and phase III (regular strong contractions at a frequency of 3 cycles per minute, propelling contents anally). This sequence is known as the migrating motor complex. Normal colonic motility comprises three components: segmentation contractions, propulsive movements, and high-amplitude propagating contractions. Physical stimulation of the intestinal lumen triggers reflexive movements (peristaltic reflex, intestino-intestinal inhibitory reflex) and visceral perception. Several methods exist for measuring intestinal motility. In this chapter, we focus on intraluminal pressure measurement and barostat techniques for assessing gastrointestinal wall movements. Intraluminal pressure measurement and barostat remain the most effective methods for the detailed evaluation of motility patterns from the upper to lower gastrointestinal tract.

T. Machida (✉)
Department of Psychosomatic Medicine, Tohoku Rosai Hospital, Sendai, Japan

Keywords

Intestinal motility · Visceral perception · Intraluminal pressure measurement · High-resolution manometry · Barostat

1 Physiology of Small Bowel and Colonic Motility

The small and large intestines possess inherent motility due to the coordinated actions of interstitial cells of Cajal, the myenteric plexus, and smooth muscle. Interstitial cells of Cajal generate pacemaker potentials through regular depolarization, serving as the origin of intestinal motility. The myenteric plexus is the primary regulator of intestinal motility, with various neurotransmitters such as acetylcholine, norepinephrine, and serotonin altering the membrane potential of smooth muscle cells to control autonomous movements.

The intestines are connected to the central nervous system via extrinsic nerves, which exert mutual influence. Extrinsic nerve fibers include sympathetic and parasympathetic nerves; sympathetic nerves release norepinephrine to inhibit intestinal motility, while parasympathetic nerves release acetylcholine to induce motility.

Normal small intestinal motility [1, 2] exhibits distinct patterns during fasting and postprandial periods. Fasting motility consists of phase I (quiescence), phase II (sporadic irregular contrac-

H. Kaneko et al. (eds.), *Disorders of Gut-Brain Interaction*,
https://doi.org/10.1007/978-981-95-6974-8_39

tions), and phase III [regular strong contractions at a frequency of 3 cycles per minute (cpm), propelling contents anally]. This sequence is known as the migrating motor complex (MMC). MMC cycles repeat every 90–160 minutes during fasting and transition rapidly to postprandial motility upon feeding, characterized by sustained irregular contractions similar to phase II. Postprandial motility persists for several hours and transitions back to fasting motility once gastric emptying is complete.

Normal colonic motility [3, 4] comprises three components: segmentation contractions forming haustra, the most frequent; propulsive movements along the colon's axis, typically anally directed in the descending and sigmoid colon but occasionally retrograde in the ascending colon; and high-pressure movements involved in defecation, known as high-amplitude propagating contractions, occurring several times daily.

2 Intestinal Motility and Perception

Physical stimulation of the intestinal lumen triggers reflexive movements (peristaltic reflex and intestino-intestinal inhibitory reflex) and visceral perception [5]. The peristaltic reflex involves acetylcholine release mediated by serotonin receptors, inducing muscle contraction and peristaltic movement upon stretch receptor stimulation. The intestino-intestinal inhibitory reflex occurs when feces or intestinal gas distends the lumen, stimulating sensory nerves in the myenteric plexus to release acetylcholine, and norepinephrine from postganglionic sympathetic neurons, relaxing smooth muscle.

Stronger distension excites sensory neurons of spinal nerves, transmitting signals to visceral somatic neurons in the spinal dorsal horn, ascending via the contralateral spinothalamic and spinoreticular tracts to the central nervous system, eliciting visceral perception.

3 Methods for Measuring Intestinal Motility

Several methods exist for measuring intestinal motility, including radioisotope and X-ray opaque marker techniques for evaluating gastrointestinal transit time, discussed in Sect. 3.2. Here, we focus on intraluminal pressure measurement and barostat techniques for assessing gastrointestinal wall movements.

3.1 Intraluminal Pressure Measurement

Intraluminal pressure measurement involves continuous recording of pressure within the gastrointestinal lumen using pressure transducers, providing quantitative analysis of gastrointestinal wall movements. Small intestinal pressure measurement [1, 6] involves inserting a nasally introduced pressure catheter into the duodenum and jejunum under fluoroscopy, recording pressure waveforms on a polygraph. Portable devices enable long-term recording during daily activities. Disorders affecting small intestinal motility often exhibit MMC abnormalities, with phase III being particularly important for clinical evaluation, including frequency, amplitude, duration, and propagation speed of contractions.

Chronic idiopathic intestinal pseudo-obstruction is a major disorder affecting small intestinal motility, characterized by weakened phase II contractions, non-propagating burst waves lasting 10–12 cpm with amplitudes over 20 mmHg for more than 2 minutes, phase III deformation, reduced frequency, decreased amplitude, prolonged contraction duration, and reduced propagation speed (Fig. 39.1).

Large intestinal pressure measurement [3, 6] involves inserting a pressure catheter via colonoscopy or sliding tube under fluoroscopy, typically measuring in the left colon from the descending colon to the sigmoid colon, though some devices

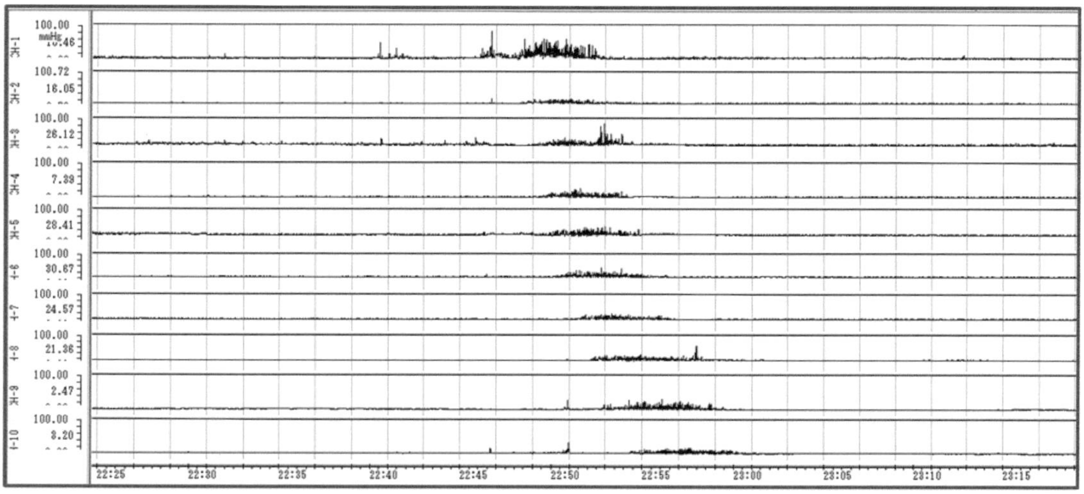

Fig. 39.1 Abnormal findings in small intestinal pressure in chronic idiopathic intestinal pseudo-obstruction. Marked low amplitude and reduced propagation speed of phase III (approximately 36 mm/min, normal 60–100 mm/min) are observed (case study, 47-year-old male)

allow measurement in the transverse and ascending colon. This technique detects contractions at multiple sites but has limitations in detecting mild contractions and colonic wall tone.

Recently, high-resolution manometry (HRM) has been applied to small and large intestinal pressure measurement, providing more detailed data compared to traditional methods with fewer pressure transducers. However, further accumulation of cases and data is needed to distinguish normal from abnormal patterns using HRM.

3.2 Barostat

The barostat involves inserting a synthetic resin bag into the colon to measure volume, pressure, and compliance [7]. The advantage of barostat lies in detecting mild contractions and colonic wall tone, which are difficult to measure with intraluminal pressure techniques, and quantitatively evaluating gastrointestinal perception [8].

Tonus measurement involves applying a constant low pressure to the colon wall using a bag. There are two methods: applying a constant pressure of approximately 10 mmHg or applying the minimum pressure required to detect respiratory fluctuations minimal distending pressure (MDP) + 2 mmHg. There are two methods for measuring colonic perception: pressure loading, which gradually increases intra-abdominal pressure, and volume loading, which gradually increases intra-abdominal volume. Both methods evaluate the level of abdominal symptoms, such as abdominal pain, that subjects perceive under various loads.

Irritable bowel syndrome (IBS) often involves enhanced colonic motility and visceral hypersensitivity, with increased segmental contractions detected by intraluminal pressure measurement and enhanced colonic tone and visceral hypersensitivity detected by the barostat (Fig. 39.2).

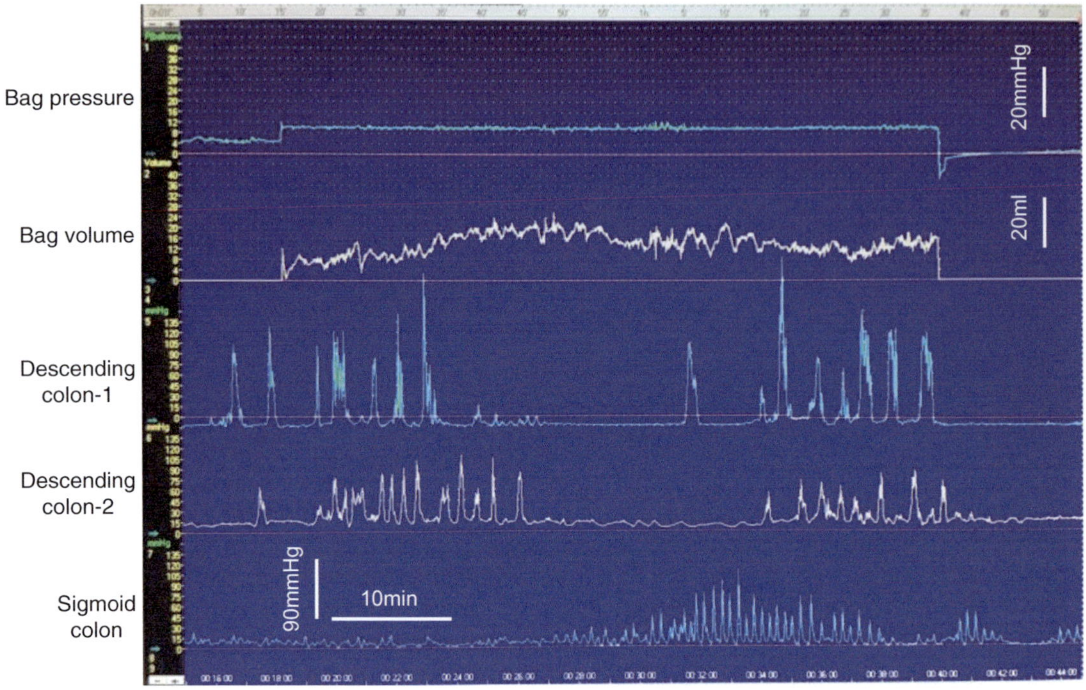

Fig. 39.2 Abnormal findings in colonic pressure and barostat in IBS. Under a constant pressure of 10 mmHg, the bag volume is 10–20 mL, indicating increased tone (normal 40–60 mL), with marked segmental contractions observed from the descending colon to the sigmoid colon (case study, 25-year-old male)

4 Conclusion

This section discusses the physiology of small and large intestinal motility and methods for measuring gastrointestinal wall movements. Despite the invasive nature of these tests, intraluminal pressure measurement and barostat remain the most effective methods for the detailed evaluation of motility patterns from the upper to lower gastrointestinal tract. Future advancements in simultaneous detection of multiple biochemical markers within the gastrointestinal lumen and concurrent motility measurement will enable more accurate and quantitative testing.

Take-Home Message
Gastrointestinal motility disorders are a major pathophysiological feature of functional gastrointestinal disorders such as IBS, as well as of conditions like chronic intestinal pseudo-obstruction. However, in daily clinical practice, reliable tools for accurately assessing gastrointestinal motility are limited. Therefore, clinicians should always keep the possibility of motility abnormalities in mind when making diagnostic and therapeutic decisions.

Competing Interests The author has no competing interests to declare that are relevant to the content of this chapter.

References

1. Kellow JE, et al. Prolonged ambulant recordings of small bowel motility demonstrate abnormalities in the irritable bowel syndrome. Gastroenterology. 1990;98:1208–18.
2. Kumar D, et al. An illustrated guide to gastrointestinal motility. 2nd ed. London: Churchil Livingstone; 1993.
3. Fukudo S, et al. Colonic motility, autonomic function, and gastrointestinal hormones under psychological stress on irritable bowel syndrome. Tohoku J Exp Med. 1987;151:373–85.
4. Rogers J, et al. Increased segmental activity and intraluminal pressures in the sigmoid colon of patients with the irritable bowel syndrome. Gut. 1989;30:634–41.

5. Mayer EA, et al. Role of visceral afferent mechanisms in functional bowel disorder. Gastroenterology. 1990;99:1688–704.
6. Fukudo S, et al. Brain-gut response to stress and cholinergic stimulation in irritable bowel syndrome. J Clin Gastroenterol. 1993;17:133–41.
7. Steadman CJ, et al. Variation of muscle tone in the human colon. Gastroenterology. 1991;101:373–81.
8. Whitehead WE, et al. Standardization of barostat procedures for testing smooth muscle tone and sensory thresholds in the gastrointestinal tract. Dig Dis Sci. 1997;42:223–41.

40 Small Bowel and Colonic Motility Test, Colonic Transit Time Testing

Takeshi Kamiya

Abstract

Colonic transit time (CTT) measurement is an objective method to evaluate colonic motility. The most useful indication of CTT is chronic constipation, particularly in cases that do not respond well to initial treatments typically provided in primary care. Chronic constipation is commonly categorized into slow transit constipation, normal transit constipation, and defecatory disorders by CTT. CTT measurement is a necessary test for classifying chronic constipation by pathophysiology and selecting appropriate treatment methods. There are several methods for measuring CTT. The radiopaque marker method involves orally ingesting a capsule containing radiopaque markers coated with barium, followed by tracking the markers with plain abdominal X-rays. This is the simplest and most cost-effective method for measuring CTT. The radioisotope (RI) method involves ingesting a test meal mixed with an RI-labeled compound, followed by counting the radiation activity in the colon over time using a gamma camera to measure CTT. Internationally, CTT measurement using wireless capsules is also performed. In Japan, measuring CTT tests are not yet performed in daily clinical practice. The widespread use of these tests in daily clinical practice in Japan is strongly desired in the future.

Keywords

Colonic motility · Colonic transit time · Chronic constipation · Radiopaque marker · Radioisotope · Wireless capsule

1 Concept

Among the measurements of transit time in the small and large intestines, the measurement of colonic transit time (CTT) is clinically useful and necessary. CTT measurement is an objective method to evaluate colonic peristalsis and motor function, and it is indicated for patients suspected of having disorders of colonic motility, including chronic constipation. There are several methods for measuring CTT [1], but all methods essentially measure the total gastrointestinal transit time from oral ingestion to anal excretion. Therefore, when evaluating CTT, it is assumed that the gastric emptying and the motility of the upper gastrointestinal tract and small intestine are normal.

T. Kamiya (✉)
Department of Medical Innovation, Nagoya City University Graduate School of Medical Sciences, Gastroenterology, Internal Medicine, Regulatory Science, Nagoya, Japan
e-mail: tmkamiya@mediacat.ne.jp

H. Kaneko et al. (eds.), *Disorders of Gut-Brain Interaction*,
https://doi.org/10.1007/978-981-95-6974-8_40

Table 40.1 Classification of chronic constipation

Reduced bowel movement frequency type	Slow transit constipation
	Normal transit constipation
Defecation difficulty type	Defecatory disorders

2 Indications

The indications for CTT measurement include all disorders presenting with colonic motility dysfunction. The most useful indication is chronic constipation, particularly in cases that do not respond well to initial treatments typically provided in primary care (dietary therapy, lifestyle guidance including exercise, and pharmacotherapy with one or two laxatives).

Chronic constipation is classified based on its cause and symptoms, and internationally, it is commonly classified by CTT [2, 3]. Based on pathophysiology, chronic constipation is categorized into slow transit constipation, normal transit constipation, and defecatory disorders (Table 40.1). CTT measurement is a useful and necessary test for classifying chronic constipation by pathophysiology and selecting appropriate treatment methods. It is also used to determine the appropriateness of total colectomy for colonic inertia.

3 Radiopaque Marker Method

The radiopaque marker method involves orally ingesting a capsule containing 24 radiopaque markers coated with barium, followed by tracking the markers with plain abdominal X-rays. This is the simplest and most cost-effective method for measuring CTT. Historically, it was developed by Hinton et al. in 1969 [4], and in the United States, these markers have been approved as medical devices by the U.S. Food & Drug Administration. Hinton et al. proposed two criteria for normal CTT: (1) the first marker appears in the stool within 3 days of ingestion, and (2) more than 80% of the markers are excreted by the fifth day. These criteria are still widely used today. The marker method is the most widely used method for measuring CTT internationally. However, as of 2025, these radiopaque markers are not approved in Japan, and thus, their use is limited to research purposes in select facilities.

A simple and representative protocol within the radiopaque marker method is the 5-day method [5]. In the 5-day method, the subject discontinues medications (laxatives) that affect bowel motility as much as possible, ingests one capsule containing 20 radiopaque markers with an appropriate amount of water, and undergoes a plain abdominal X-ray 5 days (120 hours) later (Fig. 40.1). The number of markers remaining in the intestines is counted, and if four or more markers (20%) remain, the patient is diagnosed with delayed slow transit type chronic constipation. If many markers remain in the rectum, defecatory disorders are suspected (Fig. 40.2). This method allows differentiation between delayed colonic transit type and normal colonic transit type with a single ingestion of markers and X-ray, minimizing patient time commitment and radiation exposure. However, it does not measure the exact CTT.

The 3-day method simplifies the 5-day method further, with the subject ingesting one capsule of markers and undergoing a plain abdominal X-ray 3 days (72 hours) later. If 10 or more markers (40%) remain, the patient is diagnosed with slow colonic transit type chronic constipation. The 3-day method is easier to perform as a screening test due to the shorter patient time commitment compared to the 5-day method. However, since it has been less frequently performed globally compared to the 5-day method, further evaluation is needed.

The Japanese Society of Neurogastroenterology has created a schema for the radiopaque marker method for general practitioners to promote the future use of CTT measurement in daily clinical practice (Fig. 40.3). Both the 5-day and 3-day methods are recommended. Considering that the target patients are those with chronic constipation unresponsive to initial treatment, discontinuation of medications (laxatives) affecting bowel motility is not required.

While the 5-day and 3-day methods are simple and can be performed in primary care, several

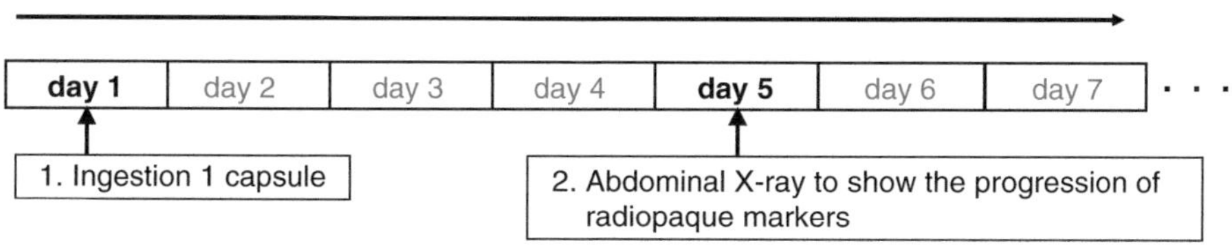

Fig. 40.1 Measurement of colonic transit time (5-day method)

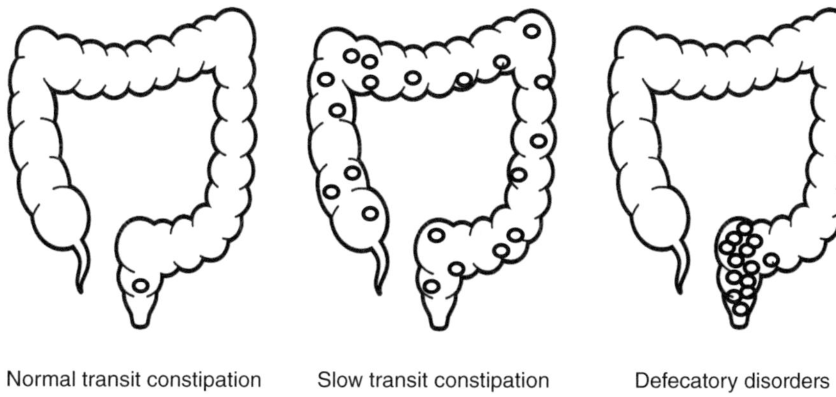

Fig. 40.2 Classification of chronic constipation using the radiopaque marker method

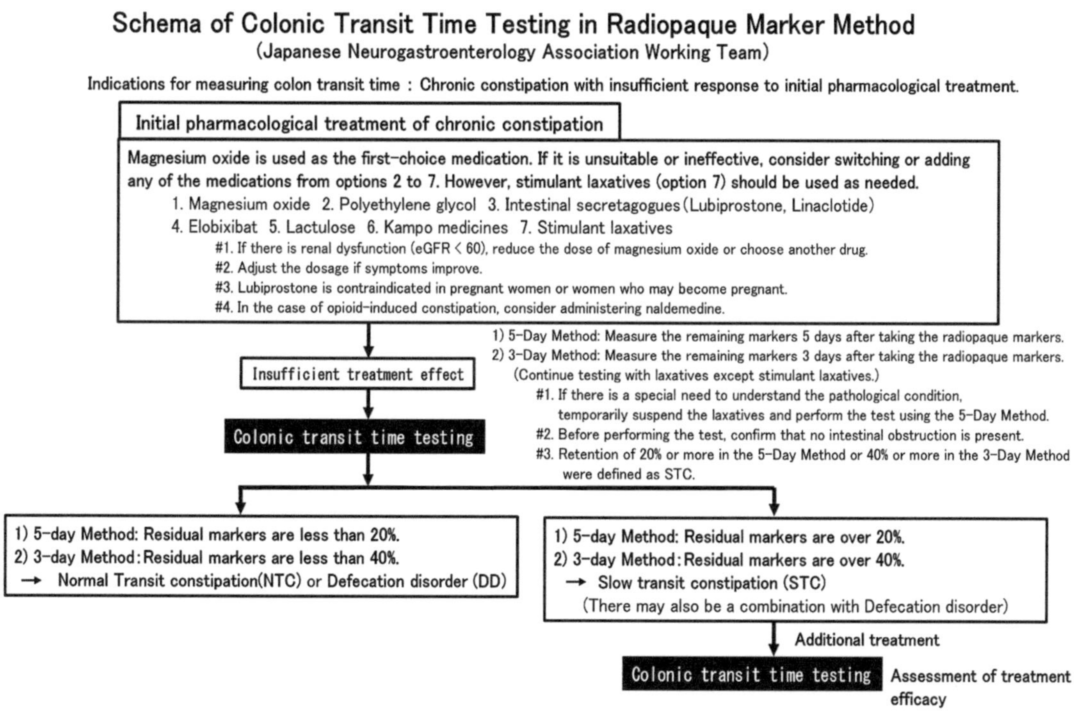

Fig. 40.3 Schematic of colonic transit time measurement using radiopaque marker examination

protocols have been reported for more detailed evaluation of CTT. Metcalf et al.'s method [6] involves ingesting one capsule containing different-shaped radiopaque markers on the mornings of days 1, 2, and 3, followed by plain abdominal X-rays on the mornings of days 4 and 7. The abdomen is divided into three regions on the X-ray: "right side," "left side," and "sigmoid colon/rectum," and the transit times for the entire colon, right colon, left colon, and sigmoid colon/rectum are measured to identify the site of delayed transit. This method allows differentiation between defecation disorder, where the sigmoid colon/rectum transit time is the longest, and slow colonic transit type, where transit is delayed throughout the colon. Another method involves ingesting one capsule each day for 6 days and taking a plain abdominal X-ray on the 7th day to measure the transit times of various colonic regions based on the distribution of markers.

4 Radioisotope Method

The radioisotope (RI) method involves ingesting a test meal mixed with an RI-labeled compound, followed by counting the radiation activity in the colon over time using a gamma camera to measure CTT [7]. ^{111}Indium is commonly used as a radiopharmaceutical. The RI method was originally developed to measure gastric emptying and is widely used internationally as the gold standard for gastric emptying tests. However, measuring CTT with this method is more complex and challenging compared to gastric emptying tests. For gastric emptying, the region of interest is limited to the stomach, allowing for the creation of an emptying curve by measuring radiation activity. In contrast, for the colon, the region of interest must be set at five to seven locations along the entire abdominal course of the colon (Fig. 40.4), making the creation and evaluation of emptying curves more complex. Additionally,

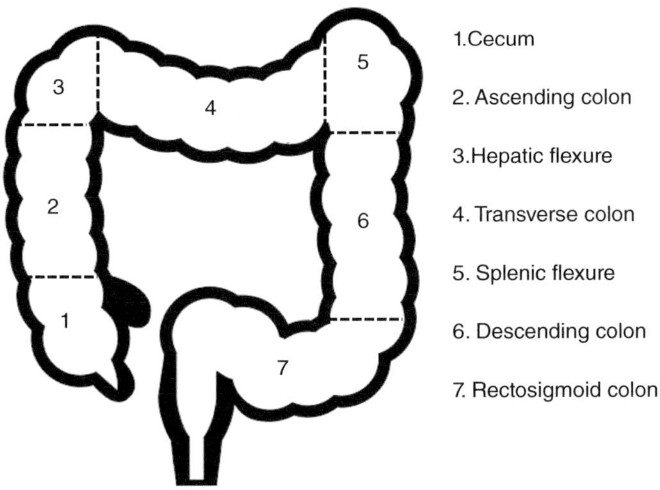

Fig. 40.4 Areas of interest in the colon using the RI method. 1: Cecum, 2: Ascending colon, 3: Hepatic flexure, 4: Transverse colon, 5: Splenic flexure, 6: Descending colon, and 7: Rectosigmoid colon

issues such as radiation exposure, handling of RI compounds, the need for large-scale testing facilities, and high costs present significant challenges, and this method is rarely performed in Japan.

5 Wireless Capsule Method

Internationally, CTT measurement using wireless capsules is also performed [8, 9]. Currently, two types of capsules are developed for transit time measurement: the Smart Pill and the Motilis 3D-Transit System. The Smart Pill senses pH, pressure, and temperature within the gastrointestinal lumen, transmitting this data in real-time to an external receiver. The capsule's position is estimated from these data, and the transit times of various gastrointestinal regions, including the colon, are measured. The Motilis 3D-Transit System tracks the capsule's position by detecting electromagnetic waves emitted by the ingested capsule with external sensors, measuring CTT. The capsules are over 2 cm in size and are contraindicated in cases of gastrointestinal obstruction, requiring a check of gastrointestinal patency similar to capsule endoscopy. The usefulness of these wireless capsule methods has been evaluated, and their correlation with the marker method has been demonstrated [1]. However, the Smart Pill emits radio frequencies that are not permitted for use in Japan, and thus, wireless capsules are not used in Japan.

It is also possible to measure CTT using capsule endoscopy by analyzing the time the capsule endoscope passes through the ileocecal valve and reaches the anus. However, this is off-label use and not the intended purpose of capsule endoscopy.

6 Conclusion

Measuring CTT is clinically very important, and several methods have been developed. However, in Japan, these tests are not yet performed in daily clinical practice, and the radiopaque marker method is only conducted for research purposes in some facilities. The widespread use of these tests in daily clinical practice in Japan is strongly desired in the future.

Take-Home Message
Internationally, chronic constipation is commonly classified by CTT. CTT measurement is an essential test for objectively evaluating colonic motility and understanding the pathophysiology of diseases with colonic motility disorders, including chronic constipation. However, in Japan, CTT measurement is currently performed only for research purposes in some facilities. The widespread use of CTT measurement in daily clinical practice in Japan is strongly desired in the future.

Competing Interests The author has no competing interests to declare that are relevant to the content of this chapter.

References

1. Bharucha AE, et al. More Movement with evaluating colonic transit in humans. Neurogastroenterol Motil. 2019;31:e13541.
2. Lembo A, et al. Chronic constipation. N Engl J Med. 2003;349:1360–8.
3. Bharucha AE, et al. American gastroenterological association technical review on constipation. Gastroenterology. 2013;144:218–38.
4. Hinton JM, et al. A new method of studying gut transit times using radiopaque markers. Gut. 1969;10:842–7.
5. Abe T, et al. Clinical evaluation of colonic transit time testing in the diagnosis of constipation. J Jpn Soc Coloproctol. 2020;73:237–43. (in Japanese).
6. Metcalf AM, et al. Simplified assessment of segmental colonic transit. Gastroenterology. 1987;92:40–7.
7. Krevsky LS, et al. Colonic transit scintigraphy. A physiologic approach to the quantitative measurement of colonic transit in humans. Gastroenterology. 1986;91:1102–12.
8. Rao SC, et al. Investigation of colonic and whole-gut transit with wireless motility capsule and radiopaque markers in constipation. Clin Gastroenterol Hepatol. 2009;7:537–44.
9. Camilleri M, et al. Wireless pH-motility capsule for colonic transit: prospective comparison with radiopaque markers in chronic constipation. Neurogastroeterol Motil. 2010;22:874–e233.

41 Small Bowel and Colonic Motility Test, Cine-MRI

Hidenori Ohkubo

Abstract

Abdominal bloating is one of the most common symptoms we encounter in daily clinical practice. When no organic cause is observed, functional constipation or irritable bowel syndrome (IBS) is primarily considered; however, chronic intestinal pseudo-obstruction (CIPO), a life-threatening motility disorder, may also be included. Conventional abdominal CT or plain X-ray exams can only evaluate the gastrointestinal tract with "static images." Cine-MRI (CMRI) is an emerging technique that allows observation of the organ movement as "videos" with a temporal resolution of <1 second. In 2013, a pilot study comparing the small intestinal motility between patients with CIPO, IBS, and healthy individuals by CMRI and evaluating its usefulness was performed. In this study, small intestinal motility was quantitatively assessed by mean luminal diameter (MLD), contraction rate (CR), and contraction cycle, using 30 coronal frames over 15 seconds with T2-weighted images. As a result, CMRI clearly detected contractility impairments, including especially marked dilatation of MLD and extremely low CR in CIPO patients.

CMRI is a useful modality that allows direct assessment of the actual "movement" of the intestines without radiation exposure. In clinical practice, CMRI is expected to be widely used for diagnosing CIPO, evaluating the effects of therapeutic interventions, and follow-up.

Keywords

Observation of the organ movement as "videos," · T2-weightend images · Mean luminal diameter · Contraction rate · Contraction cycle · Chronic intestinal pseudo-obstruction (CIPO)

1 Introduction

Symptoms such as abdominal pain, abdominal bloating, and bowel movement disorders are among the most frequently encountered clinical manifestations. However, there are many cases in which no abnormalities are found in the gastrointestinal tract by endoscopic examination. In such cases, irritable bowel syndrome (IBS) or functional constipation (FC), representative of disorders of gut–brain interaction (DGBI), are primarily considered. However, severe gastrointestinal motility disorders such as chronic intestinal pseudo-obstruction (CIPO) may also be included. Unlike DGBI, CIPO is a life-threatening

H. Ohkubo (✉)
Gastroenterology Division, Sagami Rinkan Hospital, Sagamihara, Japan
e-mail: ohkuboh@yokohama-cu.ac.jp

H. Kaneko et al. (eds.), *Disorders of Gut-Brain Interaction*,
https://doi.org/10.1007/978-981-95-6974-8_41

disease, making its differentiation extremely important [1].

CT scans are crucial for differentiating these conditions. CIPO can be relatively easily distinguished from DGBI by the presence of an air-fluid level and intestinal dilation. However, CT scans are essentially evaluations of "static images." Is there no method to directly capture the actual "movement of the intestines" in diseases characterized by "extremely severe motility disorders" like CIPO?

1.1 What Is Cine-MRI?

Cine-MRI (CMRI) is a method that directly captures the actual peristalsis of the gastrointestinal tract. CMRI is a recently developed modality that allows observation of organ movement as "videos" with a fine temporal resolution of less than 1 second. Although it has been actively applied in the cardiovascular field, such as in the diagnosis of acute myocarditis [2], recent reports have highlighted its various utilities in evaluating gastrointestinal motility. Specifically, Wakamiya et al. evaluated small intestinal motility in healthy individuals [3], and Baba et al. assessed gastric emptying movements [4], reporting that CMRI is a useful modality for evaluating gastrointestinal motility.

The settings and imaging conditions vary slightly depending on the equipment, but typically, images are captured at a speed of about two frames per second for several tens of seconds. The obtained images are continuously played back using dedicated software, allowing evaluation as videos, similar to cinema. We operate with a protocol that captures 30 images over 15 seconds. Figure 41.1 shows actual CMRI images. This is the small intestine of a healthy individual, where the small intestine, filled with intestinal fluid, is depicted as a clear high-signal area (T2-weighted image), and the temporal changes in each region are evident (arrow).

In 2013, we performed CMRI on IBS patients, who are very common in daily clinical practice,

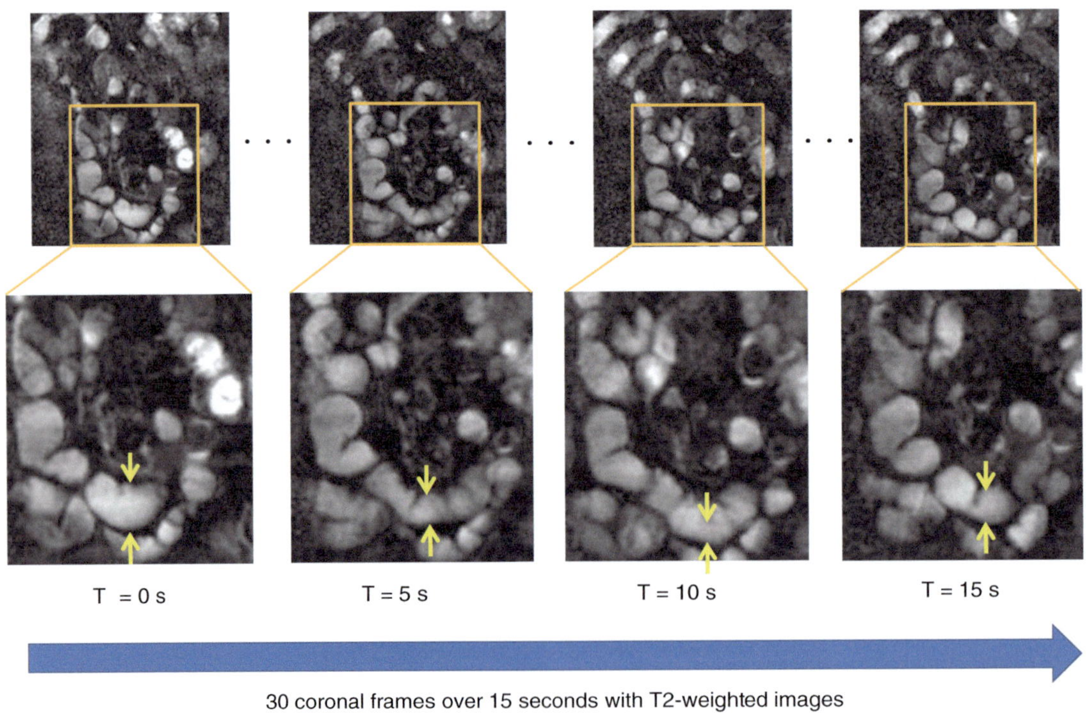

Fig. 41.1 CMRI images of the small intestine in healthy individuals

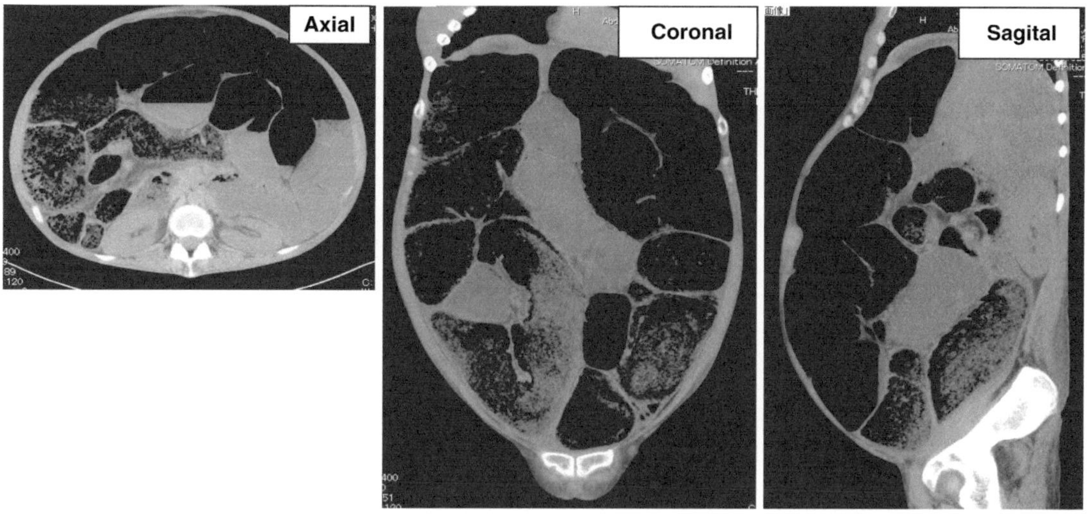

Fig. 41.2 Typical CT images of CIPO

and CIPO patients, who show the most severe motility impairment, comparing their peristaltic movements with those of the small intestine in healthy individuals [5]. In the following, we introduce the research content and discuss the latest findings.

1.2 Evaluation of Small Intestinal Motility Using CMRI

1.2.1 What Is CIPO?

First, an overview of CIPO is provided. CIPO is a rare and intractable gastrointestinal disorder characterized by chronic or recurrent symptoms of intestinal obstruction over many years. The fundamental cause is severely impaired intestinal peristalsis, leading to the accumulation of large amounts of gas and intestinal fluids, primarily in the small intestine. CT scans show pathological dilation of the small intestine and an air-fluid level, where the boundary between intestinal fluid and gas becomes linear, resembling typical intestinal obstruction (ileus). However, it is distinguished from mechanical obstruction by the absence of organic causes and from paralytic ileus by its chronic/persistent nature. Due to the potential for life-threatening complications such as nutritional disorders and bacteremia, it is a rare but critical disease that must not be overlooked. Figure 41.2 shows typical images.

CIPO is a collective term for a series of disease states presenting a similar phenotype, with a diverse range of pathologies. It can be secondary to collagen diseases such as systemic sclerosis, neurological disorders, and endocrine diseases, or it can occur idiopathically without these underlying conditions.

1.2.2 CMRI Protocol

We enrolled 12 healthy individuals, 12 IBS patients meeting the Rome criteria, and 12 CIPO patients meeting the diagnostic criteria of the Ministry of Health, Labour and Welfare (Table 41.1), and performed CMRI on each in the coronal plane. The imaging conditions were standardized according to the protocol shown in Table 41.2, with a shooting speed of one frame every 0.5 seconds and a shooting time of 15 seconds (30 images per coronal plane). To obtain clear images, healthy individuals and IBS patients underwent a water load of 1000 mL 30 minutes before the examination. In contrast, CIPO patients did not undergo a water load due to the pathologically pre-existed intestinal fluid.

Generally, in a normal small intestine, peristalsis should always be present if there are contents such as intestinal fluid. Conversely, even in

Table 41.1 Diagnostic criteria for CIPO by the Ministry of Health, Labour and Welfare Research Group [6, 7]

Diagnostic criteria:
CIPO is diagnosed when all of the following criteria are met:
1. Chronic intestinal obstruction symptoms have been present for more than 6 months.
2. Abdominal bloating or abdominal pain has been present for the last 3 months.
3. Abdominal plain X-ray, endoscopic examination, or abdominal CT shows intestinal dilation and/or air-fluid level.
4. Organic causes are excluded by gastrointestinal X-ray imaging, endoscopic examination, and so on.

Table 41.2 Controls and methods

	Healthy individuals (n = 12)	IBS patients (n = 12)	CIPO patients (n = 12)
Preprocedure	Water load: 1000 mL (30 minutes before imaging)		No water load
Imaging conditions	Common protocol b-TFE sequence, coronal plane, TR 4.1 ms, TE 2.0 ms, flip angle 80° Slice thickness 10 mm, matrix 256, FOV 380 mm Imaging interval: 0.5 seconds/frame, imaging time: 15 seconds (30 frames per coronal slice)		
Evaluation items	1. MLD (mm) 2. CR (= amplitude*/maximum dilation diameter) (%) *: Amplitude = maximum dilation diameter − maximum contraction diameter 3. Contraction cycle (seconds)		

a normal small intestine, peristalsis may cease if there are no contents. Therefore, the presence of reduced peristalsis despite the presence of intestinal contents is considered an abnormal finding.

Figure 41.3 shows typical CMRI images of each group (due to space constraints, only four images at 5-second intervals are displayed). Since these are T2-weighted images, the intestinal fluid is depicted as high-signal areas. The small intestine of healthy individuals shows no intestinal dilation and exhibits active peristaltic movements over 15 seconds (top row). Similarly, the small intestine of IBS patients shows no pathological dilation and maintains good peristalsis (middle row). In contrast, the small intestine of CIPO patients is markedly dilated compared to healthy individuals and IBS patients due to the stagnation of contents, and there is very little temporal change in the intestinal luminal diameter (bottom row). Thus, CMRI is an examination that allows for the visual assessment of small intestinal peristalsis.

1.2.3 Evaluation Method: How to Quantitatively Assess

First, for each case, three well-depicted intestinal segments were arbitrarily selected from the obtained coronal sections (measurement points), and the intestinal diameter (short axis) at each measurement point was measured for 30 frames.

Next, we created graphs as shown in Fig. 41.4 and calculated the following for each measurement point:

1. Mean luminal diameter (MLD) (mm)
2. Contraction rate (CR) (= amplitude/maximum dilation diameter) (%)
   - Amplitude = maximum dilation diameter − maximum contraction diameter
3. Contraction cycle (seconds)

Finally, for each case, the average values of the three measurement points were calculated to reduce selection bias, and these were compared between the groups.

1.2.4 Results and Discussion

Figure 41.5 shows quantitative analysis on CMRI in healthy individuals, patients with IBS, and those with CIPO. The CIPO group had a significantly larger mean intestinal diameter and a significantly lower CR compared to the healthy and IBS groups. There were no significant differences in contraction cycles between the groups. On the other hand, there were no significant differences in any of the parameters (MLD, CR, and contraction cycle) between the IBS and healthy groups.

CMRI is a useful modality that can quantitatively and visually demonstrate the reduced peristalsis of the small intestine in CIPO.

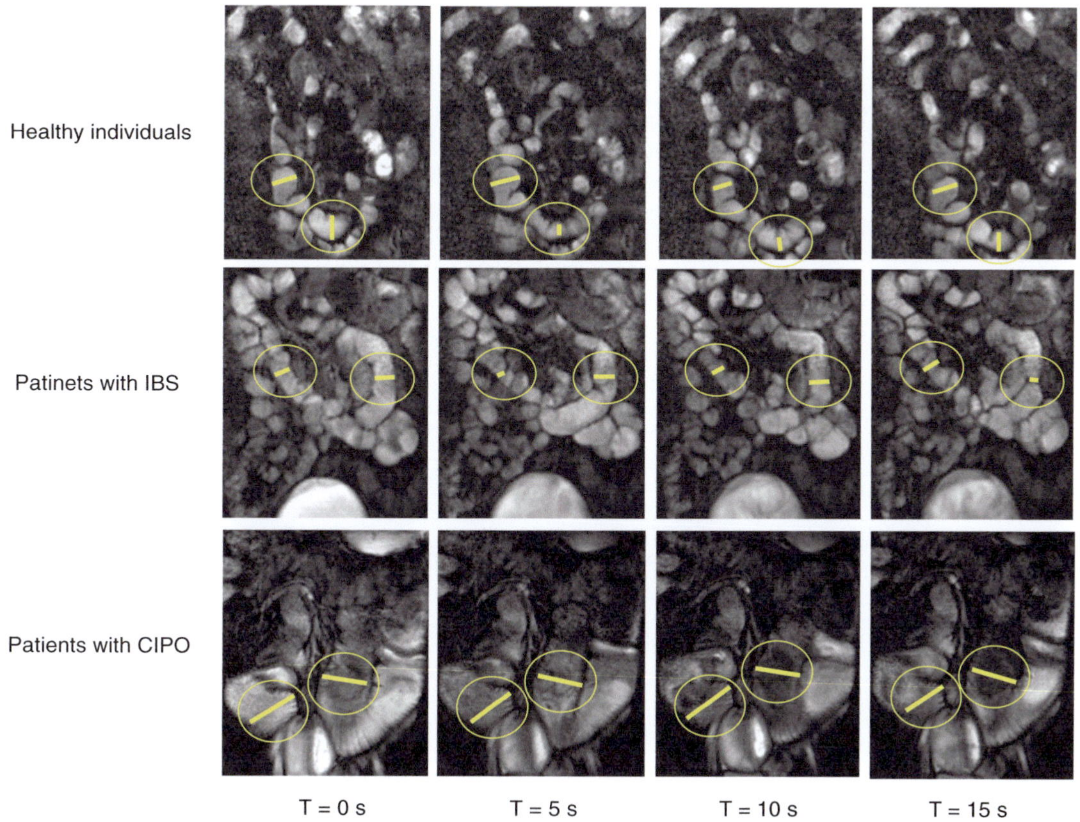

Fig. 41.3 Temporal changes and measurement points in each group using CMRI. (Modified from Ref. [5]). For each case, three measurement points were arbitrarily selected, and the luminal diameter was measured (only two points are shown in the figure: yellow circles)

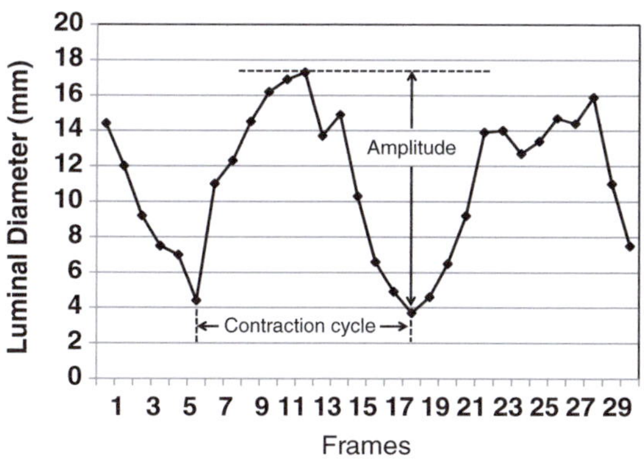

Fig. 41.4 Temporal changes in luminal diameter at measurement points. (Created from Ref. [5])

1.3 Latest Findings

Recently, van Rijn et al. in the Netherlands compared the differences in small intestinal peristalsis in CIPO patients during fasting and postprandial states using CMRI [8]. Although their protocol differed slightly from ours, such as using a b-FFE sequence and a shooting time of 20 seconds, they also evaluated in the coronal plane at a shooting speed of one frame every 0.5 seconds, resulting in almost equivalent videos. However, their measurement method differed significantly, as they used a system that automatically scores the strength of small intesti-

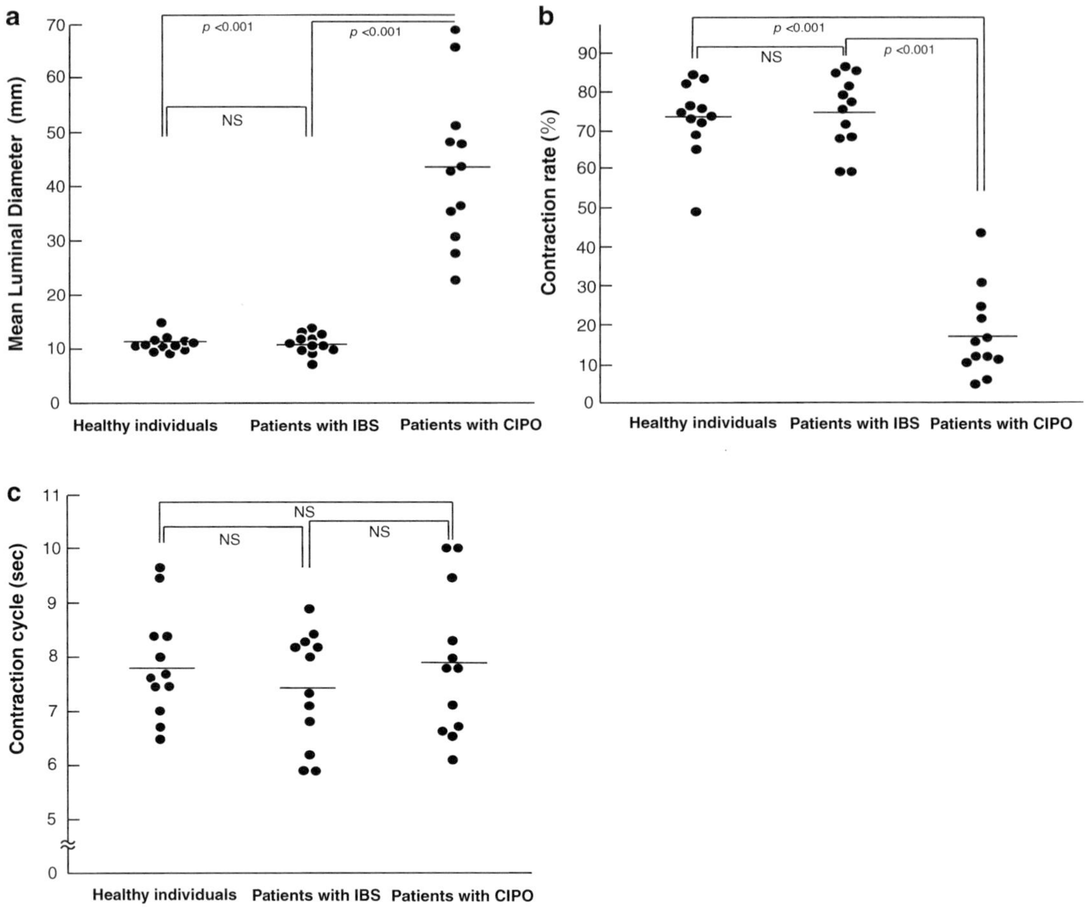

Fig. 41.5 Quantitative analysis on CMRI in healthy individuals, patients with IBS, and those with CIPO

nal peristalsis in the entire region of interest (motility score) once the region of interest is extracted. This method provides continuous and comprehensive data, which is superior to our method, but it also requires more specialized analytical knowledge.

They performed CMRI on 16 healthy individuals and 8 CIPO patients during fasting and immediately after, and 20 minutes after the administration of a nutritional supplement (300 kcal/200 mL). As a result, almost all healthy individuals showed increased small intestinal peristalsis postprandially compared to fasting. In contrast, in CIPO patients, half showed weakly increased small intestinal peristalsis postprandially, while the other half showed decreased small intestinal peristalsis.

In other words, in CIPO patients, there was no consistent trend in postprandial small intestinal peristalsis, and it varied from case to case. Although the number of cases is small, further data accumulation is expected to elucidate the pathophysiology.

1.4 Clinical Significance of CMRI in Gastroenterology

CMRI is a useful modality that allows direct assessment of the actual "movement" of the intestines without radiation exposure, unlike conventional abdominal CT or plain X-ray examinations. Additionally, compared to manometry, which is popular in Europe and the United States,

CMRI has the advantage of not requiring the insertion of pressure sensor catheters into the gastrointestinal tract, thus reducing patient burden and allowing continuous evaluation of the entire small intestine. Therefore, CMRI is expected to be widely used in clinical practice, not only for diagnosing CIPO but also for evaluating the effects of therapeutic interventions and follow-up. Furthermore, there are reports that surgery (intestinal resection) is not desirable for CIPO cases involving the small intestine [9], and CMRI, which excels in evaluating small intestinal motility, is considered very useful for considering surgical indications. Moreover, as recent reports suggest, CMRI is expected to be highly beneficial in research for elucidating pathophysiology.

Take-Home Message

- CMRI is a useful examination that can directly evaluate organ movement as "videos."
- The presence of reduced peristalsis despite the presence of intestinal contents is considered an abnormal finding.
- In CIPO, CMRI can clearly exhibit the pathological intestinal dilation (accumulation of intestinal contents) and a significant reduction in peristalsis.
- CMRI is expected to be utilized in clinical practice for "evaluating the effects of therapeutic interventions" and "follow-up."

Competing Interests The author has no competing interests to declare that are relevant to the content of this chapter.

References

1. Stanghellini V, et al. Natural history of chronic idiopathic intestinal pseudo-obstruction in adults: a single center study. Clin Gastroenterol Hepatol. 2005;3:449–58.
2. Deux JF, et al. Acute myocarditis: diagnostic value of contrast-enhanced cine steady-state free precession MRI sequences. Am J Roentgenol. 2011;197:1081–7.
3. Wakamiya M, et al. Assessment of small bowel motility function with cine-MRI using balanced steady-state free precession sequence. J Magn Reson Imaging. 2011;33:1235–40.
4. Baba S, et al. Assessment of gastric motor function by cine magnetic resonance imaging. J Gastroenterol Hepatol. 2009;24:1401–6.
5. Ohkubo H, et al. Assessment of small bowel motility in patients with chronic intestinal pseudo-obstruction using Cine-MRI. Am J Gastroenterol. 2013;108:1130–9.
6. Nakajima A, et al. Heisei 23 year Ministry of Health, Labour and Welfare Research Grant for overcoming intractable diseases. In: Epidemiological, Diagnostic, and Therapeutic Research Group on Chronic Idiopathic Intestinal Pseudo-obstruction in Japan. 1st ed. Sanno Printing; 2012. (in Japanese).
7. Ohkubo H, et al. An epidemiologic survey of chronic intestinal pseudo-obstruction and evaluation of the newly proposed diagnostic criteria. Digestion. 2012;86:12–9.
8. van Rijn KL, et al. Fasted and fed small bowel motility patterns at cine-MRI in chronic intestinal pseudo-obstruction. Neurogastroenterol Motil. 2021;33:e14062.
9. Masaki T, et al. Nationwide survey on adult type chronic intestinal pseudo-obstruction in surgical institutions in Japan. Surg Today. 2012;42:264–71.

Small Bowel and Colonic Function Test, Methods of Examinations for Intestinal Mucosal Permeability

42

Eikichi Ihara

Abstract

Dysfunction of the mucosal barrier, characterized by increased intestinal mucosal permeability, is implicated in the pathogenesis of not only local intestinal diseases but also systemic diseases, including metabolic syndrome, cardiovascular diseases, and neurodegenerative disorders. Therefore, the development and standardization of reliable methods for evaluating intestinal mucosal permeability are of great importance. This chapter has provided an overview of current methods for assessing intestinal mucosal permeability, including the short-circuit current method using the Ussing chamber, the lactulose/mannitol permeability test, and endoscopic intestinal mucosal permeability testing using a tissue conductance meter. The short-circuit current method is valuable for basic research using animal models; it is not suitable for routine clinical testing due to its requirement for multiple biopsy specimens and its procedural complexity. The lactulose/mannitol permeability test is clinically useful; however, it does not allow for distinction between the relative contribution of the small intestine and colon to overall mucosal permeability. In contrast, endoscopic intestinal mucosal permeability testing using a tissue conductance meter enables real-time evaluation of intestinal mucosal permeability in specific intestinal regions during endoscopy. Among the available methods, the tissue conductance meter, allowing in vivo, real-time, site-specific assessment during routine endoscopic procedures, is expected to gain broader application in clinical practice.

Keywords

Intestinal mucosal permeability · Short-circuit current method · Lactulose/mannitol method · Endoscopic intestinal mucosal permeability testing · Tissue conductance meter

1 Introduction

The epithelial lining of the intestinal tract serves as a mucosal barrier, demarcating the "internal exterior" of the intestinal lumen from the internal environment of the body. One of the primary mechanisms regulating this mucosal barrier function is the tight junction proteins between epithelial cells, which include transmembrane molecules such as ZO-1, occludin, and a series of claudins. Dysfunction of the mucosal barrier,

E. Ihara (✉)
Department of Medicine and Bioregulatory Science, Graduate School of Medical Sciences, Kyushu University, Fukuoka, Japan
e-mail: ihara.eikichi.167@m.kyushu-u.ac.jp

H. Kaneko et al. (eds.), *Disorders of Gut-Brain Interaction*,
https://doi.org/10.1007/978-981-95-6974-8_42

characterized by increased intestinal mucosal permeability, is implicated in the pathogenesis of local inflammation observed in conditions such as Crohn's disease and celiac disease, as well as the microinflammation seen in irritable bowel syndrome (IBS). Furthermore, increased intestinal mucosal permeability allows microorganisms and dietary antigens from the intestinal lumen to enter the systemic circulation via the portal vein, potentially leading to chronic inflammation that is not limited to local inflammation in the digestive tract but also affects various organs throughout the body, and contributing to the pathogenesis of numerous diseases, including metabolic syndrome, cardiovascular diseases, and neurodegenerative disorders. Therefore, evaluating intestinal mucosal permeability is important. This chapter provides an overview of methods for assessing intestinal mucosal permeability, including the use of the short-circuit current method, the lactulose/mannitol mucosal permeability test, and endoscopic intestinal mucosal permeability testing using a tissue conductance meter.

1.1 Intestinal Mucosal Permeability Testing Using the Short-Circuit Current Method

The epithelial lining of the intestinal tract is capable of conducting both active and passive transport of various electrolytes, regulated by ion channels, ion exchangers, and membrane transporters. The short-circuit current method, also known as the Ussing chamber technique, named after its developer, is an electrophysiological method used to measure electrolyte transport across the mucosal epithelium. This technique expresses the electrochemical properties of epithelial transport in terms of electrical circuit parameters, such as current, electromotive force, and electrical resistance, by representing epithelial transport as an electrical equivalent circuit [1]. The apparatus for the short-circuit current measurement consists of a chamber with two compartments separated by a small window onto which the mucosal epithelium is mounted. The solutions in the two compartments are in contact with the luminal and basolateral sides of the epithelium, respectively. Electrodes for measuring potential difference and short-circuit current are connected via salt bridges (Fig. 42.1). Typically, 3 M KCl solidified with 2–4% agar is used for the salt bridges. The resistance of mucosal epithelium can be calculated from the transepithelial potential difference and short-circuit current using Ohm's law. Additionally, changes in epithelial resistance can be assessed by monitoring changes in voltage and current. Drug-induced changes in electrolyte transport can also be recorded as changes in the short-circuit current. Figure 42.2 illustrates the measurement of Cl^- current following misoprostol stimulation in the mucosal epithelium of the mouse small intestine. This change in short-circuit current was abolished by pretreatment with an EP4 receptor antagonist or by the removal of Cl^- from the bathing solution.

While the short-circuit current method is useful for basic research using animal models, it is not suitable for routine clinical testing of intestinal mucosal permeability. The technique requires multiple biopsy specimens and involves a complex measurement procedure. Given the balance between invasiveness and practicality, it is unlikely that intestinal mucosal permeability testing using the short-circuit current method will become widely adopted in routine clinical practice.

1.2 Intestinal Mucosal Permeability Testing Using the Lactulose/Mannitol Test

The lactulose/mannitol test is widely used to assess the mucosal permeability of both the small intestine and colon. This test measures the absorption of lactulose, a disaccharide, and mannitol, a monosaccharide, which reflect paracellular and transcellular permeability of mucosal epithelium, respectively. Damage to mucosal epithelium or dysfunction of tight junctions leads to

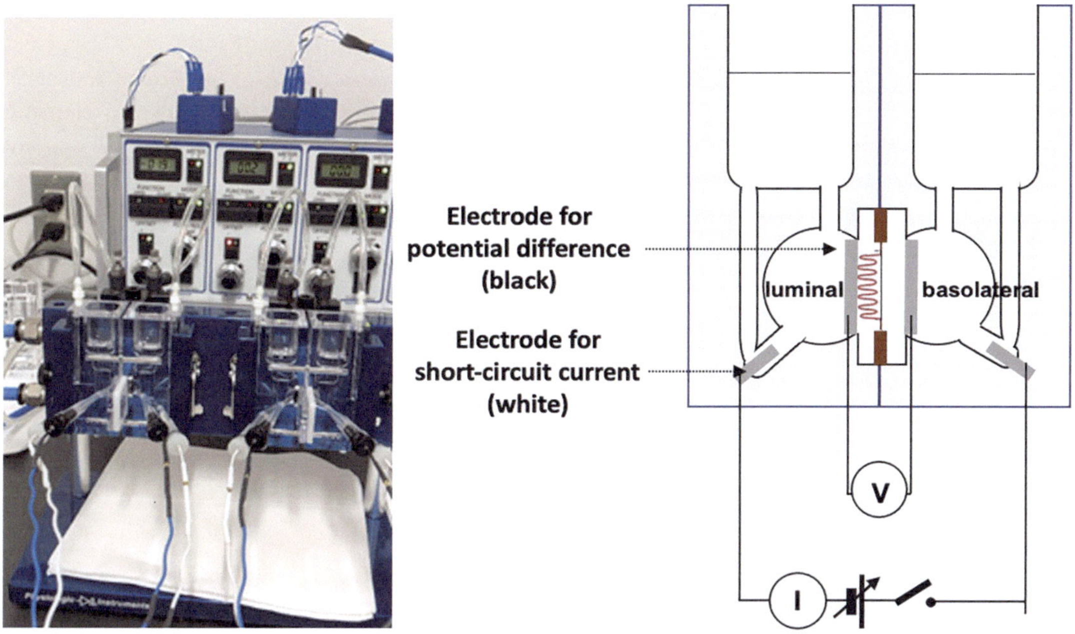

Fig. 42.1 Representative Ussing chamber system for measuring short-circuit current (Isc)

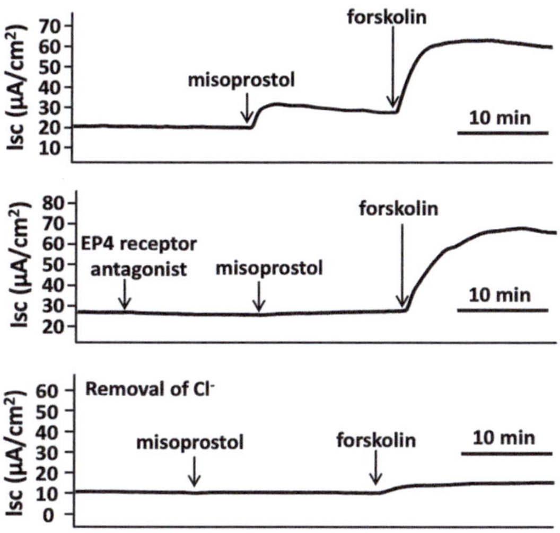

Fig. 42.2 Short-circuit current (Isc) induced by misoprostol measured using the Ussing chamber. EP4 receptor prostaglandin E receptor 4, Cl^- free treatment chloride ion-free treatment

increased lactulose absorption and decreased mannitol absorption, resulting in an elevated urinary lactulose/mannitol ratio. Urinary concentrations of lactulose and mannitol are measured using enzyme assays, gas chromatography with flame ionization detection, or tandem mass spectrometry (MS/MS) with high-performance liquid chromatography (HPLC) [2].

Although no standardized protocol has been universally adopted, one study reported a method involving a 12-hour fast followed by urination, ingestion of a sugar solution containing 10 g of lactulose and 5 g of mannitol dissolved in 400 mL of water, additional intake of 200 mL of water, and subsequent collection of urine over a 4-hour period. The collected urine samples were then frozen and analyzed by HPLC-MS/MS [3]. Other studies have used urine collection periods of 5 or 6 hours [4]. It has been reported that the collection intervals of 0–3 hours, 3–5 hours, and 5–24 hours reflect the mucosal permeability of the proximal small intestine, distal small intestine, and colon, respectively. However, it has also been shown that even the 0–2 hour collection period partially reflects colonic mucosal permeability, indicating that the 0–5 hour urine sample does not exclusively represent small intestinal mucosal permeability. Therefore, results must be interpreted with caution [5]. In some protocols, rhamnose is used instead of mannitol as the monosaccharide probe [4].

1.3 Endoscopic Intestinal Mucosal Permeability Testing Using a Tissue Conductance Meter

Recent development of the tissue conductance meter (TCM AS-TC100, Nihon Asch Co., Ltd., Tokyo, Japan) has enabled real-time evaluation of intestinal mucosal permeability in specific intestinal regions during endoscopy. The measurement probe, which can be inserted through the endoscope's forceps channel, theoretically allows evaluation of all accessible intestinal mucosa. This method uses a rod-shaped electrode sensor with a diameter of 1.9 mm to measure the electrical impedance of the intestinal mucosa.

The procedure is outlined as follows: electrodes are attached to the flexor side of both forearms, and the rod-shaped electrode sensor is introduced via the endoscope's forceps channel. Alternating currents of 320 Hz and 30.7 kHz are applied at a constant voltage of 12.5 mV, and the electrical impedance of intestinal mucosa is measured by placing the electrode tip in contact with the target intestinal mucosa for 3 seconds [6] (Fig. 42.3). Electrical impedance reflects the resistance of biological tissues [7], which can be modeled as a parallel circuit consisting of resistance and capacitance [8]. Both the resistance and capacitance vary according to homeostatic status and water content of the mucosal epithe-

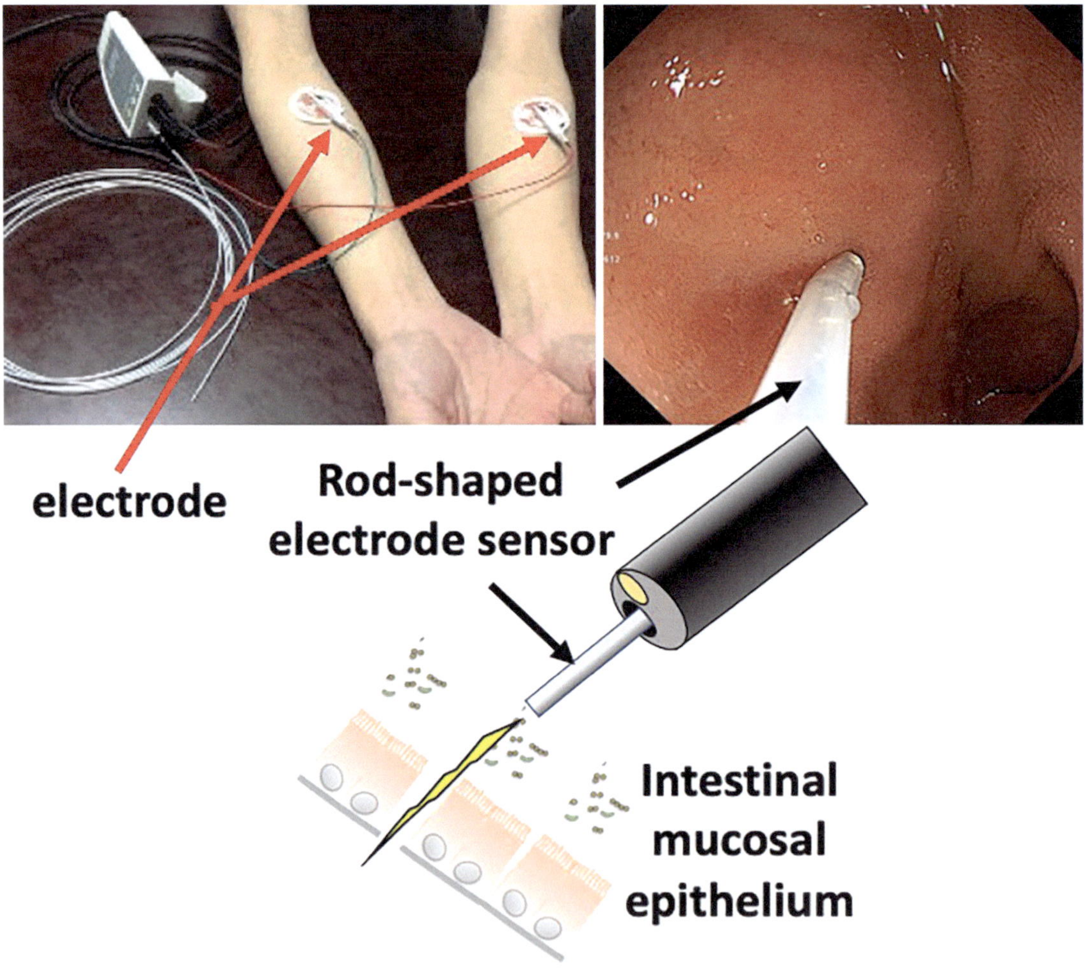

Fig. 42.3 Endoscopic mucosal permeability testing using a tissue conductance meter

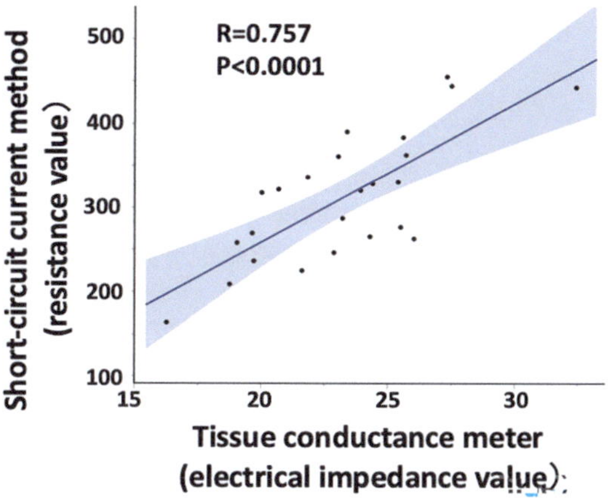

Fig. 42.4 Correlation between electrical impedance values measured by the tissue conductance meter and resistance values obtained using the short-circuit current method

lium [9]. In this parallel-circuit model, the absolute value of electrical impedance (|Z|) is theoretically calculated using the following formula:

$$|Z| = 1/\sqrt{1/R^2 + C^2\omega^2}$$

where R is the resistance, C is the capacitance, and ω is the angular frequency of the applied alternating current. When ω is sufficiently small, |Z| approximates R. Therefore, using a low frequency of 320 Hz, [R] can be reasonably estimated from |Z|. Thus, intestinal mucosal permeability (mucosal barrier function) can be assessed from the electrical impedance values obtained at this low frequency. Our studies using clinical specimens have shown a strong correlation between electrical impedance values measured by the tissue conductance meter and resistance values obtained using the short-circuit current method (Fig. 42.4). Using this device, we have demonstrated that one of the major pathophysiological features of functional dyspepsia (FD), a type of disorder of gut-brain interaction (DGBI), is increased duodenal mucosal permeability (i.e., decreased mucosal barrier function). Furthermore, in patients with FD, increased duodenal mucosal permeability has been found to be associated with reduced expression of ZO-1 and increased expression of IL-1β [6].

2 Conclusion

This chapter has provided an overview of methods for assessing intestinal mucosal permeability, including the short-circuit current method, the lactulose/mannitol permeability test, and endoscopic mucosal permeability testing using a tissue conductance meter. It has become increasingly evident that the integrity of the intestinal mucosal barrier is associated not only with local intestinal diseases but also with the pathogenesis of systemic diseases. Therefore, the development and standardization of reliable methods for evaluating intestinal mucosal permeability are of great importance. Among the available methods, the tissue conductance meter, which allows real-time in vivo measurement of intestinal mucosal permeability during widely used endoscopic procedures, is expected to gain broader application in clinical practice.

Take-Home Message

- When evaluating intestinal mucosal barrier function using a tissue conductance meter during endoscopy, it is essential to position the measurement probe as perpendicular as possible to the mucosal surface to obtain stable values.
- With the advancement of mucosal barrier function testing methods during endoscopy, as described in this chapter, we are entering an era in which DGBIs, such as FD and IBS, may be objectively diagnosed by endoscopy in routine clinical practice.

Competing Interests The author has no competing interests to declare that are relevant to the content of this chapter.

References

1. Karaki S, et al. Electrophysiological measurement of electrolyte transport in epithelial membranes: short-circuit current method. Nippon Yakurigaku Zasshi. 2004;123:211–8. (in Japanese).

2. Gervasoni J, et al. Validation of UPLC-MS/MS method for determination of urinary lactulose/mannitol. Molecules. 2018;23:2705.
3. Kato T, et al. Lubiprostone improves intestinal permeability in human, a novel therapy for the leaky gut: a prospective randomized pilot study in healthy volunteers. PLoS One. 2017;12:e0175626.
4. Zuhl M, et al. The effects of acute oral glutamine supplementation on exercise-induced gastrointestinal permeability and heat shock protein expression in peripheral blood mononuclear cells. Cell Stress Chaperones. 2015;20:85–93.
5. Maxton DG, et al. L-rhamnose and polyethyleneglycol 400 as probe markers for assessment in vivo of human intestinal permeability. Clin Sci (Lond). 1986;71:71–80.
6. Komori K, et al. The altered mucosal barrier function in the duodenum plays a role in the pathogenesis of functional dyspepsia. Dig Dis Sci. 2019;64:3228–39.
7. Koizumi H, et al. Increased permeability of the epithelium of middle ear cholesteatoma. Clin Otolaryngol. 2015;40:106–14.
8. Yamamoto T, et al. Electrical properties of the epidermal stratum corneum. Med Biol Eng. 1976;14:151–8.
9. Lawrence JN. Electrical resistance and tritiated water permeability as indicators of barrier integrity of in vivo human skin. Toxicol In Vitro. 1997;11:241–9.

Part VII

Small Bowel and Colon, Practical Edition

Diagnosis and Treatment of DGBI of the Small Bowel and Colon, Introduction

43

Shin Fukudo

Abstract

Symptoms suggesting diseases of small and/or large intestine include abdominal pain, diarrhea, constipation, abdominal bloating, hematochezia, fever, weight loss, and/or others. It is important to analyze the predominant symptoms to avoid missing organic diseases. These symptoms reflect gastrointestinal sensation, motility, secretion, absorption, mucosal permeability, bacterial overgrowth in the lumen, and/or presence of organic diseases. The Bristol Stool Form Scale (BSFS) classifies stool shapes into seven types, from type 1 to type 7, to determine the presence of bowel abnormalities. Type 4 represents normal stool and is associated with the most comfortable defecation. Changes in BSFS numbers correlate more sensitively with gastrointestinal transit time than defecation frequency. Consequently, in the Rome III, Rome IV, and coming Rome V criteria for bowel disorders in disorders of gut-brain interaction (DGBI), a state where the proportion of BSFS type 1 or 2 exceeds 25% is considered constipation, and a state where the proportion of BSFS type 6 or 7 exceeds 25% is considered diarrhea. BSFS together with other patient-reported outcome (PRO) is not only useful for diagnosing and classifying the disease types of bowel disorders of DGBI but also serves as an evaluation method for determining treatment efficacy.

Keywords

Abdominal pain · Diarrhea · Constipation · Abdominal bloating · Bristol Stool Form Scale (BSFS) · Disorders of gut-brain interaction (DGBI) · Patient-reported outcome (PRO) · Gastrointestinal sensation · Gastrointestinal motility · Mucosal permeability

1 Concept

Symptoms suggesting diseases of small and/or large intestine include abdominal pain, diarrhea, constipation, abdominal bloating, hematochezia, fever, weight loss, and/or others [1]. It is important to analyze the predominant symptoms to avoid missing organic diseases. When encountering symptoms such as mucous stools, bloody stools, fever, and weight loss, differential diagnosis with diseases such as colorectal cancer, inflammatory bowel disease, ischemic colitis,

S. Fukudo (✉)
Department of Behavioral Medicine, Graduate School of Medicine, Research Center for Accelerator and Radioisotope Science, Tohoku University, Sendai, Japan

Japanese Red Cross Ishinomaki Hospital, Ishinomaki, Japan
e-mail: shin.fukudo.c6@tohoku.ac.jp

H. Kaneko et al. (eds.), *Disorders of Gut-Brain Interaction*,
https://doi.org/10.1007/978-981-95-6974-8_43

Table 43.1 Symptoms suggestive of diseases of small and large intestine

Element	Symptom type	Description
Gastrointestinal sensation	Abdominal pain Abdominal discomfort Abdominal bloating	Dull pain, colicky pain, intermittent pain Unpleasant sensation, not painful Full sensation in the abdomen
	Urge to defecate Sensation of incomplete evacuation Difficult defecation	Urgency to defecate Reduced urge to defecate Loss of urge to defecate
Gastrointestinal motility	Diarrhea Constipation Alternating bowel habits Abdominal pain Abdominal distension Borborygmi Flatulence	Increased defecation frequency, watery stools, mushy stools Decreased defecation frequency, pellet-like stools, pellet-clustered stools Mixed loose and hard stools, symptomatic change by period Palpable spastic colon Visible changes in waist circumference Increased bowel sound Increased gas evacuation
Gastrointestinal secretion	Diarrhea Mucus	Increased stool volume Mucus discharge, stool hardening
Gastrointestinal absorption	Diarrhea	Increased stool volume, lactose or bile acid malabsorption
Mucosal permeability	Abdominal pain Diarrhea Constipation	Increased permeability Increased permeability Increased permeability
Bacterial overgrowth	Abdominal pain, distention, diarrhea	Fecal putrid odor, increased intestinal gas
Organic diseases	Tarry stool Mucous bloody stools Bloody stools Fever Weight loss Steatorrhea Extreme diarrhea Extreme constipation	Upper GI bleeding Suggesting inflammatory bowel disease Lower GI bleeding Suggesting infection or inflammation Suggesting serious diseases Suggesting pancreatic diseases DGBI unlikely DGBI unlikely

and colonic diverticulitis is necessary [2]. The presence of tarry stools, acholic stools, and steatorrhea should prompt consideration of upper gastrointestinal, hepatobiliary, and pancreatic diseases. The more frequent symptoms of diseases of small and/or large intestine are sensory and motor symptoms [3]. Sensory symptoms are subjective (Table 43.1). It is essential to quantify their nature, duration, severity, frequency, and factors that exacerbate or alleviate them as much as possible. Motor symptoms, while having subjective elements, are accompanied by objective findings (signs), allowing for quantitative analysis of their physical characteristics.

2 Bristol Stool Form Scale

The Bristol Stool Form Scale (BSFS) classifies stool shapes into seven types, from type 1 to type 7, to determine the presence of bowel abnormalities (Fig. 43.1) [4]. Type 4 represents normal stool and is associated with the most comfortable defecation. Changes in BSFS numbers correlate more sensitively with gastrointestinal transit time than defecation frequency [5]. Consequently, in the Rome III and Rome IV criteria for bowel disorders in disorders of gut-brain interaction (DGBI), a state where the proportion of BSFS type 1 or 2 exceeds 25% is

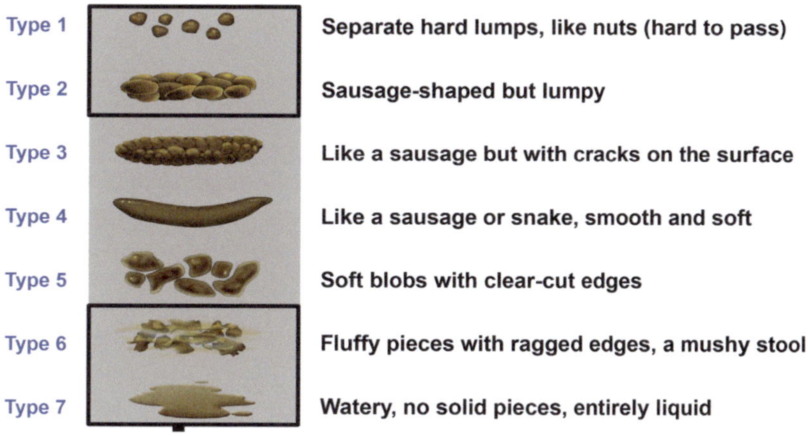

Fig. 43.1 Bristol Stool Form Scale. Type 4 represents normal stool. Types 1 and 2 indicate constipation, while types 6 and 7 indicate diarrhea

considered constipation, and a state where the proportion of BSFS type 6 or 7 exceeds 25% is considered diarrhea [4].

Subsequent research has revealed that in Asian countries, many people perceive types 1–3 as constipation and types 5–7 as diarrhea [6]. Additionally, the quality of life (QOL) of patients with chronic constipation is best for those with type 4 stools, and it deteriorates with both lower and higher BSFS numbers [7]. Furthermore, there are reports that BSFS is related to the composition of the gut microbiota [8].

From the above, BSFS is not only useful for diagnosing and classifying the disease types of bowel disorders of DGBI but also serves as an evaluation method for determining treatment efficacy. However, it should be noted that BSFS is a patient-reported outcome (PRO), inherently including recall bias. Moreover, BSFS is often calculated as integers because it is a numerical rating (ordinate) scale with values ranging from 1 to 7. It should be remembered that the intervals between numbers are defined as integers by researchers.

3 Toward the Scientific Approach in Clinical Practice

Despite the aforementioned limitations, PROs for DGBI can be referenced for diagnosis. Scales that have been validated for reliability and validity can also be used to determine treatment efficacy, particularly for gastrointestinal sensory symptoms such as abdominal pain. The Rome Committee provides internationally applicable modules. For usage, refer to the Rome Committee website [9].

Competing Interests The author(s) has no competing interests to declare that are relevant to the content of this manuscript.

References

1. Enck P, et al. Irritable bowel syndrome (IBS). Nat Rev Dis Primers. 2016;2:16014.
2. Fukudo S, et al. Evidence-based clinical practice guidelines for irritable bowel syndrome 2020. J Gastroenterol. 2021;56:193–217.
3. Fukudo S, et al. Characteristics of disorders of gut-brain interaction in the Japanese population in the Rome Foundation Global Epidemiological Study. Neurogastroenterol Motil. 2023;35:e14581.
4. Lacy BE, et al. Bowel disorders. Gastroenterology. 2016;150:1393–407.
5. Lewis SJ, et al. Stool form scale as a useful guide to intestinal transit time. Scand J Gastroenterol. 1997;32:920–4.
6. Gwee KA, et al. Asian consensus on irritable bowel syndrome. J Gastroenterol Hepatol. 2010;25:1189–205.
7. Ohkubo H, et al. Relationship between stool form and quality of life in patients with chronic constipation: an internet questionnaire survey. Digestion. 2021;102:147–54.
8. Tanabe A, et al. Gut environment and dietary habits in healthy Japanese adults and their association with bowel movement. Digestion. 2020;101:706–16.
9. The Rome Foundation. https://theromefoundation.org.

Diagnosis and Treatment of DGBI of the Small Bowel and Colon, Irritable Bowel Syndrome

44

Shin Fukudo

Abstract

Irritable bowel syndrome (IBS) is a prototype of disorders of gut–brain interaction, which is characterized by chronic abdominal pain associated with bowel movement, changes in stool consistency, and/or changes in frequency of defecation. Subtypes of IBS are identified as IBS with predominant constipation, with predominant diarrhea, with mixed bowel habits, and unclassified. Prevalence of IBS in the general population of the world/Japan is 4.1%/2.2% with dominance in females and younger age. The exact cause of IBS remains unknown. However, research suggests that environmental factors, including acting on individuals with susceptibility genes, lead to the onset of IBS. Pathophysiology of IBS is summarized as brain–gut interactions, which include abnormal stress responses, increased lower gastrointestinal motility, visceral hypersensitivity, and psychological abnormalities, such as anxiety, depression, and somatization. Gut microbiota abnormalities, increased mucosal permeability, and mucosal microinflammation are upstream factors. Diagnosis is based on the Rome IV criteria, which will be updated to the Rome V criteria. Clinical practice guidelines recommend a step-wise approach. The initial step is gut-targeted therapy with behavioral modification, including diet and exercise, probiotics, polycarbophil, and visceral neuromodulators. The second step is neuropharmacological treatment using central neuromodulators. The third step is brain–gut behavioral therapies. Further advancement of the clinical practice of IBS is warranted.

Keywords

Brain–gut interaction · Stress · Mucosal permeability · Gut microbiota · Brain–gut behavioral therapy · Low fermentable oligosaccharides, disaccharides, monosaccharides, and polyols (FODMAP) diet · Neuromodulators · 5-HT$_3$ antagonist · Intestinal secretagogue · Probiotics · Clinical practice guidelines

S. Fukudo (✉)
Department of Behavioral Medicine, Graduate School of Medicine, Research Center for Accelerator and Radioisotope Science, Tohoku University, Sendai, Japan

Japanese Red Cross Ishinomaki Hospital, Ishinomaki, Japan
e-mail: shin.fukudo.c6@tohoku.ac.jp

1 Concept

Irritable bowel syndrome (IBS) is a pathological condition characterized by abdominal pain associated with abnormal bowel habits [1]. These

H. Kaneko et al. (eds.), *Disorders of Gut-Brain Interaction*,
https://doi.org/10.1007/978-981-95-6974-8_44

symptoms are not caused by organic lesions detectable by standard clinical tests. Organic lesions include conditions such as colorectal cancer, inflammatory bowel disease (IBD), collagenous colitis, and colonic diverticulitis. However, high-precision research-level tests beyond standard clinical examinations can detect abnormalities in IBS patients [2]. IBS was the first disease conceptualized as one of the disorders of gut–brain interaction (DGBI).

2 Epidemiology

In Japan, the prevalence of IBS is 2.2% of the population according to the strict diagnostic criteria of Rome IV [3, 4]. Using the more lenient Rome III criteria, the prevalence is 9.8% [4]. The annual incidence rate is 1–2%, and IBS accounts for 31% of gastroenterology outpatient visits [2]. Globally, the prevalence of IBS is 10.1% according to the Rome III criteria, but it is 4.1% according to the Rome IV criteria. Among these, IBS with predominant constipation (IBS-C) accounts for 1.3%, IBS with mixed bowel habits (IBS-M) for 1.3%, IBS with predominant diarrhea (IBS-D) for 1.2%, and IBS unclassified (IBS-U) for 0.3% [4]. The prevalence of IBS is higher in women than in men, with a ratio of 1.8:1 [4]. The prevalence decreases with age [4].

3 Etiology and Pathophysiology

The exact cause of IBS remains unknown. However, research suggests that environmental factors acting on individuals with susceptibility genes lead to the onset of IBS. Polymorphisms in genes such as interleukin (IL)-6, Toll-like receptor (TLR)-9, and E-cadherin (CDH)-1 are mediators of susceptibility when individuals suffer from infectious enterocolitis [4]. Gut microbiota diversity changes under stress, and stress increases mucosal permeability, leading to visceral hypersensitivity [4]. This pathophysiology is summarized as the "brain–gut interactions" [2, 5]. Emphasizing the importance of signals from the gut to the brain, it is sometimes referred to as the gut–brain interaction, although the signaling is bidirectional.

Classically, the pathophysiology of IBS includes abnormal stress responses, increased lower gastrointestinal motility, visceral hypersensitivity, and psychological abnormalities such as anxiety, depression, and somatization [4]. Additionally, risk genes, gut microbiota abnormalities, increased mucosal permeability, and low-grade inflammation of the mucosa are upstream factors (Fig. 44.1) [4].

Psychosocial stressors are factors in the onset and exacerbation of IBS [5]. IBS patients show a higher correlation between stress load and worsening gastrointestinal symptoms compared to healthy individuals. Mediators include neurotransmitters like serotonin and brain–gut peptides such as corticotropin-releasing hormone (CRH) [5]. Brain imaging studies have shown activation of the anterior cingulate cortex, amygdala, and midbrain, and decreased activation of the medial and lateral prefrontal cortex in IBS patients in response to colonic stimulation [5]. Additionally, IBS patients have reduced volumes of the dorsolateral prefrontal cortex, which does not activate sufficiently under stress [6].

Prospective observations of patients with acute infectious enterocolitis show that IBS develops at a rate six to seven times higher than in individuals who did not suffer from infectious enterocolitis. This is known as post-infectious IBS [4]. Numerous reports indicate that the gut microbiota of IBS patients differs from that of healthy individuals [7]. Systematic reviews show a decrease in *Bifidobacterium* and *Faecalibacterium*, and an increase in Lactobacillaceae, *Bacteroides*, and Enterobacteriaceae [8]. Organic acids and other gut microbiota products also affect the IBS pathology [7]. IBS symptoms worsen with food intake [2]. Foods high in carbohydrates or fats, spices, alcohol, and coffee exacerbate symptoms.

Non-specific low-grade inflammation in IBS patients is not to the extent seen in patients with IBDs. In the colonic mucosa of IBS patients, increased mast cells close to enteric neurons are

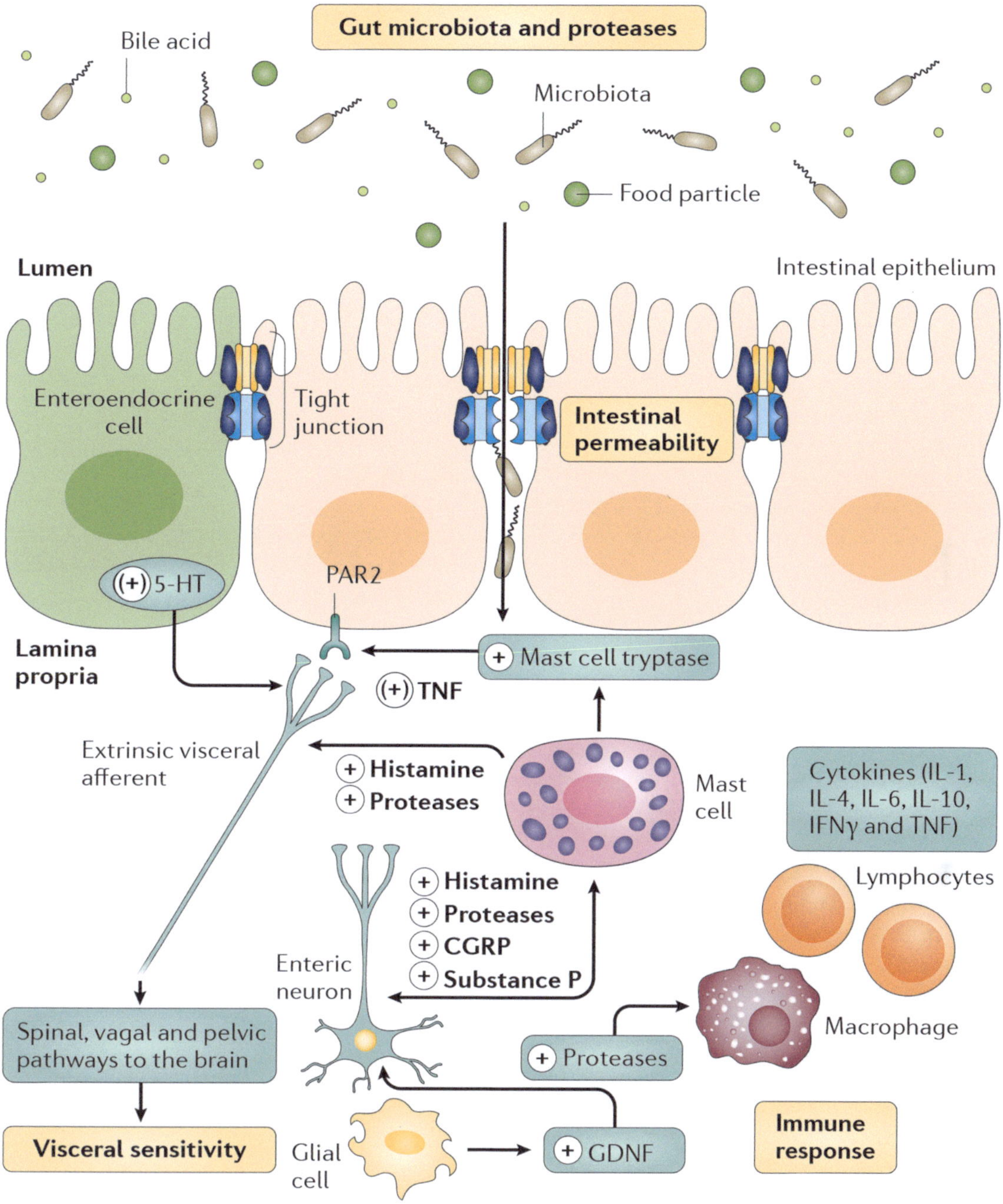

Fig. 44.1 Pathophysiology of IBS from peripheral to central. In the gastrointestinal lumen of IBS patients, gut microbiota interact with food molecules to produce metabolites. Stress, along with bacterial components, increases mucosal permeability, leading to mucosal low-grade inflammation and neural sensitization. Sensitized sensory nerve signals and inflammatory mediators alter the central nervous system. (Reproduced with permission from Ref. [4])

observed [4]. Mucosal permeability is increased in IBS [4]. IBS is considered a polygenic disorder. Analysis of 6060 twin pairs has demonstrated the heritability of IBS [2]. The concordance rate for IBS is 8.4% in dizygotic twins, but it is 17.2% in monozygotic twins. Genetic polymorphisms associated with IBS include serotonin transporter, CRH-R1 receptor, CRH-R2 receptor, CRH-binding protein, IL-10, IL-6, TLR-9, and CDH-1 genes [4]. Mutations in the *SCN5A* gene, which codes for the Na channel Nav1.5, are found in 2.2% (13 cases) of 584 IBS patients [4]. Genome-wide association studies have identified mutations in the tumor necrosis factor *TNFSF15* gene and the KDEL endoplasmic reticulum protein retention receptor 2 (*KDELR2*) and glutamate receptor, ionotropic, delta 2 (Grid2) interacting protein (*GRID2IP*) genes on chromosome 7p22.1 [4].

Table 44.1 Rome IV diagnostic criteria for IBS

Recurrent abdominal pain, on average, at least 1 day per week in the last 3 months, associated with two or more of the following:
1. Related to defecation
2. Associated with a change in the frequency of stool
3. Associated with a change in the form (appearance) of stool
*Criteria should be fulfilled for the last 3 months with symptom onset at least 6 months prior to diagnosis

Referred from Ref. [3]

4 Diagnostic Criteria and Tests

Diagnosis follows the IBS clinical practice guidelines published by the Japanese Society of Gastroenterology [2]. Essentially, it is based on the international diagnostic criteria of Rome IV (Table 44.1) [3]. Additionally, IBS is classified into four subtypes based on the frequency of stool forms according to the Bristol Stool Form Scale (refer to Fig. 44.1 in the Introduction): IBS-C, IBS-D, IBS-M, and IBS-U (Fig. 44.2) [3]. When encountering patients with persistent abdominal pain and abnormal bowel habits over the past 3 months, if all warning symptoms/signs, risk factors, and test findings described below are negative, the condition is a DGBI. IBS is then diagnosed based on the Rome IV criteria (Fig. 44.3) [2]. If the symptom pattern does not meet the Rome IV criteria for IBS, it is another DGBI [1]. There are several DGBI similar to IBS, and these disorders are interrelated and treated with common therapies. Rome IV is currently being revised to Rome V based on accumulated evidence, and switching to Rome V after revision is appropriate according to international medical trends.

Before diagnosing IBS, evaluate the presence of warning symptoms/signs and risk factors, and perform a colonoscopy or barium enema if present [2]. Warning symptoms/signs suggest organic diseases and include unexpected weight loss of more than 3 kg within 6 months, fever, blood and mucus in stools, joint pain, and abnormal physical findings (palpable abdominal mass, fluctuation, blood or palpable mass on rectal examination) [2]. Risk factors include onset or patient age over 50 years, and a history or family history of colorectal organic diseases. If the patient requests a detailed gastrointestinal examination, conduct it according to clinical necessity. Even in the absence of warning symptoms/signs and risk factors, exclude organic diseases through blood biochemical tests, complete blood counts, inflammatory markers, thyroid-stimulating hormone, urinalysis, fecal occult blood tests, and plain abdominal X-rays [2].

Depending on the clinical diversity, upper gastrointestinal endoscopy or upper gastrointestinal barium studies, abdominal ultrasound, abdominal computed tomography, abdominal magnetic resonance imaging, stool bacterial tests, stool ova tests, capsule endoscopy, small bowel imaging, and lactose tolerance tests may be necessary in some cases.

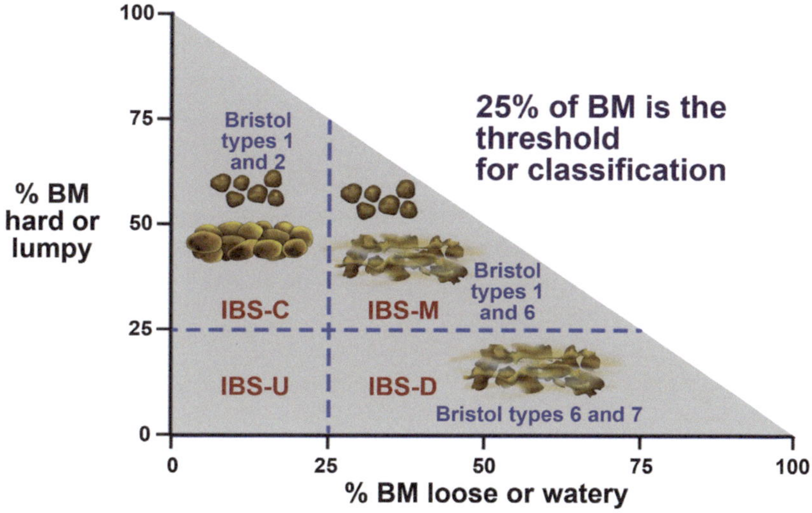

Fig. 44.2 Subtypes of IBS in Rome IV criteria. C with predominant constipation, D with predominant diarrhea, M with mixed bowel habits, U unclassified. (Reproduced with permission from Ref. [3])

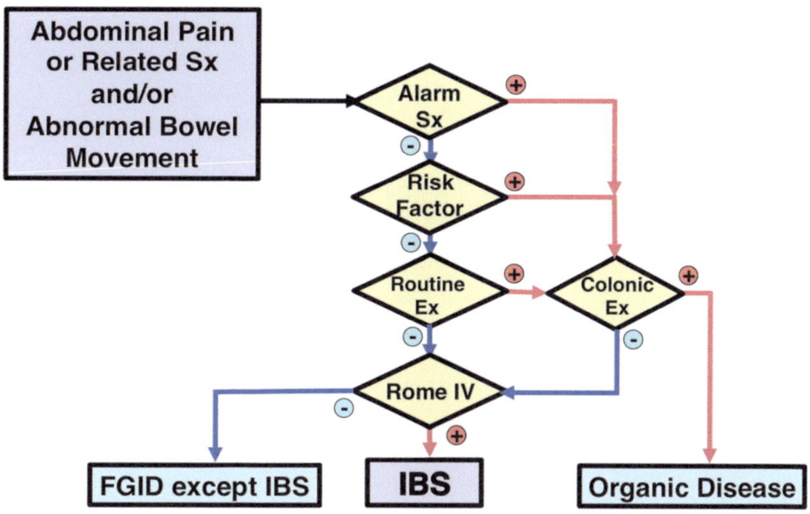

Fig. 44.3 Diagnostic algorithm for IBS. (Reproduced with permission from Ref. [2])

5 Differential Diagnosis and Complications

The critical diseases to be differentiated and excluded include gastrointestinal cancers, such as colorectal cancer, and IBD [2]. Other conditions to consider include collagenous colitis, lactose intolerance, chronic idiopathic pseudo-obstruction, and colonic inertia. Bile acid diarrhea, while potentially part of the pathophysiology of IBS-D, is increasingly recognized as a distinct disease group [9]. Systemic diseases, including thyroid disorders, also require early differentiation. Conditions frequently comorbid with IBS include functional dyspepsia (FD), gastroesophageal reflux disease, functional anorectal pain, overactive bladder, fibromyalgia, temporomandibular joint disorder, migraine, depression, and anxiety [2].

6 Treatment

Treatment follows the clinical practice guidelines for IBS published by the Japanese Society of Gastroenterology [2]. Initially, assess the patient's lifestyle and encourage improvements if IBS exacerbating factors are identified. Risk factors for gastrointestinal symptoms of IBS include an unbalanced diet, irregular meal times, lack of sleep, and psychosocial stress. Exercise therapy is also effective. Dietary therapy involves transitioning from a low-residue diet to a high-fiber diet and avoiding spices, alcohol, and specific foods that significantly exacerbate symptoms. The low FODMAP diet, which restricts fermentable oligosaccharides, disaccharides, monosaccharides, and polyols, is gaining attention as a dietary therapy for IBS [2, 4].

Initial pharmacotherapy for IBS involves medications that regulate gastrointestinal function, such as trimebutine and polycarbophil (Fig. 44.4) [2]. Probiotics are also noted for their potential to mitigate low-grade inflammation in IBS. *Bifidobacterium*, for example, normalizes the decreased anti-inflammatory/inflammatory cytokine (IL-10/12) ratio in IBS.

Pharmacotherapy tailored to IBS subtypes is efficient. For IBS-D, the 5-HT3 receptor antagonist ramosetron is indicated [10]. For IBS-C, the secretagogue (epithelial function modulator) and guanylate cyclase-C agonist linaclotide is used [11]. Linaclotide increases cyclic guanosine monophosphate in mucosal epithelial cells, which opens the cystic fibrosis transmembrane conductance regulator chloride channel, leading to Cl^- ion secretion and water secretion, and suppresses visceral hypersensitivity. Similar drugs approved for chronic constipation include the secretagogue and Cl^- channel-2 activator lubiprostone [12] and the ileal bile acid transporter inhibitor elobixibat [2]. Globally, drug development for chronic constipation, including IBS, continues, with reports on the efficacy of sodium-glucose cotransporter 1 inhibitors [13].

If abdominal pain persists with monotherapy, anticholinergics, magnesium oxide, or picosulfate for constipation, and loperamide for diarrhea are used [2]. For IBS-C with comorbid FD, serotonin 5-HT4 receptor agonist mosapride, dopamine D2 receptor antagonist and cholinesterase inhibitor itopride, and cholinesterase inhibitor acotiamide can be used [2].

When gut-targeted treatments are ineffective, antidepressants or azapirone (non-benzodiazepine) anxiolytics may be used with caution (Fig. 44.5) [2]. Brain–gut behavioral therapies, including autogenic training, hypnosis, and cognitive-behavioral therapy, have been scientifically proven to be effective for patients with refractory IBS (Fig. 44.6) [2].

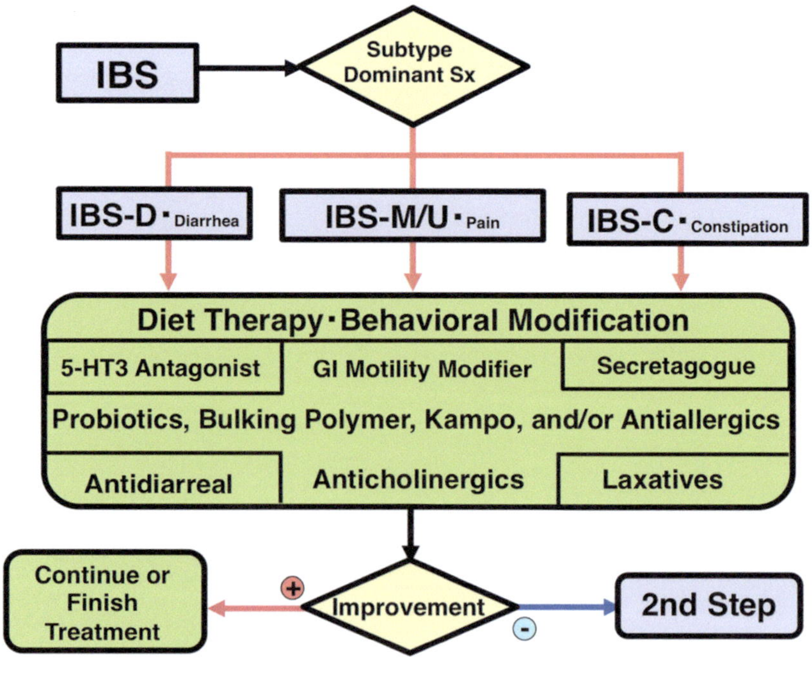

Fig. 44.4 The first-step treatment in guidelines for IBS. (Reproduced with permission from Ref. [2])

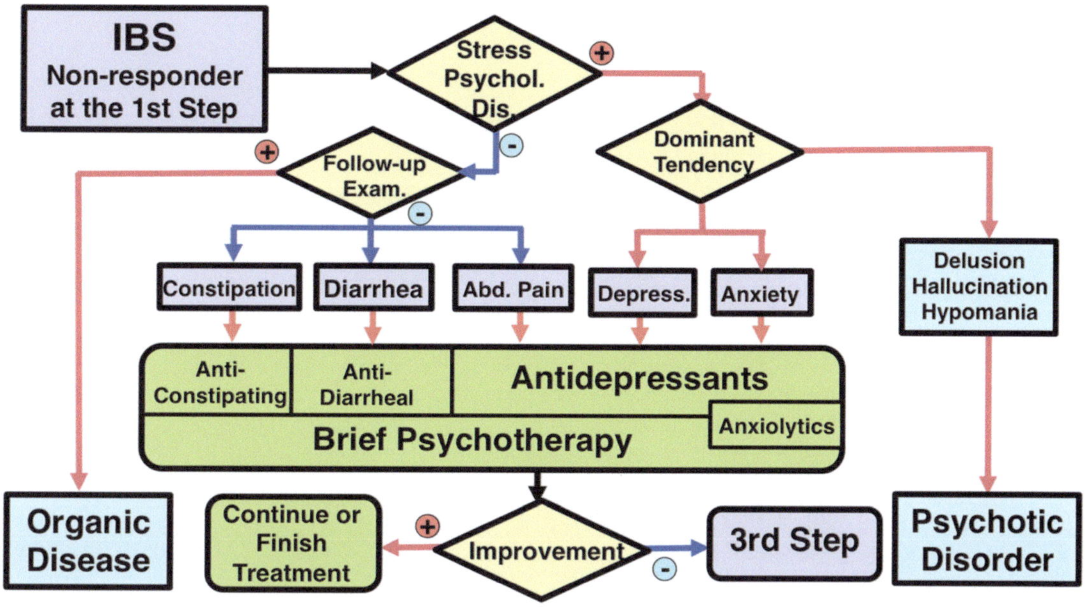

Fig. 44.5 The second-step treatment in guidelines for IBS. (Reproduced with permission from Ref. [2])

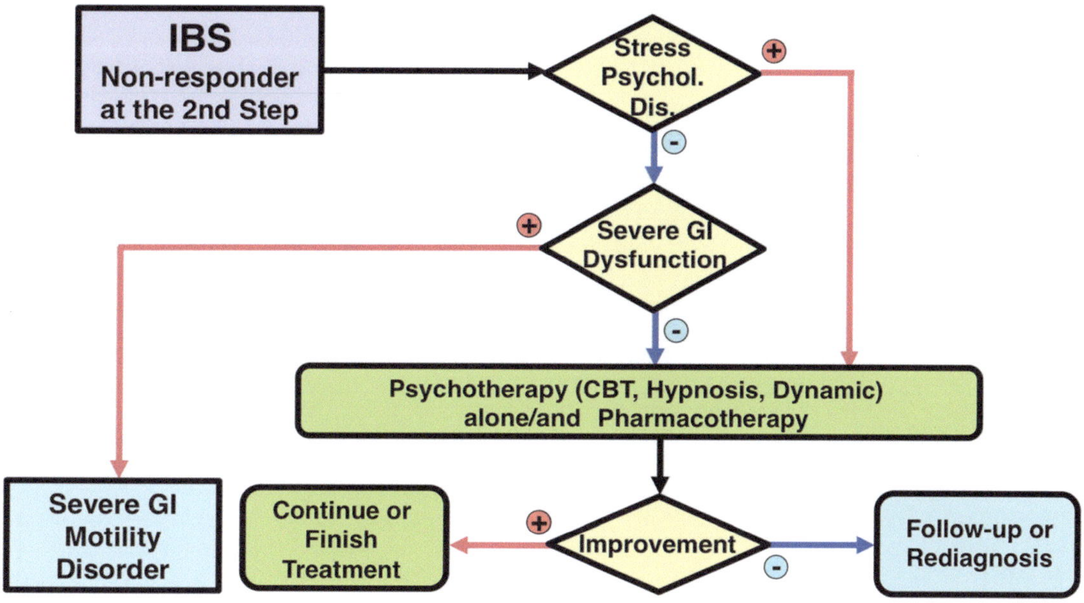

Fig. 44.6 The third-step treatment in guidelines for IBS. (Reproduced with permission from Ref. [2])

7 Prognosis

The quality of life of IBS patients is reduced [2, 4]. IBS patients frequently exhibit habitual absenteeism, disease behavior such as frequent calls to physicians, and psychological abnormalities correlated with IBS severity [2]. In the U.S. managed care population, direct costs for IBS patients are approximately 50% higher than for non-IBS individuals. The rate of cholecystectomy in IBS patients is three times higher than in non-IBS patients, appendectomy and hysterectomy are twice as high, and the incidence of back surgery is 1.5 times higher [2]. IBS has a high comorbidity rate with anxiety and depression, necessitating appropriate treatment before severe progression [2, 14]. Pediatric IBS or recurrent abdominal pain often transitions to adult IBS. Epidemiological studies suggest IBS as a risk factor for Parkinson's disease and dementia [2].

8 Conclusion

IBS patients often seek complete symptom resolution, but the treatment goal should be self-management of daily life. Physicians should explain the pathophysiology of IBS in understandable terms and diagrams, discuss lifestyle and stressors with acceptance and empathy, and suggest feasible stress-relief methods.

Take-Home Message
A frequent issue in IBS management is differentiating and overlapping with organic diseases. In Western countries, performing colonoscopy, abdominal CT, and capsule endoscopy for all IBS cases is considered excessive. Mild elevations in blood highly sensitive C-reactive protein (HS-CRP) or fecal calprotectin are observed in some IBS patients. Rationally, clinical tests should be conducted when warning factors or findings exceeding IBS are present. Diseases to be differentiated include bile acid diarrhea (malabsorption), symptomatic uncomplicated diverticular disease, food allergies, eosinophilic gastroenteritis, collagenous colitis, lymphocytic colitis, abdominal migraine, and abdominal epilepsy. However, the concept of comorbidities like IBD-IBS may become more prevalent in the future.

Competing Interests The author has no competing interests to declare that are relevant to the content of this chapter.

References

1. Drossman DA, Rome IV. Functional GI disorders: disorders of gut-brain interaction. Gastroenterology. 2016;150:1257–61.
2. Fukudo S, et al. Evidence-based clinical practice guidelines for irritable bowel syndrome 2020. J Gastroenterol. 2021;56:193–217.
3. Lacy BE, et al. Bowel disorders. Gastroenterology. 2016;150:1393–407.
4. Enck P, et al. Irritable bowel syndrome (IBS). Nat Rev Dis Primers. 2016;2:16014.
5. Fukudo S. IBS: autonomic dysregulation in IBS. Nat Rev Gastroenterol Hepatol. 2013;10:569–71.
6. Aizawa E, et al. Altered cognitive function of prefrontal cortex during error feedback in patients with irritable bowel syndrome, based on fMRI and dynamic causal modeling. Gastroenterology. 2012;143:1188–98.
7. Tana C, et al. Altered profiles of intestinal microbiota and organic acids may be the origin of symptoms in irritable bowel syndrome. Neurogastroenterol Motil. 2010;22:512–9.
8. Pittayanon R, et al. Gut microbiota in patients with irritable bowel syndrome: a systematic review. Gastroenterology. 2019;157:97–108.
9. Camilleri M, et al. Comparison of biochemical, microbial and mucosal mRNA expression in bile acid diarrhoea and irritable bowel syndrome with diarrhoea. Gut. 2023;72:54–65.
10. Fukudo S, et al. Ramosetron reduces symptoms of irritable bowel syndrome with diarrhea and improves quality of life in women. Gastroenterology. 2016;150:358–66.
11. Fukudo S, et al. A randomized controlled and long-term linaclotide study of irritable bowel syndrome with constipation patients in Japan. Neurogastroenterol Motil. 2018;30:e13444.
12. Fukudo S, et al. Lubiprostone increases spontaneous bowel movement frequency and quality of life in patients with chronic idiopathic constipation. Clin Gastroenterol Hepatol. 2015;13:294–301.
13. Fukudo S, et al. Safety and efficacy of the sodium-glucose cotransporter 1 inhibitor mizagliflozin for functional constipation: a randomised, placebo-controlled, double-blind phase 2 trial. Lancet Gastroenterol Hepatol. 2018;3:603–13.
14. Barbara G, et al. Rome Foundation Working Team Report on overlap in disorders of gut-brain interaction. Nat Rev Gastroenterol Hepatol. 2025;22:228–51.

45 Diagnosis and Treatment of DGBI of the Small Bowel and Colon, Functional Constipation

Motoyori Kanazawa and Shin Fukudo

Abstract

Chronic constipation may require careful examination and treatment. The significance of managing functional constipation lies in first differentiating secondary chronic constipation, including drug-induced constipation, and then aiming to improve the quality of life. Additionally, it is crucial to avoid cardiovascular risk factors. Utilizing treatment methods based on clinical practice guidelines is beneficial for treating patients with functional constipation. Initial treatment for chronic constipation involves dietary, exercise, and defecation environment adjustments. As pharmacotherapy for chronic constipation, osmotic laxatives (e.g., magnesium oxide), stimulant laxatives (e.g., senna), epithelial function modifiers (e.g., lubiprostone and linaclotide), ileal bile acid transporter inhibitors (e.g., elobixibat), and some kinds of Kampo medicine are currently available in Japan. Healthcare providers should carefully evaluate the potential pathologies underlying the constipation symptoms and select appropriate treatments.

M. Kanazawa (✉) · S. Fukudo
Department of Behavioral Medicine, Tohoku University Graduate School of Medicine, Sendai, Japan
e-mail: motoyori.kanazawa.d4@tohoku.ac.jp

Keywords

Functional constipation · Pathophysiology · Assessment · Diagnosis · Treatment · Quality of life (QOL)

1 Introduction

Defecation habits vary among individuals, and the term "constipation" can mean various symptoms related to bowel movement for each patient. Medically, constipation is defined as "a condition in which stool that should normally be excreted from the body cannot be expelled in sufficient quantity and comfortably" [1]. Additionally, "constipation" as a disease refers to cases where symptoms are due to abnormal bowel movement and require examination and treatment. These symptoms include those related to decreased defecation frequency (e.g., abdominal pain and abdominal bloating), hard stools (e.g., difficult defecation and excessive straining), and defecation disorders (e.g., difficulty defecating even with soft stools, excessive straining, sensation of incomplete evacuation, and frequent defecation due to this sensation) [1].

Constipation symptoms, which include decreased defecation frequency, hard stools, and defecation disorders, are diverse. Various problems related to defecation lead to a decreased quality of life (QOL) for patients complaining of

H. Kaneko et al. (eds.), *Disorders of Gut-Brain Interaction*,
https://doi.org/10.1007/978-981-95-6974-8_45

constipation symptoms [2]. This chapter provides an overview of the key points in the diagnosis and treatment of chronic constipation, particularly functional constipation.

2 Pathophysiology Classification of Chronic Constipation

When considering treatment strategies for constipation symptoms that can affect daily life, it is necessary to classify chronic constipation based on etiology and pathophysiology. Chronic constipation can be broadly divided into primary (idiopathic) constipation and secondary constipation caused by organic abnormalities in the colon and anus (e.g., colorectal cancer, inflammatory bowel disease, and rectocele: organic), underlying other diseases (symptomatic), or pharmacotherapy (drug-induced) [1, 3].

Underlying other diseases causing secondary constipation include endocrine and metabolic disorders such as diabetes, hypothyroidism, and chronic kidney disease; neurological disorders such as cerebrovascular disease, Parkinson's disease, and spinal cord injury; collagen diseases such as progressive sclerosis (scleroderma); degenerative diseases such as amyloidosis; and psychiatric disorders such as depression. Severe intestinal motility disorders, such as chronic pseudo-obstruction, megacolon, and Hirschsprung's disease, also present with significant gastrointestinal motility dysfunction, leading to severe constipation symptoms.

Many drugs can cause chronic constipation, particularly anticholinergic drugs, including anti-Parkinsonian drugs, opioids (narcotics), and psychotropic drugs [1].

Understanding the functional pathology involves focusing on colonic transit time and anorectal evacuation function. Primary chronic constipation, where the cause is not identified, is classified into "slow transit constipation," "normal transit constipation," and "defecation disorders" based on the presence or absence of delayed colonic transit and abnormal defecation (Fig. 45.1) [3]. It is important to note that some

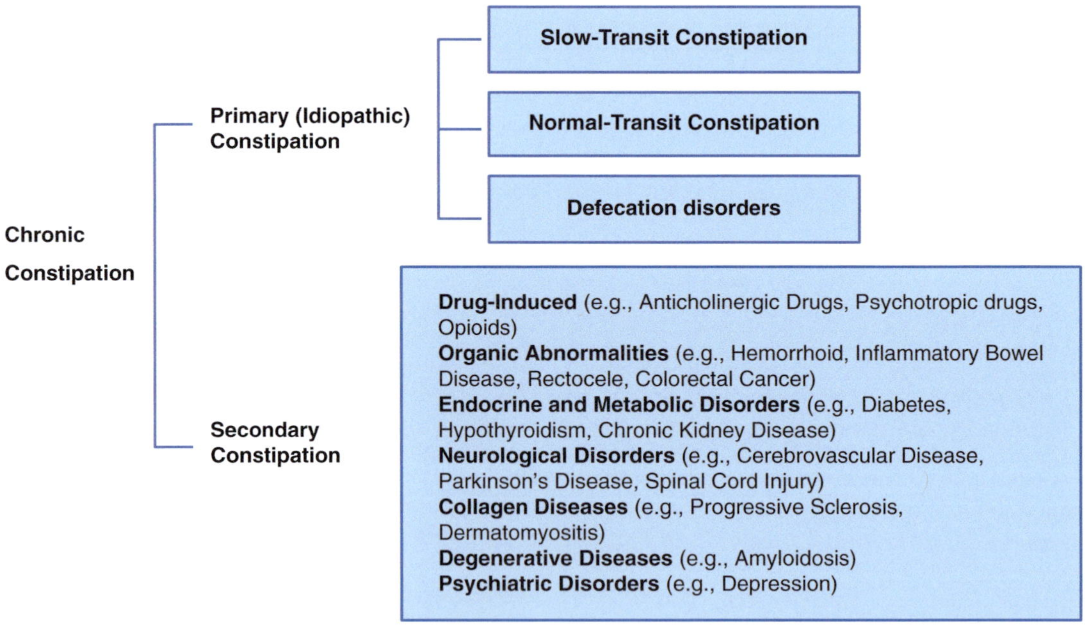

Fig. 45.1 Classification of chronic constipation [3]. Primary chronic constipation is broadly classified into slow transit constipation, normal transit constipation, and defecatory disorders. On the other hand, secondary constipation can be caused not only by drug-induced factors and organic diseases of the colon but also by underlying other conditions such as endocrine and metabolic disorders, neurological disorders, collagen diseases, degenerative diseases, and psychiatric disorders

patients may have combined pathologies of delayed colonic transit and abnormal defecation. Treatment selection based on these major pathologies is required in management for chronic constipation.

3 Colorectal and Anorectal Function Tests

Colorectal and anorectal function tests related to the pathophysiology of chronic constipation can evaluate colonic transit time and anorectal evacuation function [1]. Objective measurement tests for colonic transit time include tracking of radiopaque markers, scintigraphy with the use of radioisotopes, and tracking of the movement of a wireless motility capsule. Objective anorectal function tests include defecography, anal electromyography, anorectal manometry, and the rectal balloon expulsion test.

Even if these specialized function tests are difficult to perform, detailed medical history taking, physical findings, and clinical laboratory tests can help understand the potential abnormal colorectal or anorectal function in patients complaining of constipation in clinical practice.

4 Evaluation of Colorectal and Anorectal Function in Clinical Practice

Few medical facilities have a sufficient gastrointestinal function testing system, and non-insurance-covered tests are often limited to research purposes with ethics committee approval. Therefore, it is not easy to use various gastrointestinal function tests to evaluate the pathophysiology of chronic constipation in general clinical practice. However, detailed medical history taking, physical findings, and simple abdominal X-ray imaging can provide sufficient clues to infer each patient's problem.

4.1 Bristol Stool Form Scale

The colon plays an important role in regulating intestinal fluid and electrolytes, reabsorbing 1–2 L of water daily. The longer the stool stays in the colon, the lower the water content in the stool. It has been confirmed that the shape of the stool reflects colonic transit time [4]. Using the Bristol Stool Form Scale (see Chap. 43, Fig. 43.1), the specific hardness of the stool is obtained from the patient. Previous research has shown an inverse correlation between the average stool form score and total gastrointestinal or colonic transit time, with harder stools (lower score types) associated with delayed colonic transit time. On the other hand, while defecation frequency decreases with delayed gastrointestinal transit time, no significant correlation was found between colonic transit time and defecation frequency in chronic constipation patients [5].

4.2 Physical Findings

Palpation of the abdomen may reveal an enlarged colon, suggesting not only organic diseases such as colorectal tumors but also gas or stool retention. Digital rectal examination can differentiate organic diseases such as rectal prolapse, rectocele, and rectal cancer, which can cause defecation disorders, and estimate changes in anal pressure during straining or voluntary anal contraction [6]. If the anus does not relax properly or contracts paradoxically (paradoxical contraction) during straining, defecation disorders are suspected.

4.3 Simple Abdominal X-ray Imaging

Simple abdominal X-ray imaging can help differentiate organic diseases and estimate gastrointestinal function. It has been shown that the more gas retained in the intestines, the more likely patients are to complain of subjective abdominal bloating [7]. However, it should be noted that gastrointestinal hypersensitivity is also related to abdominal bloating, and not all patients with functional gastrointestinal disorders complaining of abdominal bloating have gas retention in the colon. Additionally, it has been reported that the amount of gas in the intestines does not necessarily correlate with gastrointestinal transit time [7].

5 Diagnosis of Functional Constipation

When it is necessary to strictly define chronic constipation for research purposes, the internationally widely used Rome diagnostic criteria are used to diagnose "functional constipation." The Rome IV diagnostic criteria were created as the revised fourth edition in 2016 [8]. According to these criteria, constipation is defined as having fewer than three spontaneous bowel movements per week, straining due to difficult defecation, hard or lumpy stools, sensation of incomplete evacuation, sensation of anorectal obstruction, or manual maneuvers to facilitate defecation, with at least two of these symptoms present for more than one-fourth of defecations (Table 45.1) [8]. Chronicity is defined as symptoms appearing at least 6 months before diagnosis and persisting for the past 3 months. However, in daily clinical practice, the definition of "chronic" is not necessarily limited to the above period and is respected by the physician examining the patient.

The Rome IV diagnostic criteria exclude irritable bowel syndrome (IBS), which has abdominal pain as the main symptom, from functional constipation [8]. However, in actual clinical practice, it is reasonable to treat IBS (especially constipation-predominant IBS) with common pathologies as "chronic constipation" without strictly distinguishing it from functional constipation.

Epidemiological surveys of various disorders of gut–brain interaction (DGBI) have been conducted worldwide based on the Rome IV diagnostic criteria. As a result, the prevalence of functional constipation was 11.7%, and IBS was 4.1% among 54,127 adults worldwide [9]. In a survey of 2,504 cases in Japan, the prevalence of functional constipation was 16.6%, and IBS was 2.2% [9]. Therefore, even considering the survey results using strict diagnostic criteria for functional constipation, the prevalence of chronic constipation in Japan is very high.

Table 45.1 Diagnostic criteria for functional constipation[a] (Rome IV)

1. Must include two or more of the following:[b]
(a) Straining during more than 25% of defecations
(b) Lumpy or hard stools in more than 25% of defecations
(c) Sensation of incomplete evacuation in more than 25% of defecations
(d) Sensation of anorectal obstruction/blockage in more than 25% of defecations
(e) Manual maneuvers to facilitate more than 25% of defecations (e.g., digital evacuation and support of the pelvic floor)
(f) Fewer than three spontaneous bowel movements per week
2. Loose stools are rarely present without the use of laxatives
3. Insufficient criteria for IBS

Adapted from Ref. [8]

[a]Criteria fulfilled for the last 3 months with symptom onset at least 6 months prior to diagnosis

[b]For research studies, patients meeting criteria for opioid-induced constipation should not be given a diagnosis of functional constipation because it is difficult to distinguish between opioid side effects and other causes of constipation. However, clinicians recognize that these two conditions may overlap

6 Significance of Constipation Management

Chronic constipation, particularly functional constipation, is classified as one of DGBI according to the Rome diagnostic criteria. Traditionally, DGBI have been understood as conditions that significantly reduce QOL but do not affect life expectancy. However, recent epidemiological studies have revealed that chronic constipation patients have poorer life expectancy outcomes.

A 15-year follow-up study comparing constipation patients with non-constipation patients showed that constipation patients had significantly worse life expectancy outcomes [10]. Various reasons can be considered for this, one of which is the increased risk of cardiovascular events due to excessive circulatory system load from straining during defecation. Epidemiological studies in Japan have also reported a significant increase in cardiovascular events as defecation frequency decreases [11]. Therefore, when controlling blood pressure in constipation patients, it is important to be aware that defecation events may trigger cardiovascular events as well as heat shock.

Furthermore, in elderly individuals, the decline in gastrointestinal physiological function due to aging increases the frequency of constipation symptoms. These constipation symptoms can lead to decreased food intake, causing nutritional disorders, sarcopenia, and frailty. These conditions can further exacerbate constipation symptoms, creating a vicious cycle.

Given these facts, constipation management is considered very important not only for patients whose QOL is reduced due to symptoms but also for elderly patients and those with cardiovascular risk factors.

7 Treatment of Functional Constipation

Based on clinical practice guidelines, the following describes commonly used treatments for chronic constipation, including functional constipation, in daily practice [1]. Note that explanations of surgical treatments or specialized treatments such as biofeedback therapy are deferred to other chapters.

7.1 Lifestyle Guidance

Initial treatment for chronic constipation involves dietary, exercise, and defecation environment adjustments. In elderly patients and some others, dietary fiber intake and fluid intake may be low, which can reduce stool volume and affect stool hardness. Aerobic exercise and stretching have been shown to improve constipation. Further guidance includes going to the toilet at a set time or when feeling the urge to defecate without holding back, and adopting a forward-leaning posture during defecation. Elderly patients often have diminished rectal sensation [12], making it difficult to feel the urge to defecate even when the rectum is filled with stool. Therefore, it is crucial to attempt defecation at set times, such as after breakfast or immediately when feeling the urge. The ideal defecation posture is squatting, as in Japanese-style toilets, but in Western-style toilets, leaning forward and contracting the abdominal muscles can facilitate defecation. Additionally, repeated straining due to incomplete defecation can increase the risk of cardiovascular events due to elevated blood pressure. In elderly patients or those with cardiovascular risk factors who frequently strain due to defecation difficulties, appropriate pharmacotherapy should be promptly administered.

7.2 Pharmacotherapy

Until about a decade ago, the main pharmacotherapy for chronic constipation in Japanese medical institutions involved magnesium oxide and anthraquinone stimulant laxatives. In other words, due to the limited types of constipation treatment drugs available at that time, patient satisfaction with treatment and medication compliance were not necessarily sufficient.

However, since the release of the new constipation treatment drug, lubiprostone, in Japan in 2012, several new constipation treatment drugs have been launched. Consequently, the range of drug options available in Japanese clinical practice has expanded.

Furthermore, in 2017, the Japanese Society of Gastroenterology's Chronic Constipation Diagnosis and Treatment Research Group created clinical practice guidelines for chronic constipation tailored to the current situation in Japan. These guidelines indicate the strength of recommendations and evidence levels for each constipation treatment method [1]. Below are representative constipation treatment drugs:

7.2.1 Osmotic Laxatives (Strong Recommendation, High-Quality Evidence)

Osmotic laxatives can be broadly divided into saline laxatives, sugar laxatives, infiltrative laxatives, and high-molecular compounds. These laxatives utilize osmotic gradients to induce water secretion in the intestines, softening stools and increasing defecation frequency.

Magnesium oxide, a commonly used saline laxative in Japan, reacts with gastric acid to form magnesium chloride ($MgCl_2$), which then becomes magnesium bicarbonate [$Mg(HCO_3)_2$] or magnesium carbonate ($MgCO_3$) in the intestines, drawing water from the intestinal wall through osmotic pressure and softening intestinal contents.

Sugar laxatives exert their effects through the osmotic properties of non-absorbable monosaccharides and disaccharides, such as lactulose, mannitol, and sorbitol.

Infiltrative laxative dioctyl sodium sulfosuccinate reduces stool surface tension through surfactant action, allowing water to penetrate and soften the stool.

Polyethylene glycol, a high-molecular compound with a polymerized ethylene glycol structure, is available in Japan with added electrolytes such as sodium chloride to maintain electrolyte balance in the intestines.

7.2.2 Stimulant Laxatives (Weak Recommendation, Moderate-Quality Evidence)

Stimulant laxatives include anthraquinone derivatives (senna, sennosides, and rhubarb) and diphenyl derivatives (bisacodyl and sodium picosulfate). Both are inactive glycosides when ingested but are hydrolyzed by intestinal bacteria or gastrointestinal enzymes into active forms, acting on the myenteric plexus of the colon to promote peristalsis and inhibit water absorption from the intestines, exerting a laxative effect.

Stimulant laxatives show effects within hours of ingestion but can cause electrolyte abnormalities, abdominal pain, and dehydration, leading to watery diarrhea. Long-term use can lead to tolerance and dependence, so they should be prescribed sparingly, preferably for short-term or as-needed use.

7.2.3 Epithelial Function Modifiers (Strong Recommendation, High-Quality Evidence)

Lubiprostone, a prostaglandin derivative, activates ClC-2 chloride channels on the luminal side of the small intestine, promoting osmotic water secretion into the intestines, softening stools, enhancing stool transport, and facilitating defecation. This drug is contraindicated in pregnant women, and attention should be paid to the nausea side effects, which are common in young women.

Linaclotide is a guanylate cyclase-C receptor agonist on intestinal epithelial cells. Activation of this receptor increases intracellular cyclic guanosine monophosphate (cGMP) levels, leading to activation and opening of cystic fibrosis transmembrane conductance regulator chloride channels. This action promotes chloride ion secretion into the gastrointestinal lumen, along with water secretion, exerting a laxative effect. Additionally, cGMP is secreted from the basal side of epithelial cells, inhibiting visceral sensory nerves in the gastrointestinal mucosa, improving visceral hypersensitivity.

7.2.4 Ileal Bile Acid Transporter Inhibitors (Not Included in 2017 Clinical Practice Guidelines)

Elobixibat, launched in Japan in 2018, inhibits bile acid transporters at the terminal ileum, partially suppressing bile acid reabsorption, increasing bile acid levels in the intestines. As a result, bile acids promote water secretion and peristalsis in the intestines, increasing defecation frequency and improving stool form.

7.2.5 Kampo Medicine (Weak Recommendation, Low-Quality Evidence)

Kampo medicine is composed of combinations of multiple herbal medicines, with effects varying based on the included herbs and their proportions. Herbal medicines with intestinal motility-enhancing effects include rhubarb and zanthoxylum. Rhubarb contains sennosides, so its side effects should be considered similar to stimulant laxatives.

7.2.6 Other Pharmacotherapies

Other pharmacotherapies include probiotics, prokinetics, enemas, suppositories, manual disimpaction, and retrograde colonic irrigation. Although high-quality evidence is not sufficiently reported for these treatments, they are confirmed to be useful for constipation symptoms and should be appropriately implemented. However, caution should be exercised to avoid repeated use of enemas and suppositories due to the risk of rectal perforation or habituation.

8 Conclusion

The goal of treating functional constipation is to achieve and maintain a satisfactory state of spontaneous defecation (without a sensation of incomplete evacuation) and improve QOL [13]. If sufficient treatment does not improve defecation abnormalities or associated symptoms, reconsideration of the differential diagnosis and consultation with a specialist for objective evaluation of colorectal and anorectal function should be considered. Healthcare providers should carefully evaluate the potential pathologies underlying the constipation symptoms reported by patients and select appropriate treatments without dismissing the symptoms.

Take-Home Message

The significance of managing functional constipation lies in first differentiating secondary chronic constipation, including drug-induced constipation, and then aiming to improve the QOL of patients who feel distressed by defecation-related symptoms. Additionally, it is crucial to avoid cardiovascular risk factors. Utilizing treatment methods based on clinical practice guidelines is beneficial for treating patients with functional constipation.

Competing Interests The authors have no competing interests to declare that are relevant to the content of this manuscript.

References

1. Japanese Society of Gastroenterology Chronic Constipation Diagnosis and Treatment Research Group, editor. Chronic constipation clinical practice guidelines 2017. Nankodo; 2017. (in Japanese).
2. Belsey J, et al. Systematic review: impact of constipation on quality of life in adults and children. Aliment Pharmacol Ther. 2010;31:938–49.
3. Lembo A, et al. Chronic constipation. N Engl J Med. 2003;349:1360–8.
4. Lewis SJ, et al. Stool form scale as a useful guide to intestinal transit time. Scand J Gastroenterol. 1997;32:920–4.
5. van der Sijp JR, et al. Radioisotope determination of regional colonic transit in severe constipation: comparison with radio opaque markers. Gut. 1993;34:402–8.
6. Bremmer S, et al. Simultaneous defecography and perioneography in defecation disorders. Dis Colon Rectum. 1995;38:969–73.
7. Reiner CS, et al. MR defecography in patients with dyssynergic defecation: spectrum of imaging findings and diagnostic value. Br J Radiol. 2011;84:136–44.
8. Lacy BE, et al. Bowel disorders. Gastroenterology. 2016;150:1393–407.
9. Sperber AD, et al. Worldwide prevalence and burden of functional gastrointestinal disorders, results of Rome Foundation global study. Gastroenterology. 2021;160:99–114.
10. Sumida K, et al. Constipation and risk of death and cardiovascular events. Atherosclerosis. 2019;281:114–20.
11. Honkura K, et al. Defecation frequency and cardiovascular disease mortality in Japan: the Ohsaki cohort study. Atherosclerosis. 2016;246:251–6.
12. Lagier E, et al. Influence of age on rectal tone and sensitivity to distension in healthy subjects. Neurogastroenterol Motil. 1999;11:101–7.
13. Tack J, et al. Association between health-related quality of life and symptoms in patients with chronic constipation: an integrated analysis of three phase 3 trials of prucalopride. Neurogastroenterol Motil. 2015;27:397–405.

Diagnosis and Treatment of DGBI of the Small Bowel and Colon, Functional Diarrhea

46

Ken Sato

Abstract

Functional diarrhea (FDr) is one of Disorders of gut-brain interaction (DGBI) characterized by recurrent loose or watery stools without predominant abdominal pain or bloating. It is distinct from Irritable bowel syndrome with diarrhea (IBS-D), which includes abdominal pain as a key diagnostic criterion. FDr is diagnosed using the Rome IV criteria, requiring symptoms for at least six months and excluding IBS-D. Epidemiological studies report prevalence rates ranging from 1.5% to 17%, but research on its pathophysiology remains limited. Potential mechanisms include gut-brain axis dysfunction, bile acid levels, and psychosocial factors, though these are less pronounced compared to IBS-D.

Differential diagnosis is essential to exclude conditions such as infections, inflammatory bowel disease, celiac disease, food intolerances, and bile acid malabsorption. Diagnostic tools include stool tests, endoscopy, and biochemical evaluations. Treatment options are limited and often align with IBS-D management strategies, including dietary modifications like a low-FODMAP diet, probiotics, Loperamide, and Ramosetron. Antibiotics such as Rifaximin may also be effective.

Given the overlap in symptoms between FDr and IBS-D, treatments for IBS-D may be applicable to FDr. However, further research is needed to better understand its pathophysiology and develop targeted therapies. Comprehensive differential diagnosis remains essential for accurate identification and management.

Keywords

Functional diarrhea · FDr · IBS-D · Rome IV · Chronic diarrhea · A low-FODMAP diet · Ramosetron · Loperamide

1 Concept

Functional diarrhea (FDr) is one of the disorders of gut–brain interaction (DGBI) in the lower gastrointestinal tract, characterized by recurrent episodes of loose and watery stools. Although the symptoms are similar to those of irritable bowel syndrome with predominant diarrhea (IBS-D), the diagnostic criteria for IBS include recurrent abdominal pain associated with abnormal bowel movements. In contrast, FDr is primarily characterized by recurrent diarrhea, without abdominal pain and abdominal bloating. Even if they are

K. Sato (✉)
Hirosaki University, Health Service Center/Graduate School of Gastroenterology, Hematology and Clinical Immunology, Hirosaki, Japan
e-mail: kenjirou@hirosaki-u.ac.jp

H. Kaneko et al. (eds.), *Disorders of Gut-Brain Interaction*,
https://doi.org/10.1007/978-981-95-6974-8_46

present, they will be mild. Given that diarrhea is a symptom observed in many gastrointestinal diseases, differential diagnosis is essential to exclude malignant diseases, inflammatory bowel disease, infections, pancreatic dysfunction, microscopic colitis, food-related conditions, malabsorption, and other disorders.

2 Epidemiology

Epidemiological studies on FDr are limited. However, a study conducted on randomly selected subjects from the general population in five cities in China reported a prevalence of 1.54% [1]. Other studies have reported varying prevalence rates, ranging from 1.5% to approximately 17% [2–5].

3 Pathophysiology and Disease Characteristics

Research on the pathophysiology of FDr is sparse. Similar to other DGBI, it is unlikely that a single etiology or pathophysiological mechanism is responsible for the onset of FDr; rather, multiple factors are presumed to be involved. In IBS, pathophysiological mechanisms include gastrointestinal motility disorders, visceral hypersensitivity, psychological abnormalities, preceding infectious gastroenteritis, genetic factors, gut microbiota alterations, increased mucosal permeability, and microscopic inflammation. The interaction of these factors, known as the "gut–brain axis," is crucial in the pathophysiology of IBS and is also suggested to be relevant in FDr [6]. A study comparing 100 patients with FDr and IBS-D found no significant difference in the frequency of diarrhea between the two groups. However, patients with IBS-D experienced more discomfort related to urgency and more severe abdominal pain, while there was no significant difference in anxiety, depression, or sleep disturbances between the two groups [7]. In another study, patients with IBS, FDr, and functional constipation (FC) were compared using the Hospital Anxiety and Depression Scale (HADS), the Patient Health Questionnaire (PHQ-12), and physical symptoms such as abdominal pain. The results showed that IBS patients had significantly higher scores on the HADS and PHQ-12, as well as higher levels of depression, anxiety, and somatization compared to FDr/FC patients. Additionally, IBS patients reported more frequent abdominal pain and somatic symptoms [8], suggesting a stronger involvement of psychosocial factors in IBS compared to FDr. There was no significant difference in psychosocial factors between the FDr and FC groups.

Early-life traumatic experiences, such as those in childhood, have been reported to be associated with the pathophysiology of DGBI. In a pig model of early weaning stress, chronic diarrhea, increased intestinal mucosal permeability, and increased mast cells were observed [9], suggesting a link to chronic diarrhea symptoms.

Similar to IBS, there are reports on the efficacy of probiotics in improving symptoms of FDr. A small randomized controlled trial in FDr patients reported that 2 months of *Lactiplantibacillus plantarum* CJLP243 intake resulted in a reduction in the frequency of loose stools compared to pre-intake levels [11].

Recent studies have also examined the relationship between bowel movements and bile acid levels in stool. Comparisons between DGBI groups and control groups revealed that the bile acid profiles in stool were similar between FDr and IBS-D, and between FC and IBS-C. FDr and IBS-D groups, which primarily exhibit diarrhea, had significantly higher levels of primary bile acids such as cholic acid and chenodeoxycholic acid compared to FC, IBS-C, and control groups [10]. This suggests a potential link between bile acid levels and stool forms in FDr. However, research on the pathophysiology of FDr remains limited compared to IBS, necessitating further investigation for a clearer understanding of the disease.

4 Diagnostic Criteria

FDr is diagnosed using the Rome criteria, the international standard for DGBI. Previously, the Rome III diagnostic criteria (Table 46.1) were

Table 46.1 Rome III diagnostic criteria for FDr [11]

More than 75% of bowel movements are loose (mushy) or watery stools without abdominal pain.
Symptoms have been present for at least 6 months, and the above criteria have been met for the past 3 months.

Table 46.2 Rome IV diagnostic criteria for FDr [12]

Loose or watery stools in more than 25% of bowel movements without predominant abdominal pain or bothersome abdominal bloating.
Symptoms have been present for at least 6 months, and the above criteria have been met for the past 3 months.
Cases meeting the diagnostic criteria for IBS-D are excluded.

Table 46.3 Differential diagnosis of FDr

Food-related causes
Food intolerance: Lactose intolerance, fructose intolerance, and sorbitol intolerance
Food allergy
Inflammatory Bowel Disease
Crohn's disease and ulcerative colitis
Endocrine disorders
Hyperthyroidism and diabetes mellitus
Tumor-related disorders
WDHA syndrome and carcinoid syndrome
Celiac disease
Microscopic colitis
Collagenous colitis and lymphocytic colitis
Malabsorption syndromes
Protein-losing gastroenteropathy
Amyloidosis

used, but the Rome IV criteria (Table 46.2) were published in 2016 and are currently used internationally. The Rome III criteria defined FDr as having no abdominal pain, whereas the Rome IV criteria allow for the presence of abdominal pain or abdominal bloating, provided that these are not predominant symptoms. In IBS, abdominal pain is a diagnostic criterion, but in DGBI, abdominal pain is often accompanied by abdominal bloating. Therefore, according to the Rome IV criteria, even if abdominal pain or discomfort is present, it is not considered a predominant symptom, and FDr is defined as the presence of soft or watery stools at a frequency of 25% or higher. Additionally, the Rome III criteria required loose stools in more than 75% of bowel movements, but this was revised to "more than 25%" based on accumulated data. The exclusion of IBS is also noted in the criteria.

Future epidemiological studies will be necessary, but the change in abdominal symptoms and the proportion of diarrhea may lead to an increase in cases diagnosed as FDr.

5 Examination and Differential Diagnosis

For the diagnosis of FDr, a thorough medical history, current symptoms, and physical examination are crucial. Diarrhea is a common symptom indicative of various gastrointestinal diseases, including endocrine and metabolic disorders, infections, food allergies, and food intolerances, necessitating a broad differential diagnosis.

Diarrhea should be evaluated based on stool forms rather than the frequency of bowel movements. The Bristol Stool Form Scale and a bowel movement diary are useful diagnostic tools [12]. In addition to lactose intolerance caused by dairy product consumption, diarrhea following the consumption of lactose, sorbitol, or fructose contained in certain fruits, candies, gum, and other sweeteners is a sign of food intolerance. Such food-induced diarrhea is often overlooked, so careful questioning is necessary.

Warning signs such as unexpected weight loss, awakening due to diarrhea, antibiotic use preceding diarrhea, bloody stools, large volumes of diarrhea, and frequent bowel movements suggest organic diseases. In particular, large volumes of watery diarrhea may indicate watery diarrhea hypokalemia and achlorhydria (WDHA) syndrome caused by vasoactive intestinal peptide-producing tumors, primarily in the pancreas. A family history of colorectal cancer, inflammatory bowel disease, or celiac disease warrants careful examination (Table 46.3).

Peripheral blood biochemical tests should be performed on all patients to differentiate conditions such as hyperthyroidism and diabetes. In cases of suspected carcinoid syndrome, characterized by increased intestinal secretion due to serotonin, blood serotonin and urinary 5-hydroxyindole acetic acid levels should be measured. Malnutrition, weight loss, anemia, and electrolyte abnormalities suggest malabsorption, necessitating differential diagnosis for celiac disease, giardiasis, and tropical sprue, particularly in relevant regions. Celiac disease, caused by abnormal intestinal permeability and immune response to gluten, requires testing for celiac-related antibodies and duodenal biopsy via upper gastrointestinal endoscopy.

Stool tests, including stool culture for infection diagnosis and fecal calprotectin for screening inflammatory bowel disease, are useful. Steatorrhea indicates malabsorption syndrome, requiring investigation of pancreaticobiliary diseases via CT, MRI, and gastrointestinal examinations.

Lower gastrointestinal endoscopy should be performed in cases with warning signs or family history suggesting gastrointestinal malignancies or inflammatory bowel disease. Even in the absence of such findings, empirical treatment failure for chronic diarrhea warrants endoscopy. All chronic diarrhea cases in patients over 50 years of age should be examined [12]. Microscopic colitis, including collagenous colitis and lymphocytic colitis, causes chronic watery diarrhea and requires biopsy for diagnosis. Medications such as proton pump inhibitors, nonsteroidal anti-inflammatory drugs, and selective serotonin reuptake inhibitors may be associated with chronic diarrhea, making a detailed medication history essential.

Bile acid diarrhea, caused by excessive bile acid entering the colon due to bile acid malabsorption, is a potential cause of refractory chronic diarrhea. The SeHCAT scan, measuring the absorption state of orally ingested ^{75}Selenium homotaurocholic acid (SeHCAT), is reported to be useful [13].

6 Treatment

Research on the treatment of FDr is limited, and there is a lack of robust evidence. Consequently, the treatment of FDr is often considered in line with the treatment for IBS-D, which presents similar symptoms. Dietary guidance to avoid foods that can induce diarrhea, such as fats, caffeine, and spices, is recommended. Additionally, foods containing fermentable oligosaccharides, disaccharides, monosaccharides, and polyols (collectively known as FODMAPs) are poorly digested and absorbed in the small intestine. These foods are fermented and broken down by gut microbiota in the colon, increasing osmotic pressure and drawing water into the intestinal lumen. A low-FODMAP diet has been shown to improve symptoms of IBS [14]. Considering the mechanism of action, it may also be effective for FDr, although current evidence is insufficient.

Pharmacological treatments that may be beneficial include probiotics, the 5-HT_3 antagonist ramosetron, and the peripheral μ-opioid agonist loperamide. Loperamide has been shown to improve stool frequency, stool consistency, and fecal urgency in patients with FDr and IBS-D [15]. The efficacy of antibiotics such as rifaximin, which have been effective in IBS, may also be promising for FDr.

Take-Home Message

Given the multitude of diseases that can cause chronic diarrhea, it is crucial to understand the potential underlying conditions thoroughly and perform appropriate differential diagnoses before diagnosing FDr using the Rome IV criteria. Although research on FDr is limited and evidence regarding its pathophysiology and treatment is scarce, similarities in chronic diarrhea symptoms between FDr and IBS-D suggest that treatments for IBS-D may be applicable to FDr.

Competing Interests The author has no competing interests to declare that are relevant to the content of this chapter.

References

1. Zhao YF, et al. Epidemiology of functional diarrhea and comparison with diarrhea-predominant irritable bowel syndrome: a population-based survey in China. PLoS One. 2012;7:e43749.
2. Roshandel D, et al. Symptom patterns and relative distribution of functional bowel disorders in 1,023 gastroenterology patients in Iran. Int J Colorectal Dis. 2006;21:814–25.
3. Schmulson M, et al. Frequency of functional bowel disorders among healthy volunteers in Mexico City. Dig Dis. 2006;24:342–7.
4. Sorouri M, et al. Functional bowel disorders in Iranian population using Rome III criteria. Saud J Gastroenterol. 2010;16:154–60.
5. Chang F-Y, et al. Prevalence of functional gastrointestinal disorders in Taiwan: questionnaire-based survey for adults based on the Rome III criteria. Asia Pac J Clin Nutr. 2012;21:594–600.
6. Tack J. Functional diarrhea. Gastroenterol Clin North Am. 2012;41:629–37.
7. Singh P, et al. Similarities in clinical and psychological characteristics of functional diarrhea and irritable bowel syndrome with diarrhea. Clin Gastroenterol Hepatol. 2020;18:399–405.
8. Shiha MG, et al. Increased psychological distress and somatization in patients with irritable bowel syndrome compared with functional diarrhea or functional constipation, based on Rome IV criteria. Neurogastroenterol Motil. 2021;33:e14121.
9. Pohl CS, et al. Early weaning stress induces chronic functional diarrhea, intestinal barrier defect, and increased mast cell activity in a porcine model of early life adversity. Neurogastroenterol Motil. 2017;29:e13118.
10. James SC, et al. Concentrations of fecal bile acids in participants with functional gut disorders and healthy controls. Metabolites. 2021;11(9):612.
11. Longstreth GF, et al. Functional bowel disease. Gastroenterology. 2006;130:1480–91.
12. Lacy BE, et al. Bowel disorders. Gastroenterology. 2016;150:1393–407.
13. Gracie DJ, et al. Prevalence of, and predictors of, bile acid malabsorption in outpatients with chronic diarrhea. Neurogastroenterol Motil. 2012;24:983–e538.
14. Halmos EP, et al. A diet low in FODMAPs reduces symptoms of irritable bowel syndrome. Gastroenterology. 2014;146:67–75.
15. Efskind PS, et al. A double-blind placebo-controlled trial with loperamide in irritable bowel syndrome. Scand J Gastroenterol. 1996;31:463–8.

47 Diagnosis and Treatment of DGBI of the Small Bowel and Colon, Functional Abdominal Bloating

Mitsuru Moriya

Abstract

Abdominal bloating is a common symptom, newly defined in the Rome IV criteria as recurrent sensations of bloating, pressure, and gas retention lasting at least six months. It often coexists with mild pain and bowel irregularities, particularly in patients with constipation predominant IBS and functional constipation. Epidemiologically, 16–31% of the general population experience bloating, with women more affected than men. Symptoms significantly impair quality of life for many patients. The pathophysiology is multifactorial: increased gastrointestinal contents (gas, stool, liquid, fat), motility disorders, abnormal viscerosomatic reflexes causing muscle relaxation, and visceral hypersensitivity possibly influenced by hormones and psychological factors. Gas accumulation is linked to swallowing air, fermentation, and bacterial overgrowth like small intestinal bacterial overgrowth (SIBO). Stool retention, liquid presence after meals, and fat accumulation also contribute. Diagnosis follows Rome IV criteria, requiring symptom duration and frequency. Warning signs warrant exclusion of organic disease through tests. Treatment includes lifestyle modifications such as a low-FODMAP diet, exercise to strengthen abdominal muscles, and pharmacotherapy including probiotics, herbal medicines, simethicone, and sometimes antibiotics or antidepressants. Psychological therapies like cognitive-behavioral therapy are also tried. While not life-threatening, functional abdominal bloating reduces quality of life. Tailored treatment and a positive therapeutic relationship improve outcomes.

M. Moriya (✉)
Health Sciences University of Hokkaido, Sapporo, Japan
e-mail: mmoriya@hoku-iryo-u.ac.jp

H. Kaneko et al. (eds.), *Disorders of Gut-Brain Interaction*,
https://doi.org/10.1007/978-981-95-6974-8_47

Keywords

Abdominal bloating · Rome IV · Pharmacotherapy · Kampo medicines · Psychotherapy · Dietary adjustments · Exercise

1 Concept

Abdominal bloating is a common complaint encountered in daily clinical practice. The revision from Rome III to Rome IV international diagnostic criteria describes functional abdominal bloating as characterized by recurrent sensations of abdominal bloating, abdominal pressure, and the feeling of gas retention. Additionally, mild abdominal pain and mild bowel movement abnormalities may co-occur, with symptoms present for at least 6 months and the main symptom (abdominal bloating) observed over the past 3 months [1].

Among patients with disorders of gut–brain interaction (DGBI), those with constipation-predominant irritable bowel syndrome (IBS) and functional constipation tend to experience abdominal bloating [1], necessitating differential diagnosis.

2 Epidemiology

The incidence of functional abdominal bloating has not been evaluated in large-scale prospective studies [1]. However, the prevalence of abdominal bloating in the general population is reported to be between 16% and 31% [2]. Women are more likely to report abdominal bloating than men (19.2% vs. 10.5%), and they tend to perceive it as more severe [1]. Among patients with bloating (without a diagnosis of IBS), 75% rate the severity of their symptoms as moderate to severe, and 50% report that their daily life is restricted by the symptoms [3].

3 Etiology and Pathophysiology

Various theories have been proposed regarding the pathophysiology of abdominal bloating [1]. These can be categorized into four main factors: increased gastrointestinal contents (gas, stool, liquid, fat) [2], gastrointestinal motility disorders [3], abnormal viscerosomatic reflexes leading to abdominal muscle relaxation [4], and visceral hypersensitivity and psychological factors (Fig. 47.1) [4].

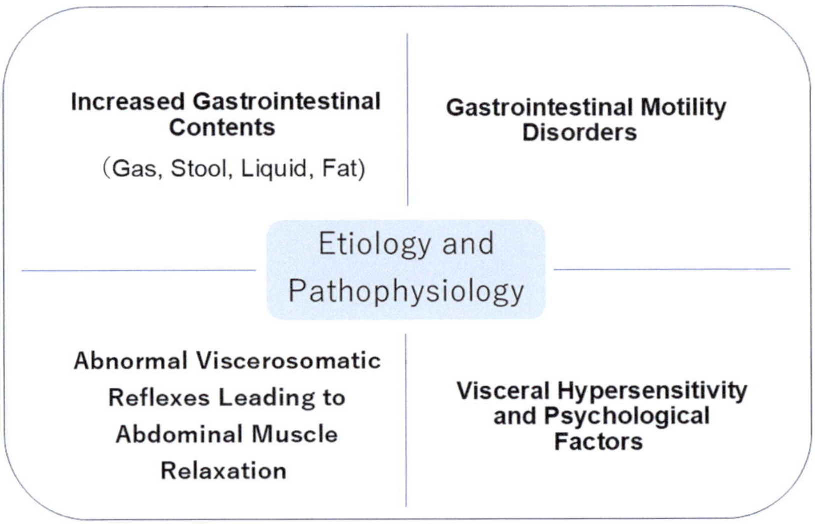

Fig. 47.1 Etiology and pathophysiology of abdominal bloating [4]

3.1 Increased Gastrointestinal Contents

(i) *Gas:* Abdominal bloating is thought to result from increased intra-abdominal contents, with symptoms changing rapidly, suggesting dependence on gas. The homeostasis of intestinal gas relies on the balance between its production and expulsion. Gas production results from swallowed air, chemical reactions (especially neutralization of acids and alkalis in the upper gastrointestinal tract), diffusion from the bloodstream, and fermentation by gut microbiota. Gas expulsion occurs through gastrointestinal motility, absorption into the bloodstream, bacterial consumption, and expulsion via the anal sphincter. Aerophagia, one of the DGBI, involves frequent and large amounts of air swallowing, causing symptoms of abdominal bloating. Resistant starches (partially broken down by amylase in the small intestine and reaching the colon), oligosaccharides, and dietary fibers are incompletely absorbed in the small intestine, entering the colon and fermenting, leading to secondary bacterial overgrowth. Carbohydrate intolerance, such as lactose and fructose intolerance, is associated with small intestinal bacterial overgrowth, which can cause abdominal bloating [2]. Excessive bacteria in the small intestine ferment carbohydrates, producing gas and causing symptoms due to intestinal distension.

(ii) *Stool:* Bloating is frequently reported by patients with constipation. Stool retained in the rectum can cause delayed transit in the small and large intestines, worsening bloating in patients with constipation. Rectal dysfunction underlying functional constipation may be a significant factor in the onset of bloating. There are currently no direct studies on the relationship between functional abdominal bloating and gut microbiota.

(iii) *Liquid:* After meals, food is diluted by large amounts of gastric juice, breaking down solids and promoting digestion and absorption. Generally, patients with bloating report symptoms shortly after meals rather than when fasting. Therefore, stimulation of the proximal small intestine by liquid is suspected to cause bloating symptoms. Additionally, liquid fat infusion in patients with bloating has been shown to slow intestinal movement.

(iv) *Fat:* Meta-analysis has shown no correlation between abdominal bloating and body mass index (BMI) [5]. However, there is a potential link between weight gain and bloating. Approximately 40% of individuals reporting bloating also report weight gain at the onset of symptoms [6]. Thus, recent increases in abdominal fat may contribute to the onset of bloating.

3.2 Gastrointestinal Motility Disorders

There are no direct studies on gastrointestinal motility in functional abdominal bloating, but the relationship between bloating and gastrointestinal motility has been reported in other diseases such as gastroparesis, chronic intestinal pseudo-obstruction, and scleroderma. A prospective study of over 2000 patients with functional constipation and constipation-predominant IBS found that more than 90% reported bloating, with those having longer colonic transit times experiencing more severe bloating.

3.3 Abnormal Viscerosomatic Reflexes Leading to Abdominal Muscle Relaxation

One hypothesis for the onset of bloating is that it results from the displacement of visceral organs due to increased gas rather than increased intra-abdominal contents. The abdominal cavity is bounded by the vertebrae and defined by the posterior abdominal wall, the diaphragm, and the abdominal muscles of the anterior abdominal wall. In healthy individuals, increased intestinal gas triggers normal viscerosomatic reflexes, causing diaphragm relaxation and abdominal muscle contraction, preventing bloating. In patients with bloating, abnormal viscerosomatic reflexes cause diaphragm contraction and abdominal muscle relaxation, leading to bloating [7].

3.4 Visceral Hypersensitivity and Psychological Factors

(i) *Visceral Hypersensitivity:* Abdominal bloating is associated with visceral hypersensitivity, with hormonal roles also hypothesized. Approximately 40–75% of women with IBS report worsening bloating and bowel movements around menstruation. Hormonal influences related to menstruation are thought to alter intestinal sensitivity, though the involvement of estrogen is debated.

(ii) *Psychological Factors:* The role of psychological factors in the etiology and pathophysiology of bloating remains debated. Although there are reports of strong associations between psychological stress symptoms, such as depression, and bloating, these associations have not been sufficiently confirmed by other researchers.

4 Diagnostic Criteria and Examination

The Rome IV diagnostic criteria for functional abdominal bloating are shown in Fig. 47.2 [1]. Strictly speaking, these criteria are for functional abdominal bloating/distention, but distinguishing between the two is challenging, so they are collectively referred to as functional abdominal bloating.

Criteria fulfilled for the last 3 months with symptom onset at least 6 month prior to diagnosis

Must include both of following

1. Recurrent bloating and/or distension occurring, on average, at least 1 day per week; abdominal bloating and/or distension predominates over other symptoms.
   (Mild pain related to bloating may be present as well as minor bowel movement abnormalities)
2. There are insufficient criteria for a diagnosis of irritable bowel syndrome, functional constipation, functional diarrhea, or postprandial distress syndrome

Fig. 47.2 Roma IV diagnostic criteria for functional abdominal bloating [1]

5 Differential Diagnosis and Complications

Figure 47.3 shows the diagnostic and treatment algorithm for abdominal bloating [8]. If warning symptoms (e.g., bloody stools, anemia, fever, weight loss, and abdominal masses) are present, organic diseases should be suspected, and blood tests, endoscopy, and imaging should be promptly performed. Even in the absence of warning symptoms, these tests should be conducted as much as possible to rule out organic diseases. If the diagnostic criteria for DGBI, such as IBS or functional dyspepsia, are met, treatment should follow those guidelines. If the criteria are not met, the diagnostic criteria for functional abdominal bloating (symptoms present for at least 6 months, with recurrent bloating at least one day per week over the past 3 months) should be considered. If met, a diagnosis of functional abdominal bloating is made, but treatment remains the same even if the criteria are not fully met for functional abdominal bloating.

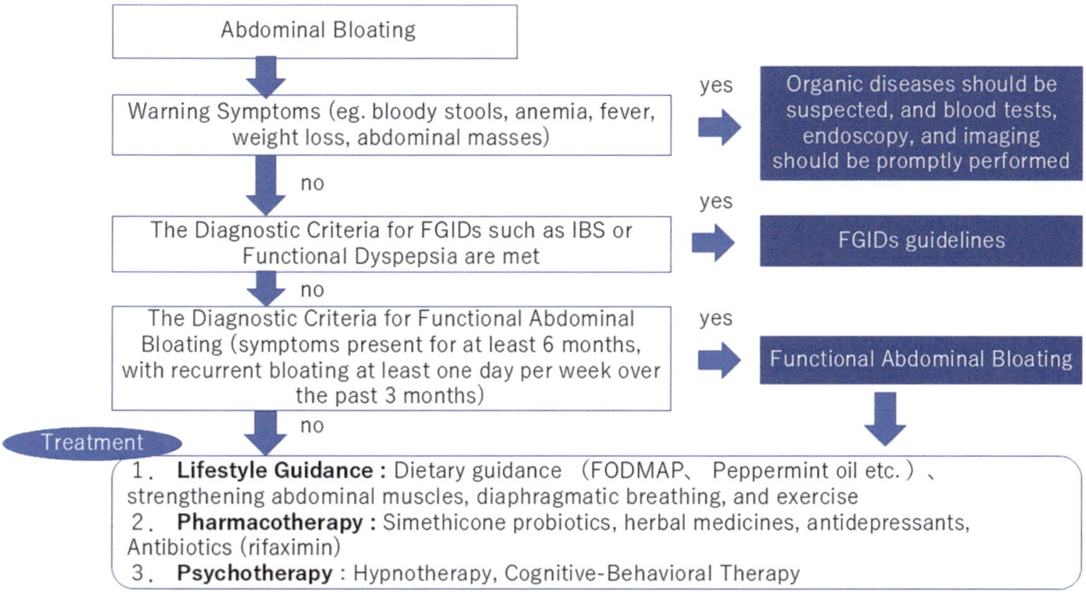

Fig. 47.3 Diagnostic and treatment algorithm for abdominal bloating [2, 8]

6 Treatment

1. *Lifestyle Guidance*
   Dietary guidance [1, 8] emphasizes low-FODMAP foods, such as rice and buckwheat, which are less fermented by gut microbiota [9]. FODMAP stands for fermentable oligosaccharides (fructans and galactooligosaccharides), disaccharides (lactose), monosaccharides (fructose), and polyols (sorbitol, mannitol, isomalt, xylitol, and glycerol). Peppermint oil has also been reported to be effective. Some patients exhibit abdominal muscle relaxation, and strengthening abdominal muscles through compression garments, diaphragmatic breathing, and exercise is recommended [10]. Although a small RCT reported no significant improvement in bloating with 10–15 minutes of walking after each meal [11], another study found significant improvement with 20 minutes of aerobic exercise three times a week [12]. From a pathophysiological perspective, exercises that strengthen the abdominal muscles, such as resistance training, are also considered beneficial. Exercise is beneficial for improving bowel movements and reducing fat, potentially improving bloating and associated depression in the long term.
2. *Pharmacotherapy:* Alpha-glucosidase inhibitors used in the treatment for diabetes mellitus increase intestinal gas and should be discontinued if prescribed. Simethicone (Gascon®) is considered useful. Treatments with probiotics, herbal medicines (such as Daikenchuto and Tokito), and antidepressants have been attempted. Antibiotics (rifaximin) have been reported to be effective in some patients.
3. *Psychotherapy:* Hypnotherapy and cognitive-behavioral therapy have been attempted.

7 Prognosis

Functional abdominal bloating, like IBS, does not directly threaten life but is considered a disease that reduces quality of life.

8 Conclusion

Functional abdominal bloating is an independent concept within DGBI according to the Rome IV diagnostic criteria. The etiology is diverse, and treatment should be tailored to the specific causes.

Take-Home Message

The etiology of functional abdominal bloating is diverse, and treatment involves a combination of pharmacotherapy, including Kampo medicines, psychotherapy, dietary adjustments, and exercise. In clinical practice, treatment is often tailored to the patient's preferences through trial and error. A positive attitude toward these treatments can foster a good patient–physician relationship and sometimes lead to unexpectedly favorable outcomes.

Competing Interests The author has no competing interests to declare that are relevant to the content of this chapter.

References

1. Lacy BE, et al. Bowel disorders. Gastroenterology. 2016;150:1393–407.
2. Lacy BE, et al. Management of Chronic Abdominal Distension and Bloating. Clin Gastroenterol Hepatol. 2021;19:219–31.
3. Sandler RS, et al. Abdominal pain, bloating, and diarrhea in the United States: prevalence and impact. Dig Dis Sci. 2000;45:1166–71.
4. Iovino P, et al. Bloating and functional gastro-intestinal disorders: where are we and where are we going? World J Gastroenterol. 2014;20(39):14407–19.
5. Eslick GD. Gastrointestinal symptoms and obesity: a meta-analysis. Obes Rev. 2012;13:469–79.
6. Sullinan SN. A prospective study of unexplained visible abdominal bloating. N Z Med J. 1994;107:428–30.
7. Villoria A, et al. Abdomino-phrenic dyssynergia in patients with abdominal bloating and distension. Am J Gastroenterol. 2011;106:815–9.
8. Mari A, et al. Bloating and Abdominal Distension: Clinical Approach and Management. Adv Ther. 2019;36:1075–84.
9. Pessarelli T, et al. The low-FODMAP diet and the gluten free diet in the management of functional abdominal bloating and distension. Front Nutr. 2022;8:1–8.
10. Sullivan SN. Functional abdominal bloating with distention. ISRN Gastroenterol. 2012;2012:721820.
11. Hosseini-Asl MK, et al. The effect of a short-term physical activity after meals on gastrointestinal symptoms in individuals with functional abdominal bloating: a randomized clinical trial. Gastroenterol Hepatol Bed Bench. 2021;14:59–66.
12. Dehnavi ZM, et al. The effect of 8 weeks aerobic exercise on severity of physical symptoms of premenstrual syndrome: a clinical trial study. BMC Womens Health. 2018;18:80.

48 Diagnosis and Treatment of Motility Disorder of the Small Bowel and Colon, Chronic Intestinal Pseudo-Obstruction

Hidenori Ohkubo

Abstract

Chronic intestinal pseudo-obstruction (CIPO) is a rare and life-threatening digestive disorder characterized by significantly reduced intestinal peristalsis, leading to the pathological intestinal dilatation and persistent obstructive symptoms without any mechanical cause. Etiologically, CIPO is classified into idiopathic and secondary. In cases with secondary CIPO, systemic sclerosis is the most common cause. Medication is the primary treatment; however, management is generally difficult. In severe cases, nutritional therapy and decompression therapy play a key role. Percutaneous endoscopic gastrojejunostomy has recently been in the spotlight, in that this method allows for on-demand decompression at home without nasal tube insertion, reducing patients' burden and improving quality of life. Conversely, intestinal resection should be avoided, except in emergencies such as strangulation, because it often causes postoperative dilatation of the small bowel and further progression of malnutrition due to short bowel syndrome. Prognosis is generally poor, with a 5-year survival rate of 78% and a 10-year survival rate of 75% in adult cases requiring home intravenous hyperalimentation, extremely low for a non-malignant disease. Better prognosis is reported for cases with preserved oral intake and younger onset (under 20 years), while secondary CIPO with systemic sclerosis has a poorer prognosis. Appropriate management is crucial, and recognition of this disease is essential.

Keywords

Severely impaired peristalsis · Small intestinal bacterial overgrowth (SIBO) · Intestinal sterilization therapy · Nutritional therapy · Decompression therapy · Percutaneous endoscopic gastrojejunostomy (PEG-J)

1 Introduction

Chronic intestinal pseudo-obstruction (CIPO) is a rare and severe disorder characterized by significantly reduced intestinal peristalsis, leading to the stagnation of intestinal contents, pathological intestinal dilation, and persistent symptoms of intestinal obstruction throughout life [1].

Historically, even gastroenterologists and general physicians often failed to diagnose CIPO, with many unaware of the disease itself, leading to an average of eight years to reach a definitive diagnosis [2]. However, recent advancements in research have gradually improved disease recognition, and new treatments have been developed. This section provides an overview of the history,

H. Ohkubo (✉)
Gastroenterology Division, Sagami Rinkan Hospital, Sagamihara, Japan
e-mail: ohkuboh@yokohama-cu.ac.jp

H. Kaneko et al. (eds.), *Disorders of Gut-Brain Interaction*,
https://doi.org/10.1007/978-981-95-6974-8_48

diagnosis, epidemiology, pathophysiology, treatment, and prognosis of CIPO.

2 History

CIPO was first reported by Dudley in 1958 [3]. At that time, it was considered a "mysterious intestinal obstruction," and patients were frequently subjected to exploratory laparotomies. In Japan, the first report appeared in 1979, but the disease name and concept remained inconsistent, and the disease itself was not well recognized.

Gradually, the concept of "chronic intestinal obstruction without organic cause" and the term "pseudo-obstruction" became established, primarily in Western countries. However, in Japan, the recognition and establishment of the disease concept and nomenclature lagged behind Western countries, with low awareness even after 2000. Since 2009, comprehensive research by the Ministry of Health, Labour and Welfare (led by Nakajima A et al.) has advanced, leading to a better understanding and increased recognition of the disease in Japan [4].

3 Disease Concept

CIPO is a collective term for a condition that presents as a series of symptoms and includes a variety of pathophysiological states. Rather than being a single "disease," it represents a "state" resulting from different underlying conditions that cause significant intestinal dilation and chronic, irreversible intestinal obstruction. Secondary CIPO can be caused by collagen diseases (such as systemic sclerosis and Sjögren's syndrome), neurological disorders (such as Parkinson's disease and mitochondrial encephalomyopathy), and endocrine disorders (such as hypothyroidism), among others, with systemic sclerosis being the most common. Conversely, idiopathic CIPO occurs without these underlying conditions [chronic idiopathic intestinal pseudo-obstruction (CIIP)] [4].

Initially, CIPO patients may not experience significant symptoms and can lead normal lives, but symptoms become apparent over time. The most common symptom is abdominal bloating, observed in almost all cases [5]. Idiopathic cases often manifest suddenly due to biological stressors such as abdominal surgery (e.g., ileocecal surgery) or childbirth, while secondary cases gradually become apparent with the progression of the underlying disease. Once symptoms become apparent, they are irreversible and persist for life. CIPO primarily affects the small intestine, leading to malabsorption and various deficiency symptoms (small intestinal dysfunction). While abdominal bloating symptoms appear relatively early, small intestinal dysfunction typically occurs after significant disease progression. The period during which small intestinal absorption is preserved despite bloating is termed the "compensated phase," while the onset of small intestinal dysfunction marks the "decompensated phase."

Typical images of CIPO are shown in Fig. 48.1. The small intestine is mainly affected, and there are also patterns accompanied by dilation of the upper digestive tract, such as the esophagus and stomach. When only the large intestine is dilated, this is called megacolon and is classified separately from CIPO [1].

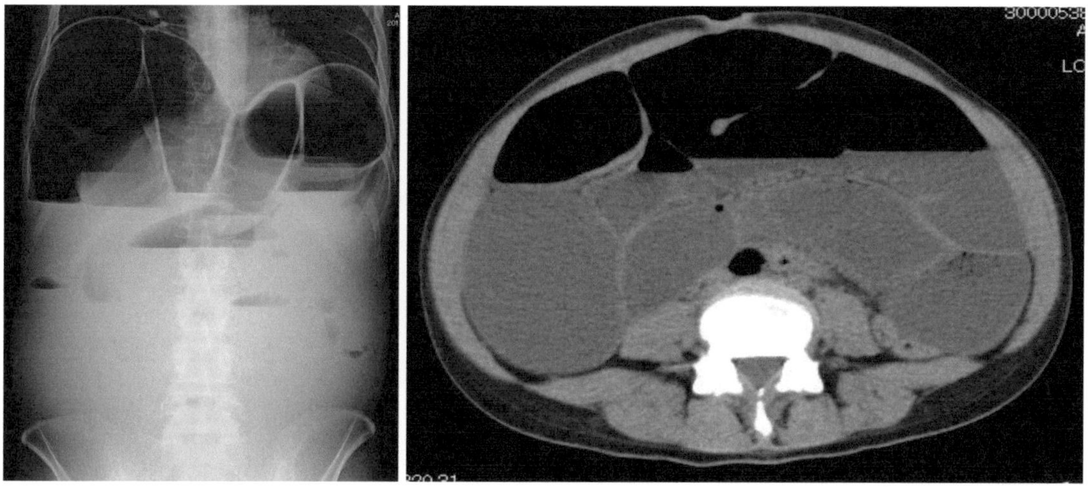

Fig. 48.1 Typical images of CIPO. (Left) Abdominal plain X-ray (standing position), (Right) Abdominal CT (axial section)

4 Diagnosis

Historically, the concept of chronic intestinal obstruction without organic cause, accompanied by chronic abdominal bloating and air-fluid level on imaging, existed primarily in Western countries, but clear diagnostic criteria were lacking. Diagnosis often requires specialized procedures such as manometry (evaluating peristaltic patterns by inserting a catheter with pressure sensors into the gastrointestinal tract) and full-thickness biopsy (pathological evaluation of a wedge-shaped resection of the gastrointestinal wall from mucosa to serosa), making diagnosis challenging.

In 2009, the Ministry of Health, Labour and Welfare research group (led by Nakajima A et al.) established the world's first clear diagnostic criteria [5]. The criteria include:

1. Symptoms persisting for more than 6 months
2. Abdominal pain or bloating present for the past 3 months
3. Significant intestinal dilation and air-fluid level formation on imaging
4. Absence of organic causes

These criteria are simple and do not require specialized tests such as manometry or full-layer biopsy, making diagnosis possible even for non-gastroenterologists.

Subsequent research has reported that cine MRI (3-2-3 cine MRI examination) is useful for evaluating small intestinal peristalsis and differentiating similar diseases [6]. Cine MRI is non-invasive, radiation-free, and allows observation of the entire small intestine, making it an excellent modality (see Chap. 41).

CIPO can also occur in children and adolescents. In pediatric cases, it is considered a Hirschsprung disease-related disorder, but seamless management from childhood to adulthood is necessary. Taguchi et al. have developed guidelines for the management of Hirschsprung disease-related disorders [7], including revised diagnostic criteria shown in Table 48.1. Cine MRI can substitute for manometry and full-thickness biopsy, which are limited to certain facilities in Japan.

CIPO was newly recognized as a designated intractable disease by the Ministry of Health, Labour and Welfare in January 2015.

Table 48.1 Diagnostic criteria for CIIP [7]

The following seven criteria must all be met:
1. Persistent or recurrent severe intestinal obstruction symptoms, such as abdominal bloating, nausea/vomiting, and abdominal pain, require hospitalization
2. Disease duration of at least 2 months for neonatal onset and at least 6 months for onset after infancy
3. Imaging shows gastrointestinal dilation and an air-fluid level[a]
4. No organic lesions causing gastrointestinal obstruction
5. No morphological abnormalities in the nerve plexus on HE staining of full-thickness intestinal biopsy[b]
6. Exclusion of megacystis-microcolon-intestinal hypoperistalsis syndrome and segmental dilatation of the intestine in pediatric cases
7. Exclusion of secondary CIPO

[a]In neonates, an air-fluid level on a standing abdominal plain X-ray is not necessarily required
[b]If a full-thickness intestinal biopsy is not available, cine MRI or gastrointestinal manometry demonstrating clear motility abnormalities centered on the small intestine can be used

5 Epidemiology

According to a nationwide survey by Iida et al. [8], the prevalence of CIPO in Japan is extremely low, with 1.0 males and 0.8 females per 100,000 population, with no gender difference. The average age at diagnosis is 63 years for males and 59 years for females, but the onset age is unclear due to the long time to definitive diagnosis.

6 Pathophysiology

In CIPO, gastrointestinal (especially small intestinal) peristalsis is severely impaired, leading to the stagnation of intestinal contents such as intestinal fluids and gas. Concurrently, intestinal bacteria settle and overgrow in the small intestine [small intestinal bacterial overgrowth (SIBO)]. Normally, intestinal bacteria convert carbohydrates into short-chain fatty acids, producing gases such as carbon dioxide, hydrogen, and methane. Excessive gas production due to SIBO further stagnates contents, increasing intestinal pressure and causing pathological dilation. This results in symptoms such as abdominal bloating and pain. This state can lead to extensive digestive and absorption disorders (small intestinal dysfunction) and sometimes bacterial translocation into the bloodstream, causing severe conditions such as malnutrition, dehydration, electrolyte abnormalities, and bacteremia, which can be fatal if not properly managed. Excessive weight loss and cachexia require careful attention (Fig. 48.2).

Gastrointestinal peristalsis is controlled by the contraction of intestinal smooth muscles via the autonomic nervous system (vagus nerve) and the activity of pacemaker cells (interstitial cells of Cajal) within the intestinal smooth muscle. Pathologically, abnormalities in these components have been reported in CIPO [9], categorized into three types: myogenic, neurogenic, and mesenchymopathic (interstitial cells of Cajal-related) (Fig. 48.3). These often overlap.

1. *Myogenic:* Atrophy, degeneration, and vacuolation of intestinal smooth muscle
2. *Neurogenic:* Reduction and degeneration of the myenteric (Auerbach) plexus (a layer of nerve cells between the inner circular and outer longitudinal muscle layers)
3. *Mesenchymopathic (interstitial cells of Cajal-related):* Reduction and disappearance of interstitial cells of Cajal

However, it remains unclear whether these pathological findings are the cause or result of the clinical picture.

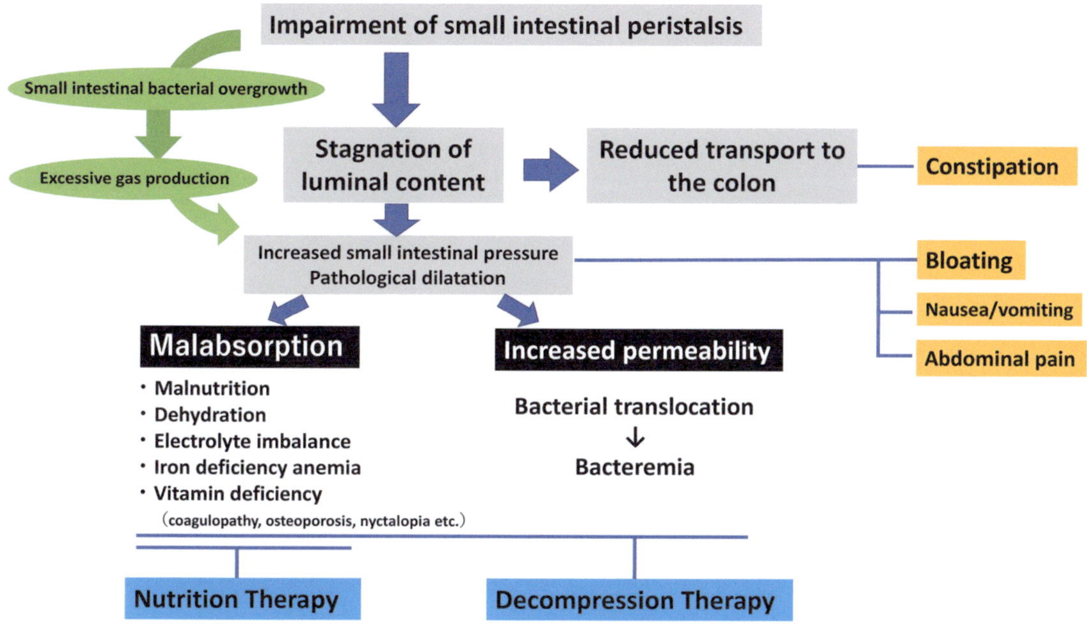

Fig. 48.2 Pathophysiology of CIPO

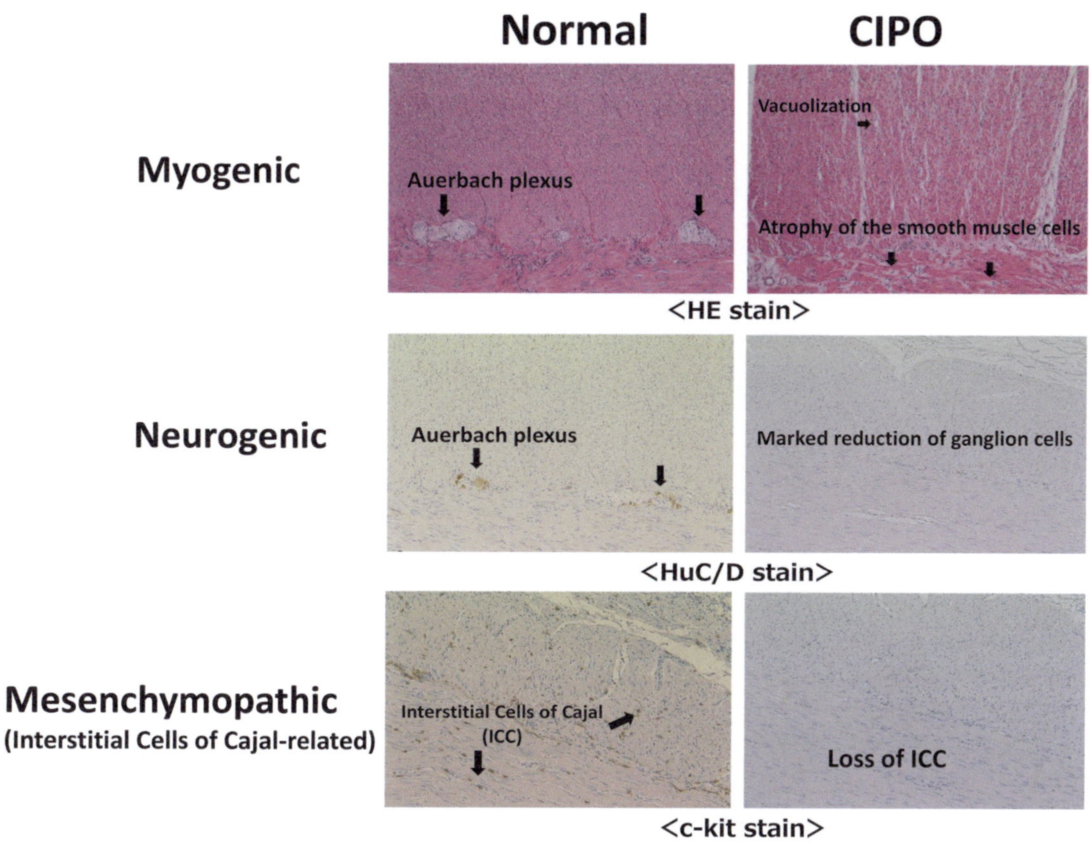

Fig. 48.3 Typical pathological findings of CIPO

7 Treatment

In cases of CIPO involving the small intestine, intestinal resection is generally contraindicated [10]. This is because resecting the dilated intestine often leads to postoperative dilation of the remaining small intestine and further progression of malnutrition due to short bowel syndrome. Therefore, except in emergencies such as strangulation, medical treatment is the primary approach.

1. Prokinetic Agents
   Initially, various gastrointestinal prokinetic agents and laxatives are used to control bowel movements. Specific medications include mosapride, Daikenchuto, metoclopramide, pantothenic acid, and senna-based preparations. However, these are often insufficient.
2. Nutritional Therapy
   During the compensated phase, oral intake is often possible, but a low-residue diet is preferable to minimize the burden on the gastrointestinal tract. In the decompensated phase, elemental nutrition (e.g., Elental®) is introduced. In cases of severe abdominal bloating or significant malnutrition, intravenous hyperalimentation (IVH) is necessary. However, attention must be paid to risks such as catheter infections, venous thrombosis, fatty liver, and cirrhosis.
3. Intestinal Sterilization Therapy
   Methane and hydrogen produced by SIBO are major causes of intestinal dilation and abdominal bloating. Therefore, non-absorbable antibiotics are used to control intestinal bacteria. Rifaximin, metronidazole, and fluoroquinolones have been reported to be effective against SIBO [11], and significant improvement in small intestinal gas has been observed in several cases (Fig. 48.4). However, these are off-label uses in Japan.
4. Decompression Therapy
   Traditionally, ileus tubes and decompression jejunostomy were common. However, ileus tubes cause significant patient discomfort and can only be temporarily placed during hospitalization, while jejunostomy cannot control the amount of drainage, posing major issues. In 2017, the author reported the usefulness of percutaneous endoscopic gastrojejunostomy (PEG-J) for decompression therapy in CIPO [12] (Fig. 48.5). This involves creating a gastrostomy and placing a decompression tube in the jejunum through the gastrostomy. This method allows for on-demand decompression at home without nasal tube insertion, reducing patient burden and improving quality of life.

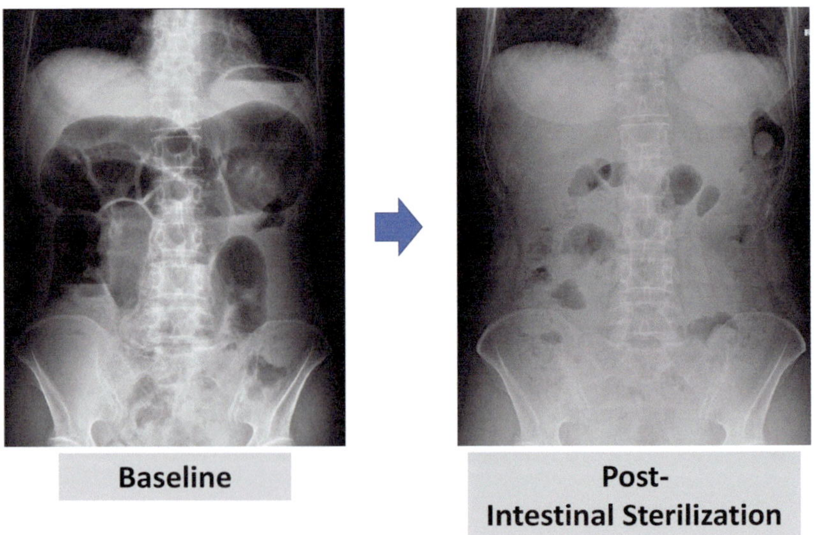

Fig. 48.4 Intestinal sterilization therapy with metronidazole

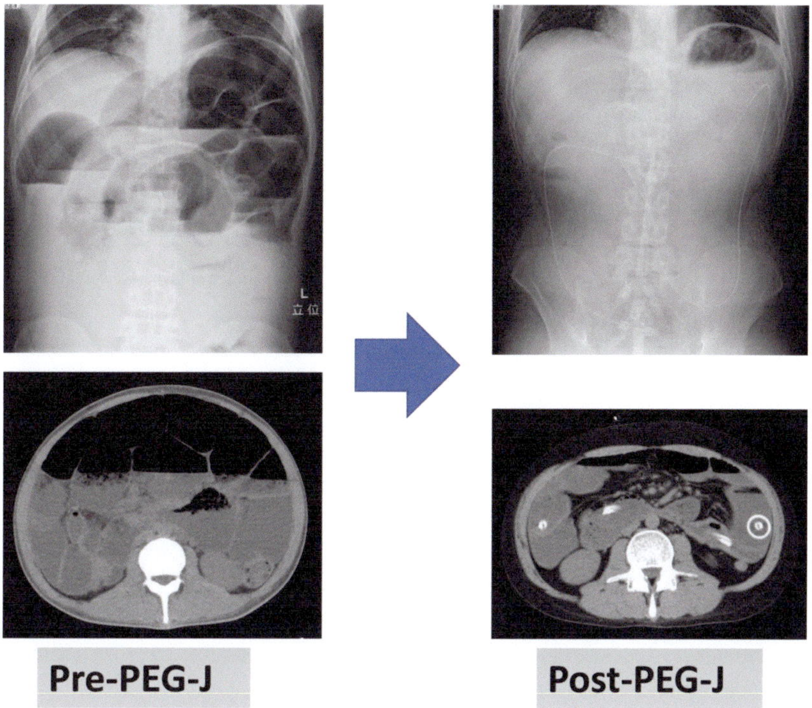

Fig. 48.5 PEG-J for decompression

Oral intake is possible even with PEG-J, but proper management of drainage is necessary, and it often causes chemical dermatitis around the stoma, requiring regular tube replacement and outpatient follow-up.

8 Prognosis

In 2009, Amiot et al. reported that the 5-year survival rate for adults with CIPO requiring home IVH was 78%, and the 10-year survival rate was 75% [13]. These figures are extremely low for a non-malignant disease. Better prognosis is reported for cases with preserved oral intake and younger onset (under 20 years), while secondary CIPO associated with systemic sclerosis has a poorer prognosis.

9 Conclusion

CIPO significantly impairs patients' activities of daily living throughout their lives and can be life-threatening. Therefore, appropriate management is crucial, and it is essential to be aware of the disease and consult specialized facilities when in doubt about treatment.

Take-Home Message

- CIPO is a designated intractable disease caused by a significant reduction in small

intestinal peristalsis, leading to chronic paralytic ileus, which can sometimes be fatal.
- Treatment primarily involves nutritional therapy and decompression therapy, with intestinal sterilization being effective in some cases.
- CIPO can cause pneumatosis cystoides intestinalis and free intraperitoneal gas, but unlike gastrointestinal perforation, it does not present with peritonitis, making differentiation relatively easy. Avoiding unnecessary laparotomy is crucial as it often exacerbates symptoms.

Competing Interests The author has no competing interests to declare that are relevant to the content of this chapter.

References

1. Stanghellini V, et al. Chronic intestinal pseudo-obstruction: manifestations, natural history and management. Neurogastroenterol Motil. 2007;19:440–52.
2. Stanghellini V, et al. Natural history of chronic idiopathic intestinal pseudo-obstruction in adults: a single center study. Clin Gastroenterol Hepatol. 2005;3:449–58.
3. Dudley HA, et al. Intestinal pseudo-obstruction. J R Coll Surg Edinb. 1958;3:206–17.
4. Nakajima A, et al. Chronic Intestinal Pseudo-obstruction (CIPO): Clinical Practice Guidelines. Ministry of Health, Labour and Welfare Research Project on Overcoming Intractable Diseases (Research Group on the Epidemiology, Diagnosis, and Treatment of Chronic Idiopathic Intestinal Pseudo-obstruction in Japan). 1st ed. Sanno Printing; 2012. (in Japanese)
5. Ohkubo H, et al. An epidemiologic survey of chronic intestinal pseudo-obstruction and evaluation of the newly proposed diagnostic criteria. Digestion. 2012;86:12–9.
6. Ohkubo H, et al. Assessment of small bowel motility in patients with chronic intestinal pseudo-obstruction using cine-MRI. Am J Gastroenterol. 2013;108:1130–9.
7. Taguchi T. Guidelines for the Management of Hirschsprung Disease-Related Disorders: Practical Edition. Ministry of Health, Labour and Welfare Research Project on Establishing Guidelines for Rare and Intractable Gastrointestinal Diseases from Childhood to Adulthood; 2017. (in Japanese)
8. Iida H, et al. Epidemiology and clinical experience of chronic intestinal pseudo-obstruction in Japan: a nationwide epidemiologic survey. J Epidemiol. 2013;23:288–94.
9. Amiot A, et al. The role of immunohistochemistry in idiopathic chronic intestinal pseudo-obstruction (CIPO): a case-control study. Am J Surg Pathol. 2009;33:749–58.
10. Masaki T, et al. Nationwide survey on adult type chronic intestinal pseudo-obstruction in surgical institutions in Japan. Surg Today. 2012;42:264–71.
11. Rao SSC, et al. Small intestinal bacterial overgrowth: clinical features and therapeutic management. Clin Transl Gastroenterol. 2019;10:e00078.
12. Ohkubo H, et al. Efficacy of percutaneous endoscopic gastro-jejunostomy (PEG-J) decompression therapy for patients with chronic intestinal pseudo-obstruction (CIPO). Neurogastroenterol Motil. 2017;29:e13127.
13. Amiot A, et al. Long-term outcome of chronic intestinal pseudo-obstruction adult patients requiring home parenteral nutrition. Am J Gastroenterol. 2009;104:1262–70.

49 Diagnosis and Treatment of Motility Disorders of the Small Bowel and Colon, Megacolon

Akiko Fuyuki

Abstract

Megacolon is a state of pathological dilatation of the colon without mechanical causes, including malignancy, volvulus, and strangulation. It is classified as "acute" or "chronic" based on clinical course. Acute megacolon includes acute colonic pseudo-obstruction and toxic megacolon. Chronic megacolon is further classified as "idiopathic" or "secondary" based on the absence or presence of underlying causes. Treatment and prognosis vary depending on the pathology. For acute colonic pseudo-obstruction, neostigmine administration and endoscopic decompression are effective. If the small intestine is not involved, total colectomy may be successful. It is generally transient with a relatively good prognosis. In toxic megacolon, surgical treatment is absolutely indicated in cases of perforation, uncontrollable bleeding, or organ failure. Even if surgical treatment is not indicated, bowel rest and decompression are necessary with systemic monitoring in preparation for potential surgical intervention. Prognosis is generally poor, with a mortality rate of 19–45% in cases with ulcerative colitis, and 38–80% in those with pseudomembranous colitis. For chronic megacolon, dietary and pharmacological therapies are fundamental. Surgical treatment is indicated for cases with insufficient response to conservative therapies or recurrent sigmoid volvulus. While refractory, prognosis is good if defecation control is achieved or surgical treatment is successful.

Keywords

Acute megacolon · Acute colonic pseudo-obstruction (Ogilvie syndrome) · Toxic megacolon · Chronic megacolon · Decompression therapy · Total colectomy

1 Concept

Megacolon refers to a pathological dilation of the colon without organic causes such as malignancy, volvulus, or strangulation. It is classified as "acute" or "chronic" based on clinical course, but in daily clinical practice, megacolon often refers to a chronic state of colonic dilation. This condition is distinct from chronic intestinal pseudo-obstruction, which primarily affects the small intestine. Megacolon lacks specific clinical symptoms and often presents with common symptoms such as abdominal bloating and chronic constipation.

A. Fuyuki (✉)
Department of Palliative Care, Shin-yurigaoka General Hospital, Kawasaki, Japan
e-mail: fuyukia@yokohama-cu.ac.jp

H. Kaneko et al. (eds.), *Disorders of Gut-Brain Interaction*,
https://doi.org/10.1007/978-981-95-6974-8_49

Table 49.1 Classification of megacolon

Acute	Acute colonic pseudo-obstruction Toxic megacolon
Chronic	Megacolon (idiopathic, secondary)

2 Classification

Megacolon is classified as "acute" or "chronic" based on clinical course. Acute megacolon includes acute colonic pseudo-obstruction (Ogilvie syndrome) and toxic megacolon, which arises from chronic inflammation such as inflammatory bowel disease or infections like pseudomembranous colitis. Especially, toxic megacolon is a severe, emergent condition. Chronic megacolon is further classified as "idiopathic" or "secondary" based on the presence or absence of underlying causes (Table 49.1).

3 Epidemiology

The lifetime incidence of toxic megacolon in patients with ulcerative colitis is reported to be 1.0–2.5% [1], and the incidence associated with pseudomembranous enterocolitis is reported to be 0.4–3.0% [2]. Recently, there has been a notable increase in *Clostridioides difficile* infections due to the use of broad-spectrum antibiotics, drawing attention to toxic megacolon caused by pseudomembranous enterocolitis. The detailed epidemiology of other forms of megacolon remains unclear. Idiopathic chronic megacolon is reported to have no gender differences.

4 Etiology and Pathophysiology

Acute colonic pseudo-obstruction often follows various systemic diseases, particularly postoperative conditions (Table 49.2). It is presumed to involve autonomic nervous system dysregulation in the colon, but the details remain unclear. In toxic megacolon, conditions listed in Table 49.3 are causative.

Table 49.2 Background diseases and triggers of acute megacolon

Cardiovascular diseases	Myocardial infarction, heart failure, and post-cardiopulmonary resuscitation
Metabolic disorders	Electrolyte imbalance (especially hypokalemia), liver failure, renal failure, and alcohol intoxication
Drug-induced	Phenothiazines, antidepressants, opioids, anti-Parkinson drugs, and lead poisoning
Infections	Sepsis, pneumonia, pancreatitis, herpes zoster, acute appendicitis, meningitis, and pleuritis
Tumors	Leukemia and retroperitoneal tumors
Postoperative	Post-kidney transplant, post-cesarean section, post-abdominal surgery, post-pelvic surgery, and post-gynecological surgery
Trauma	Under mechanical ventilation, spinal cord injury, pelvic injury, and femoral injury

Table 49.3 Background diseases and triggers of toxic megacolon

Inflammation	Ulcerative colitis Crohn's disease Behçet's disease
Infections	Bacteria (Salmonella, Shigella, Campylobacter, Yersinia, *Clostridioides difficile*) Parasites (e.g., Amoeba)
	Viruses (cytomegalovirus and HIV)
Others	Barium enema X-ray Colonoscopy
	Administration of bowel motility inhibitors Drugs (antidiarrheals, narcotics, anticholinergics)

Chronic inflammation or infection leads to significant mucosal epithelial damage, resulting in the loss of normal gastrointestinal absorption function. This leads to electrolyte imbalances such as hypokalemia, which further impairs gastrointestinal motility, contributing to megacolon. Additionally, the spread of inflammation to the intestinal muscle layer and nitric oxide produced by inflammatory cells causes strong smooth muscle relaxation. The breakdown of

Table 49.4 Background diseases and triggers of secondary megacolon

Neurological diseases	Adult Hirschsprung disease Ganglion cell reduction syndrome Parkinson's disease Recklinghausen disease
Muscular diseases	Myotonic dystrophy
Endocrine disorders	Hypothyroidism Diabetes Pheochromocytoma
Malignant tumors	Retroperitoneal malignant tumors
Others	Cathartic syndrome (laxative abuse) Psychiatric disorders Drug-induced

the epithelial barrier allows toxins and gut microbiota to enter the bloodstream, causing systemic toxic symptoms. Conversely, the cause of idiopathic chronic megacolon remains unknown. Secondary chronic megacolon can be caused by neurological diseases (e.g., adult Hirschsprung disease and Parkinson's disease), myotonic dystrophy, endocrine disorders (e.g., hypothyroidism, diabetes, and pheochromocytoma), psychiatric disorders, laxative abuse, and medications (Table 49.4). The pathophysiology is largely unexplained but often involves rectal relaxation, functional impairment, and sensory disturbances, leading to defecation difficulties and delayed colonic transit time. Symptoms overlap with chronic constipation, but chronic functional constipation does not develop pathological colonic dilation. Histopathologically, it is classified as myogenic (degeneration and inflammatory cell infiltration of intestinal smooth muscle), neurogenic (degeneration and reduction of autonomic nerve cells), or mesenchymopathic (interstitial cells of Cajal-related)(reduction of pacemaker cells independent of the autonomic nervous system), but these categories often overlap, and details remain unclear [3].

5 Diagnostic Criteria and Tests

There are no clear diagnostic criteria for megacolon other than toxic megacolon, but generally, a cecal diameter of 12 cm or more, an ascending colon diameter of 8 cm or more, and a rectosigmoid colon diameter of 6.5 cm or more are considered indicative of megacolon [4].

Abdominal CT and plain abdominal X-rays are useful for diagnosis, with pathological colonic dilation being a key finding after excluding organic diseases (Figs. 49.1 and 49.2). If exclusion of organic diseases is difficult with CT and plain X-rays alone, gastrointestinal contrast studies with iodinated contrast agents (Gastrografin) and colonoscopy may be considered. Clinical symptoms include constipation, abdominal bloating, abdominal pain, nausea, and vomiting, but these are not specific to this condition. Diagnostic criteria for toxic megacolon are listed in Table 49.5 [5].

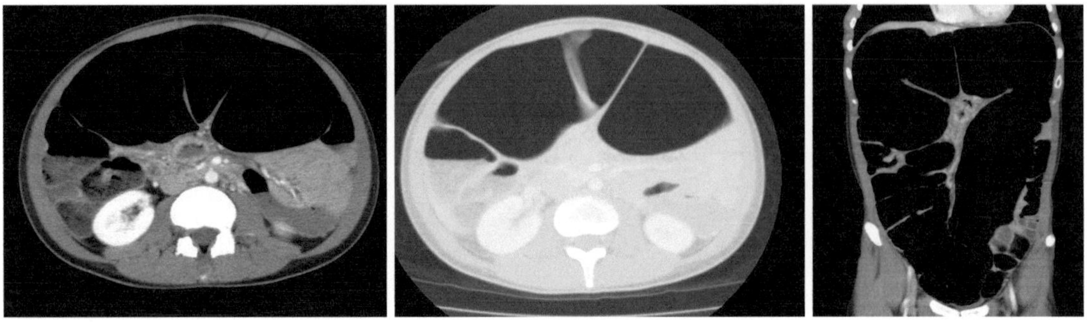

Fig. 49.1 Plain abdominal X-ray. Demonstrates the formation of air-fluid levels and pathological bowel dilation

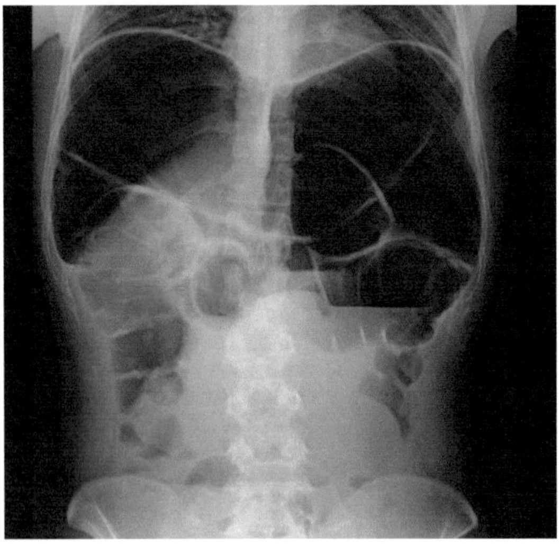

Fig. 49.2 CT scan. Left and middle: Axial CT images. Right: Coronal CT image. All images show pathological bowel dilation

Table 49.5 Diagnostic criteria for toxic megacolon

1. Radiographic evidence of colonic dilation (transverse or ascending colon diameter ≥ 6 cm on imaging)
2. Fulfillment of three or more of the following criteria:
1. Fever ≥ 38 °C
2. Heart rate ≥ 120 beats per minute
3. Leukocytosis (white blood cell count > 10,500 × 10^3/μL)
4. Anemia
3. Fulfillment of one or more of the following criteria:
1. Dehydration
2. Altered mental status
3. Electrolyte imbalance
4. Hypotension

6 Treatment

For acute megacolon, the efficacy of neostigmine has been demonstrated in overseas controlled trials. Endoscopic decompression is effective in some cases. If the affected area is limited to the colon, total colectomy may be successful.

In toxic megacolon, surgical treatment is absolutely indicated in cases of perforation, uncontrollable bleeding, organ failure, or shock. Subtotal colectomy with ileostomy is often chosen due to lower complication and mortality rates compared to total colectomy. If surgical treatment is not indicated, bowel rest and decompression are necessary, including fasting, central venous management, and placement of a nasogastric or ileus tube, with early systemic management and monitoring in preparation for potential surgical intervention. Additionally, controlling the underlying disease is essential, with steroid administration for inflammatory bowel disease and antibiotics for infections to reduce inflammation. Anticholinergic drugs, barium enema, and endoscopy are contraindicated. For chronic megacolon, dietary and pharmacological therapies are fundamental [4] (Fig. 49.3). Biofeedback therapy, a pelvic floor muscle training, is also attempted to improve defecation function [6]. Surgical treatment is indicated for cases with insufficient response to Internal medicine treatment or recurrent sigmoid volvulus. In secondary megacolon, controlling the underlying disease in addition to managing abdominal symptoms is crucial.

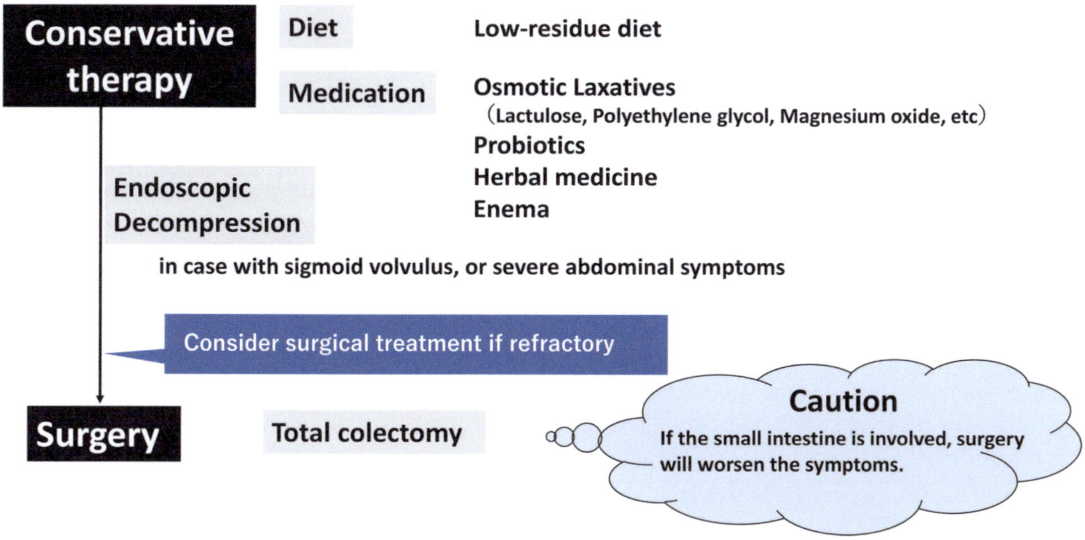

Fig. 49.3 Treatment of chronic megacolon

(i) Dietary Therapy: Low-residue diet is recommended. While dietary fiber intake is generally effective for improving constipation, in megacolon, fiber intake may increase stool volume and exacerbate abdominal symptoms.
(ii) Pharmacological Therapy: To control defecation, osmotic laxatives (polyethylene glycol, lactulose, and magnesium sulfate), probiotics, and enemas are selected. Long-term pharmacological therapy is often necessary due to difficulty in symptom control. Even if symptoms improve, normalization of the dilated bowel is considered difficult.
(iii) Decompression Therapy: In cases of severe abdominal bloating and pain due to bowel dilation, endoscopic decompression may be performed, but it is only a temporary relief of symptoms.
(iv) Surgical Treatment: Surgical treatment is indicated for cases with poor response to medical treatment or recurrent sigmoid volvulus due to pathological dilation. The general surgical procedure is total colectomy with ileorectal anastomosis [7]. Partial resection of only the dilated bowel can highly lead to residual colonic dilation [8]. If the small intestine is also affected, colectomy is associated with post-operative recurrence and exacerbation of the small intestine, requiring thorough preoperative evaluation. In such cases, cine MRI is useful for evaluating small bowel peristalsis. In cases of long-term laxative use leading to anal dysfunction, improvement in quality of life after the surgical intervention is considered unlikely.

Adult Hirschsprung disease is characterized by congenital absence of the myenteric (Auerbach) and submucosal (Meissner) plexuses, resulting in narrowing of the affected area and dilation of the proximal segment. If the area of nerve plexus absence is small, control with enemas and laxatives may be possible, but many cases require surgical treatment [9]. Appropriate diagnosis and treatment lead to a relatively good prognosis, making differentiation from other chronic megacolon conditions important.

7 Prognosis

Acute megacolon is generally transient with a good prognosis, but there is a risk of cecal and right-sided colonic perforation, which carries a mortality rate of approximately 50%, making it a severe condition. Toxic megacolon generally has a poor prognosis, although this varies slightly depending on the underlying disease. In cases of ulcerative colitis, the mortality rate ranges from 19% to 45%, with particularly poor outcomes in cases of perforation. Even when conservative treatment leads to improvement, the long-term prognosis is poor, with a high recurrence rate reported. In cases of pseudomembranous colitis, the prognosis is extremely poor, with a mortality rate of 38–80%.

Chronic megacolon, while refractory, has a relatively good prognosis if defecation control is achieved or if surgical treatment is successful.

8 Conclusion

Megacolon often presents with common abdominal symptoms such as constipation and abdominal bloating in daily clinical practice, but it is a rare disease with very low awareness, leading to cases where appropriate diagnosis and treatment are not provided. With an aging society, this condition is expected to become clinically significant, particularly in association with Parkinson's disease and disuse syndrome. Recognizing the pathophysiology is essential, and further appropriate differentiation, diagnosis, and treatment selection are required.

Take-Home Message
The course and treatment options for megacolon vary depending on the pathology, but there are no established diagnostic criteria for conditions other than toxic megacolon, leading to frequent cases of inappropriate diagnosis and treatment selection. It is crucial to first become familiar with this condition. Chronic megacolon, in particular, causes refractory constipation and abdominal bloating, and symptoms often do not improve when treated as ordinary chronic constipation. If defecation control is difficult despite the absence of organic causes, this condition should be actively considered in the differential diagnosis.

Competing Interests The author has no competing interests to declare that are relevant to the content of this chapter.

References

1. Autenrieth DM, et al. Toxic megacolon. Inflamm Bowel Dis. 2012;18:584–91.
2. Earhart MM. The identification and treatment of toxic megacolon secondary to pseudomembranous colitis. Dimens Crit Care Nurs. 2008;27:249–54.
3. Ohkubo H, et al. Histopathologic findings in patients with idiopathic megacolon: a comparison between dilated and non-dilated loops. Neurogastroenterol Motil. 2014;26:571–80.
4. Gattuso JM, et al. Clinical features of idiopathic megarectum and idiopathic megacolon. Gut. 1997;41:93–9.
5. Jalan KN, et al. An experience of ulcerative colitis. I. Toxic dilation in 55 cases. Gastroenterology. 1969;57:68–82.
6. Gladman MA, et al. Novel concepts in the diagnosis, pathophysiology, and management of idiopathic megabowel. Colorectal Dis. 2008;10. 531–538; discussion 538–540
7. Marc A, et al. Systematic review of surgical options for idiopathic megarectum and megacolon. Ann Surg. 2005;241:562–74.
8. Masaki T, et al. Nationwide survey of chronic intestinal pseudo-obstruction in surgical institutions in Japan. Surg Today. 2012;42:264–71.
9. Nakajima A, et al. Chronic Intestinal Pseudo-obstruction (CIPO). 1st ed. Tokyo: Sanno Printing; 2012. (in Japanese)

50 Case Discussion, Constipation

Ryuji Sakakibara

Abstract

Autonomic nervous system disorders of the bowel cause constipation, which not only affects the quality of life but also leads to emergency intestinal pseudo-obstruction. Diseases affecting gut innervation include diabetic neuropathy, dementia with Lewy bodies/Parkinson's disease, and multiple system atrophy. Here, we focus on typical such cases and discuss their pathophysiology and proper management.

Keywords

Parkinson's disease · Multiple system atrophy · Neurogenic gastrointestinal dysfunction · Constipation · Autonomic dysfunction · Autonomic failure

1 Introduction

Autonomic nervous system disorders, such as constipation and ileus (colonic inertia) requiring emergency visits, increase with age, and peripheral nerve disorders have become recognized as the responsible lesions [1, 2]. Patients with constipation and ileus often simultaneously experience symptoms such as indigestion. Among the causes of idiopathic upper gastrointestinal symptoms (gastroparesis), diabetes was reported to be the most common, accounting for 37–50%. Similarly, among the causes of idiopathic lower gastrointestinal symptoms (constipation), dementia with Lewy bodies (DLB) and Parkinson's disease (PD) were reported in 3% and diabetes in 4–19% of cases [3, 4].

2 Case Presentation

Case: A 67-year-old male presented with constipation and loud vocalizations at night, accompanied by his wife.

History of Present Illness: The patient had experienced constipation (difficulty in defecation and reduced frequency of defecation [once a week]) for the past year and a half. During the same period, he began to vocalize loudly at night. An MRI of the brain was performed by the previous physician, which showed no abnormalities. Recently, the patient noticed a slight tremor in his left hand and experienced forward falls while walking downhill.

Medical History: No notable conditions.

Family History: No notable conditions.

Current Symptoms: Height: 172 cm, weight: 67 kg, temperature: 36.5 °C, pulse: 78/min, regular, and blood pressure: 114/80 mmHg (sitting). Consciousness is alert. No abnormalities

R. Sakakibara (✉)
Neurology Clinic Tsudanuma and Dowakai Chiba Hospital, Funabashi, Japan

H. Kaneko et al. (eds.), *Disorders of Gut-Brain Interaction*,
https://doi.org/10.1007/978-981-95-6974-8_50

were found in cranial nerves. Tendon reflexes were normal, and no pathological reflexes were observed. Sensory systems were normal. Muscle tone in the limbs was normal, but a mild resting tremor was noted in the left hand, along with mild bradykinesia during repetitive alternating movements of the left hand. Autonomic nervous system symptoms included constipation and nocturia (twice per night). According to the patient's wife, the loud vocalizations at night involved shouting as if fighting or being attacked in a dream, accompanied by arm flailing and kicking. When awakened by his wife, the patient reported, "I was dreaming."

Key Points of Case 1

Rapid Eye Movement (REM) Sleep Behavior Disorder (RBD): The loud vocalizations and arm flailing or kicking motions at night are not hallucinations but rather RBD, where muscle tone does not decrease during REM sleep, causing dream experiences to manifest as vocalizations and movements (sleep enactment). RBD is associated with lesions in the brainstem's locus coeruleus and raphe nuclei. Constipation, from a neurological perspective, is linked to peripheral nerve lesions, including the enteric nervous system. Additionally, the resting tremor and bradykinesia in the left hand suggest lesions in the substantia nigra-striatum pathway (Parkinsonian syndrome).

Key Points of Case 2

Differential Diagnosis of Parkinsonian Syndrome: Conditions causing Parkinsonian syndrome include silent cerebral infarction (white matter multiple cerebral infarction), normal pressure hydrocephalus, PD, progressive supranuclear palsy, multiple system atrophy, corticobasal degeneration, and drug-induced Parkinsonian syndrome (antipsychotics, antidepressants, antiemetics [e.g., metoclopramide], and gastrointestinal motility drugs [e.g., sulpiride and itopride]).

Key Points of Case 3

MRI Findings: The previous physician performed an MRI of the brain, which showed no abnormalities. Neurological diseases generally have a detection rate of approximately 60% on brain MRI. This is intermediate between neurosurgical diseases (almost 100%) and psychiatric diseases (almost 0%). PD is one of the representative diseases that can be difficult to detect on MRI. Among the Parkinsonian syndromes mentioned above, silent cerebral infarction, normal pressure hydrocephalus, progressive supranuclear palsy, multiple system atrophy, and corticobasal degeneration show abnormalities on brain MRI, whereas PD and drug-induced Parkinsonian syndrome do not.

Key Points of Case 4

PD: In PD, not only are lesions found in the substantia nigra-striatum pathway, but Lewy bodies and Lewy neurites are also observed in the locus coeruleus, raphe nuclei, and enteric nervous system. The diagnosis for the patient is PD, which is considered a systemic disease affecting peripheral nerves, including the enteric nervous system.

Key Points of Case 5

Lewy Body Constipation (LBC): Recently, constipation preceding PD (often accompanied by RBD) has come to be known as LBC [4]. In such patients, myocardial metaiodobenzylguanidine (MIBG) scintigraphy (evaluation of peripheral norepinephrine [sympathetic] nerves) and DAT scan (evaluation of central dopamine nerves) have shown abnormalities, and this case also demonstrated abnormalities in these neuroimaging studies (Fig. 50.1). Lewy body diseases, including PD and DLB, are reported to be present in 7–8% of the general population in their 80s, warranting attention.

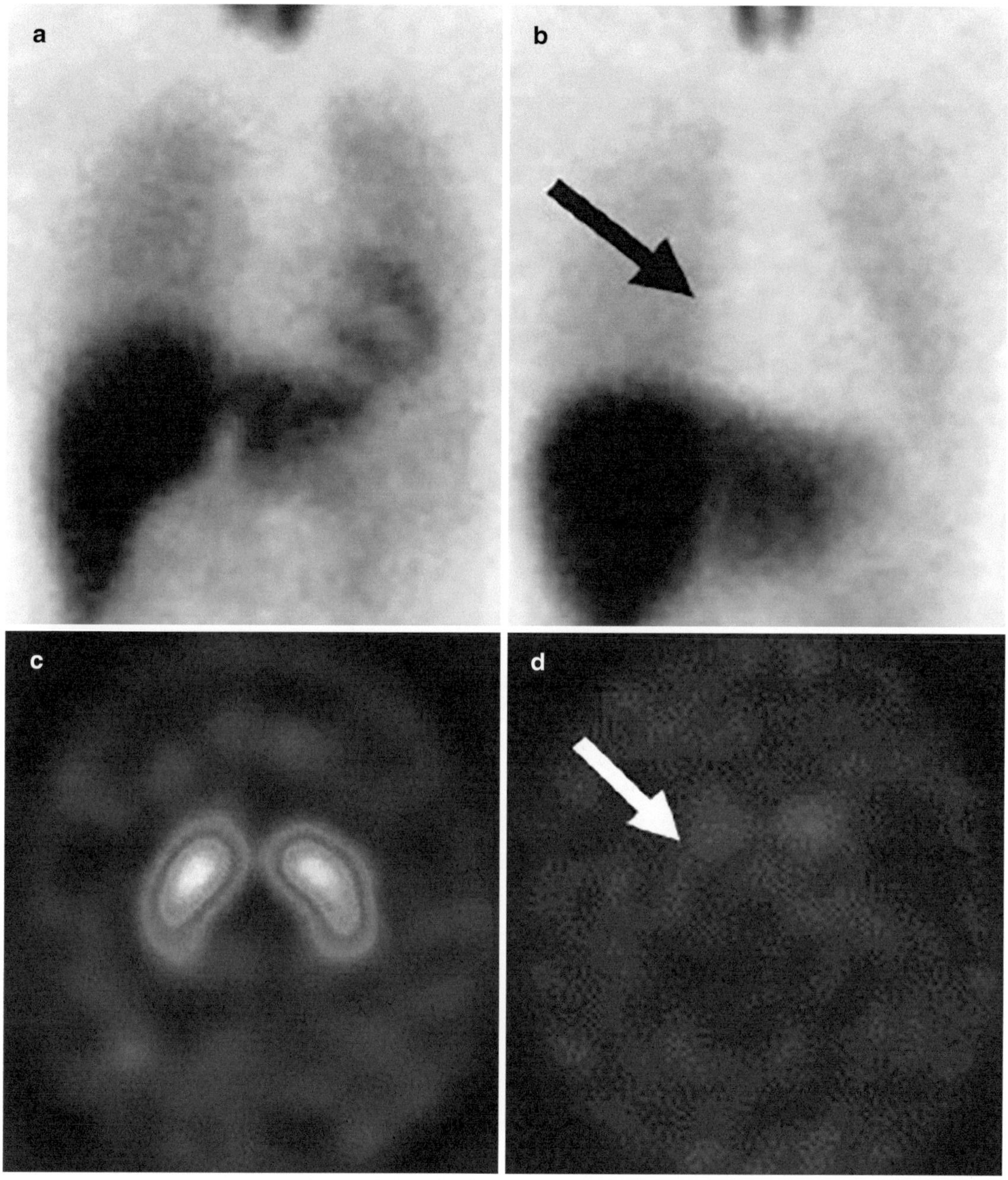

Fig. 50.1 Imaging studies in PD. Myocardial MIBG scintigraphy: (**a**) Normal late image value of heart–mediastinum ratio (HMratio). (**b**) Peripheral norepinephrine denervation (arrow). *Brain DAT Scan:* (**c**) Normal specific binding ratio (SBR), (**d**) central dopamine denervation (arrow), DAT scan (normal >2.0), and MIBG SBR normal >3.0

3 Clinical Course

Initially, the patient was treated with osmotic laxatives and epithelial function-modifying drugs, starting with a small dose of lubiprostone (12 μg, bid) to prevent nausea, followed by the usual dose (24 μg, bid), resulting in some improvement. The patient requested additional treatment, and a Kampo medicine (daikenchuto, 15 g/day, tid) with serotonin $5HT_3$ receptor-stimulating effects was initiated, leading to a reduction in difficulty defecating and an increase in defecation frequency to three to five times per week. Measurement of total colonic transit time (CTT) before and after the combination therapy showed improvement from 82 to 32 h (normal upper limit <39 h) (Fig. 50.2a), significantly enhancing patient satisfaction. Videomanometry was also effective in the detailed examination of the pathology (Fig. 50.2b) [1, 2].

Key Points of Case 6

Treatment of Constipation in the Elderly: For elderly patients with constipation, exercise and dietary fiber intake are recommended first. Pharmacotherapy should start with bulk-forming agents (polycarbophil) or osmotic laxatives (magnesium preparations, macrogol 14000) and epithelial function-modifying drugs (lubiprostone, linaclotide, and elobixibat). If these are insufficient, gastrointestinal motility drugs such as peripheral cholinergic agents (nizatidine), selective serotonin $5HT_4$ receptor agonists (mosapride), and Kampo medicine (daikenchuto with $5HT_3$-stimulating effects) can be added (Fig. 50.3).

Key Points of Case 7

Objective Gastrointestinal Function Tests: Objective tests for gastrointestinal function include the radiopaque marker method (CTT) (Fig. 50.2a). This test evaluates the transport function from the proximal colon to the rectum and is simple, correlating well with direct evaluation using radioactive isotopes. Specifically, a test capsule containing 20 radiopaque, non-absorbable ring markers (Sitzmarks, Konsyl Pharmaceuticals Inc., Edison, NJ, USA) is ingested every morning for 6 days, followed by a plain abdominal X-ray on the seventh day to count the remaining markers along the intestines. During the test period, normal diet, hydration, and exercise are maintained, but laxatives and enemas are generally avoided. There are no specific contraindications. The number of markers multiplied by 1.2 is considered the

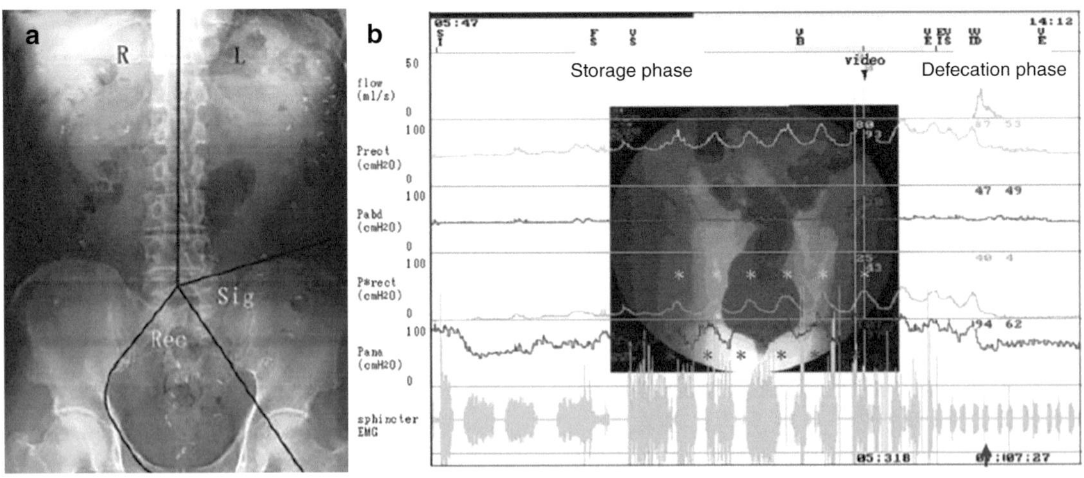

Fig. 50.2 CTT in healthy individuals (**a**) and rectoanal videomanometry (**b**). *Prect:* rectal pressure, *Pabd:* abdominal pressure, *P*rect:* rectal muscle pressure, *Pana:* anal sphincter pressure, and *Sphincter EMG:* sphincter electromyography

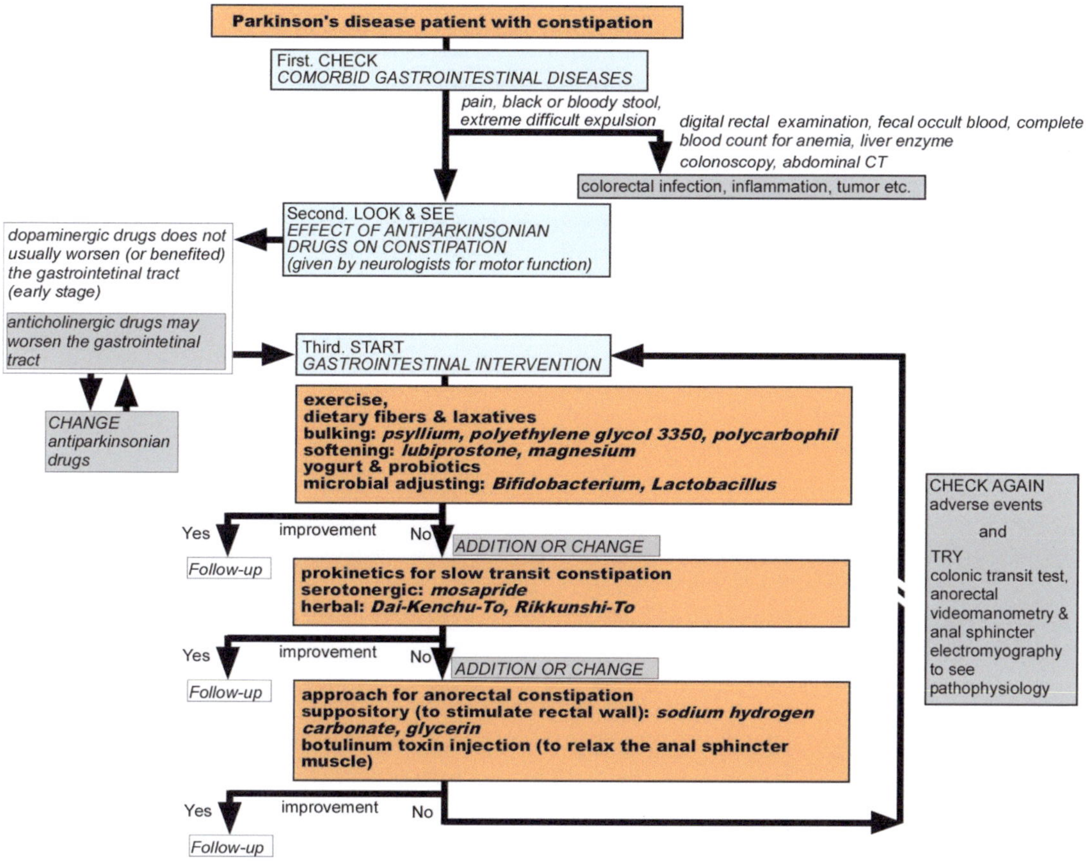

Fig. 50.3 Treatment of LBC and gastrointestinal symptoms in PD/DLB

CTT. In healthy individuals, the total colonic CTT is 39 h. Note that this method is not covered by insurance, and ethical committee approval and individual importation of Sitzmarks are required for use.

4 Discussion

In PD/DLB, Lewy bodies appear not only in the central nervous system but also in peripheral nerves, including the gastrointestinal tract. Gastrointestinal dysfunction in PD/DLB can lead to decreased absorption of levodopa, resulting in malignant syndrome, paralytic ileus (pseudo-obstruction), intestinal intussusception, volvulus, and fecal impaction ulcers requiring emergency visits. Recently, it has been clarified that Lewy body pathology in PD/DLB patients precedes in the intestines rather than the brain. The mechanisms reported include the following:

1. Honolulu Heart Program Study: Comparing individuals who defecate more than twice a day with those who defecate less than once a day, the latter group had a fourfold higher risk of developing PD. Constipation may lead to future motor symptoms, with an onset period of 10–20 years [5].
2. Braak's Hypothesis: According to Braak, Lewy body pathology in PD appears first in the dorsal motor nucleus of the vagus nerve, which is involved in autonomic functions, rather than in the substantia nigra, which is involved in motor functions [6].
3. Clinical Epidemiology: Exposure to environmental toxins (e.g., pesticides) may alter the gut microbiota, leading to Lewy body pathol-

ogy in the enteric nervous system [7]. Genome-wide association studies and microRNA analyses have highlighted substances such as GTP cyclohydrolase 1 (rotenone and paraquat) as being involved in both environmental toxins and PD pathology [8]. Changes in gut microbiota in PD include increased *Akkermansia* and decreased *Faecalibacterium* and *Roseburia*, although these changes are also observed in idiopathic constipation patients [9].

4. Prion-Like Neuroinfectivity: Aggregates of α-synuclein in the enteric nervous system exhibit prion-like neuroinfectivity, potentially ascending to the brainstem via sympathetic (thoracolumbar sympathetic trunk) and parasympathetic (vagus nerve, pelvic nerve, and spinal cord) pathways. Moderate impairment of the vagus nerve may promote both anterograde and retrograde transmission of α-synuclein from the gastrointestinal tract to the brain [10].

   Regarding the possibility of diagnosing such ultra-early stage patients, recent reports have indicated that among 18 patients diagnosed with LBC through neuroimaging, five progressed to PD/DLB, and myocardial MIBG scintigraphy showed a significantly higher positivity rate compared to DAT scans [4].

   Gastrointestinal motility is primarily regulated by the enteric nervous system, with parasympathetic acetylcholine (M_3 receptor) inducing contraction, serotonin (5-HT_4) promoting motility, and dopamine (D_2) inhibiting it (based on knockout mouse studies). Central nervous system regulation is also involved. In PD/DLB patients, upper gastrointestinal abnormalities include delayed gastric emptying (gastric emptying test) and abnormal electrogastrograms. Lower gastrointestinal abnormalities include prolonged CTT (slow-transit constipation), decreased rectal contraction as observed in rectoanal videomanometry, reduced abdominal pressure, and paradoxical sphincter contraction during defecation (PSD, anismus) (rectal constipation) [4]. These are primarily attributed to Lewy body pathology in the enteric nervous system, with central lesions also contributing to reduced abdominal pressure and PSD. Additionally, decreased levels of the gastrointestinal hormone ghrelin are observed in PD [11].

Gastrointestinal symptoms are known to worsen the prognosis of PD/DLB [12], likely reflecting complications such as ileus due to decreased gastrointestinal motility, drug resistance in motor symptoms (delayed-on, no-on), and malignant syndrome. Treatment of gastrointestinal symptoms in PD/DLB should follow general constipation treatment guidelines, minimizing emergency visits [4]. The treatment flow is shown in Fig. 50.3. Symptoms suggesting LBC in constipation patients include RBD (often referred to as adult sleep-talking, where muscle tone is not suppressed during sleep, leading to loud vocalizations and limb movements during dream experiences) and frontal lobe symptoms (selfish/unrestrained personality changes, absent-mindedness).

First, check for coexisting organic gastrointestinal diseases. Next, if motor symptoms are present, assess whether treatment for motor symptoms (e.g., levodopa) improves constipation. Levodopa may centrally improve gastrointestinal motility (deep brain stimulation can improve gastric emptying). Anticholinergic drugs are not recommended due to concerns about reducing gastrointestinal motility. If these measures are insufficient, start with exercise and toilet modifications [13, 14]. Then, use bulk-forming agents (which stretch the intestinal wall and gastrointestinal motility agent: e.g., psyllium, polyethylene glycol 3350, and polycarbophil) [8], stool softeners (e.g., lubiprostone, linaclotide [15], elobixibat, and magnesium), yogurt, and probiotics are used.

If these are still insufficient, use prokinetic agents for slow-transit constipation (e.g., prokinetics, Ach agents like nizatidine, serotonin 5-HT_4 agents like mosapride, and Kampo medicines like Rikkunshito and Daikenchuto) and rectal stimulants for rectoanal constipation (e.g., lecithin/carbonate suppositories and glycerin enemas). In Western countries, botulinum toxin injections are used for PSD/anismus.

Given that PD/DLB patients often initially present to gastroenterology, early intervention through collaboration between gastroenterology and neurology is crucial.

Competing Interests The author has no competing interests to declare that are relevant to the content of this chapter.

References

1. Sakakibara R, et al. Review of Autonomic Nervous System Function Tests for the Gastrointestinal Tract. Autonomic Nervous System Function Tests, 5th Edition (Japanese Society of Autonomic Nervous System). Bunkodo; 2015: 342–344. (in Japanese)
2. Sakakibara R, et al. Gastrointestinal disorders due to neurological and psychiatric diseases: bedside manual. Chugai Igakusha. 2019;(in Japanese)
3. Coon EA, et al. Predicting phenoconversion in pure autonomic failure. Neurology. 2020;95:e889–97.
4. Sakakibara R, et al. Lewy body constipation. J Anus Rectum Colon. 2019;3:10–7.
5. Abbott RD, et al. Frequency of bowel movements and the future risk of Parkinson's disease. Neurology. 2001;57:456–62.
6. Gelpi E, et al. Multiple organ involvement by alpha-synuclein pathology in lewy body disorders. Mov Disord. 2014;29:1010–8.
7. Yan D, et al. Pesticide exposure and risk of Parkinson's disease: dose-response meta-analysis of observational studies. Regul Toxicol Pharmacol. 2018;96:57–63.
8. Aloizou AM, et al. Parkinson's disease and pesticides: are micrornas the missing link? Sci Total Environ. 2020;744:140591. Epub 2020 Jun 29.
9. Nishiwaki H, et al. Meta-analysis of gut dysbiosis in Parkinson's disease. Mov Disord. 2020; Online ahead of print.
10. Del Tredici K, et al. To stage, or not to stage. Curr Opin Neurobiol. 2020;61:10–22.
11. Pietraszko W, et al. Assessments of plasma acyl-ghrelin levels in Parkinson's disease patients treated with deep brain stimulation. Peptides. 2020;128:170299. Epub 2020 Apr 16.
12. Wu YH, et al. Premotor symptoms as predictors of outcome in Parkinson's disease: a case-control study. PLoS One. 2016;11:e0161271. eCollection 2016.
13. Rao SS, et al. Effects of acute graded exercise on human colonic motility. Am J Physiol. 1999;276(5 Pt 1):G1221–6.
14. Sakakibara R, et al. Influence of body position on defecation in humans. Low Urin Tract Symptoms. 2010;2:16–21.
15. Freitas ME, et al. Linaclotide and prucalopride for management of constipation in patients with Parkinsonism. Mov Disord Clin Pract. 2018;5:218–20.

51 Case Discussion, Diarrhea

Yoshihisa Urita

Abstract

Diarrhea resistant to many medications and abdominal pain that worsen after meals often interfere with daily life. Malabsorption is an important cause of chronic diarrhea, whereas clinical diagnosis is difficult, especially when using an insurance-covered diagnostic method. In addition, the clinical diagnosis of a digestive disorder, which frequently induces malabsorption, is more difficult. Bile acid malabsorption may cause a digestive disorder, resulting in chronic diarrhea. However, there is no diagnostic method for bile acid malabsorption in clinical practice in Japan. Diarrhea following terminal ileum surgery, cholecystectomy, or upper gastrointestinal surgery also suggests bile acid diarrhea that does not improve with antidiarrheal medications. Bile acids are essential for micelle formation in fat digestion and are reabsorbed at the terminal ileum for reuse after fat absorption. If not reabsorbed and reaching the colon, bile acids activate cyclic AMP-dependent Cl^- channels in the colon, moving Cl^- ions into the lumen. Na^+ ions follow through intercellular spaces, increasing luminal osmolarity and causing water movement into the intestines, resulting in diarrhea. Cholestyramine, an anion exchange resin, binds bile acids by replacing Cl^- ions with bile acid COO^- ions, excreting bile acids in feces, effectively treating bile acid malabsorption-induced diarrhea. Cholestyramine is useful for diagnostic treatment.

Keywords

Irritable bowel syndrome (IBS) · Bile acid malabsorption · Cholestyramine · Terminal ileum surgery · Cholecystectomy · Upper gastrointestinal surgery · Dyslipidemia

1 Introduction

The causes of chronic diarrhea are diverse, but many patients are treated for irritable bowel syndrome (IBS). Treatments include serotonin receptor-3 antagonists (ramosetron), polycarbophil, anticholinergic drugs, as well as antidiarrheal medications such as loperamide and tannic acid albumin. While these treatments often control bowel movements and minimize impact on daily life, some patients do not respond at all. In such cases, treatment for psychiatric disorders is sometimes considered, but often without effect. Due to the ineffectiveness of various treatments, patients may become anxious and seek care from multiple medical institutions.

Y. Urita (✉)
Urita Clinic, General Medicine, Aomori, Japan
e-mail: foo@med.toho-u.ac.jp

H. Kaneko et al. (eds.), *Disorders of Gut-Brain Interaction*,
https://doi.org/10.1007/978-981-95-6974-8_51

2 Case Presentation (Bile Acid Malabsorption)

Case: A 64-year-old male.
Chief Complaint: Diarrhea.
Medical History: Appendectomy at age 9; bipolar disorder treated at a psychiatric clinic since age 39.
Family History: No notable conditions.
Allergy History: No notable conditions.
Smoking History: None.
Alcohol Consumption: Occasional drinking.
History of Present Illness: The patient has experienced sudden diarrhea for 20 years, particularly after breakfast. Diarrhea is rare in the evening and at night. Although he has an appetite, he has started to eat less due to concerns about diarrhea, resulting in a weight loss of 1–2 kg over the past year. He visited a nearby clinic and underwent upper and lower endoscopy, abdominal CT, and abdominal ultrasound, but no abnormalities were found. He was treated for diarrhea-predominant IBS with ramosetron, polycarbophil calcium, and loperamide, but his symptoms did not improve, affecting his ability to commute. He visited three other medical institutions without improvement and was referred to our department.
Physical Examination: No anemia in the palpebral conjunctiva, no jaundice in the bulbar conjunctiva. Chest: clear heart sounds, no rales. Abdomen: surgical scar in the lower right abdomen, no tenderness, normal bowel sounds.

3 Clinical Course

Multiple upper and lower endoscopies were performed previously, all showing no significant abnormalities. Therefore, a gastrointestinal function test, the ^{13}C-acetate breath test [1], was conducted (Fig. 51.1).

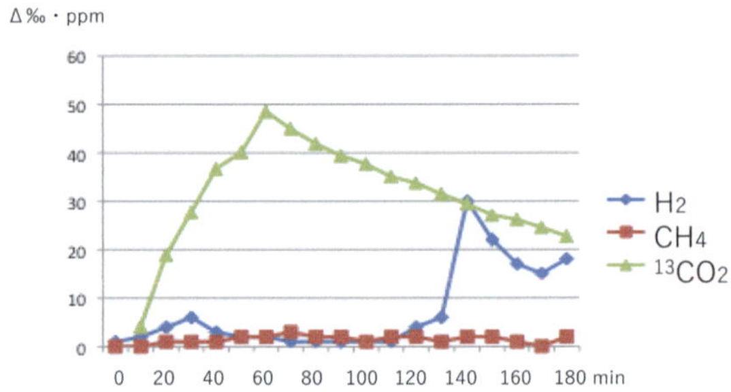

Fig. 51.1 Excretion curve of ^{13}C-acetate and hydrogen breath test in the healthy volunteer

A stable isotope, ^{13}C, was used in the form of 100 mg of ^{13}C-acetate, combined with 20 mL of lactulose (an osmotic laxative), and mixed into 200 mL of Racol NF™ enteral nutrition (200 kcal). The patient ingested this mixture, and hydrogen, methane, and $^{13}CO_2$ levels in the breath were measured over time to create a $^{13}CO_2$ excretion curve. Acetate is rapidly absorbed after gastric emptying and metabolized in the liver, with $^{13}CO_2$ excreted in the breath, reflecting gastric emptying dynamics. The peak time is crucial as an indicator of gastric emptying, and in this case, it was 60 min, within the normal range (40–80 min) [1]. Lactulose is not absorbed in the small intestine and reaches the colon, where it is broken down by intestinal bacteria through fermentation, producing short-chain fatty acids, hydrogen, and methane in patients with methane-producing bacteria.

The time when hydrogen and methane levels rise in the breath indicates the arrival of food in the colon, typically within 100–160 min. In this case, hydrogen gas levels rose above 10 ppm at 140 min, indicating no shortening or delay in small intestinal transit time. If small bowel bacterial overgrowth (SIBO) were present, early elevation of hydrogen and methane would be observed. Thus, gastrointestinal motility was normal, and SIBO was ruled out.

Given the patient's history of appendectomy at age 9, it was considered that the function of the terminal ileum, the site of bile acid reabsorption, might be affected. Additionally, the ineffectiveness of many medications suggested bile acid malabsorption-induced diarrhea. Therefore, 500 mg of cholestyramine (an anion exchange resin) was administered four times daily, resulting in the complete resolution of diarrhea that had persisted for over 20 years.

4 Discussion

When imaging and endoscopic examinations show no morphological abnormalities, chronic diarrhea is often treated as a psychiatric disorder by internists and gastroenterologists, with antidepressants and benzodiazepines frequently prescribed. However, at this stage, responses to SIBO, malabsorption, and bile acid malabsorption are often inadequate. Increased food intake in the small intestine enhances absorption, leading to elevated blood glucose and insulin secretion. In cases of overeating, absorption cannot keep up, resulting in relative malabsorption. An increase in carbohydrates in the intestines promotes the proliferation of intestinal bacteria that use them as an energy source. The short-chain fatty acids produced by this fermentation process stimulate the secretion of incretins, which inhibit gastrointestinal motility while increasing the movement of water to the intestines, causing diarrhea (Fig. 51.2).

SIBO can occur when bacteria proliferate in the small intestine for some reason. SIBO can occur due to various causes, including post-gastrectomy, diabetes-induced gastrointestinal motility disorders, and idiopathic cases. Hydrogen breath tests are useful for diagnosis but are not covered by insurance, so clinical diagnosis often relies on symptom improvement with antibiotics. Early elevation of hydrogen in breath tests indicates SIBO, but in this case, early elevation was absent, ruling out SIBO.

Malabsorption is easily associated with exocrine pancreatic insufficiency, particularly in chronic pancreatitis cases, but less so in other conditions. Digestion requires contact between digestive enzymes and food, so if the timing of food entry into the intestines and enzyme secretion is mismatched, malabsorption occurs. Besides chronic pancreatitis, malabsorption can result from gastrointestinal surgery, cholecystectomy, gallbladder dysfunction, and gastrointestinal motility disorders. Malabsorption leads to prolonged food retention in the intestines, creating an environment conducive to bacterial overgrowth, potentially resulting in SIBO. High-potency digestive enzymes like pan-

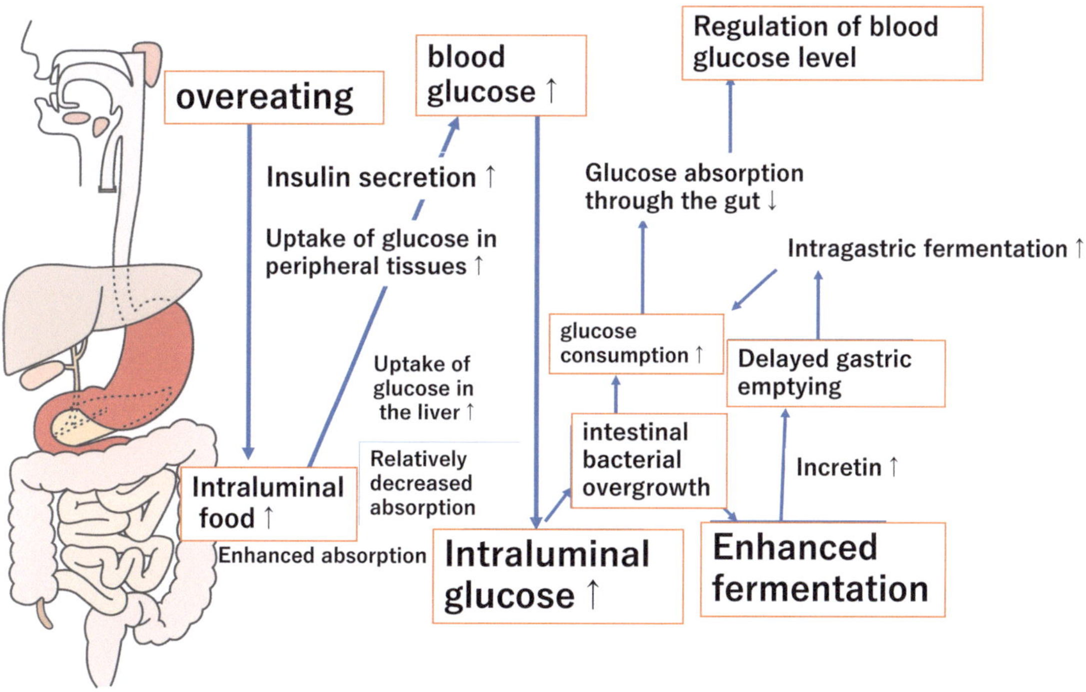

Fig. 51.2 Relative malabsorption and gastrointestinal function

crelipase are standard for exocrine pancreatic insufficiency, with a daily dose of 12 tablets, but diarrhea due to enzyme-food mismatch often improves with half this dose. Conversely, standard digestive enzyme medications may require three to five times the usual dose to ensure adequate contact with food.

In a study of 210 IBS patients with chronic diarrhea, ^{13}C-acetate breath tests were conducted to assess gastrointestinal motility and SIBO. Results showed SIBO in 51.0%, gastrointestinal motility disorders in 18.6% (gastric emptying disorders in 10.4% and small intestinal motility disorders in 9.0%), and no abnormalities in 38.1%. More than one-third of chronic diarrhea cases showed no significant differences in gastrointestinal motility or gut bacteria compared to normal, strongly suggesting bile acid malabsorption as a cause (Table 51.1).

Bile acids are essential for micelle formation in fat digestion and are reabsorbed at the terminal ileum for reuse after fat absorption. If not reabsorbed and reaching the colon, bile acids activate cyclic AMP-dependent Cl^- channels in the colon, moving Cl^- ions into the lumen. Na^+ ions follow through intercellular spaces, increasing luminal osmolarity and causing water movement into the intestines, resulting in diarrhea. This often occurs in patients with a history of terminal ileum resection for intussusception or appendectomy during childhood. This case's history of childhood appendectomy strongly suggested bile acid diarrhea. Early post-appendectomy occurrence is rare, likely due to changes in the intestinal environment and infections over time.

Several diagnostic methods for bile acid malabsorption have been reported (Table 51.1). None are covered by insurance in Japan, so the actual diagnosis is often exclusionary. Reports using the selenium-homocholic acid taurine test have examined the severity of bile acid malabsorption. Oral administration of Se-labeled bile acids and measurement of whole-body radioactivity at 3 h and 7 days post-administration diagnose bile acid malabsorption if residual radioactivity is less than 15%, with severe cases diagnosed at less than 5%. Severe bile acid malabsorption is found in 4–13% of chronic diarrhea cases, and moderate cases in 12–65%, indicating a surprisingly high frequency [3]. Fibroblast growth factor 19, produced in the ileum, suppresses bile acid synthesis in the liver, and its decreased production can cause bile acid diarrhea [2].

Cholestyramine is originally a cholesterol-lowering agent used to treat hypercholesterolemia. It works by disrupting the enterohepatic circulation of bile acids, thereby reducing the pool of bile acids, promoting bile acid synthesis, increasing cholesterol demand in the liver, and inducing LDL receptors. As a result, it helps lower cholesterol levels and is administered at a dose of six tablets per day. Cholestyramine, an anion exchange resin, binds bile acids by replacing Cl^- ions with bile acid COO^- ions, excreting bile acids in feces, effectively treating bile acid malabsorption-induced diarrhea. For diarrhea, a daily dose of four tablets is often sufficient, with patients frequently reporting noticeable changes in bowel movements the day after administration. Cholestyramine is also effective in cases of

Table 51.1 Diagnosis of bile acid malabsorption [2]

Method	Criteria	Advantages	Disadvantages
Fecal bile acid measurement	>1.2 mmol/day	Accurate	Time-consuming, requires stool collection
SeHCAT	>15%	Reproducible	Not available in Japan
Fecal ^{14}C-bile acid	–	–	Not available in Japan
7α-Hydroxy-4-cholesten-3-one (C4)	>25 ng/mL	Blood test indicates bile acid synthesis	–
FGF19	<120 pg/mL	Blood test indicates bile acid synthesis	Diurnal variation

SeHCAT Selenium-homocholic acid taurine test, *FGF19* Fibroblast growth factor 19

impaired bile secretion, such as insufficient gallbladder contraction observed in postprandial CT or abdominal ultrasound, or post-cholecystectomy due to bile acid–intestinal circulation mismatch. In clinical practice, cholestyramine's effectiveness often leads to a diagnosis of bile acid malabsorption (diagnostic treatment).

5 Conclusion

Abdominal pain and diarrhea that worsen after meals, especially breakfast, and improve in the evening suggest bile acid malabsorption. Diarrhea resistant to many medications often responds well to cholestyramine, an anion exchange resin. Diarrhea following terminal ileum surgery, cholecystectomy, upper gastrointestinal surgery, or long-standing diabetes also suggests bile acid diarrhea. Cases with insufficient gallbladder contraction postprandially or low bile storage in the gallbladder during fasting also indicate bile acid diarrhea. Diagnosing bile acid malabsorption is challenging in Japan, but cholestyramine is useful for diagnostic treatment and should be considered for chronic diarrhea treatment. However, insurance coverage for cholestyramine is limited to cases of bile acid malabsorption with dyslipidemia.

Take-Home Message
Diarrhea that does not improve with antidiarrheal medications such as loperamide, ramosetron, polycarbophil calcium, and tannic acid albumin may be due to bile acid diarrhea, and cholestyramine may be effective. It is important to check the timing of diarrhea onset in relation to meals and the patient's surgical history.

Competing Interests The author has no competing interests to declare that are relevant to the content of this chapter.

References

1. Urita Y, et al. Efficacy of lactulose plus 13-C-acetate breath test in the diagnosis of gastrointestinal motility disorders. J Gastroenterol. 2002;373:442–8.
2. Johnston I, et al. New insights into bile acid malabsorption. Curr Gastroenterol Rep. 2011;13:418–25.
3. Wedlake L, et al. Systematic review: the prevalence of idiopathic bile acid malabsorption as diagnosed by SeHCAT scanning in patients with diarrhoea-predominant irritable bowel syndrome. Aliment Pharmacol Ther. 2009;30:707–17.

Case Discussion, Abdominal Pain

52

Taisuke Nomura

Abstract

Abdominal pain is a frequent clinical complaint, ranging from mild to severe causes. When organic disease is excluded, persistent pain lasting over 3 months is classified as functional abdominal pain. Under Rome III, such pain without bowel habit changes was termed functional abdominal pain syndrome, later renamed centrally mediated abdominal pain syndrome (CAPS) in Rome IV, emphasizing central hypersensitivity and psychosocial factors.

A 24-year-old male student developed abdominal pain, appetite loss, and weight loss during exam stress in 2020. Extensive gastrointestinal and neurological investigations revealed no organic disease. Despite nutritional recovery, abdominal pain persisted, and dizziness later developed. At our hospital, workup again excluded organic causes. Stress, study difficulties, and anxiety were significant, with psychological testing showing moderate depression. Prior gastrointestinal therapies were ineffective, so treatment with antidepressants, lifestyle guidance, dietary counseling, and pain coping strategies was initiated. Within 2 weeks, abdominal symptoms, appetite mood, and weight improved.

Discussion highlights the overlap of CAPS with conditions such as abdominal epilepsy, abdominal migraine, and somatic symptom disorder, reflecting central nervous system involvement. Genetic susceptibility, stress, and environmental triggers contribute. Effective management requires addressing the brain–gut axis, central hypersensitivity, psychiatric symptoms, and psychosocial context.

Keywords

Brain-gut ineration · Functional abdominal pain · Central visceral hypersensitivity · Environmental factor · Psychological factor

1 Introduction

Abdominal pain is one of the most common symptoms encountered in outpatient and emergency care, with causes ranging from mild to severe and urgent conditions. It is essential for gastroenterologists, general internists, and emergency physicians to differentiate between diseases and assess severity. To exclude organic diseases in cases of acute abdominal pain, blood, urine, fecal occult blood tests, abdominal ultrasound, abdominal CT, gastroscopy, and colonoscopy are performed. Chronic abdominal pain

T. Nomura (✉)
NOMURA Internal and Psychosomatic Medicine, Sendai, Japan
e-mail: office@nomura-psm.net

H. Kaneko et al. (eds.), *Disorders of Gut-Brain Interaction*,
https://doi.org/10.1007/978-981-95-6974-8_52

persisting for more than three months, excluding organic diseases, is defined as functional abdominal pain, is also recognized. According to the international diagnostic criteria for functional gastrointestinal disorders, Rome III [1], chronic abdominal pain without bowel movement abnormalities is defined as functional abdominal pain syndrome (FAPS), with an estimated prevalence of about 2% in adults. In 2016, the Rome III criteria were revised to Rome IV [2], renaming FAPS to centrally mediated abdominal pain syndrome (CAPS), emphasizing the significant involvement of central nervous system hypersensitivity and psychosocial factors.

2 Case Presentation (Centrally Mediated Abdominal Pain Syndrome)

Case: A 24-year-old male university student.

Chief Complaint: Abdominal pain, difficulty eating, weight loss, dizziness.

History of Present Illness: In 2020, during his fourth year of university, the patient experienced stress related to exams and progression, leading to loss of appetite and abdominal pain, resulting in significant weight loss (4 kg in 1 month). He was hospitalized for 2 months at a nearby clinic, where gastrointestinal examinations revealed no organic diseases. His weight recovered with enteral nutrition, and he returned to school. However, abdominal pain persisted, and in 2022, he developed dizziness. He visited the neurosurgery and otolaryngology departments, underwent a brain MRI, but no abnormalities were found. Suspecting psychological factors, he was referred to our hospital.

3 Clinical Course

At the initial visit, a detailed medical interview regarding abdominal pain, bowel movement abnormalities, and loss of appetite was conducted. Physical examination revealed tenderness in the periumbilical and epigastric regions. Blood tests, including inflammatory markers, were normal, and previous gastrointestinal examinations showed no abnormalities. Brain MRI and otolaryngological examinations also showed no abnormalities, excluding organic diseases. Long-term abdominal pain and associated difficulty eating and weight loss often lead to anxiety and depression, so stress factors triggering the symptoms were assessed. Current stressors included abdominal pain and difficulty eating, leading to weight loss and inability to concentrate on studies, causing significant anxiety about promotion and graduation. Psychological tests indicated moderate depression (SDS: 51). Regarding abdominal pain, previous treatments from the gastroenterology department included proton pump inhibitors, gastrointestinal function regulators, antispasmodics, and diarrhea was treated with a high-molecular-weight *polymer* and a serotonin receptor antagonist. However, symptoms did not improve. Therefore, antidepressants (escitalopram + sulpiride) were prescribed for anxiety and depression associated with abdominal pain. To further improve lifestyle habits, the patient was guided to regulate sleep, exercise, and meal times, and received dietary counseling. The patient was also instructed to record abdominal pain symptoms and was taught coping strategies for pain, with the aim of promoting behavioral changes in daily life. Two weeks after starting treatment, abdominal symptoms gradually improved, appetite and weight increased, and anxiety and depression symptoms improved.

4 Discussion

Many hypotheses have been tested regarding the causes and management of abdominal pain symptoms without organic diseases, and the pathophysiology has been extensively studied. For example, abdominal epilepsy [3], a condition characterized by recurrent abdominal pain and abnormal electroencephalogram (EEG) findings such as slow waves and spikes, has been reported since the 1950s as an example of abdominal pain in which involvement of the central nervous system was suspected. The international classification of epileptic seizures (1981) included “partial seizures: autonomic seizures” [4]. Reports on EEG findings and abdominal pain are also found [5–7]. Additionally, recurrent abdominal pain strongly associated with migraines was classified as abdominal migraine in the International Classification of Headache Disorders in 2014 [8]. Furthermore, in cases where depression and anxiety symptoms associated with abdominal pain are central, the diagnosis of somatic symptom disorder (formerly pain disorder) in the DSM-5 [9], which is the diagnostic criteria of the American Psychiatric Association, is consistent with the symptoms of CAPS.

Thus, abdominal pain without organic diseases can be diagnosed differently depending on whether the focus is on gastrointestinal symptoms, neurological perspective, or psychiatric symptoms, but the underlying pathophysiology is thought to be very similar. Central visceral hypersensitivity is hypothesized to link these conditions, and research on the pathophysiology of central nervous system sensitization in visceral pain, including abdominal pain, is ongoing [10]. Genetic susceptibility differences among individuals, along with environmental factors such as stress and infections, are being elucidated as triggers for abdominal pain symptoms. Psychological factors and changes in central nervous system sensitivity play important roles in abdominal pain, and a multifaceted approach is required for abdominal pain without organic abnormalities. Depression and anxiety associated with abdominal symptoms are associated with changes in brain cognitive functions (altered pain sensitivity, fixing abdominal pain symptoms). This gut–brain axis indicates that central nervous system changes affect abdominal pain. Therefore, in refractory abdominal pain, addressing central nervous system changes and psychiatric symptoms related to gastrointestinal symptoms is crucial for improving abdominal symptoms. In parallel with physical examination, it is important to investigate various background factors, recording and evaluating the nature, intensity, duration, and triggers of abdominal pain, and identifying inappropriate behavior patterns or excessive pain responses.

Take-Home Message

When considering functional abdominal pain, it is essential to consider the involvement of the central nervous system in gastrointestinal symptoms from the perspective of the brain-gut interaction. This requires addressing central nervous system symptoms such as headaches, nausea, dizziness, and psychiatric symptoms such as anxiety, tension, depression, and insomnia that occur alongside abdominal pain, considering psychological and social backgrounds.

Competing Interests The author has no competing interests to declare that are relevant to the content of this chapter.

References

1. Drossman DA, et al. Rome III: the functional gastrointestinal disorders. McLean, VA: Degnon Associates; 2006.
2. Rome Foundation. Rome IV diagnostic criteria for functional gastrointestinal disorders. Raleigh, NC: Rome Foundation; 2016.
3. Moore MT. Paroxysmal abdominal pain: a form of focal symptomatic epilepsy. JAMA. 1944;124:561–3.
4. Commission on Classification and Terminology of the International League Against Epilepsy (No authors listed). Proposal for revised clinical and electroencephalographic classification of epileptic seizures. Epilepsia. 1981;22:489–501.
5. American Academy of Pediatrics Subcommittee on Chronic Abdominal Pain, North American Society for Pediatric Gastroenterology Hepatology, and Nutrition. Chronic abdominal pain in children. Pediatrics. 2005;115:e370–81.
6. Sagami Y, et al. A case of temporal lobe epilepsy with abdominal symptoms recognized as visceral hypersensitivity in gastrointestinal function tests. J Psychosomatic Gastroenterol. 2005;12:78–9. (in Japanese)
7. Zinkin NT, et al. Abdominal epilepsy. Best Pract Res Clin Gastroenterol. 2005;19:263–74.
8. Japanese Headache Society, International Headache Classification Committee. International Classification of Headache Disorders, 3rd Edition Beta Version. Igaku-Shoin; 2014. p. 14. (in Japanese)
9. American Psychiatric Association. Diagnostic and Statistical Manual of Mental Disorders, 5th ed (DSM-5). 2013.
10. Fukudo S. Psychosomatic correlation in central nervous system sensitization pathology. J Psychosomatic Med. 2021;61:177–85. (in Japanese)

53 Topics, Opioid-Induced Constipation/Narcotic Bowel Syndrome

Takaomi Kessoku

Abstract

Opioid-induced constipation (OIC) is one of the most frequent and distressing adverse effects of opioid therapy. Unlike other opioid-related side effects that improve with tolerance, OIC persists and significantly impairs quality of life, treatment adherence, and health economics. In Japan, the incidence of OIC has been reported at 40–65%, highlighting its clinical burden. Preventive strategies, including prophylactic laxatives and peripherally acting μ-opioid receptor antagonists such as naldemedine, are recommended to reduce its impact. Tapentadol, with its dual mechanism of action, may also lower the risk of constipation. In contrast, narcotic bowel syndrome (NBS) is a less recognized but clinically important manifestation of opioid-induced bowel dysfunction, characterized by chronic or recurrent abdominal pain that paradoxically worsens with continued or escalated opioid use. NBS often mimics functional or obstructive gastrointestinal disorders, leading to diagnostic delay and inappropriate dose escalation. Early recognition, structured opioid tapering, symptomatic pharmacologic therapy, and psychological support are essential for management. As opioid prescriptions increase beyond cancer-related pain to chronic nonmalignant conditions, greater clinical awareness of both OIC and NBS is crucial. Optimized diagnosis, prevention, and treatment strategies are indispensable to improve patient outcomes and ensure safe opioid use.

Keywords

Opioid-induced constipation · Prophylactic therapy · Naldemedine · Narcotic bowel syndrome · Opioid · Pain · Laxative

1 Opioid-Induced Constipation

1.1 Definition

Opioid-induced constipation (OIC) is one of the most common adverse effects experienced by patients receiving opioid analgesics. It results from the activation of μ-opioid receptors within the enteric nervous system. Unlike other opioid-related side effects such as drowsiness or nausea—which tend to improve within approximately

T. Kessoku (✉)
Department of Palliative Medicine and Gastroenterology, International University Health and Welfare Narita Hospital, Narita, Japan

Department of Gastroenterology, International University Health and Welfare Graduate School of Medicine, Narita, Japan

Department of Gastroenterology and Hepatology, Yokohama City University Graduate School of Medicine, Yokohama, Japan

H. Kaneko et al. (eds.), *Disorders of Gut-Brain Interaction*,
https://doi.org/10.1007/978-981-95-6974-8_53

10 days due to the development of tolerance—OIC rarely shows tolerance, necessitating early diagnosis and appropriate treatment.

1.2 Epidemiology

In Japan, a 2012 retrospective study reported that OIC occurred in approximately 40% of patients taking opioids, with an incidence of 34% in those receiving prophylactic laxatives and 55% in those without such prophylaxis [1]. A 2019 prospective observational study found a higher incidence of 56%, increasing to 65% in patients not receiving preventive treatment [2]. Internationally, the prevalence varies widely, with reports ranging from 32% to 87% in Europe [3] and 5% to 97% in the Netherlands [4].

1.3 Pathophysiology

Opioids exert analgesic effects by binding to central μ-opioid receptors, which constitute about 80% of the total, while 20% are found in the gastrointestinal (GI) tract. Activation of these receptors in the gut reduces GI secretions and peristalsis, delays intestinal transit, and increases anal sphincter tone, leading to OIC [5].

1.4 Diagnostic Criteria and Evaluation

The Rome IV criteria are widely used for diagnosing disorders of gut–brain interaction [6]. Functional constipation is defined under Criterion C2, while OIC is specifically defined under Criterion C6—highlighting its clinical importance. According to Rome IV, OIC is diagnosed when constipation newly develops or worsens following the initiation, change, or increase in opioid therapy, and two or more of the following symptoms are present (Fig. 53.1):

1. Straining during defecation.
2. Lumpy or hard stools.
3. Sensation of incomplete evacuation.
4. Sensation of anorectal obstruction/blockage.
5. Manual maneuvers to facilitate defecation.
6. Fewer than three spontaneous bowel movements per week.

Importantly, only item 6 addresses defecation frequency, while the others reflect defecatory difficulty [6] (Table 53.1).

	Oxycontine	Tapentadol	Hydromorphonne	Fentanyle	Morphine
Pros	Older people and first time ○ Most frequently used	**Few digestive symptoms neuropathic pain**○	Once-daily formulation available Smaller doses available Dyspnoea○	Less constipation and drowsiness Paste available Severe renal dysfunction○	Various methods of administration Respiratory distress○
Cons	Renal dysfunction △ Drug interactions noted	Large tablets. Beware of serotonin syndrome.	Renal dysfunction △	Principle first choice× Beware of serotonin syndrome Beware of drug interactions	Renal dysfunction× Strong side effects
Number of times taken internally	2 times/day	2 times/day	1 times/day	No oral formulation	2 times/day
drug formulation	Tablets, capsules Dispersions, injections	Tablets (no rescue)	Tablets, injections	Patch, injection (tablets for rescue only)	Tablets, fine granules, suppositories Oral solutions, injections, etc.
Metabolic pathway	CYP3A4 CYP2D6	Glucuronide conjugation	Glucuronide conjugation	CYP3A4	Glucuronide conjugation
Concurrent medications to be aware of (changes in blood levels of opioids)	Antifungals (↑) Macrolides (↑) Antiepileptics (↓) Anticancer drugs	SSRIs, SNRIs, MAO inhibitors (serotonin syndrome)	None	Antifungals (↑) Macrolides (↑) Antiepileptic drugs (↓) SSRIs, SNRIs, MAO inhibitors (serotonin syndrome) Anticancer drugs	None

Fig. 53.1 Characteristics of various opioid preparations

Table 53.1 Diagnostic criteria for narcotic bowel syndrome (NBS) [19]

Pain worsens or disappears incompletely with continued or increased narcotic administration
Gastrointestinal pain that worsens markedly when narcotic doses are decreased and improves when narcotics are restarted ("soar and crash")
Progression in frequency, duration and intensity of episodes of gastrointestinal pain
The nature and intensity of the pain cannot be explained by other known diagnoses

1.5 Differential Diagnosis and Comorbidities

Although OIC is commonly suspected in patients using opioids, especially those with cancer, it is crucial to recognize that chronic idiopathic constipation may coexist. If patients do not respond to standard OIC treatments, clinicians should consider underlying functional constipation.

1.6 Prevention

1.6.1 Selection of Opioid Agents with Minimal GI Side Effects

Tapentadol, which acts via both μ-opioid receptor agonism and norepinephrine reuptake inhibition (dual mechanism), is associated with a lower incidence of OIC. In a Japanese multicenter retrospective study ($n = 906$), only 0.1% of patients discontinued tapentadol due to constipation [7]. Co-administration of naldemedine (NAL) significantly reduced treatment discontinuation due to adverse events (odds ratio: 5.1) [7]. At our institution, we recommend tapentadol as the first-line opioid for patients at high risk of OIC, particularly those with pre-existing chronic constipation or difficulty achieving pain control (Fig. 53.2).

1.6.2 Use of Prophylactic Laxatives

With the approval of NAL in Japan, the therapeutic landscape for OIC has changed. Although off-label, NAL and traditional laxatives are often prescribed concurrently with opioids. The Japanese clinical guidelines for cancer pain management (2020 edition) recommend the prophylactic use of osmotic and stimulant laxatives based on clinical experience, safety profile, and cost-effectiveness. Prophylactic laxative use significantly reduces OIC incidence. Recent randomized trials have also demonstrated that while NAL and magnesium oxide achieve similar bowel movement frequencies, NAL better maintains bowel-related quality of life [8].

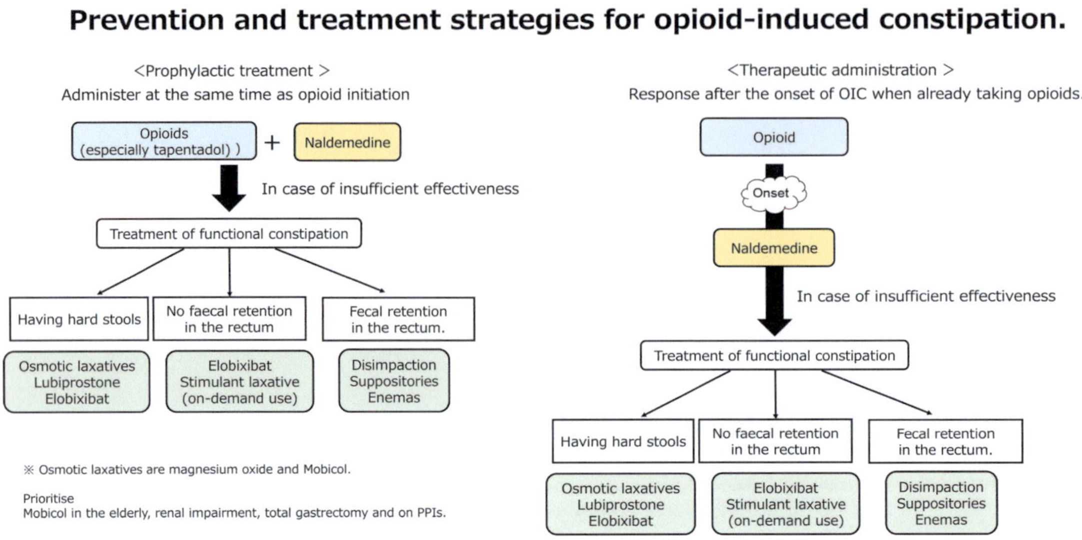

Fig. 53.2 Characteristics of various opioid preparations. Prevention and treatment strategies for opioid-induced constipation

1.7 Prognosis

OIC negatively impacts patient outcomes in several ways [9–13]:

1. Reduced quality of life.
2. Increased healthcare costs.
3. Discontinuation or modification of analgesics in one-third of cases.

From both a clinical and a health economics standpoint, proactive identification and management of OIC are critical.

2 Narcotic Bowel Syndrome

2.1 Definition

Narcotic bowel syndrome (NBS) is a subset of opioid-induced bowel dysfunction characterized by chronic or recurrent abdominal pain that worsens with continued or increased opioid use. Though underrecognized, NBS is gaining attention, especially in the context of increasing opioid prescriptions for chronic nonmalignant pain. First reported in the United States over 20 years ago [14–16] and later in China [17], NBS represents a maladaptive response to prolonged opioid exposure.

2.2 Epidemiology

The estimated prevalence of NBS is 4.2–6.4% among chronic opioid users [18].

2.3 Pathophysiology

NBS may develop in opioid-naïve individuals post-surgery or following acute pain episodes, or in patients with underlying functional GI disorders. The proposed mechanisms include:

- Activation of excitatory pain pathways in the biphasic opioid control system.
- Facilitation of pain transmission via the rostral ventral medulla and dynorphin/CCK pathways.

Morphine tolerance and hyperalgesia mediated by glial cell activation.

2.4 Diagnosis

NBS presents with colicky abdominal pain that intensifies as the opioid effect wanes. Although initially relieved by opioids, the pain-free interval shortens with time, leading to escalating opioid use. Associated symptoms include nausea, bloating, intermittent vomiting, and constipation. Patients may develop "sitophobia" (fear of eating) due to pain exacerbation after meals, leading to mild weight loss.

Diagnostic imaging may mimic partial bowel obstruction but typically reflects adynamic ileus or pseudo-obstruction. Fecal loading is common. Laboratory tests are usually unremarkable. The diagnostic hallmark is recognition that continued opioid use perpetuates or worsens symptoms, rather than alleviating them [19].

2.5 Clinical Characteristics

NBS remains underdiagnosed due to limited awareness of opioid-induced visceral pain and motility disorders. Clinicians may misinterpret opioid efficacy, thereby escalating doses and perpetuating the pain–opioid cycle. Patients often relapse shortly after discharge, necessitating repeat emergency visits or hospitalizations.

2.6 Management

Effective NBS treatment requires early recognition, a strong therapeutic alliance, structured opioid tapering protocols, symptomatic pharmacologic management (e.g., antidepressants, benzodiazepines, and clonidine), laxative therapy, and cognitive behavioral therapy.

3 Conclusion

While opioids have traditionally been used for cancer-related pain, their use is expanding in Japan to include non-cancer conditions such as chronic back pain, heart failure, and interstitial lung disease. As opioid prescriptions increase, heightened clinical attention to OIC and NBS is essential for optimizing patient outcomes.

Competing Interests The author has no competing interests to declare that are relevant to the content of this chapter.

References

1. Ishihara M, et al. Japanese Study Group for the relief of opioid-induced gastrointestinal dysfunction. A multi-institutional study analyzing effect of prophylactic medication for prevention of opioid-induced gastrointestinal dysfunction. Clin J Pain. 2012;28:373–81.
2. Tokoro A, et al. Incidence of opioid-induced constipation in Japanese patients with cancer pain: a prospective observational cohort study. Cancer Med. 2019;8(10):4883–91.
3. Larkin PJ, et al. The management of constipation in palliative care: clinical practice recommendations. Palliat Med. 2008;22(7):796–807.
4. Oosten AW, et al. A systematic review of prospective studies reporting adverse events of commonly used opioids for cancer-related pain: a call for the use of standardized outcome measures. J Pain. 2015;16(10):935–46.
5. Camilleri M, et al. Emerging treatments in neurogastroenterology: a multidisciplinary working group consensus statement on opioid-induced constipation. Neurogastroenterol Motil. 2014;26(10):1386–95.
6. Lacy BE, et al. Bowel Disorders. Gastroenterology. 2016;150:1393–407.
7. Kessoku T, et al. Tapentadol safety and patient characteristics associated with treatment discontinuation in cancer therapy: a retrospective multicentre study in Japan. Pain Ther. 2021;28
8. Kessoku T, et al. Effectiveness of naldemedine compared with magnesium oxide in preventing opioid-induced constipation: a randomized controlled. Trial Cancers (Basel). 2022;14(9):2112.
9. Kalso E, et al. Opioids in chronic non-cancer pain: systematic review of efficacy and safety. Pain. 2004;112(3):372–80.
10. Panchal SJ, et al. Opioid-induced bowel dysfunction: prevalence, pathophysiology and burden. Int J Clin Pract. 2007;61(7):1181–7.
11. Timothy JB, et al. The prevalence, severity, and impact of opioid-induced bowel dysfunction: results of a US and European patient survey (PROBE 1). Pain Med. 2009;10(1):35–42.
12. Tuteja AK, et al. Opioid-induced bowel disorders and narcotic bowel syndrome in patients with chronic non-cancer pain. Neurogastroenterol Motil. 2010;22(4) 424–30, e96.

13. Hjalte F, et al. The direct and indirect costs of opioid-induced constipation. J Pain Symptom Manag. 2010;40(5):696–703.
14. Sandgren JE, et al. Narcotic bowel syndrome treated with clonidine. Ann Intern Med. 1984;101:331–4. [PubMed: 6147108]
15. Rogers M, Cerda JJ. Editorial: the narcotic bowel syndrome. J Clin Gastroenterol. 1989;11:132–5.
16. Wong V, et al. A case of narcotic bowel syndrome successfully treated with clonidine. Postgrad Med J. 1994;70:138–40. [PubMed: 7909601]
17. Chen J, et al. Heroin addiction and surgical abdominal pain: report of three cases. Chin J Internal Med. 1995;34:46–8.
18. Kurlander JE, Drossman DA. Diagnosis and treatment of narcotic bowel syndrome. Nat Rev Gastroenterol Hepatol. 2014;11(7):410–8.
19. Grunkemeier DM, et al. Clin Gastroenterol Hepatol. 2007;5:1126–39.

Topics, Gut Microbiota and Functional Bowel Disorders

54

Tatsuhiro Masaoka

Abstract

Gut microbiota play several physiological and pathophysiological roles. Dysbiosis, a state of altered gut microbiota, has been increasingly recognized for its association with various diseases. In line with this trend, functional bowel disorders, which are disorders of gut-brain interaction in the lower gastrointestinal tract, are influenced by gut microbiota. As treatments of functional bowel disorders targeting gut microbiota include probiotics, low fermentable oligosaccharides, disaccharides, monosaccharides, and polyols diets, non-absorbable antibiotics, and fecal microbiota transplantation are known. However, the optimal treatment strategy in this area is not established yet. Further research is required to investigate these issues.

Keywords

Functional bowel disorders · Irritable bowel syndrome · Functional constipation · Gut microbiota · Dysbiosis · Probiotics · Low FODMAP diets · Antibiotics · Fecal microbiota transplantation

1 Introduction

The lower gastrointestinal tract, unlike the upper gastrointestinal tract, where gastric acid and bile acids are secreted, allows for the reabsorption of bile acids at the terminal ileum, creating an environment conducive to bacterial colonization and the formation of gut microbiota. The total weight of the gut microbiota is estimated to be 1–2 kg. Approximately 99% of the gut microbiota consists of bacteria belonging to the phyla Firmicutes, Actinobacteria, Bacteroidetes, and Proteobacteria. Gut microbiota play roles in the metabolism of dietary fibers that human digestive enzymes cannot degrade, the production of short-chain fatty acids, defense against pathogens, and the synthesis of vitamins. Dysbiosis, a state of altered gut microbiota, has been increasingly recognized for its association with various diseases such as cancer, inflammatory diseases, and metabolic disorders. In line with this trend, functional bowel disorders, which are disorders of gut–brain interaction (DGBI) in the lower gastrointestinal tract, are influenced by gut microbiota. This chapter provides an overview of the role of gut microbiota in the pathophysiology of functional bowel disorders and the treatment strategies targeting gut microbiota.

T. Masaoka (✉)
Kawasaki Municipal Hospital, Kawasaki, Japan
e-mail: tmasaoka@mbr.nifty.com

H. Kaneko et al. (eds.), *Disorders of Gut-Brain Interaction*,
https://doi.org/10.1007/978-981-95-6974-8_54

2 Gut Microbiota and Functional Bowel Disorders

There have been numerous reports on the presence of dysbiosis in irritable bowel syndrome (IBS), a representative functional bowel disorder. Meta-analyses of gut microbiota in IBS have shown a decrease in genus *Bifidobacterium* and genus *Faecalibacterium*, and an increase in family *Lactobacillaceae*, genus *Bacteroides*, and family *Enterobacteriaceae* [1]. In Japan, studies have reported an increase in *Lactobacillus* and *Veillonella* in the fecal gut microbiota of IBS patients, along with elevated concentrations of acetate, propionate, and total organic acids in fecal metabolites, which correlate with IBS symptoms [2]. These findings suggest that gut microbiota and their metabolites are involved in the pathophysiology of IBS. The Japanese Society of Gastroenterology's "Evidence-based clinical practice guidelines for Irritable Bowel Syndrome 2020," commented as "Gut microbiota, increased mucosal permeability, and low-grade inflammation are associated with the pathophysiology of IBS" for the background question "Are gut microbiota, increased mucosal permeability, and low-grade inflammation associated with the pathophysiology of IBS?" [3]. In functional constipation, another functional bowel disorder, the presence of dysbiosis has also been reported [4].

Post-infectious IBS (PI-IBS) is a subgroup of IBS patients who develop the condition following acute gastroenteritis. The concept of PI-IBS was proposed following a cohort study in Spain, where the prevalence of IBS increased among individuals who contracted infectious gastroenteritis caused by *Salmonella enteritidis* [5]. Dysbiosis triggered by infection is thought to induce IBS-like symptoms. Meta-analyses reported an odds ratio of 5.86 (95% confidence interval: 3.60–9.54) for PI-IBS following acute infection, indicating an increased risk of IBS development for several years post-infection [6].

3 Treatment of Functional Bowel Disorders Targeting Gut Microbiota

In clinical practice, IBS treatment often involves symptomatic therapies such as antispasmodics, antidiarrheals, and laxatives for abdominal pain, diarrhea, and constipation, respectively. Treatments targeting gut microbiota as one of the pathophysiology of IBS include probiotics, low fermentable oligosaccharides, disaccharides, monosaccharides, and polyols (FODMAP) diets, non-absorbable antibiotics, and fecal microbiota transplantation (FMT) [7].

In Japan, probiotics are covered by insurance and are used as pharmacological therapy for IBS regardless of the subtype. Probiotics are microorganisms considered beneficial for human health. Related terms include prebiotics, which are indigestible food components that promote the growth of beneficial gut microbiota, and synbiotics, which combine probiotics and prebiotics. Numerous intervention trials and meta-analyses have confirmed the efficacy of probiotics such as *Bifidobacterium infantis* in IBS [8]. The mechanisms of efficacy include the antibacterial properties of administered bacteria against pathogenic bacteria, regulation of tight junctions in intestinal epithelial cells to maintain intestinal permeability, normalization of intestinal motility to reduce visceral hypersensitivity, and balancing the production of interleukin (IL)-10 and IL-12 in the intestine [9]. Probiotics are not only effective but also superior in terms of safety and cost. However, the optimal types and doses of probiotics for IBS treatment remain unclear. Recent studies have shown that specific strains such as *Bifidobacterium infantis* and *Lactobacillus reuteri* are effective in improving IBS symptoms [10, 11], warranting further investigation. Probiotics have also been reported to be effective in functional constipation, another functional bowel disorder, in studies conducted in Japan [12].

The efficacy of low FODMAP diets for IBS has been reported from Western countries. These short-chain carbohydrates are poorly absorbed in the small intestine, rapidly fermented and metabolized by gut bacteria, producing hydrogen and methane gases, and drawing water into the intestinal lumen due to their high osmolarity. Low FODMAP diets have been reported to improve symptoms in 50–80% of IBS patients, with the mechanism thought to involve changes in gut microbiota and metabolites [13, 14]. Thus, low FODMAP diets are considered treatments targeting gut microbiota. However, the optimal duration for maintaining a low FODMAP diet is not established yet. Data on the efficacy of low FODMAP diets for IBS patients in Japan are currently lacking, and further data collection is demanded to determine the feasibility of introducing strict dietary restrictions in clinical practice.

The efficacy of non-absorbable antibiotics, particularly rifaximin, for IBS has been reported from Western countries. In 2011, a study involving around 300 patients in each group (rifaximin and placebo) was published in the New England Journal of Medicine [15]. Under physiological conditions, the presence of bile acids keeps bacterial counts low in the small intestine. However, in small intestinal bacterial overgrowth (SIBO), characterized by abnormal proliferation of bacteria such as *Escherichia coli* and *Clostridium perfringens*, increased production of hydrogen and methane gases, intestinal motility disorders, malabsorption, and intestinal mucosal inflammation occur [16]. Some IBS patients diagnosed based on symptoms may have SIBO, and the mechanism by which non-absorbable antibiotics are effective for IBS is thought to involve normalization of gut microbiota and suppression of SIBO [17]. In the United States, rifaximin is approved for use in diarrhea-predominant IBS patients, and its use is strongly recommended in the 2021 revised guidelines of the American College of Gastroenterology (ACG) [18]. Rifaximin is available but is only covered by Japanse health insurance system for hyperammonemia in hepatic encephalopathy, and further investigation into its efficacy for IBS patients in Japan is anticipated.

4 Fecal Microbiota Transplantation

FMT is a treatment that transplants the gut microbiota from a donor into the recipient's alimentary tract. The first report of FMT for IBS was published in 2014, showing symptom improvement in 9 out of 13 cases (70%), with only one case of increased flatulence as an adverse event [19]. In Japan, FMT using colonoscopy was performed on 10 IBS patients (eight with diarrhea-predominant IBS) resistant to medical treatment for over a year based on Rome III criteria, resulting in normalization of stool consistency in 6 out of 10 cases, improvement in abdominal symptoms, and increased gut microbiota diversity [20]. No severe adverse events were observed in this study. Johnsen et al. conducted a randomized controlled trial (RCT) comparing self-administered stool with FMT, reporting a symptom improvement rate of 65% (36 out of 55 cases) in the treatment group versus 43% (12 out of 28 cases) in the control group 3 months post-FMT, indicating that the improvement rate was significantly higher in the treatment group [21]. Mazzawi et al. performed FMT using upper gastrointestinal endoscopy on 13 IBS patients based on Rome III criteria, observing symptom improvement in eight cases, which was maintained throughout the 20- or 28-week observation period [22].

Conversely, some reports indicate no clear efficacy. Halkjaer et al. conducted a randomized double-blind placebo-controlled trial administering stool capsules or a placebo for 12 days to IBS patients, finding significant symptom improvement in both the treatment and placebo groups 3 months post-administration, despite improved gut microbiota diversity in the treatment group [23]. A meta-analysis of RCTs on FMT for IBS showed that symptom improvement 3 months post-FMT was comparable to placebo. The ACG guidelines state that evidence for the efficacy of FMT for IBS is lacking, and it is not recommended at present. Recently, long-term outcomes of FMT for IBS have been reported, showing symptom improvement, enhanced quality of life, and improved dysbiosis in the donor stool group, with no long-term adverse events [24].

Thus, the efficacy of FMT for IBS remains inconclusive and requires further investigation. Factors influencing study design include the route of administration (endoscopy, enema, stool capsules), the state of the stool (freshly collected or frozen), the setting of control groups, the origin of donor stool, and the frequency of administration. Further research is needed, including considerations of study design.

5 Conclusion

The role of gut microbiota in the pathophysiology of functional bowel disorders is well-established. However, how to leverage this knowledge for treatment and management remains an area for further investigation. Further research is required to investigate these issues.

Take-Home Message
In the treatment of functional bowel disorders targeting gut microbiota, the most practical therapy in clinical practice is considered to be the administration of probiotics. As mentioned above, the types and optimal doses of effective probiotics are not yet clear, but it is recommended to start with formulations available at the reader's facility.

Competing Interests The author has no competing interests to declare that are relevant to the content of this chapter.

References

1. Pittayanon R, et al. Gut microbiota in patients with irritable bowel syndrome—a systematic review. Gastroenterology. 2019;157:97–108.
2. Tana C, et al. Altered profiles of intestinal microbiota and organic acids may be the origin of symptoms in irritable bowel syndrome. Neurogastroenterol Motil. 2010;22(512–519):e114–5.
3. Fukudo S, et al. Evidence-based clinical practice guidelines for irritable bowel syndrome 2020. J Gastroenterol. 2021;56:193–217.
4. Parthasarathy G, et al. Relationship between microbiota of the colonic mucosa vs feces and symptoms, colonic transit, and methane production in female patients with chronic constipation. Gastroenterology. 2016;150:367–79.
5. Mearin F, et al. Dyspepsia and irritable bowel syndrome after a salmonella gastroenteritis outbreak: one-year follow-up cohort study. Gastroenterology. 2005;129:98–104.
6. Thabane M, et al. Systematic review and meta-analysis: the incidence and prognosis of post-infectious irritable bowel syndrome. Aliment Pharmacol Ther. 2007;26:535–44.
7. Masaoka T, et al. Latest findings on the treatment of irritable bowel syndrome (current status and future prospects of irritable bowel syndrome treatment). J Japan Soc Gastroenterol. 2019;116:570–5. (in Japanese)
8. O'Mahony L, et al. Lactobacillus and bifidobacterium in irritable bowel syndrome: symptom responses and relationship to cytokine profiles. Gastroenterology. 2005;128:541–51.
9. Abbas Z, et al. Cytokine and clinical response to Saccharomyces boulardii therapy in diarrhea-dominant irritable bowel syndrome: a randomized trial. Eur J Gastroenterol Hepatol. 2014;26:630–9.
10. Yuan F, et al. Efficacy of Bifidobacterium infantis 35624 in patients with irritable bowel syndrome: a meta-analysis. Curr Med Res Opin. 2017;33:1191–7.
11. Hojsak I. Probiotics in disorders of gut-brain interaction. Adv Exp Med Biol. 2019;1125:121–37.
12. Fuyuki A, et al. Efficacy of bifidobacterium bifidum G9-1 in improving quality of life in patients with chronic constipation: a prospective intervention study. Biosci Microbiota Food Health. 2021;40:105–14.
13. Staudacher HM, et al. The low FODMAP diet: recent advances in understanding its mechanisms and efficacy in IBS. Gut. 2017;66:1517–27.
14. McIntosh K, et al. FODMAPs alter symptoms and the metabolome of patients with IBS: a randomised controlled trial. Gut. 2017;66:1241–51.
15. Pimentel M, et al. Rifaximin therapy for patients with irritable bowel syndrome without constipation. N Engl J Med. 2011;364:22–32.
16. Rezaie A, et al. How to test and treat small intestinal bacterial overgrowth: an evidence-based approach. Curr Gastroenterol Rep. 2016;18:8.
17. Pimentel M. Review of rifaximin as treatment for SIBO and IBS. Expert Opin Investig Drugs. 2009;18:349–58.
18. Lacy BE, et al. ACG clinical guideline: management of irritable bowel syndrome. Am J Gastroenterol. 2021;116:17–44.

19. Pinn DM, et al. Is fecal microbiota transplantation the answer for irritable bowel syndrome? A single-center experience. Am J Gastroenterol. 2014;109:1831–2.
20. Mizuno S, et al. Bifidobacterium-rich fecal donor may be a positive predictor for successful fecal microbiota transplantation in patients with irritable bowel syndrome. Digestion. 2017;96:29–38.
21. Johnsen PH, et al. Faecal microbiota transplantation versus placebo for moderate-to-severe irritable bowel syndrome: a double-blind, randomised, placebo-controlled, parallel-group, single-Centre trial. Lancet Gastroenterol Hepatol. 2018;3:17–24.
22. Mazzawi T, et al. The kinetics of gut microbial community composition in patients with irritable bowel syndrome following fecal microbiota transplantation. PLoS One. 2018;13:e0194914–04.
23. Halkjær SI, et al. Faecal microbiota transplantation alters gut microbiota in patients with irritable bowel syndrome: results from a randomised, double-blind placebo-controlled study. Gut. 2018;67:2107–15.
24. El-Salhy M, et al. Efficacy of fecal microbiota transplantation for patients with irritable bowel syndrome at 3 years after transplantation. Gastroenterology. 2022;163:982–994.e14.

55 Topics, Scientific Significance of the Bristol Stool form Scale

Yuji Naito

Abstract

The Bristol Stool Form Scale (BSFS) is a diagnostic tool that classifies stool shape and consistency into seven categories and is widely used as a criterion for diagnosing constipation and diarrhea. Among constipation patients, the strongest factors associated with decreased Patient Assessment of Constipation Quality of Life (QOL) scores (indicating better QOL) were "normal stool form" (BSFS Type 4) and "bowel movements more than three times per week." The relationship between gut microbiota and BSFS is also updated.

Keywords

Bristol Stool Form Scale · Chronic constipation · Quality of life · Gut microbiota

1 What Is the Bristol Stool Form Scale?

The Bristol Stool Form Scale (BSFS) (see Fig. 43.1, in Chap. 43) was proposed in 1997 by Heaton from the University of Bristol, UK. It is a diagnostic tool that classifies stool shape and consistency into seven categories and is widely used as a criterion for diagnosing constipation and diarrhea [1]. While the BSFS relies on patient-reported subjective information, recent advancements have introduced artificial intelligence (AI) applications, including smartphone-based analyses [2]. AI-based stool characteristic analysis showed a stronger correlation with diarrhea severity scores than patient reports, suggesting that it could provide a more objective measure of stool characteristics for future clinical research.

Y. Naito (✉)
Department of Human Immunology and Nutrition Science, Kyoto Prefectural University of Medicine, Kyoto, Japan
e-mail: ynaito@koto.kpu-m.ac.jp

H. Kaneko et al. (eds.), *Disorders of Gut-Brain Interaction*,
https://doi.org/10.1007/978-981-95-6974-8_55

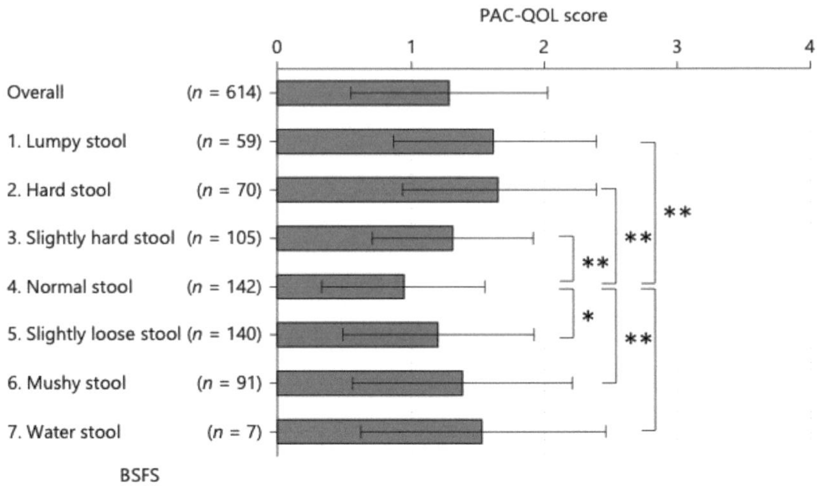

Fig. 55.1 Relationship between BSFS and the Japanese version of the PAC-QOL. Statistically significant differences were observed between BSFS type 4 and all the other types except Type 7 ($^*p < 0.05$ and $^{**}p < 0.01$)

2 BSFS and Chronic Constipation

The BSFS is recognized as a reflection of colonic transit time [3, 4]. Alongside bowel movement frequency, it serves as a valuable indicator of intestinal motility. Numerous studies suggest that Types 1 and 2 are indicative of delayed colonic transit constipation. However, in an Asian study utilizing radiopaque markers for colonic transit time analysis, BSFS Types 3 and below were found to be better predictors of delayed colonic transit than Type 2 or lower [5].

According to the Rome IV diagnostic criteria for chronic constipation, a diagnosis requires the presence of at least two out of six specified criteria, one of which is "Lumpy or hard stools (BSFS 1-2) more than one-fourth (25%) of defecations." Similarly, the "Chronic Constipation Treatment Guidelines" published in Japan include "stools presenting as Type 1 or 2 in more than one-fourth of defecations" as a diagnostic criterion [6].

3 BSFS and Quality of Life

A study conducted in Japan involving 614 adult patients diagnosed with chronic constipation and receiving prescribed medications (306 men and 308 women) examined the relationship between BSFS and QOL [7]. QOL was assessed using the Japanese version of the Patient Assessment of Constipation Quality of Life (PAC-QOL), a self-report evaluation tool consisting of 28 questions using a 5-point Likert scale.

The most commonly used laxatives before the survey were magnesium oxide-based osmotic laxatives (64.8%), followed by stimulant laxatives (26.4%), Kampo medicines (19.9%), suppositories/enemas (8.6%), and other medications (17.6%). The mean PAC-QOL score was 1.29 ± 0.74, with the lowest score (indicating the highest QOL) being 0.94 ± 0.61, except for Type 7, aged 65 years or older; Type 4 BSFS was observed regardless of age. Statistically significant differences were observed between BSFS type 4 and all the other types except Type 7 (Fig. 55.1).

Key factors influencing QOL in constipation patients included stool form, bowel movement frequency, history of anxiolytic or antidepressant use, age, gender, and treatment duration. Among these, the strongest factors associated with decreased PAC-QOL scores (indicating better QOL) were "normal stool form" (BSFS Type 4) and "bowel movements more than three times per week."

Yamada et al. [8] conducted a treatment satisfaction survey among 167 patients with chronic constipation and found that 60% were dissatisfied with their treatment. Additionally, factors associated with treatment satisfaction included "less than three bowel movements per week" (odds ratio: 0.376, 95% CI: 0.156–0.904, $P = 0.029$) and "BSFS Type 3" (odds ratio: 0.401, 95% CI: 0.170–0.946, $P = 0.037$). These findings suggest that, in Japan, Type 3 stool, traditionally considered normal, may not be perceived as satisfactory.

4 BSFS and Gut Microbiota

Many studies have investigated the relationship between gut microbiota and constipation, and analysis of BSFS and the gut microbiota is ongoing. Vandeputte et al. [9] reported that in individuals with hard stools (Types 1 and 2), indicative of functional constipation and delayed colonic transit, microbial diversity (richness and evenness) was increased, with a notable decrease in Prevotella species. Their study, which focused on young to middle-aged Western women, highlights the necessity of considering racial and geographical variations in microbiota composition.

Takagi et al. [10] conducted a 16S rRNA V3-V4 sequencing analysis on the gut microbiota of 277 healthy Japanese individuals and reported findings related to BSFS. Gender differences were observed in microbial diversity (β-diversity), in genus-level analysis, with men exhibiting higher levels of Prevotella, Megamonas, Fusobacterium, and Megasphaera, while women had higher levels of Bifidobacterium, Ruminococcus, and Akkermansia. Recent shotgun metagenomic analyses have further confirmed age- and sex-related microbiota variations. Contributing factors may include differences in phages that control the bacterial flora.

The analysis of the relationship between the gut microbiota and BSFS revealed no significant differences in diversity between men and women based on stool consistency. Genus-level analysis revealed that Fusobacterium and Bilophila were significantly increased in men with softer stools (BSFS Types 5 and 6), whereas Oscillospira was more abundant in those with harder stools (BSFS Types 1 and 2). Bifidobacterium, a beneficial bacterium commonly found in Japanese women, accounting for an average of 10% of the total, was more prevalent in individuals with harder stools, with this trend being more pronounced in women.

5 Conclusion

BSFS is a useful tool for maintaining a positive patient–physician relationship related to stool form-related interventions, and more objective assessment methods utilizing image analysis are currently being developed. Patient satisfaction surveys conducted in Japan indicate that BSFS Type 4 is associated with the highest satisfaction levels. This differs from the Western perspective, where Types 3, 4, and 5 are considered normal, and therefore further consideration is required in future responses.

Take-Home Message
The BSFS is an essential clinical tool for diagnosing chronic constipation, assessing QOL, and understanding constipation pathophysiology. In Japan, BSFS Type 4 is particularly associated with higher patient satisfaction in QOL assessments.

Competing Interests The author has no competing interests to declare that are relevant to the content of this chapter.

References

1. Mearin F, et al. Bowel disorders. Gastroenterology. 2016;150:1393–407.
2. Pimentel M, et al. A smartphone application using artificial intelligence is superior to subject self-reporting when assessing stool form. Am J Gastroenterol. 2022;117:1118–24.
3. Degen LP, et al. How well does stool form reflect colonic transit? Gut. 1996;39:109–13.
4. Longstreth GF, et al. Functional bowel disorders. Gastroenterology. 2006;130:1480–91.
5. Jaruvongvanich V, et al. Prediction of delayed colonic transit using Bristol stool form and stool

frequency in eastern constipated patients: a difference from the west. J Neurogastroenterol Motil. 2017;23:561–8.
6. Japanese Society of Gastroenterology. Chronic Constipation Treatment Guidelines 2017 (Chronic Constipation Diagnosis and Treatment Research Group). Nankodo; 2017. (in Japanese)
7. Ohkubo H, et al. Relationship between stool form and quality of life in patients with chronic constipation: an internet questionnaire survey. Digestion. 2021;102:147–54.
8. Yamada E, et al. Positioning of Bristol stool form scale type 3 in constipation treatment satisfaction: a multicenter study in Japan. J Gastroenterol Hepatol. 2021;36:2125–30.
9. Vandeputte D, et al. Stool consistency is strongly associated with gut microbiota richness and composition, enterotypes, and bacterial growth rates. Gut. 2016;65:57–62.
10. Takagi T, et al. Differences in gut microbiota associated with age, sex, and stool consistency in healthy Japanese subjects. J Gastroenterol. 2019;54:53–63.

Part VIII

Anorectum, Basic Edition

Anorectum, Anatomy

56

Shingo Tsujinaka

Abstract

This chapter outlines the anatomy, epithelium, vasculature, musculature, and innervation of the rectum and anal canal. The rectum extends from the sacrum to the upper edge of the puborectalis muscle attachment, harboring mucus-secreting columnar epithelium. The (surgical) anal canal, 4–5 cm long, is defined as the tubular part extending from the upper edge of the puborectalis muscle attachment to the anal verge and comprises transitional epithelium, anal epithelium, and stratified squamous epithelium to the boundary of anal skin. Muscular components, including the levator ani muscles, conjoined longitudinal muscle, and internal/external sphincters, support fecal continence and defecation. Arterial supply derives from superior, middle, and inferior rectal arteries, whereas venous plexuses drain into the portal and systemic systems. Neural regulation involves sympathetic and parasympathetic fibers from splanchnic and pelvic nerves, as well as somatic innervation via the pudendal and levator ani nerves, facilitating coordinated motor and sensory control. These structures mutually contribute to the functional and surgical relevance of anorectal anatomy.

Keywords

Columnar epithelium · Transitional zone epithelium · Stratified squamous epithelium · Levator ani muscle · Internal anal sphincter · External anal sphincter · Conjoined longitudinal muscle · Superior and inferior hypogastric plexuses · Pelvic splanchnic nerves · pudendal nerve

1 Rectum and Anal Canal

1.1 Rectum

The large intestine is approximately 1.5 m long (Fig. 56.1), with the rectum being the most distal part. The terminal portion of the rectum is expanded, forming the ampulla. The rectum is defined as extending from the level of the sacrum to the upper edge of the attachment of the puborectalis muscle, ending at the anal canal [1]. The longitudinal muscle bands of the colon, known as taeniae, are absent in the rectum, where they merge to form a continuous longitudinal muscle layer. Therefore, the boundary between the colon and rectum can also be defined by the termination of the taeniae [2]. The rectum is approximately 15–20 cm in length and is further

S. Tsujinaka (✉)
Tohoku Medical and Pharmaceutical University, Sendai, Japan
e-mail: tsujinakas@tohoku-mpu.ac.jp

H. Kaneko et al. (eds.), *Disorders of Gut-Brain Interaction*,
https://doi.org/10.1007/978-981-95-6974-8_56

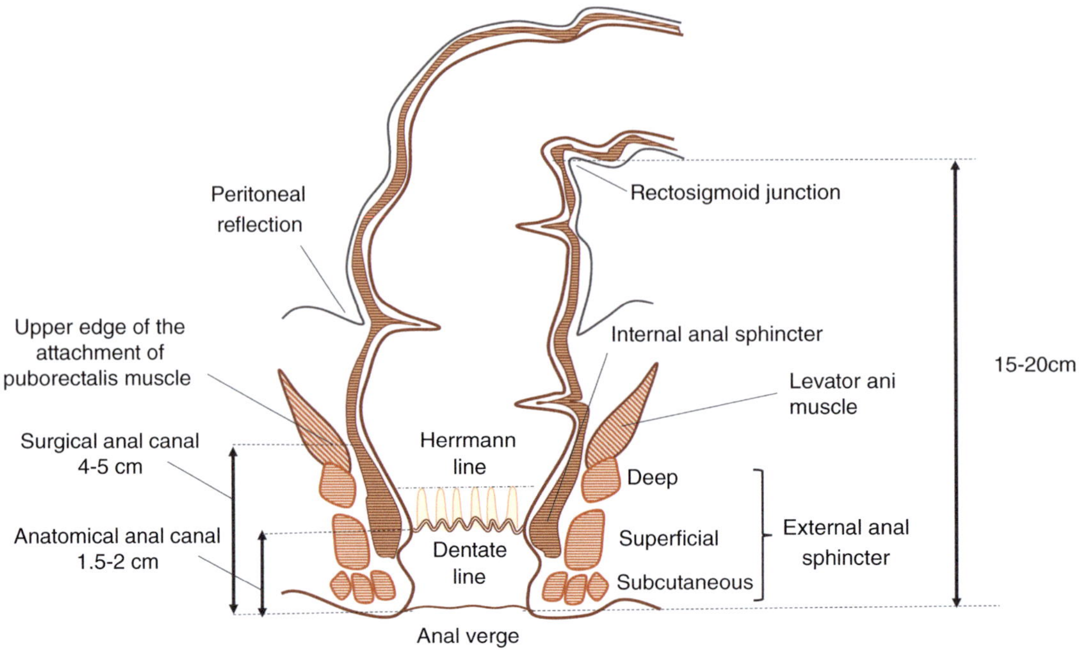

Fig. 56.1 Rectum and anal canal

subdivided into the rectosigmoid junction (from the promontory to the lower edge of the second sacral vertebra), the upper rectum (from the second sacral vertebra to the peritoneal reflection), and the lower rectum (from the peritoneal reflection to the upper edge of the attachment of the puborectalis muscle) [1].

1.2 Anal Canal

The anus is the terminal part of the digestive tract and serves as the outlet for feces (Fig. 56.1). The anal verge is defined as the boundary between the external opening of the anus and the perianal skin, visible during anal inspection, although its exact range is not clearly defined [3]. The anal canal is defined in the "Japanese Classification of Colorectal Carcinoma" as the tubular part extending from the upper edge of the attachment of the puborectalis muscle to the anal verge [1], also referred to as the surgical anal canal (length 4–5 cm) [2]. Approximately 1.5–2 cm above the anal verge is the dentate line, which marks the junction between the rectum (derived from the endoderm) and the anus (derived from the ectoderm) [3, 4]. The portion from the dentate line to the anal verge is referred to as the anatomical anal canal, while the part enclosed by the upper and lower edges of the internal and external anal sphincters is referred to as the histological anal canal [3].

2 Epithelium of the Rectum and Anus

2.1 Columnar Epithelium

The epithelium of the rectum, like other parts of the digestive tract, consists of simple columnar epithelium (Fig. 56.2). The mucosal surface is covered with villi, and between their bases are tubular invaginations known as crypts, which are predominantly occupied by goblet cells in the rectum [5]. Therefore, the rectal mucosa secretes a large amount of mucus, facilitating the smooth passage of feces.

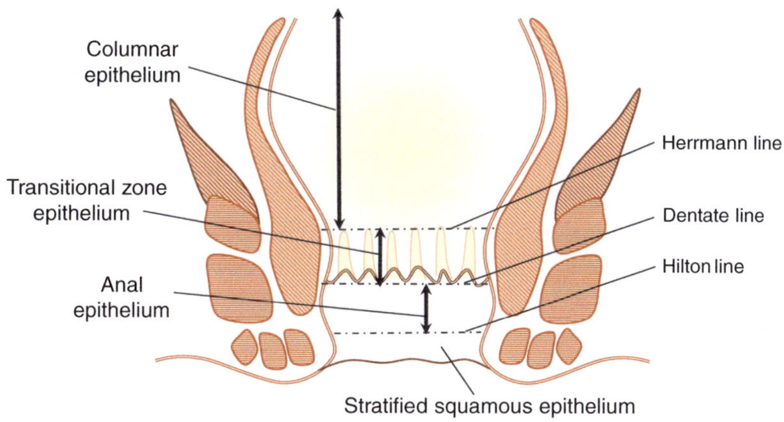

Fig. 56.2 Epithelium of the rectum and anus

2.2 Transitional Zone Epithelium

The upper third of the surgical anal canal, starting from the upper edge of the attachment of the puborectalis muscle, transitions from mucosa to skin and is referred to as the transitional zone epithelium (Fig. 56.2). This boundary line is known as Hermann's line, coinciding with the upper edge of the attachment of the puborectalis muscle. The transitional zone epithelium extends to the dentate line and consists of a mixture of columnar, cuboidal, and stratified squamous epithelium. The transitional zone epithelium features 8–14 longitudinal folds known as anal columns [6, 7]. The grooves between the anal columns are called anal sinuses. The lower ends of the anal columns form small elevations known as anal papillae, while the lower ends of the anal sinuses form depressions known as anal crypts, where anal ducts open and lead to anal glands. The circular line connecting the anal papillae and anal crypts is the dentate line.

2.3 Stratified Squamous Epithelium

Below the dentate line, the epithelium transitions to stratified squamous epithelium, which lacks skin appendages such as sebaceous and sweat glands and does not have a keratinized layer (Fig. 56.2). This is referred to as anal epithelium, which appears white-yellow due to the low melanin content and extends to the Hilton's line, the boundary with normal skin [7]. Hilton's line corresponds to the intermuscular groove between the internal and external anal sphincters.

3 Musculature of the Rectum and Anus

3.1 Levator Ani Muscle

The lesser pelvis consists of the pelvic inlet, pelvic walls, and pelvic outlet (Fig. 56.3). The pelvic outlet is closed by the pelvic floor, which is referred to as the pelvic diaphragm. The pelvic diaphragm is composed of the levator ani muscle, piriformis muscle, and coccygeus muscle, which elevate the anal canal. The levator ani muscle is a collective term for the puborectalis muscle, pubococcygeus muscle, and iliococcygeus muscle, which are striated muscles innervated by somatic nerves and deeply involved in defecation. The puborectalis muscle originates and attaches to the posterior surface of the pubis, forming a U-shaped sling on both sides that encircles the rectum. Contraction of the puborectalis muscle pulls the rectum anteriorly and superiorly, creating an acute anorectal angle that closes the anal canal. The pubococcygeus muscle originates from the body of the pubis and runs posteriorly to attach to the anococcygeal ligament. The iliococcygeus

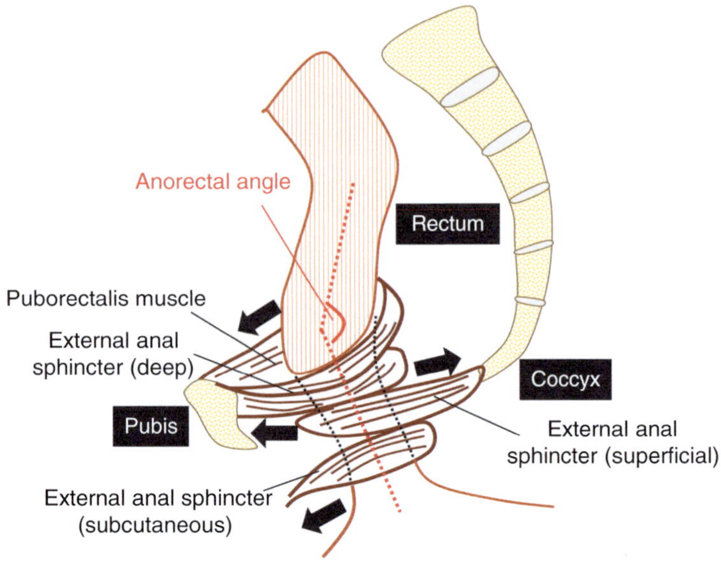

Fig. 56.3 Contraction directions of the puborectalis muscle and external anal sphincter

muscle originates from the obturator internus muscle fascia and the ischial spine, attaching to the anococcygeal ligament [8].

3.2 Internal Anal Sphincter

The internal anal sphincter is a smooth muscle that develops and thickens in the anal canal portion of the circular muscle (proper muscular layer) of the intestinal wall. It is an involuntary muscle controlled by the autonomic nervous system. Continuous contraction of the internal anal sphincter keeps the anal canal closed at rest.

3.3 External Anal Sphincter

The external anal sphincter is a striated muscle derived from the neuroectoderm, functioning voluntarily (Fig. 56.3). Contraction of the external anal sphincter actively closes the anal canal. The external anal sphincter is divided into subcutaneous, superficial, and deep parts. The subcutaneous part is a circular muscle located beneath the skin near the anal verge, closing the anus. Contraction of the subcutaneous part pulls the anus anteriorly. The superficial part is the largest and most powerful muscle of the external anal sphincter, encircling the anus, spindle-shaped from both sides [6]. The muscle bundles attach anteriorly to the central tendon of the perineum and posteriorly to the anococcygeal ligament (coccygeal-sacral ligament), attaching to the coccyx [3, 6]. Therefore, contraction of the superficial part pulls the anus posteriorly. The deep part encircles the upper part of the anal canal, closing it. The deep part merges with the puborectalis muscle, oral-posteriorly, forming a unified structure. Together with the puborectalis muscle, the deep part pulls the anal canal anteriorly.

3.4 Conjoined Longitudinal Muscle

The conjoined longitudinal muscle is a fibrous smooth muscle tissue running longitudinally between the internal and external anal sphincters, formed by the fusion of the longitudinal muscle of the rectum and the fibers of the levator ani muscle (Fig. 56.3) [3]. The branches of the conjoined longitudinal muscle are broadly divided into internal and external branches. The internal branches penetrate the internal anal sphincter near the dentate line, forming the mucosal support ligament and connective tissue network (Treitz ligament), fixing the muscle layer and hemorrhoidal venous plexus to the epithelium [3,

6, 7]. The external branches penetrate and disperse the muscle bundles of the subcutaneous part of the external anal sphincter, attaching to the perianal skin. Additionally, the fibers running between the subcutaneous and superficial parts of the external anal sphincter form the transverse septum, constituting the floor of the ischiorectal fossa [6, 9].

4 Vasculature of the Rectum and Anus

4.1 Arteries

The rectum and anus are supplied by the superior rectal artery, middle rectal artery, and inferior rectal artery (Fig. 56.4). The superior rectal artery branches from the inferior mesenteric artery, dividing into two branches at the level of the third sacral vertebra and descending within the rectal wall, with terminal branches extending to the level of the internal anal sphincter, where they anastomose with branches of the middle and inferior rectal arteries [10]. The middle rectal artery branches from the internal iliac artery, distributing to the rectal wall from the anterolateral side at the level of the lateral ligament. The inferior rectal artery branches from the internal pudendal artery, a branch of the internal iliac artery, exiting the pelvic cavity below the piriformis muscle, traversing the ischioanal fossa and external anal sphincter to reach the perineum, distributing to the anal canal and perianal skin [4, 8].

4.2 Veins

The veins of the rectum and anus accompany the corresponding arteries (Fig. 56.4). Within the pelvic cavity, these veins intercommunicate, forming venous plexuses distributed on the visceral surface [8]. Most of the venous plexus of the rectum drains into the portal system via the superior rectal vein, while the venous plexus of the anal canal drains into the systemic circulation via the middle and inferior rectal veins. The rectal venous plexus around the anal canal is divided into upper and lower parts by the dentate line. The upper rectal venous plexus is located above the dentate line, between the internal anal sphincter and the anal canal epithelium, where it communicates with branches of the superior rectal artery [8]. The engorgement of this venous plexus leads to the formation of internal hemorrhoids; hence, it is also called the superior hemorrhoidal plexus [2]. Conversely, the lower rectal venous plexus is located below the dentate line, distributed in the external anal sphincter and perianal

Fig. 56.4 Vascular distribution of the rectum and anus

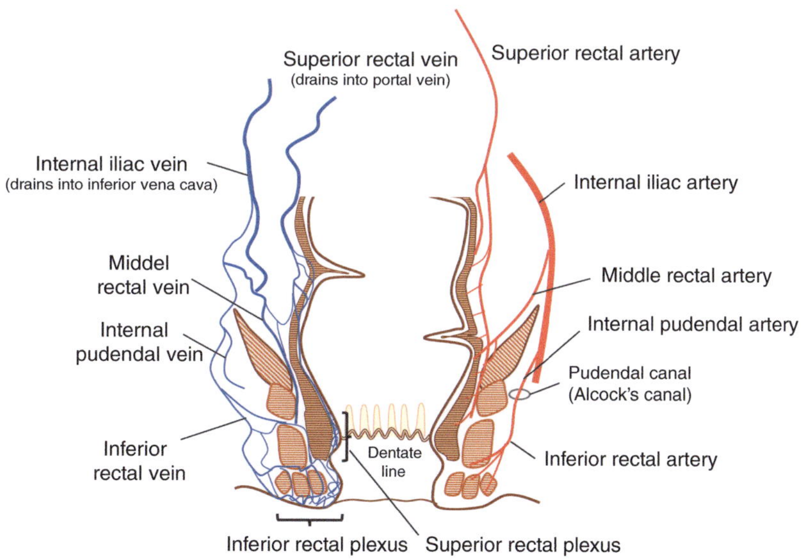

skin. The engorgement of this venous plexus leads to the formation of external hemorrhoids; hence, it is also called the inferior hemorrhoidal plexus [2].

5 Nerves of the Rectum and Anus

5.1 Sympathetic Nervous System

The rectum, being an abdominal viscus, is innervated by the visceral nerves (Fig. 56.5). The lumbar splanchnic nerves and sacral splanchnic nerves, which arise from ganglia associated with the sympathetic trunk, contain preganglionic sympathetic fibers and visceral afferent fibers, and proceed to the prevertebral plexus. The superior and inferior hypogastric plexuses, which are distal parts of the prevertebral plexus, divide into the right and left hypogastric nerves in the pelvic cavity, forming the pelvic plexus together with the pelvic splanchnic nerves [10].

5.2 Parasympathetic Nervous System

The rectum receives parasympathetic innervation from the vagus nerve and the pelvic splanchnic nerves (Fig. 56.5). The pelvic splanchnic nerves arise from the second to fourth sacral spinal segments, containing parasympathetic efferent fibers, and proceed to the pelvic plexus. The pelvic splanchnic nerves also contain visceral afferent fibers. Additionally, some fibers of the pelvic splanchnic nerves ascend along branches of the inferior mesenteric artery, providing parasympathetic innervation to that region [10].

5.3 Somatic Nervous System

The anal canal is innervated by the somatic nervous system. The pudendal nerve arises from the second to fourth sacral spinal segments, exits the pelvic cavity, and travels through the pudendal canal within the obturator internus muscle fascia

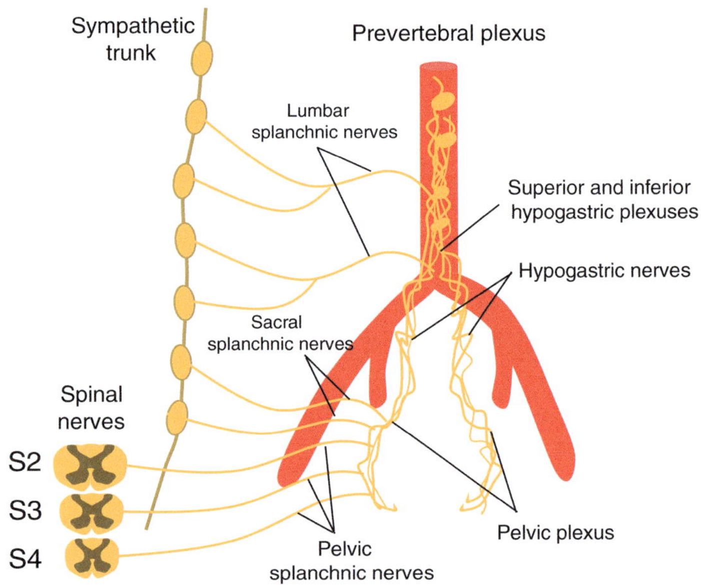

Fig. 56.5 Autonomic nervous system of the rectum and anal canal

(accompanied by the internal pudendal artery) to reach the perineum. The pudendal nerve divides into three terminal branches: the inferior rectal nerve, the perineal nerve, and the dorsal nerve of the penis or clitoris. The inferior rectal nerve innervates the external anal sphincter and levator ani muscle and provides sensory innervation to the perianal skin. The perineal nerve innervates the skeletal muscles of the perineal region and provides sensory innervation to the scrotum or labia. The dorsal nerve of the penis or clitoris provides sensory innervation to those regions [10]. Recently, there have been reports suggesting the existence of the levator ani nerve, which arises from the anterior branch of the second sacral spinal segment, directly innervating the coccygeus and levator ani muscles from the lumbosacral plexus, and controlling their motor function [10, 11].

Competing Interests The author has no competing interests to declare that are relevant to the content of this chapter.

References

1. Japanese Society for Cancer of the Colon and Rectum, ed. Japanese classification of colorectal carcinoma. 9th ed. Kanehara & Co., Ltd; 2018. p. 7–9. (in Japanese)
2. Townsend CN, editor. Sabiston textbook of surgery, 20th ed. Elsevier. 2017:1312–23.
3. Fujiwara M. Anatomical terminology of the anus and anal canal. Stomach and Intestine. 2017;52:541–2. (in Japanese)
4. Townsend CN, editor. Sabiston textbook of surgery, 20th ed. Elsevier. 2017:1394–5.
5. Abe K, et al. Histology. 20th ed. Nanzando Co., Ltd; 2019. p. 327–9. (in Japanese)
6. Tsuji J, et al. Anatomy of the anus. Clin Surgery. 2022;77:894–9. (in Japanese)
7. Oki S, et al. Anatomy of the rectum and anus. Adult Dis Lifestyle-Related Dis. 2016;46:1489–96. (in Japanese)
8. Drake RL, et al. Translated by Akita K. Gray's Anatomy. 4th ed. Elsevier Japan; 2019. p. 352–442. (in Japanese)
9. Kurihara H, et al. New classification of anal fistula: clarification of posterior complex fistula and low intermuscular fistula. J Japan Soc Coloproctol. 2008;16:467–75. (in Japanese)
10. Drake RL, et al. Translated by Akita K. Gray's Anatomy. 4th ed. Elsevier Japan; 2019. p. 265–301. (in Japanese)
11. Takeyama M. Anatomy of the pelvic floor. In: Goto M et al., editors. Basics and clinical practice of excretion rehabilitation. 2nd ed. Nakayama Shoten; 2022. p. 38–46. (in Japanese)

57 Anorectum, Physiology of Defecation Mechanism (Gastrointestinal Motility)

Joji Kuromizu

Abstract

Defecation is the act of expelling feces from the digestive tract through the anus. It is an event arising from the integrated and coordinated combination of sensory-motor functions, intrinsically linked to the function of fecal continence.

The large intestine functions by transporting contents from the terminal ileum to the cecum toward the anus while absorbing water and solidifying the contents. It also stores the contents until conditions are suitable for defecation.

The most crucial factor for achieving normal bowel movements is feeling the urge to defecate; defecation begins with this sensation. The urge is triggered by high-amplitude propagated contractions that propel contents into the rectum.

When the decision to defecate is made, the contents are expelled due to increased rectal pressure and relaxation of the pelvic floor and anal canal. Defecation is thought to be brought about by both spontaneous straining and coordinated colonic contractions.

When stool is expelled, the rectum perceives emptiness, causing the external anal sphincter to contract in a reflex action known as the closure reflex, sealing the anal canal. As abdominal pressure further decreases, the pelvic floor's postural reflex reactivates, returning the anorectal angle to its baseline position, thereby concluding defecation.

Keywords

Defecation · Defecation desire · Sampling reflex · Anorectal angle · Fecal continence · Postural reflex · High-amplitude propagated contractions · Anal cushion · Recto-anal inhibitory reflex

1 Defecation

Defecation is the act of expelling feces from the gastrointestinal tract through the anus. Defecation is controlled by the central nervous system and occurs through the integrated and coordinated interaction of sensory stimuli, neural reflexes, and sensory-motor functions such as the contraction and relaxation of the colon, pelvic floor muscles, and anal sphincter muscles. This process is closely linked to the functions of fecal retention and continence. Typically, when the sensation of needing to defecate (defecation desire) is felt, one selects a suitable location and adopts a sitting

J. Kuromizu (✉)
Department of Anorectal Surgery and Anorectal Physiology, Matsushima Hospital, Coloproctology Center, Yokohama, Japan
e-mail: j.kuromizu@matsushima-hp.or.jp

H. Kaneko et al. (eds.), *Disorders of Gut-Brain Interaction*,
https://doi.org/10.1007/978-981-95-6974-8_57

or squatting posture to defecate, depending on the environment. When defecation is not possible, such as when there is no nearby toilet or while traveling, temporary restraint is possible, with the capacity and duration of restraint calculated according to the situation to maintain continence. Additionally, when rectal distension is felt, it is possible to distinguish between feces and gas, allowing for flatulence as appropriate. These abilities to restrain, tolerate, and distinguish vary under different conditions and may sometimes be lost. Although knowledge and consensus on the mechanisms of defecation and fecal continence are not yet sufficient, this section will describe defecation in four phases to facilitate understanding: the basic phase, pre-defecation phase, defecation phase, and post-defecation phase [1].

1.1 Basic Phase

Normal colon function involves transporting contents from the terminal ileum to the cecum at an appropriate speed toward the anus, absorbing water from the contents, and gradually solidifying them. The colon stores the contents until conditions are suitable for defecation. Colon motor activity increases after awakening and is higher during the day than at night, showing a circadian rhythm, and also increases after meals. Simplified, colon motor function can be divided into transit and contractile activities. The upper limit of normal colon transit time in adults is approximately 72 h, while in children, it is faster, reported to be less than 57 h. Colon motility is characterized by short-term phasic contractions and sustained contractions, with phasic contractions further classified into non-propagating or propagating contractions. Non-propagating contractions are the most common phenomenon, with frequencies of 2–4 cycles/min or 6–8 cycles/min and amplitudes of 5–50 mmHg, although the role of non-propagating activity in luminal transport is unclear.

Propagating contractions include retrograde (oral propagation) and anterograde (anal propagation), with the ratio potentially influenced by the pathophysiological mechanisms of colon transit time. High-amplitude propagated contractions (HAPCs) are well-known, with amplitudes exceeding 100 mmHg, occurring five to six times a day in adults, primarily originating from the proximal colon, with only one-third reaching the anus and the remainder converging in the rectosigmoid colon. The sigmoid colon exhibits periodic contractions important for regulating the transfer of contents to the rectum, with a mechanism where expansion leads to contraction, facilitating the progression of contents to the rectum.

Rectal motor activity is unaffected by food intake and propagates retrogradely, hypothesized to function as a mechanism to keep the rectum empty by inhibiting the influx of contents. At rest, the levator ani, puborectalis, and external anal sphincter muscles are continuously contracted, known as the "postural reflex," aiding in supporting pelvic organs. Among these, the contractile traction of the puborectalis muscle maintains the anorectal angle (see Fig. 56.3 in Chap. 56) at approximately 90°, contributing to continence.

The anal canal is typically closed by the tonic activity of the internal and external anal sphincters and the anal cushion (the anal cushion is a raised structure composed of capillaries, connective tissue, and elastic fibers between the sphincters and mucosa, rich in elasticity, aiding in closing the anal canal). Resting anal tone is 85% due to the internal anal sphincter and 15% due to the anal cushion, with the external anal sphincter also in a state of tonic activity. The anal cushion provides "sealing" that cannot be achieved by sphincter tone alone. Essential to the activity characteristics of the anal canal is the intermittent and temporary relaxation of the internal anal sphincter, which opens the upper anal canal funnel-shaped, allowing unconscious or conscious recognition of the properties of descending rectal contents. This reflex is known as the "sampling reflex," occurring approximately seven times per hour in healthy individuals.

The internal anal sphincter is almost always maximally contracted, with its main reflex being relaxation. The recto-anal inhibitory reflex (RAIR) (Note 1) occurs when rectal distension stimulates relaxation of the internal anal sphincter, observed even in patients with external anal sphincter paralysis, cauda equina lesions, and complete spinal cord injury, indicating that this reflex is not influenced by cerebral neural control. This reflex is controlled by the enteric nervous system and is absent in patients with Hirschsprung's disease.

1.2 Pre-defecation Phase

The most crucial aspect of normal defecation is the sensation of needing to defecate (defecation desire), which initiates defecation. The rectum is considered the primary site for the generation of defecation desire, with gradual rectal distension initially causing a desire to pass gas, which then transforms into a persistent defecation desire. Distension up to 15 cm from the anal verge induces defecation desire, while distension beyond the oral side of this point causes colonic-type sensations similar to suprapubic pain or abdominal bloating. In patients with a retained rectum after colectomy, balloon distension on the anal side of the anastomosis induces normal defecation desire. Defecation desire originating outside the rectum can be induced by stimulating nerve endings and stretch receptors in the pelvic floor muscles, including the puborectalis muscle. Studies in patients after rectal resection have observed that although the preoperative defecatory urge differs, the sensation of "content fullness" is maintained. Both the rectum and pelvic floor are involved in generating normal fullness and defecation desire.

Colonic motility due to HAPCs moves contents toward the anus, with sigmoid colon expansion leading to contraction, accompanied by relaxation of the rectosigmoid colon, facilitating the transfer of contents to the rectum. Rectal sensation is maintained even after bilateral pudendal nerve block, but completely disappears with high spinal anesthesia (T6-S1), including abdominal discomfort. The biomechanical characteristics of the rectal wall involve the rectum expanding in response to the inflow of contents, whereby the sensitivity of the rectum can respond to increases in volume, a phenomenon known as adaptive relaxation. This enables the rectum to function as a temporary storage organ—in other words, it possesses reservoir function. The pelvic floor maintains continuous contraction during this phase, resulting in the maintenance of continence. When defecation desire occurs and defecation is inconvenient, voluntary contraction of the pelvic floor muscles, including the external anal sphincter and puborectalis muscle, allows restraint. At this time, the anorectal angle becomes acute.

1.3 Defecation Phase

The sampling reflex (Note 2) promotes defecation desire, and when a conscious decision to defecate is made, increased rectal pressure and relaxation of the pelvic floor and anal canal result in the expulsion of contents. In healthy adults, 35–40% of all HAPCs occur during or just before defecation, associated with defecation. Straining during defecation increases intra-pelvic pressure, thereby increasing rectal pressure. Intuitively, simultaneous rectal contraction is thought to promote expulsion, but the involvement of rectal contraction has not been proven. Defecation is likely brought about by both spontaneous straining and coordinated colonic contractions. Adequate relaxation of the pelvic floor muscles, combined with increased intra-abdominal pressure, lowers the pelvic floor, accompanied by relaxation of the puborectalis muscle, straightening the anorectal angle (see Fig. 56.3 in Chap. 56). This is essential for effective defecation, and failure to achieve this can result in defecation disorders known as pelvic floor dyssynergia or dyssynergic defecation. During defecation, both the internal and external anal sphincters relax coordinately, causing relaxation of the anal canal. Relaxation of the internal anal sphincter occurs involuntarily in response to rectal distension (RAIR), proportional to rectal pressure. After adopting a suitable posture for defecation, the Valsalva maneuver is performed by closing the glottis and contracting the abdominal muscles and diaphragm. At this time, the conjoint longitudinal muscle of the anus contracts, causing flattening of the anal cushion and shortening of the anal canal. Additionally, the pressure of the incoming fecal mass further flattens the anal cushion. All these changes occur simultaneously, lowering anal pressure below rectal pressure, resulting in a pressure gradient from the rectum to the outside.

Inadequate coordination of increased intra-abdominal pressure and insufficient relaxation of the pelvic floor muscles, along with inappropriate contraction of the external anal sphincter during defecation, can lead to defecation disorders. This contraction of the external anal sphincter, known as paradoxical contraction, occurs when straining for defecation causes contraction of the puborectalis muscle and external anal sphincter, which should relax during defecation.

Once defecation begins, sensory input from the anus is assumed to maintain defecatory activity until the rectum is empty. Even in patients with spinal cord injury, defecation is almost completely performed once initiated, likely due to spinal reflexes.

1.4 Post-defecation Phase

This phase begins with the cessation of actions that increase intra-pelvic pressure and the sensation that the rectum is completely empty. It is initiated under semi-voluntary control, followed by involuntary movements of the external anal sphincter and pelvic floor muscles to close the anal canal and relieve rectal pressure. The external anal sphincter instantly closes the anal canal, a reflex known as the "closure reflex," which is crucial at the end of defecation as it allows the internal anal sphincter to recover its tone, no longer inhibited by rectal distension. This reflex appears to be cortically regulated, as it is impaired in patients with spinal cord injury. When straining ceases and intra-abdominal pressure decreases, the postural reflex of the pelvic floor reactivates, resulting in contraction of the puborectalis muscle, returning the anorectal angle to its basic state. This passive expansion of the anal cushion completely closes the anal canal.

2 Fecal Continence

Normal anal continence is maintained by the coordinated function of the pelvic floor muscles, normal recto-anal sensation and sampling reflex, appropriate rectal capacity and compliance, and normal rectal and anal canal motility, ensuring that anal pressure remains higher than rectal pressure [2]. Additionally, the anal cushion provides "sealing" that cannot be achieved by sphincter tone alone. The ability to distinguish between feces and gas, allowing for flatulence or defecation, indicates that the mechanism is not merely a simple pressure differential for retaining or expelling rectal contents. Although the mechanism of continence is complex, it is an essential function for individuals in social life.

2.1 Mechanisms of Continence

Several theories explaining the mechanisms of continence have been reported. In 1965, Phillips and Edwards proposed the flutter valve theory, similar to the mechanism preventing reflux into the esophagus, where increased intra-abdominal pressure creates a high-pressure zone in the lower rectum, preventing rectal contents from entering the anus. Parks reported the flap valve theory, suggesting that increased intra-abdominal pressure pushes the anterior rectal wall, creating an acute anorectal angle to maintain continence. Both theories explain why continence is primarily not due to the anal sphincters, as rectal pressure can be higher than anal pressure without causing fecal leakage. Parks associated incontinence with perineal descent and the obtuse anorectal angle, proposing postanal repair surgery to correct the obtuse anorectal angle.

However, in 1986, Bartolo et al. concluded that the valve mechanism was not proven by radiological examination, electromyography, or recto-anal pressure studies, and that continence was due to the anal sphincters. Duthie et al. confirmed that incontinence improved after postanal repair surgery, with significant increases in anal canal resting pressure and voluntary contraction pressure, despite no improvement in the anorectal angle. Similar results were observed after anterior sphincteroplasty or levatorplasty, suggesting that the obtuse anorectal angle in incontinent patients is due to puborectalis muscle weakness, indicating that continence is related to rectal and anal pressures.

2.2 Rectal and Anal Sensation

Normal individuals can pass gas separately from defecation, requiring the ability to distinguish between feces and gas. Rectal fullness is primarily sensed by stretch receptors in the pelvic floor muscles, while gas, which does not increase pressure as much as solid matter, is distinguished by the ability to sense differences in rectal pressure. Sensory ability also exists in the upper anal canal mucosa, with the anal sampling reflex playing a crucial role. Maintaining normal continence requires sensation and rectal compliance (Note 3), with central nervous system control essential for local action. However, the exact mechanisms maintaining normal continence remain unclear.

2.2.1 Note 1 RAIR

This reflex serves both sampling and defecation functions. When a large amount of feces accumulates in the rectum, the pressure of the relaxed internal anal sphincter does not recover, and inhibition persists. At this point, defecation can occur if desired. After defecation, the external anal sphincter closes the anal canal (closure reflex), and the internal anal sphincter recovers its tone.

2.2.2 Note 2 Sampling Reflex

The RAIR causes relaxation of the internal anal sphincter, opening the oral side of the anal canal. Rectal contents (feces or gas) enter a limited sensory area (located on the anal side of the upper closure site of the anal canal), where temperature, pain, and slight tactile sensations can be distinguished, similar to the sensation at the fingertip.

2.2.3 Note 3 Rectal Compliance

Rectal compliance is calculated as dV/dP = mL/mmHg. As the rectum fills with feces, reflex-induced rectal expansion increases compliance, allowing adaptation up to 300 mL. Beyond this volume, pressure increases, approaching the tolerance limit, resulting in a sense of urgency for defecation [3].

Take-Home Message

The defecation mechanism includes "defecation," which expels feces, and "continence," which maintains restraint to prevent leakage. During defecation, high HAPCs occur in the colon, resulting in the influx of feces into the rectum from the left colon. Rectal distension induces defecation desire, and the RAIR simultaneously identifies contents, leading to defecation. Alternatively, restraint can be exercised if defecation is inconvenient, with the degree of restraint adjusted according to the state of the rectum and colon and the characteristics of the feces. Various reflexes and sensations interact complexly to maintain delicate defecation functions.

Competing Interests The author has no competing interests to declare that are relevant to the content of this chapter.

References

1. Palit S, et al. The physiology of human defecation. Dig Dis Sci. 2012;57:1445–64.
2. Duthie GS, et al. Faecal continence and defaecation. Butterworth Heinemann: Coloproctology and the Pelvic Floor; 1992.
3. Nyam DC. The current understanding of continence and defecation. Singapore Med J. 1998;39:132–6.

58 Anorectal Function Test, Anorectal Manometry

Joji Kuromizu

Abstract

Objective methods for evaluating anorectal function include anorectal manometry, anal electromyography, and defecography. These are useful for diagnosing defecation disorders such as fecal incontinence and constipation, as well as for assessing function after treatment.

Anorectal manometry primarily measures sphincter function, including resting pressure (the contraction capacity of the internal anal sphincter for the most part), voluntary contraction pressure (the contraction capacity of the external anal sphincter), the recto-anal inhibitory reflex [1], and the cough reflex. Additionally, rectal reservoir function is assessed by inserting and retaining a balloon within the rectum, inflating it with air to expand it, and measuring the volume that induces the urge to defecate and the maximum tolerable volume.

The equipment used for inspection is expensive, and particularly, the strain gauge transducer probes require careful handling. Furthermore, calibrating the equipment according to the manufacturer's recommendations prior to inspection is crucial for accurate measurements, necessitating the acquisition of measurement techniques.

However, the current situation lacks uniformity regarding the equipment used for inspection, the implementation methods, and the interpretation of results.

This section describes the equipment used for inspection, the inspection methods and parameters, and the evaluation process.

Keywords

Anorectal functional disorders · Anorectal manometry · Defecation disorders · Fecal incontinence · Run-in period · Physiological anal canal length · Recto-anal inhibitory reflex · Cough reflex · Rectal sensation

1 Concept

Global surveys indicate that anorectal functional disorders affect 10–20% of the population, significantly impacting quality of life. Currently, various tests are available to evaluate anal function, including anorectal manometry, anal ultrasound, defecography, anal electromyography, and balloon expulsion tests. These tests provide valuable information on the pathophysiology of fecal incontinence, defecation disorders, and anal pain. Among these, anorectal manometry is widely recognized and utilized for diagnosing

J. Kuromizu (✉)
Department of Anorectal Surgery and Anorectal Physiology, Matsushima Hospital, Coloproctology Center, Yokohama, Japan
e-mail: j.kuromizu@matsushima-hp.or.jp

H. Kaneko et al. (eds.), *Disorders of Gut-Brain Interaction*,
https://doi.org/10.1007/978-981-95-6974-8_58

and evaluating the function of defecation disorders such as fecal incontinence and constipation (including delayed colonic transit and difficult defecation) [2].

2 Anorectal Manometry

2.1 Measurement Equipment

Various equipment is required to measure, record, and store anorectal pressures. The main components include probes, pressure recording devices, display devices (monitors, printers, etc.), and data storage devices (computers). Probes can be categorized into: (i) micro-balloon type, (ii) water-perfused probes, and (iii) strain gauge transducer-equipped probes (microchip transducers). Currently, type (iii) is the most commonly used, although each type has its advantages and disadvantages, and their prevalence has evolved over time from (i) to (ii) to (iii). Type (ii) is less prone to malfunction and cheaper than type (iii), but it requires a perfusion pump and is cumbersome to calibrate. Type (iii) is user-friendly and easy to handle, but it is prone to malfunction and expensive. Additionally, probes may have multiple pressure sensors along the vertical axis or circumference, requiring transducers for each channel (ch), making multi-channel probes more expensive. There are also types with balloons at the tip, indicating a lack of standardization in the equipment [3].

2.2 Measurement Method

Measurements are performed with the subject in the left lateral decubitus position, with thighs flexed at 90°. Pre-procedure preparation involves ensuring defecation before the test, avoiding laxatives or enemas immediately before the test. However, if fecal retention is observed, an enema is administered at least 30 min before the test. Before starting the test, the equipment is adjusted, particularly calibrating the recording device and probe (transducer) accurately according to the manufacturer's instructions, which is crucial for correct pressure measurement.

The probe is inserted approximately 6 cm into the rectum (with the pressure sensor at the tip positioned within the rectum). For probes with a pressure sensor in one channel or circumference, pressures are measured while withdrawing the probe from the rectum. There are two withdrawal methods: (i) station pull-through method, where the probe is withdrawn in stages of 5–10 mm to measure pressures at each site, and (ii) rapid pull-through method, where an automatic withdrawal device continuously withdraws the probe at a constant speed while measuring pressures. The recorded waveforms are stored in the recording device, with most data now stored and analyzed on computers. The author uses a one-channel probe and automatic withdrawal device to measure anorectal pressure curves when needed (e.g., measuring physiological anal canal length), and an eight-channel probe in the vertical axis direction for other measurements.

2.3 Measurement Items

Measurement items are selected based on the patient's symptoms. The probe is inserted and left in place for about 5 min to stabilize the waveform before starting measurements (run-in period). Immediately after probe insertion, the stimulus may trigger the recto-anal inhibitory reflex, causing a drop in resting pressure and waveform disturbance, necessitating waiting for pressure recovery to resting levels. With a one-channel probe, resting pressure and voluntary contraction pressure can be measured by either withdrawal method, but measuring physiological anal canal length (high-pressure zone) is preferable using anorectal pressure curves obtained by automatic withdrawal. With an eight-channel probe, after confirming waveform stability, maximum resting pressure is measured over 1 min. Next, the pressure during conscious anal contraction for 10 s is measured, with the maximum value recorded as maximum squeezing pressure. Additionally, the duration of contraction pressure exceeding 50% of maximum squeezing pressure over 30 s may be measured. Other measurement items include changes in anorectal pressure during straining for defecation and pressure during coughing (cough reflex). Subsequently, a balloon is inserted and positioned with its center 10 cm from the anal verge within the rectum, waiting for resting pressure to stabilize (with a one-channel probe, the pressure sensor is positioned at the site of maximum resting pressure). The relaxation of anal pressure upon instant injection of 30–50 mL of air indicates the recto-anal inhibitory reflex, which is assessed for its presence [4].

For rectal sensation tests, air is gradually injected into a balloon positioned 10 cm from the anal verge within the rectum, with the volume at which a slight sensation is first felt recorded as the first constant sensation volume (FCSV) (mL). Continued air injection until a strong defecation desire is felt is recorded as the desire to defecate volume (DDV) (mL). Further air injection until the sensation becomes intolerable is recorded as the maximum tolerable volume (MTV) (mL). Physiological anal canal length and maximum resting pressure primarily reflect internal anal sphincter function, while maximum anal canal squeezing pressure and cough reflex reflect external anal sphincter function. Additionally, the FCSV and DDV correlate with sensory ability, while the maximum tolerated volume correlates with fecal storage capacity. The recto-anal inhibitory reflex is used in diagnosing Hirschsprung's disease, correlating with neurological disorders. The lower the anastomosis site in rectal resection and the more extensive the lymph node dissection, the lower the reflex occurrence rate.

When performing pressure measurements, detailed inquiries about defecation, including daily defecation frequency, defecation desire, stool characteristics, presence and circumstances of incontinence (feces, mucus, gas), ability to distinguish between feces and gas, and ability to restrain defecation, are necessary.

3 Evaluation of Tests

3.1 Anal Sphincter Function

Physiological anal canal length represents the contraction activity site of the internal anal sphincter, with shortening commonly observed after ultra-low anterior resection or intersphincteric resection (ISR), and sometimes after anal fistula surgery. A decrease in maximum resting pressure indicates weakened internal anal sphincter activity, suggesting muscle damage or nerve injury. Maximum squeezing pressure is measured in the lower anal canal, approximately 5–15 mm from the anal verge, with decreases indicating external anal sphincter damage or central nervous system conduction disorders. Contraction pressure duration is considered an indicator of restraint ability. Increased pressure during coughing reflects the closure reflex of the external anal sphincter, sometimes exceeding maximum squeezing pressure, indicating poor voluntary anal contraction. Changes in pressure waveform during straining are useful for diagnosing obstructed defecation, such as functional defecation disorders. Diagnosing paradoxical contraction of the puborectalis muscle or external anal sphincter is possible, aiding in determining the suitability of biofeedback therapy [5]. The absence of the recto-anal inhibitory reflex is a well-known diagnostic criterion for Hirschsprung's disease, with the reflex considered important for recognizing rectal contents and maintaining continence. The occurrence rate of the reflex tends to decrease after ultra-low anterior resection or ISR, useful for evaluating postoperative defecation disorders.

3.2 Reservoir Function

DDV indicates rectal sensory response to distension stimuli, significantly decreasing in rectal inflammation or poor distension, leading to frequent defecatory urges. Maximum tolerable volume represents storage capacity, correlating with defecation frequency. In patients complaining of no defecatory urge, normal DDV and maximum tolerable volume suggest that feces have not reached the rectum, indicating delayed colonic transit time. Conversely, frequent defecatory urges with low FCSV, DDV, and MTV indicate hypersensitivity and reduced storage capacity. When the maximum tolerable volume exceeds 300 mL, diminished rectal sensation suggests unclear defecatory urge, useful for selecting treatment methods.

4 Conclusion

Anorectal manometry is a valuable objective tool for diagnosing anorectal functional disorders, evaluating functional recovery, and predicting functional improvement. However, this test alone cannot explain all aspects of anorectal function, necessitating comprehensive evaluation with imaging and other functional tests for an accurate understanding of the pathologic condition.

Take-Home Message

Precision is crucial in conducting tests. Test operators must thoroughly understand the test objectives, characteristics, and methods of the equipment used. Additionally, detailed explanations to subjects and obtaining their cooperation are essential. Stabilizing the subject's posture and relaxation, zero-point correction of the equipment, and stable measurement operations all contribute to the stability of measurement results, enhancing the value of the evaluation, highlighting the significance of anorectal manometry in various contexts.

Competing Interests The author has no competing interests to declare that are relevant to the content of this chapter.

References

1. Nixon HH. Anal canal pressures in the diagnosis of Hirschsprung's disease. J Pediatr Surg. 1967;2:544–52.
2. Kuromizu J. Study on postoperative anal function in sphincter-preserving surgery for lower rectal cancer. J Japan Soc Coloproctol. 1989;42:10–22. (in Japanese)
3. Rao SSC, et al. Minimum standards of anorectal manometry. Neurogastroenterol Mot. 2002;14:553–9.
4. Read NW, et al. Anorectal manometry. Coloproctology and the Pelvic Floor Butterworth Heinemann. 1992:119–45.
5. Rao SSC. Dyssynergic defecation and biofeedback therapy. Gastroenterol Clin N Am. 2008;37:569–86.

Anorectal Function Test, Anorectal Sensation Test

59

Joji Kuromizu

Abstract

Humans choose a convenient time and suitable location within tolerable limits to defecate and carry out the act. This requires recognizing the sensation of the urge to defecate beforehand and having time to prepare. Failure to perform this basic function can lead to bowel disorders such as fecal incontinence or constipation. The urge to defecate is crucial for normal bowel function, and anorectal sensory testing aids in evaluating this urge.

The most commonly performed test is the simple balloon distension test. For specific patients, the rectal barostat is useful for assessing both motor and sensory function, but facilities equipped with this device are limited, and it is not widely used.

As an evaluation of anorectal sensory testing, hypersensitivity may be associated with decreased compliance, capacity, or an exaggerated response to rectal distension. Conversely, rectal hyposensitivity (numbness) is observed in states where the urge to defecate is diminished or absent.

However, current balloon distension studies confirm that rectal volume and rectal pressure are not correlated, and that rectal pressure is the primary trigger for rectal fullness sensation. Therefore, developing a simple method to measure rectal pressure during rectal fullness sensation is necessary for accurate diagnosis of the urge to defecate.

Keywords

Bowel urgency · Fecal incontinence · Constipation · Anorectal function · Anorectal manometry · Sampling reflex · Desire to defecate · Anorectal disorders

1 Introduction

Humans possess a social behavior pattern that allows them to choose and execute defecation at a convenient time and appropriate place within acceptable limits. To achieve this, it is necessary to consciously recognize the need to defecate in advance through the sensation of bowel urgency and prepare accordingly. However, when there is a dysfunction in anorectal function, this seemingly natural behavior becomes impossible, leading to fecal incontinence, constipation, and anal pain, thereby impairing the quality of life.

Defecation status is obtained through a careful and detailed medical interview, but objective information on anorectal function requires some functional tests. The main tests include anorectal

J. Kuromizu (✉)
Department of Anorectal Surgery and Anorectal Physiology, Matsushima Hospital, Coloproctology Center, Yokohama, Japan
e-mail: j.kuromizu@matsushima-hp.or.jp

H. Kaneko et al. (eds.), *Disorders of Gut-Brain Interaction*,
https://doi.org/10.1007/978-981-95-6974-8_59

manometry, balloon expulsion test, electromyography, and pudendal nerve conduction study.

Recognition of rectal filling (bowel urgency) is crucial for normal defecation function, and anorectal sensory testing is essential for the physiological evaluation of anorectal function. The widely performed anorectal sensory test is the simple balloon distension test, usually conducted as part of the anorectal manometry procedure. For specific patients, an electronic rectal barostat, useful for evaluating both motor and sensory functions, is employed. However, facilities equipped with such devices are few, and the typical barostat protocol can take about an hour to complete, making it not widely available for routine use.

This chapter describes the balloon distension test, which is most commonly performed in daily clinical practice and recommended by the International Anorectal Physiology Working Group (IAPWG) [1].

1.1 Anorectal Sensory Function

Sensations related to defecation involve afferent nerve endings not only in the rectum but also in the upper anal canal, which must detect rectal fullness (distension or pressure) and distinguish the contents of the rectum (solid, liquid, and gas). The sampling reflex of the anal canal allows rectal contents to descend into the upper anal canal for identification, enabling the selective release of gas. The healthy anal canal has tactile, pain, and thermal sensations, with specialized sensory nerve endings such as Pacinian corpuscles (pressure), Meissner's corpuscles (vibration, dynamic two-point discrimination), Merkel cells (tactile, static two-point discrimination), Golgi-Mazzoni corpuscles (thermal), and free nerve endings (pain). These somatic nerve endings contribute to the sensory function of the distal rectum and upper anus via the pudendal nerve [2].

Testing anorectal sensation is important for both fecal incontinence and defecation disorders.

1.2 Balloon Distension Test

This test evaluates rectal sensation by perceiving rectal distension. It is performed by inflating an elastic balloon attached to a catheter placed in the rectum with air. Some types have a balloon attached to the tip of the probe used for anorectal manometry. Air is injected manually using a syringe or automatically using a continuous infusion pump. The balloon capacity must be at least 400 mL, with some researchers reporting that at least 250 mL should be injected, while others set the upper limit at 350 mL. This is because the stiffness of the balloon material affects its distensibility, with stiffer materials increasing the risk of rectal injury due to higher internal pressure. Latex-free balloons with a thickness of 0.1 mm are highly distensible (soft) and safe even with 350 mL injection.

The patient is positioned in the left lateral decubitus position with the knees and hips flexed at approximately 90°. As part of the anorectal manometry procedure, it is assumed that a digital rectal examination has confirmed the absence of fecal retention in the rectum at the start of the test.

First, explain to the subject that a balloon will be inserted through the anus, apply lubricant, and gently insert the balloon. The balloon is positioned so that its center is 10 cm from the anal verge (or 3–5 cm above the upper edge of the anal canal). Air is gradually injected into the balloon, and an injection rate of 10 mL per second is recommended. Before starting the injection, explain to the subject, "We will gradually inflate the balloon with air, so please let us know when you feel a constant sensation," "We will continue to inflate, so please let us know when you feel a strong urge to defecate," and "Next, we will inflate more air, so please let us know when you can no longer tolerate it, feel like you might leak stool, or feel pain." The volume at which the subject first feels a sensation in the rectum is the first constant sensation volume. The volume at which the subject feels a strong urge to defecate is the desire to defecate volume (DDV). The volume at which the subject can no longer tolerate it is the maximum tolerable volume (MTV). The measurement unit is mL, and each volume is recorded at the time of the subject's report. The IAPWG protocol and the London classification define standard terms for anorectal motor and sensory functions.

Balloon distension is a stimulus that induces a sensation similar to the passage of a large amount of stool through the rectum, and the DDV and MTV are reproducible.

1.3 Rectal Barostat

This test uses a non-elastic (plastic) bag, which is preferable to a balloon that requires correction for its inherent elasticity, as its characteristics do not affect internal pressure. The bag is inserted and placed in the rectum, and air is injected using an electronic device that allows precise inflation, with the volume and pressure inside the bag (rectum) recorded simultaneously. Rectal compliance can be calculated from the derived pressure–volume curve.

1.4 Evaluation of Anorectal Sensory Testing

The threshold for measuring rectal sensation can be normal, decreased (hypersensitivity), or increased (hyposensitivity) in both fecal incontinence and chronic constipation.

Rectal hypersensitivity is commonly observed in patients with diarrhea-predominant irritable bowel syndrome (IBS), ulcerative colitis, and radiation enteritis, who experience urgency and frequent bowel movements. Rectal hypersensitivity is also characteristic of urgency, urge incontinence, and low anterior resection syndrome. Such hypersensitivity may be associated with decreased compliance, excessive response to volume, or rectal distension. Normalizing sensory thresholds in hypersensitive patients is associated with positive clinical outcomes through behavioral therapy, medication, and surgical treatment, although good outcomes are not necessarily related to changes in sensory factors after intervention.

On the other hand, rectal hyposensitivity (dullness) is often observed simultaneously with weakened or absent bowel urgency in patients with chronic constipation, constipation-predominant IBS, fecal incontinence, and defecation disorders following spinal cord injury. These may be primary (direct impairment of afferent pathway function), secondary (altered biomechanical properties such as rectal distension), or both. When sensation is dull, the expected situation is that stool may leak unconsciously before the person realizes the need to respond. Retraining the sensation in such patients has been shown to improve continence by continuously training to contract the external anal sphincter in a timely manner.

The evaluation of rectal sensory function is crucial in the clinical management of patients with anorectal disorders. Nevertheless, the simple elastic balloon distension method is currently insufficiently standardized [3].

1.5 Future Challenges

Previous studies have confirmed that rectal pressure is the main trigger for the sensation of rectal fullness. However, rectal pressure and rectal volume do not correlate, functioning independently, and studies have shown that rectal fullness sensation does not decrease even if rectal volume increases without an increase in rectal pressure. Therefore, rectal hyposensitivity should be limited to patients with elevated rectal pressure thresholds rather than those with "abnormally" elevated rectal volume thresholds [4]. In other words, currently, only sensory thresholds emphasizing volume are used to test rectal fullness sensation, but if all patients with increased rectal volume are diagnosed with decreased rectal sensation, that is, rectal sensory dullness, there may be inconsistencies in clinical management. The development of a simple method to measure rectal pressure for rectal fullness sensation is desired.

Take-Home Message

Human sensations are very delicate and subtle, and the expression methods vary among individuals. Therefore, to ensure objectivity, it is necessary to explain the sensations to the patient before the test and standardize the expression methods. It is important to explain the difference between the initial sensation of a foreign body in the rectum and the urge to defecate, as well as the limits of tolerance, and to obtain the patient's understanding for stable measurements. The stability of the examiner's technique is also essential.

Competing Interests The author has no competing interests to declare that are relevant to the content of this chapter.

References

1. Carrington EV, et al. The international anorectal physiology working group (IAPWG) recommendations: standardized testing protocol and the London classification for disorders of anorectal function. Neurogastroenterol Motil. 2020;32:e13679.
2. Knowles CH. Human studies of anorectal sensory function. Ir J Med Sci. 2018;187:1143–7.
3. Carrington EV, et al. Advances in the evaluation of anorectal function. Nat Rev Gastroenterol Hepatol. 2018;15:309–23.
4. Verkuijl SJ, et al. Normal rectal filling sensations in patients with an enlarged rectum. Dig Dis Sci. 2019;64:1312–9.

60 Anorectal Function Test, Pudendal Nerve Terminal Motor Latency

Shota Takano

Abstract

Pudendal nerve terminal motor latency (PNTML) testing is a diagnostic procedure used to evaluate the conduction time of the pudendal nerve. Although PNTML testing is now rarely performed in Japan, it remains a potentially valuable tool for identifying the etiology of fecal incontinence.

Keywords

Pudendal nerve terminal motor latency (PNTML) · Electromyography (EMG) · Pudendal nerve · Fecal incontinence

1 Pudendal Nerve Terminal Motor Latency Testing

Pudendal nerve terminal motor latency (PNTML) testing is a diagnostic procedure used to evaluate the conduction time of the pudendal nerve. The test involves inserting a specially designed electrode, affixed to a gloved finger, into the rectum (Fig. 60.1). Electrical stimulation is applied to the left and right pudendal nerves, and the latency—the time from stimulation to the elicited response of the external anal sphincter—is measured via electromyography (EMG) (Fig. 60.2). A prolonged conduction time is indicative of neurogenic dysfunction; however, the specific cutoff values for abnormality may vary slightly between institutions. Generally, a latency exceeding 2.2 ms is considered abnormal [1].

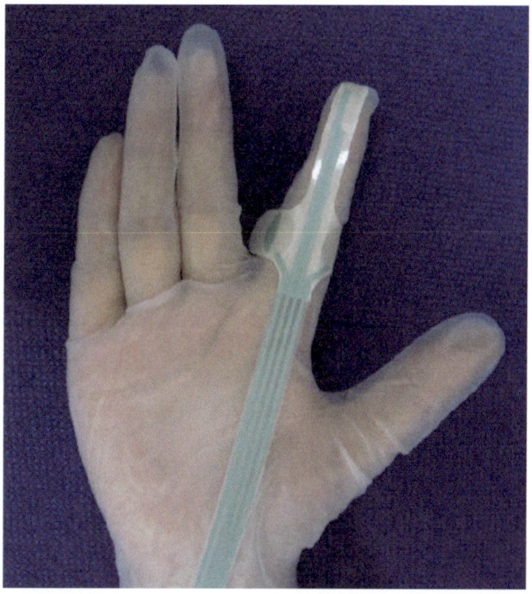

Fig. 60.1 Electrode device affixed to a glove for PNTML testing

Delayed pudendal nerve conduction is associated with perineal descent, straining-induced pelvic floor descent, and pudendal nerve injury resulting from vaginal delivery [2]. In patients

S. Takano (✉)
Department of Functional Anorectal Disorder, Coloproctology Center, Takano Hospital, Kumamoto, Japan
e-mail: micw@takano-hospital.jp

H. Kaneko et al. (eds.), *Disorders of Gut-Brain Interaction*,
https://doi.org/10.1007/978-981-95-6974-8_60

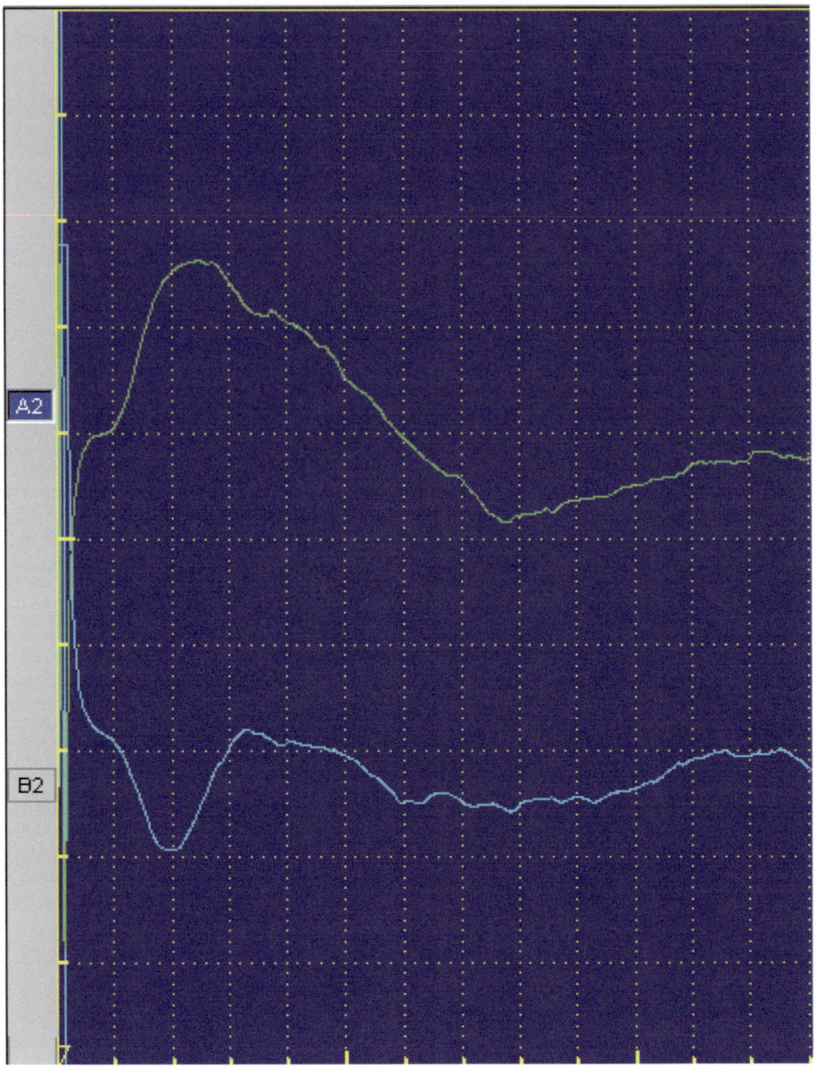

Fig. 60.2 EMG waveform used to assess conduction latency

with idiopathic fecal incontinence, PNTML is significantly prolonged compared to control groups. It has been reported that there are cases where the conduction time is prolonged on one side and cases where it is prolonged on both sides. In approximately 66% of patients with idiopathic fecal incontinence, normal conduction was observed on both sides, prolonged conduction was observed on both sides in 15% of cases, and prolonged conduction was observed on one side in 20% of cases.

Clinically, patients without conduction delay tend to respond more favorably to biofeedback therapy compared to those with delayed conduction. However, the clinical utility of this test for fecal incontinence has declined in recent years due to several limitations: lack of reproducibility, insufficient standardized normative data, and inadequate consideration of confounding factors such as age, childbirth history, and body mass index. Considering the low reliability of these findings and the possibility that pudendal nerve conduction time may not be involved in fecal incontinence, the clinical significance of PNTML is limited.

Take-Home Message
Although PNTML testing is now rarely performed in Japan, it remains a potentially valuable tool for identifying the etiology of fecal incontinence. Because the procedure involves inserting a device into the patient's anus, thorough pre-procedural explanation and gentle technique are essential to ensure patient comfort and cooperation.

Competing Interests The author has no competing interests to declare that are relevant to the content of this chapter.

References

1. The Japan Society of Coloproctology. Guidelines for the diagnosis and treatment of fecal incontinence. Tokyo: Nankodo; 2017. (in Japanese)
2. Takahashi T, et al. The Role of Each Examination on the Diagnosis of Fecal Incontinence. J Jpn Soc Coloproctol. 2015;68:940–5. (in Japanese)

61 Anorectal Function Test, Anal Electromyography

Shota Takano

Abstract

Anal electromyography (EMG) is a diagnostic technique used to assess the electrical activity of the external anal sphincter and the puborectalis muscle. In patients with fecal incontinence, the electrical activity of both the external anal sphincter and the puborectalis muscle is often reduced. As anal EMG can be applied therapeutically—particularly in biofeedback training—it is a valuable skill for clinicians to acquire. In Japan, plug-type surface EMG electrodes are commonly used.

Keywords

Anal electromyography (EMG) · External anal sphincter · Puborectalis muscle · Motor unit potentials · Biofeedback training

Anal electromyography (EMG) is a diagnostic technique used to assess the electrical activity of the external anal sphincter and the puborectalis muscle. By recording and analyzing the motor unit potentials (MUPs) generated by these muscles, EMG enables differentiation between neurogenic and myogenic etiologies of dysfunction. It is also employed to evaluate the motor behavior of the anal sphincter complex during defecation [1].

There are two primary types of EMG: needle EMG and surface EMG. The examination is typically performed with the patient in the left lateral decubitus position, using either surface electrodes or needle electrodes. In a normal EMG, a sufficient number of MUPs—defined as electrical activities with specific amplitude and duration—are observed in the external anal sphincter during voluntary contraction or straining (Fig. 61.1). During defecation, these MUPs either disappear or show a marked reduction. A decrease in electrical activity during sphincter contraction or coughing suggests possible nerve fiber injury.

In patients with fecal incontinence, the electrical activity of both the external anal sphincter and the puborectalis muscle is often reduced compared to control subjects [2]. In a study of patients with idiopathic fecal incontinence, abnormal findings were observed in 65% of external anal sphincters and 43% of puborectalis muscles [2].

Needle EMG is particularly effective in detecting denervation and can help determine whether external anal sphincter dysfunction is myogenic, neurogenic, or of mixed origin. Surface EMG, which uses plug-type or sponge electrodes inserted into the anal canal, records the EMG activity of the sphincter complex. While surface EMG correlates with sphincter pressure, it cannot

S. Takano (✉)
Department of Functional Anorectal Disorder, Coloproctology Center, Takano Hospital, Kumamoto, Japan
e-mail: micw@takano-hospital.jp

H. Kaneko et al. (eds.), *Disorders of Gut-Brain Interaction*,
https://doi.org/10.1007/978-981-95-6974-8_61

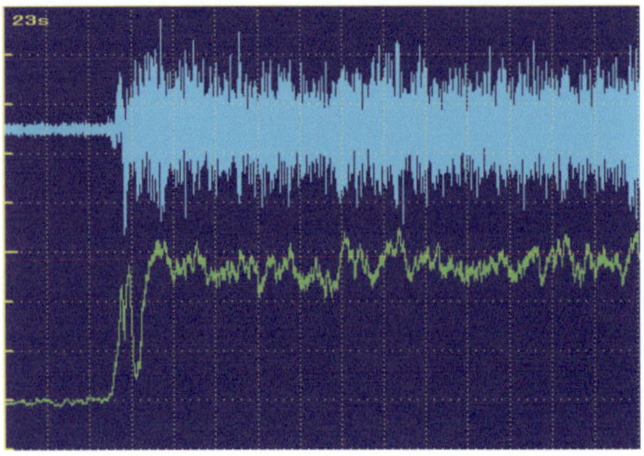

Fig. 61.1 EMG waveform of the external anal sphincter

distinguish the underlying cause of sphincter weakness. Nevertheless, surface EMG is utilized in some facilities as a component of biofeedback therapy for fecal incontinence [1].

Take-Home Message

As anal EMG can be applied therapeutically—particularly in biofeedback training—it is a valuable skill for clinicians to acquire. In Japan, plug-type surface EMG electrodes are commonly used. Gentle and careful handling techniques are necessary to avoid injuring the anus.

Competing Interests The author(s) has no competing interests to declare that are relevant to the content of this manuscript.

References

1. Takahashi T, et al. The Role of Each Examination on the Diagnosis of Fecal Incontinence. J Jpn Soc Coloproctol. 2015;68:940–5. (in Japanese).
2. The Japan Society of Coloproctology. Guidelines for the diagnosis and treatment of fecal incontinence. Tokyo: Nankodo; 2017. (in Japanese).

Anorectal Function Test, Defecography

62

Toshihiro Noake

Abstract

Defecography is a test that a viscous contrast agent is injected into the rectum, the subject is forced to perform excretion movements, and still images or videos are taken at rest, squeeze, and strain to examine defecation dynamics in a functional and morphological manner. The purpose of defecography and examination techniques is explained. The endpoints were anorectal angle, puborectal muscle length, pelvic descent, presence and size of rectocele, and expulsion rate. The pathologies that are revealed with this examination include levator ani syndrome, rectocele, rectal prolapse, rectal mucosal prolapse, and perineal descent.

Keywords

Defecography · Levator ani syndrome · Rectocele · Rectal prolapse · Perineal descent

1 Defecography

Defecography is a dynamic radiological examination used to evaluate the functional and anatomical aspects of defecation. In this procedure, a viscous contrast medium is introduced into the rectum, and the patient is instructed to perform defecatory maneuvers. Static or dynamic imaging is then performed during rest, contraction, and straining phases to assess defecatory mechanics.

1.1 Purpose

According to the *Clinical Practice Guidelines for Chronic Constipation 2017* [1], constipation is classified into organic and functional types. Functional constipation is further subdivided into infrequent bowel movements and difficult defecation. Defecography is particularly useful for dynamically diagnosing defecatory disorders in patients suspected of having difficult defecation [2]. When combined with colonic transit studies and anorectal manometry, it allows for a more comprehensive evaluation of constipation.

1.2 Examination Procedure

1. *Preparation*: Bowel preparation with laxatives is generally not required. However, if the rectum is filled with formed stool that may hinder contrast administration, enemas or suppositories may be used.
2. *Contrast preparation*: A simulated stool is prepared by mixing powdered contrast medium with carboxymethylcellulose (CMC)

T. Noake (✉)
Kurume Coloproctology Center, Coloproctology, Kurume, Japan
e-mail: kurume-hp@nifty.com

H. Kaneko et al. (eds.), *Disorders of Gut-Brain Interaction*,
https://doi.org/10.1007/978-981-95-6974-8_62

jelly to create approximately 150 g of paste (Fig. 62.1). Since viscosity is difficult to standardize, additional powdered CMC is added as needed to achieve a consistency similar to Bristol Stool Form Scale Type 5 (Fig. 62.2).
3. *Patient explanation*: As this is a unique test requiring defecation in a clinical setting, thorough explanation and patient understanding are essential. Efforts should be made to minimize anxiety and embarrassment, including the use of privacy screens.
4. *Contrast administration*: With the patient in the left lateral decubitus position, a catheter tip is gently inserted into the rectum, and 150 mL of contrast is instilled. Care must be taken to avoid perforation or anal trauma.

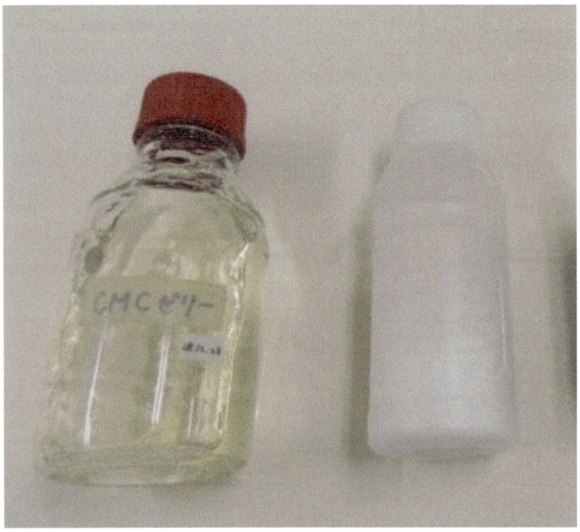

Fig. 62.1 Carboxymethylcellulose (CMC) jelly and powdered contrast medium (Barium)

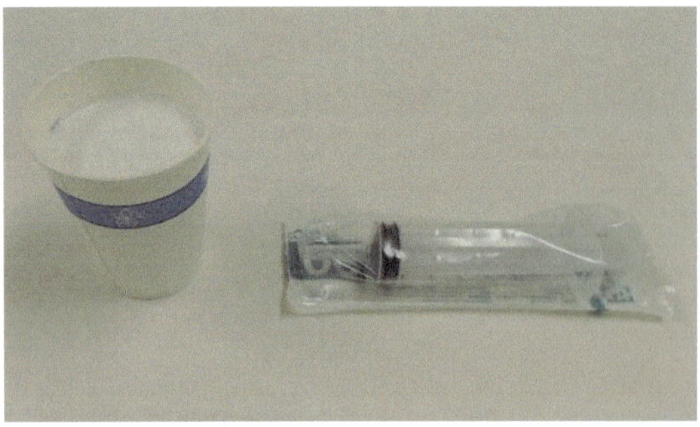

Fig. 62.2 Simulated stool and catheter tip with disposable syringe

5. *Positioning*: The patient is seated on a dedicated commode placed on a fluoroscopy table, which is gradually tilted to an upright position. Safety measures, such as handrails, should be used to prevent falls. The patient is positioned in a true lateral view, ensuring that the first sacral vertebra, coccyx, pubic symphysis, and perineum are within the field of view, and the femoral heads are superimposed (Fig. 62.3).
6. *Imaging*: Fluoroscopic images are obtained during rest, voluntary contraction (squeeze), straining, and postdefecation rest and straining. Additional frontal images are taken during rest and straining. Fluoroscopic video is recorded during straining.
7. *Postexamination interview*: After the procedure, the patient is asked about sensations of incomplete evacuation, residual stool, or discomfort.

1.3 Evaluation Criteria

Key anatomical landmarks and measurements used in defecography are illustrated in Fig. 62.4:

- *Anorectal angle (ARA)* (Angle E): Formed between the central axis of the anal canal (Line A) and a line connecting the center of the rectum to the upper edge of the anal canal (Line B).
- *Perineal descent*: Measured as the vertical distance between a line connecting the superior margin of the pubic symphysis and the tip of the coccyx (Line C) and a parallel line passing through the perineum.
- *Rectocele*: The size of rectocele is determined by the distance between the anterior wall of the anal canal and the apex of the rectocele.
- *Evacuation rate*: Calculated by comparing the volume of contrast medium before and after defecation using histogram data.

Although evacuation rate is not routinely measured, it is used at our institution to assess treatment efficacy by quantifying the expulsion of simulated stool.

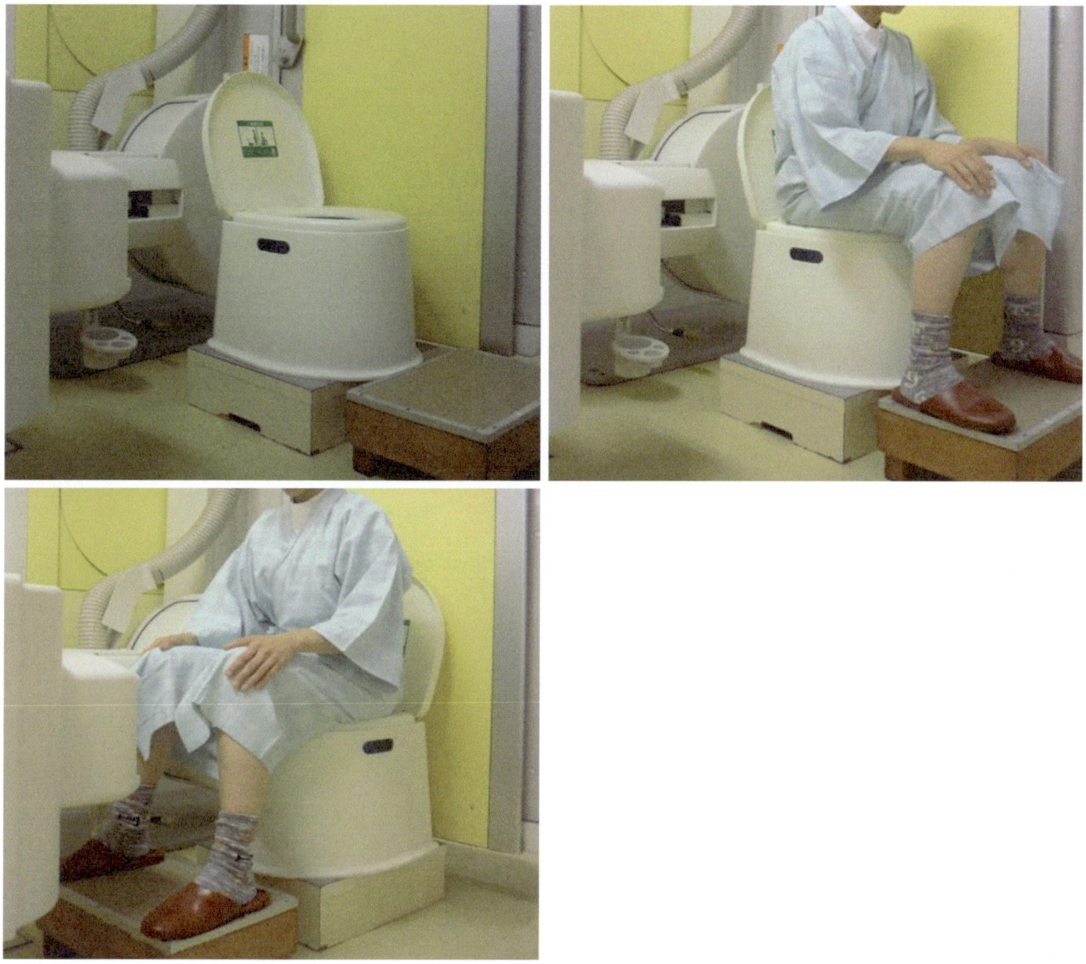

Fig. 62.3 Portable commode and imaging positions during defecography. *Top:* Portable commode mounted on the fluoroscopy table, *Middle:* Lateral seated position with static and dynamic imaging during rest, contraction, and straining, *Bottom:* Frontal seated position with static and dynamic imaging during rest and straining

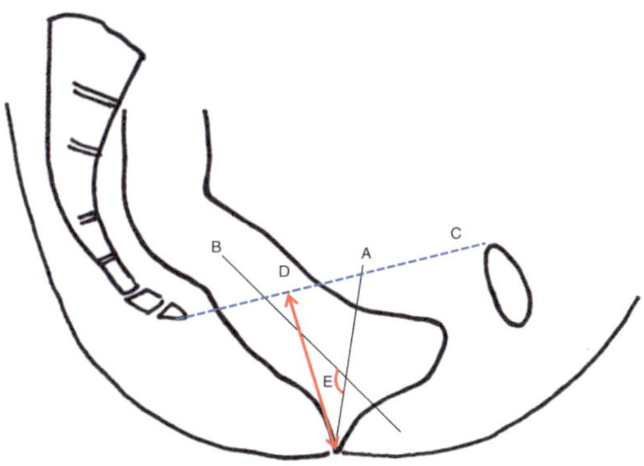

Fig. 62.4 Reference lines and anorectal angle in defecography. (**A**) Central axis of the anal canal, (**B**) central axis of the rectum, (**C**) pubococcygeal line, (**D**) perineal descent, (**E**) anorectal angle

A normal defecographic image is shown in Fig. 62.5. At rest, the simulated stool remains in the rectum without leakage. During contraction, the anorectal angle becomes more acute and the perineum elevates. During straining, the anorectal angle becomes obtuse, perineal descent of less than 2 cm occurs, and the anal canal opens during evacuation.

1.4 Pathophysiological Findings

1. *Pelvic floor dyssynergia*: Characterized by failure of the anorectal angle to become

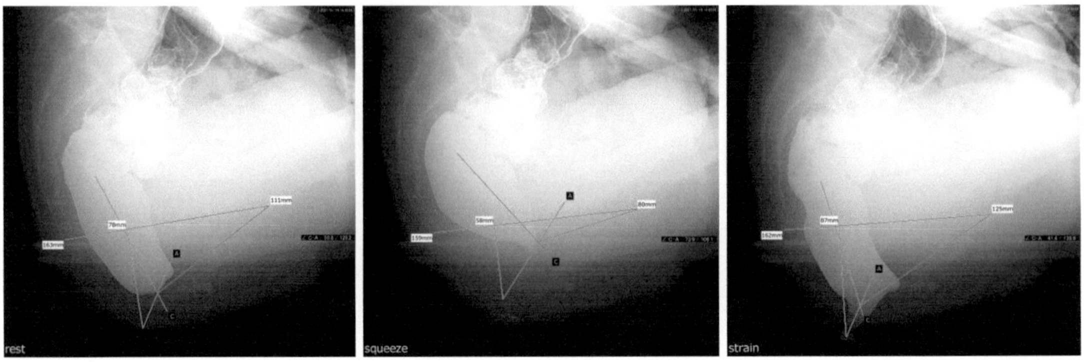

Fig. 62.5 Normal defecographic image. Left, rest; middle, squeeze; right, strain

obtuse or paradoxical narrowing during straining, resulting in difficult defecation.

2. *Rectocele*: Protrusion of the anterior rectal wall toward the vaginal side due to anteriorly directed abdominal pressure. Patients may report manual pressure on the posterior vaginal wall to aid defecation. Entrapment of formed stool within the rectocele during defecography is a characteristic finding.
3. *Rectal prolapse/intussusception*: Identified by invagination of the proximal rectum into the distal rectum during straining. If the rectum protrudes externally, it is classified as rectal prolapse; if it remains within the rectum or anal canal, it is termed rectal intussusception. Both can cause difficult defecation.
4. *Rectal mucosal prolapse*: Involves protrusion of the rectal mucosa in a lobulated pattern beyond the anal canal without intussusception. Differentiation from rectal prolapse may be difficult based on defecography alone.
5. *Perineal descent*: Diagnosed when perineal descent exceeds 2 cm during straining. The pelvic floor bulges toward the anal side, contributing to defecatory dysfunction.

Take-Home Message

While defecography can reveal various abnormalities, the ROME IV criteria [3] note that interpretation is not standardized, and similar findings may be observed in asymptomatic individuals. Therefore, standardization across institutions is needed. At a minimum, efforts should be made to unify interpretation criteria within each facility. Defecography should not be used in isolation but rather in conjunction with other diagnostic modalities for comprehensive evaluation.

Competing Interests The author(s) has no competing interests to declare that are relevant to the content of this manuscript.

References

1. Japanese Society of Gastroenterology, Research Group for the Diagnosis and Treatment of Chronic Constipation. Clinical practice guidelines for chronic constipation 2017. Tokyo: Nankodo; 2017. (in Japanese).
2. Goto HM, et al., editors. Rehabilitation of elimination: theory and clinical practice. 2nd ed. Nakayama Shoten: Tokyo; 2022. (in Japanese).
3. Drossman DA, et al. Functional gastrointestinal disorders (ROME IV). ROME Foundation; 2016.

Anorectal Function Test, Balloon Expulsion Test

63

Tatsuya Abe

Abstract

This chapter focuses on the Balloon Expulsion Test (BET), a simple and cost-effective physiological assessment used to evaluate defecatory function in patients with suspected defecation disorders, a subtype of functional constipation. BET involves inserting a balloon into the rectum, inflating it with water or air, and then attempting to expel the balloon to simulate defecation. It is particularly useful for identifying patients who may benefit from biofeedback therapy, which has shown greater efficacy than laxatives or dietary fiber in treating defecation disorders. Although there is no standardized protocol for BET, failure to expel the balloon within 1–2 minutes is generally considered abnormal. This chapter discusses the diagnostic utility of BET in comparison with anorectal manometry and defecography, highlighting its high specificity but limited sensitivity. While BET alone cannot confirm or exclude a diagnosis, it remains a valuable tool when interpreted alongside clinical symptoms and other physiological tests.

Keywords

Anorectal manometry · Biofeedback therapy · Balloon expulsion test · Defecation disorder · Defecography

1 Purpose of the Examination

The balloon expulsion test (BET) is a physiological assessment used to evaluate the ability to evacuate stool by inserting a simulated stool or balloon into the rectum and instructing the subject to expel it. This test is primarily indicated for patients suspected of having defecation disorder, a subtype of functional constipation, or for those with refractory constipation unresponsive to multiple laxatives [1]. In patients with defecation disorders, biofeedback therapy is often more effective than treatment with dietary fiber or laxatives [2]. Therefore, when symptoms suggestive of defecation disorder are present—such as excessive straining, a sensation of incomplete evacuation, or manual maneuvers to facilitate defecation—physiological tests such as BET and anorectal manometry are recommended prior to initiating pharmacologic therapy [1].

T. Abe (✉)
Department of Proctology, Kunimoto Hospital, Anorectal Surgery, Asahikawa, Japan
e-mail: t-abe@cf6.so-net.ne.jp

H. Kaneko et al. (eds.), *Disorders of Gut-Brain Interaction*,
https://doi.org/10.1007/978-981-95-6974-8_63

2 BET Procedure

Routine bowel preparation is generally unnecessary. However, if the rectum is filled with stool or if there is concern about leakage during the test, an enema or suppository may be used to empty the rectum.

One method involves the use of a simulated stool (FECOM), consisting of a silicone shell (2.4 cm in diameter, 9 cm in length) filled with barium gel. However, in most facilities, a latex balloon is used, which is inflated with water or air to perform the BET (Fig. 63.1) [3]. There is currently no standardized protocol regarding patient positioning, balloon inflation volume, or time limits for expulsion. Typically, a deflated balloon is inserted into the lower rectum with the patient in the left lateral decubitus position and then inflated with approximately 50 mL of water. The patient is then seated on a commode and instructed to strain as if defecating. Expulsion of the inflated balloon within 1–2 minutes is considered normal; failure to do so is interpreted as inability to expel (see Table 63.1).

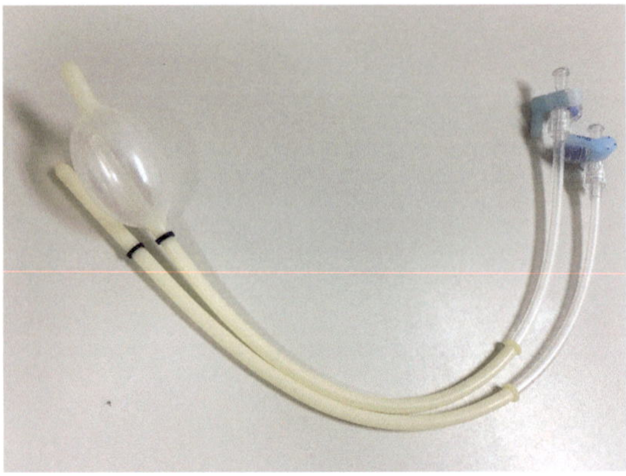

Fig. 63.1 Custom-made rectal balloon. A 14Fr Nelaton catheter fitted with a rubber cover designed for intracavitary temperature probes, secured using a hemorrhoidal ligation rubber ring

Table 63.1 Diagnostic accuracy of the balloon expulsion test (BET) for defecation disorders

Author (year)	Journal volume	Sample size	Balloon contents/ volume	Position/time limit	Sensitivity (%)	Specificity (%)
Minguez M (2004)	*Gastroenterology* 126	130	Water at 36 °C, Desire to Defecate Volume	Seated, <1 min	88	89
Bordeianou L (2011)	*Dis Colon Rectum* 54	123	Air, 60 mL	Seated, <5 min	52	85
Kassis NC (2015)	*Int Urogynecol J* 26	60 (females only)	Water, 50 mL	Seated, <2 min	33	80
Seong MK (2016)	*Ann Surg Treat Res* 90	87	Water, 60 mL	Seated, <30 sec	74	86

3 Diagnostic Utility of BET

Historically, the gold standard for diagnosing defecation disorders was defecography (see Chap. 62). Defecography allows for simultaneous evaluation of anorectal angle dynamics, evacuation rate, and the presence of structural abnormalities such as rectocele or rectal intussusception [3]. However, defecography lacks standardized methodology and interpretation criteria, requires specialized equipment, and involves radiation exposure for both patients and healthcare providers. Consequently, when defecation disorder is suspected, it is recommended to first perform anorectal manometry and BET, which are safer and more accessible [1].

Table 63.1 summarizes key studies comparing BET results with diagnoses made using defecography and anorectal manometry. While BET demonstrates relatively high specificity, its sensitivity is limited. Therefore, if a patient with symptoms of defecation difficulty is unable to expel the balloon, the likelihood of a defecation disorder is high. However, successful balloon expulsion does not definitively exclude the diagnosis [4]. Currently, no single test can accurately diagnose defecation disorders in isolation. A comprehensive diagnosis must be based on clinical symptoms in conjunction with multiple physiological assessments.

Take-Home Message

- Although the balloon expulsion test (BET) has limitations in diagnostic accuracy when used alone, it remains a valuable tool due to its low cost and simplicity.
- Even in settings where anorectal manometry or defecography cannot be performed, a diagnosis of defecation disorder can be sufficiently established by combining clinical symptoms with BET findings.
- Caution should be exercised in patients with a history of rectal surgery, as the test may place stress on the anastomotic site.

Competing Interests The author(s) has no competing interests to declare that are relevant to the content of this manuscript.

References

1. Bharucha AE, et al. American Gastroenterological Association technical review on constipation. Gastroenterology. 2013;144:218–38.
2. Abe T. Treatment of defecation disorders: biofeedback therapy and more. Gastroenterology (Shokakinaika). Igaku-Shoin. 2020:80–5. (in Japanese).
3. Abe T. Rectal balloon expulsion test. In: Goto H, et al., editors. Continence rehabilitation: theory and clinical practice. 2nd ed. Tokyo: Nakayama Shoten; 2022. p. 301–2. (in Japanese).
4. Rao SSC, et al. Clinical utility of diagnostic tests for constipation in adults: a systematic review. Am J Gastroenterol. 2005;100:1605–15.

Part IX

Anorectum, Practical Edition

64 Diagnosis and Treatment of DGBI of the anorectum, Fecal Incontinence

Toshiki Mimura

Abstract

Fecal incontinence (FI) is defined as "the involuntary or uncontrollable loss of feces through the anus." In the *2017* edition *of Japanese Clinical Guidelines for Fecal Incontinence*, its prevalence is estimated at approximately 10% in the general population. It is usually caused by multiple etiologies and factors including stool consistency, function of defecation-related musculature, anorectal sensory function, rectal pressure·capacity·compliance, colonic function, and cognitive and mobility function.

To diagnose its underlying causes, medical history taking and physical examination are essential, followed by specialized examinations including anorectal physiology examinations and endoanal ultrasonography. FI can be classified into passive and urge types based on symptoms.

After excluding organic causes, initial management should be tailored to the symptom type, underlying cause, and severity—beginning with dietary, lifestyle, and bowel habit guidance, as well as pharmacotherapy. If these initial treatments fail, referral to a specialized facility is recommended.

Specialized conservative therapies include pelvic floor muscle training, biofeedback therapy, and transanal irrigation. If these conservative therapies fail, surgery treatment should be considered. First-line surgical procedures include sacral neuromodulation and sphincteroplasty, while second-line surgical procedures include antegrade continence enema, graciloplasty, ventral rectopexy, and stoma creation. Anal sphincter regenerative therapy is emerging as a promising experimental therapy.

Keywords

Fecal incontinence · Anal incontinence · Anorectal physiology examination · Endoanal ultrasonography · Pelvic floor muscle training · Biofeedback therapy · Transanal irrigation · Sacral neuromodulation · Anal sphincteroplasty · Stoma

1 Introduction

Fecal incontinence (FI) has historically been referred to as a "silent affliction," as it is a symptom that significantly impairs daily life, yet patients often hesitate to seek help and rarely visit medical institutions on their own for exami-

T. Mimura (✉)
Division of Gastroenterological, General and Transplant Surgery, Department of Surgery, Jichi Medical University, Shimotsuke, Japan
e-mail: mimurat@jichi.ac.jp

H. Kaneko et al. (eds.), *Disorders of Gut-Brain Interaction*,
https://doi.org/10.1007/978-981-95-6974-8_64

nation or treatment. This reluctance is attributed not only to the benign nature of the disorder and the associated embarrassment but also to the limited awareness—among both patients and healthcare providers—that symptoms can potentially be improved or cured through conservative therapies or surgical treatment.

However, since sacral neuromodulation for FI was covered by national health insurance in April 2014 and the publication of the *Clinical Guidelines for Fecal Incontinence 2017* Edition (FI Guidelines) in March 2017 [1], public and media attention toward FI has increased. Furthermore, in April 2018, transanal irrigation was approved for insurance coverage for patients with refractory defecation disorders due to spinal cord injury (excluding those postrectal surgery). These developments have led to a rise in the number of patients seeking medical care for FI, necessitating that even nonspecialist healthcare providers be equipped to offer initial management. This chapter provides an overview of FI based on the FI Guidelines.

1.1 Concept and Definition

Multiple academic societies and organizations have proposed various definitions of FI, and no single universally accepted definition exists [2]. The simplest definition is provided by the *Glossary of Stoma and Continence Rehabilitation Terminology* compiled by the Japanese Society of Stoma and Continence Rehabilitation, which defines FI as the "involuntary loss of feces." Similarly, the sixth International Consultation on Incontinence (ICI) defines "fecal incontinence" as the "involuntary loss of feces" [3].

The ICI further defines flatus incontinence as the "involuntary loss of rectal gas or flatus," mucous incontinence as the "involuntary loss of mucous only (without feces)," and collectively refers to these as anal incontinence, defined as the "involuntary loss of feces and/or flatus and/or mucous."

In Japan, the FI Guidelines [1] define FI not merely as "involuntary loss of feces" but more precisely as "the involuntary or uncontrollable loss of feces through the anus." This definition encompasses two different types of FI: passive fecal incontinence, where stool leaks without the patient's awareness (i.e., unconscious leakage), and urge fecal incontinence, where the patient perceives the urge to defecate but cannot reach the toilet in time (i.e., leakage against one's will). When flatus incontinence is also present, the condition is referred to as anal incontinence.

1.2 Epidemiology

Systematic reviews report a wide variation in the prevalence of FI among the general population, ranging from 0.9% to 19.5% [2]. These discrepancies are attributed to differences in the definitions, survey methodologies, response rates, and study populations. A 2016 systematic review of studies in the general population that standardized the definition of FI as "liquid or solid stool leakage occurring at least once per month" found prevalence rates of 8.3–8.4% in interview or telephone surveys and 11.2–12.4% in anonymous postal surveys. While the results were generally consistent across survey methods, the slightly lower prevalence observed in interviews and telephone surveys is likely attributable to respondent embarrassment.

Similarly, a 2004 systematic review of 16 studies reported a prevalence range of 0.4–18%. However, when limited to three studies that minimized bias, the prevalence was estimated at 11–15%, suggesting that the true prevalence in the general population is approximately 10% [2].

In Japan, the FI Guidelines [1] report that the prevalence of FI among individuals aged 65 and older is 8.7% in men and 6.6% in women, based on a door-to-door interview study of 1405 individuals conducted by Nakanishi et al., yielding a combined prevalence of 7.5%. Another study by Mimura et al. using an anonymous postal survey of 274 employees aged 20–65 years reported a prevalence of 4% for liquid or solid FI occurring at least once per month [2]. Based on population demographics, this translates to approximately three million individuals aged 20–65 and 2.3 million individuals aged 65 and older, totaling over five million people with FI in Japan [2]. This estimate excludes residents of long-term care facilities, where prevalence rates are reported to be 50–80%. A 2019 systematic review reported a prevalence of 42.8% among institutionalized individuals aged 65 and older.

Although epidemiological studies often show no significant sex differences, approximately 70% of patients who seek medical care for FI are women [4]. This may be due to obstetric-related FI and a higher sensitivity to symptoms among women.

1.3 Etiology and Pathophysiology

The main factors involved in FI include stool consistency, function of defecation-related musculature (internal and external anal sphincters, puborectal muscle, and levator ani), anorectal sensory function, rectal pressure·capacity·compliance, colonic function, cognitive and mobility function. Numerous causes of FI can impair one or more of these six factors [5]. Often, multiple etiologies and pathophysiological mechanisms coexist [6, 7].

Below is an explanation of how dysfunction in each factor contributes to FI.

1.3.1 Soft or Liquid Stool Consistency

Stool consistency, typically assessed using the Bristol Stool Form Scale (BSFS), is a key determinant in defecation disorders. Types 6 and 7 (loose or watery stools) can cause FI on their own. In patients with passive FI due to impaired internal anal sphincter function, stool may be chronically loose (type 5 or 6) even in the absence of acute diarrheal illness.

1.3.2 Dysfunction of Defecation-Related Musculature Including Anal Sphincter

The musculature involved in FI includes the internal anal sphincter (IAS), external anal sphincter (EAS), and the levator ani muscle group, including the puborectal muscle.

The IAS is composed of smooth muscle and functions involuntarily. It contributes to more than half of the resting anal canal pressure, which typically ranges from 60 to 100 mmHg [8]. Therefore, when IAS function declines due to aging or other factors, resting pressure in the anal canal decreases. In such cases, during upright activities such as sitting or walking, gravitational force acts on rectal contents (e.g., mucus or liquid stool), allowing them to leak through the anal canal and result in passive FI. In contrast, during sleep or when lying down, gravity does not act in anal canal direction, making leakage due to IAS dysfunction rare in the supine position.

The EAS and puborectal muscle, components of the levator ani, are striated muscles under voluntary control. These muscles allow conscious contraction to maintain continence. When their contractile strength is reduced—due to obstetric injury (e.g., vaginal delivery), pudendal neuropathy, or aging—the anal canal cannot generate or sustain pressure higher than the rectal pressure that accompanies the urge to defecate. As a result, stool may be expelled before the patient reaches the toilet, leading to urge FI.

1.3.3 Impaired Anorectal Sensory Function

In cases where anorectal sensory function is diminished—due to spinal cord injury, aging, or other causes—patients may not perceive the urge to defecate even when stool moves from the sigmoid colon into the rectum via mass peristalsis. If this state persists and the patient does not attempt to defecate, a condition known as rectal fecal impaction may develop, characterized by the accumulation of a large amount of stool in the rectum. Eventually, part of this retained stool may leak out involuntarily, resulting in passive FI through a mechanism of overflow FI [9].

Unlike passive FI caused by IAS dysfunction, overflow incontinence is not dependent on gravitational forces acting on rectal contents. Therefore, it frequently occurs even in the supine position, such as during sleep. The presence or absence of nocturnal FI can thus provide clues to the underlying cause of passive FI. Importantly, rectal fecal impaction can be readily diagnosed through digital rectal examination.

1.3.4 Abnormal Rectal Pressure, Capacity, and Compliance

In patients with irritable bowel syndrome (IBS), rectal hypersensitivity may cause abnormally high rectal pressure during defecatory urge, leading to urge FI. Diarrhea-predominant IBS further increases this risk due to loose stool. Reduced rectal compliance (distensibility) in IBS can also cause excessive pressure increase with small amount of stool, leading to urge FI.

Patients who have undergone rectal resection with anus preserving operation for rectal cancer may experience low anterior resection syndrome (LARS), characterized by frequent, irregular, or urgent defecation, passive and urge FI, and difficult defecation. Reduced compliance and capacity of the neorectum are contributing factors. Persistent small-volume stool retention in the neorectum can also lead to overflow incontinence, resulting in passive FI and nocturnal FI, as well as defecation difficulty and a sensation of incomplete evacuation because small amount of stool is difficult to evacuate by straining.

1.3.5 Colonic Dysfunction

When colonic water absorption or storage capacity is impaired, diarrhea and frequent defecation occur, which can lead to FI. Such colonic dysfunction can occur not only in acute enteritis but also in IBS. In LARS, the sigmoid colon is often partially resected along with the rectum, reducing the capacity of the sigmoid colon, which normally serves as a reservoir for stool. As a result, symptoms such as frequent defecation, clustering of stool, irregular bowel movements, and urge FI may occur.

1.3.6 Cognitive and Mobility Dysfunction

Even in the absence of any impairment of colonic or anorectal function such as the defecation-related muscles or anorectal sensory function, FI can occur if cognitive or physical mobility function is impaired, preventing appropriate toileting behavior. This condition is referred to as disability associated fecal incontinence, which is broadly classified into two types: impaired cognition fecal incontinence and impaired mobility fecal incontinence.

Impaired cognition FI refers to FI that occurs due to impaired cognitive function, such as in those with dementia. These individuals may lack the social or hygienic understanding that defecation should be done in a toilet, leading to defecation in inappropriate settings, or they may forget the location of the toilet, resulting in FI.

Impaired mobility FI refers to FI that occurs in individuals with physical disabilities, such as lower limb amputation due to trauma, where mobility is impaired. In such cases, the individual may take too long to reach the toilet after feeling the urge to defecate, resulting in FI.

1.4 Diagnosis and Examination

To diagnose the underlying causes of FI, it is essential to conduct a thorough clinical evaluation that includes a detailed medical history, anorectal digital examination, anorectal physiology examinations, and endoanal ultrasonography. However, in medical facilities that do not specialize in the management of FI, it is often necessary to estimate the cause based solely on the patient's history and physical findings. Even when the precise etiology cannot be determined, as long as serious underlying conditions such as colorectal cancer or inflammatory bowel disease—which require specific treatment—are not suspected, it is appropriate to initiate initial management strategies that are feasible within the capabilities of the facility. If the patient's symptoms do not sufficiently improve with this approach, referral to a specialized center is recommended [10].

When a patient presents with symptoms of FI, the clinician should begin by obtaining a comprehensive history, including current medication use, followed by a physical examination that includes inspection and digital examination of the anorectal region. If findings suggest the presence of organic disease, such as colorectal cancer or inflammatory bowel disease, further diagnostic procedures, including colonoscopy, should be performed to confirm the diagnosis and guide appropriate treatment.

1.4.1 Medical History Taking

Key elements include bowel habits, onset and triggers of FI, symptom characteristics, past medical, surgical and obstetric history, comorbidities, and current medications. FI is categorized into passive and urge types; when both are present, it is termed mixed FI. In specialized centers, passive, urge, and mixed fecal, incontinence accounts for 49%, 16%, and 35%, respectively [4].

Scoring systems commonly used to assess the severity of FI include the Fecal Incontinence Severity Index (FISI), Cleveland Clinic Florida Fecal Incontinence Score (CCFIS), and St. Mark's Score. The LARS Score is used for low anterior resection syndrome (LARS) [1]. The Japanese version of the Fecal Incontinence Quality of Life Scale (JFIQL) is useful for evaluating FI-specific quality of life [11].

Past anorectal surgeries (e.g., for hemorrhoids, anal fistulas, and anal fissures), trauma, and obstetric history in women should be reviewed. Medication history should be scrutinized for inappropriate or unrecognized use of laxatives, because FI may occur due to diarrhea, resulting from the excessive or inappropriate use of laxatives prescribed for constipation or from unrecognized use of medications that act as laxatives [9].

1.4.2 Physical Examination

During visual inspection, the clinician should assess for the presence of scars resulting from previous anorectal surgeries. In female patients, particular attention should be paid to scars from perineal lacerations or episiotomies sustained during vaginal delivery. Digital rectal examination should be performed to evaluate for the presence of fecal impaction, masses, or blood. In addition, the resting tone of the anal sphincter and the degree of contraction of the pelvic floor and anal sphincter muscles as well as the movement of the perineum during voluntary squeeze should be assessed.

As a useful method for the subjective evaluation of anal canal tone at rest and sphincter contraction strength with digital rectoanal examination, the Digital Rectal Examination Scoring System (DRESS) is useful. It scores both resting and squeeze pressures on a six-point scale from 0 to 5 [12]. DRESS scores, when assessed by experienced clinicians, have been shown to correlate well with the results of anorectal manometry.

1.4.3 Specialized Examinations

If symptoms do not sufficiently improve with initial conservative therapy, specialized examinations should be performed to identify the underlying cause of FI and guide further treatment.

Anorectal Manometry

Anorectal manometry is used to evaluate the contractile function of the anal sphincter using a manometric catheter. The main parameters measured include functional anal canal length, maximum resting pressure, and both the absolute and incremental values of maximum voluntary squeeze pressure [8]. For detailed methodology, refer to Chap. 58.

Rectal Balloon Sensation Test

This test assesses rectal sensory function by inflating a balloon placed in the rectum with air. Key parameters include the threshold for initial sensation, the volume at which the urge to defecate is perceived, and the maximum tolerable volume. For further details, refer to Chap. 59.

As part of the national initiative to promote task-shifting/sharing under the "Work Style Reform for Physicians," a revision to the Enforcement Order of the Clinical Laboratory Technologists Act came into effect on October 1, 2021. As a result, anorectal physiology examinations, including anorectal manometry and rectal balloon sensation testing, can now be independently performed by clinical laboratory technologists under the order of a physician.

Endoanal Ultrasonography (See Fig. 64.1)

This examination is performed transanally using a dedicated anal ultrasound probe. The internal anal sphincter appears as a hypoechoic (low-echo) circular structure, while the external

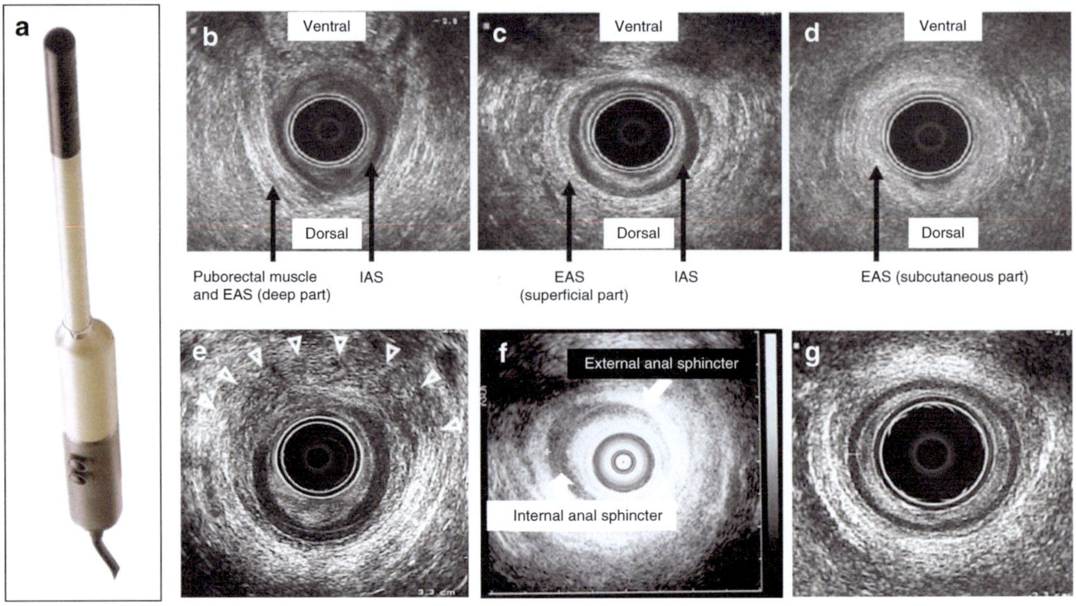

Fig. 64.1 Endoanal ultrasonography. (**a**) Transanal three-dimensional ultrasound probe (Type 2050, B-K Medical, Denmark). The probe operates at a variable frequency of 6–16 MHz and allows for three-dimensional image reconstruction. (**b**–**d**) Normal anal ultrasonographic images. Using the anal ultrasound probe, the internal and external anal sphincters are evaluated for damage at the upper (**b**), middle (**c**), and lower (**d**) levels of the anal canal. The external anal sphincter (EAS) (striated muscle) appears as a high-echogenic ring, while the internal anal sphincter (IAS) (smooth muscle) appears as a low-echogenic ring. (**e**–**g**) Pathological findings on endoanal ultrasonography. (**e**) Obstetric anal sphincter injury. Both the low-echogenic (IAS) and high-echogenic (EAS) rings are disrupted ventrally (toward the vaginal side) between the 10 and 2 o'clock positions, indicated by arrowheads. (**f**) Surgically induced sphincter injury. A case of passive fecal incontinence following hemorrhoidectomy. The IAS is absent from the 1 to 6 o'clock position on the left side, and the anterior right IAS appears relatively thickened. (**g**) Internal anal sphincter degeneration (IASD). No structural damage is observed in either sphincter, but the IAS is thinned to less than 2 mm in thickness. *Abbreviations:* IAS internal anal sphincter, EAS external anal sphincter

anal sphincter appears as a hyperechoic (high-echo) ring. The thickness and integrity of each sphincter can be evaluated separately. This modality is particularly useful for diagnosing the presence and extent of sphincter damage, which may indicate the need for sphincteroplasty.

In addition to the above, other diagnostic modalities include anal mucosal electrical stimulation testing, pudendal nerve terminal motor latency testing, anal electromyography, pelvic MRI, and defecography. Other ultrasound techniques, such as transvaginal and transperineal ultrasonography, are also available but are not commonly performed and are therefore omitted from this article.

1.5 Treatment

The flowchart for initial management, specialized diagnostic testing, and conservative therapy for FI, as outlined in the *Clinical Guidelines for Fecal Incontinence* (FI Guidelines), is presented in Fig. 64.2. The flowchart for surgical treatment is shown in Fig. 64.3. A wide range of treatment options is available, from conservative approaches to surgical interventions. Given that FI is a benign

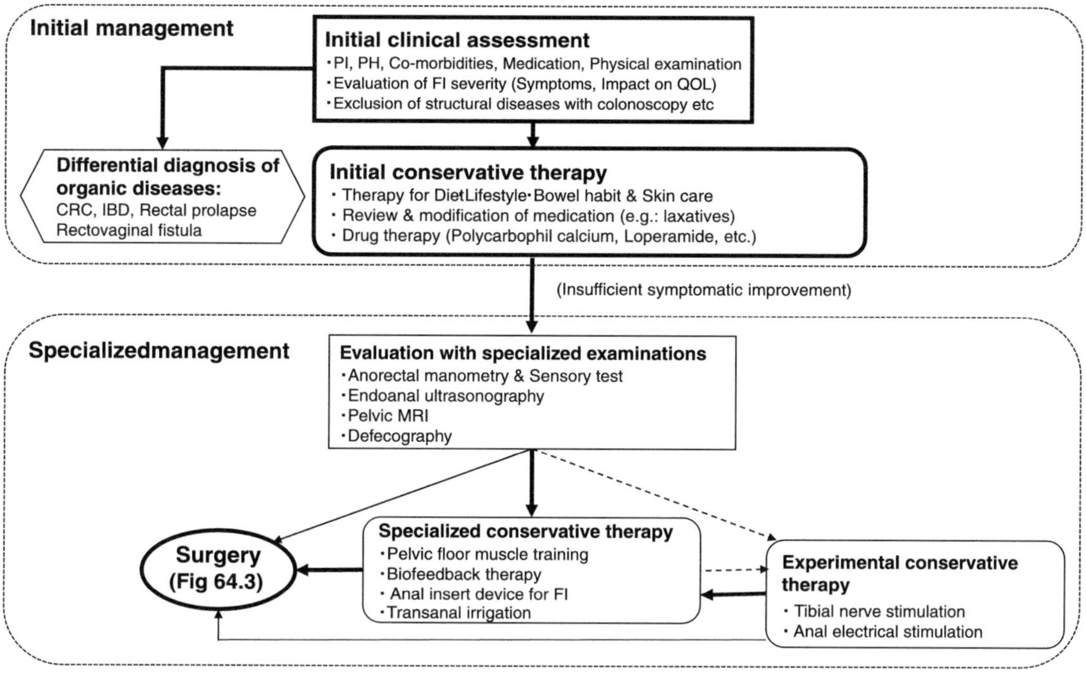

Fig. 64.2 Flowchart for initial management, specialized examinations, and conservative therapy for fecal incontinence. (cited and translated from Ref. [1]). *Abbreviations:* PI present illness, PH past history, FI fecal incontinence, QoL quality of life, CRC colorectal cancer, IBD inflammatory bowel disease

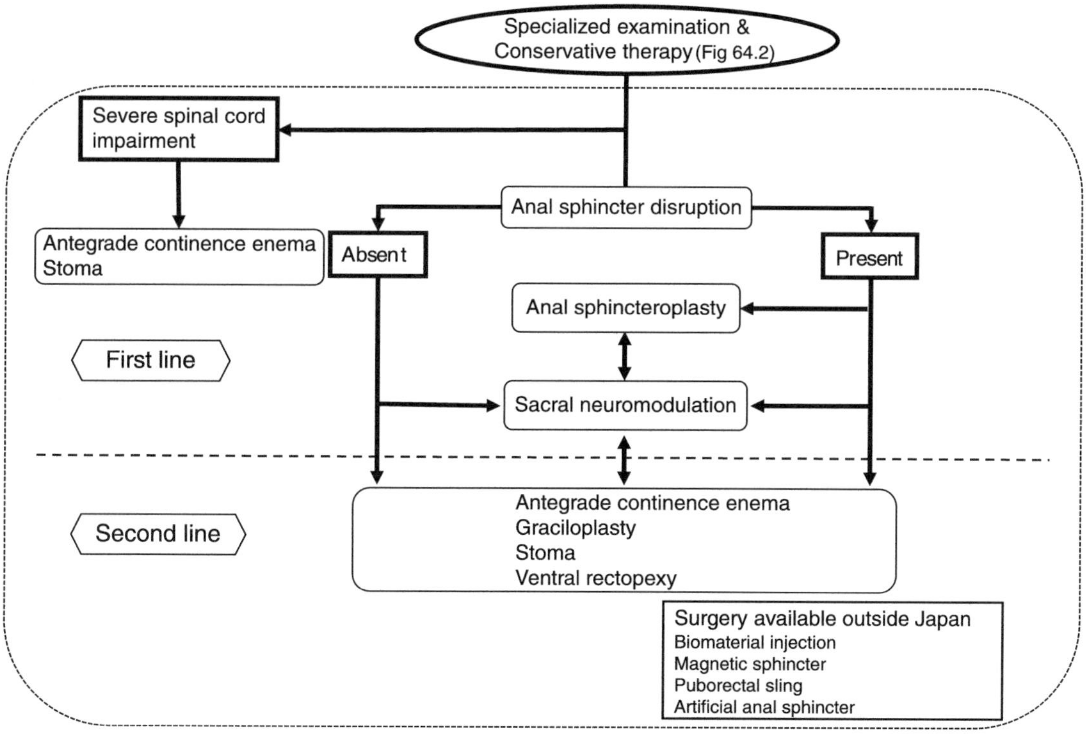

Fig. 64.3 Flowchart for surgical treatment of fecal incontinence. (cited and translated from Ref. [1])

condition, the general principle is to begin with the least invasive therapies. Even when surgery is indicated, it is recommended to start with the least invasive surgical techniques [10, 13].

1.5.1 Differentiation and Treatment of Organic Diseases

If the initial clinical evaluation reveals conditions such as colorectal cancer, inflammatory bowel disease, rectal prolapse, rectovaginal fistula, or significant anal sphincter injury, the primary disease should be addressed first. Surgical intervention should be considered as necessary based on the underlying pathology.

1.5.2 Initial Conservative Therapy (Fig. 64.2)

If organic disease is ruled out, the next step is to provide the patient and caregivers with education and information about FI. Management should begin by addressing modifiable factors that are relatively easy to correct. This includes evaluating and improving access to toilet facilities in the living environment and reviewing medications, particularly the inappropriate or excessive use of laxatives.

Dietary, Lifestyle, and Bowel Habit Guidance and Skincare

For FI associated with loose stools, the FI Guidelines [1] recommend the intake of dietary fiber with a recommendation grade of A (meaning strong recommendation based on high-level evidence with complete consensus among the guideline committee members). Additionally, bowel habit training and skincare are recommended for the prevention and treatment of incontinence-associated dermatitis (IAD) due to FI with a grade of B (meaning moderate recommendation based on lower-level evidence but with consensus).

To prevent and improve defecation disorders, including both FI and constipation, it is important to enjoy a varied and balanced diet rich in fermented foods and dietary fiber, to consume moderate amounts of coffee and alcohol as preferred, to maintain adequate hydration without becoming dehydrated, to lead a regular and low-stress lifestyle, to ensure sufficient and consistent sleep, and to engage in moderate physical activity such as walking or light exercise [14].

Pharmacotherapy

Many patients with FI, regardless of the underlying cause, present with mild, frequent loose stools. In such cases, oral administration of calcium polycarbophil often improves stool consistency and, consequently, FI. If calcium polycarbophil alone is insufficient, loperamide hydrochloride may be added. However, initiating treatment with the standard 1 mg capsule formulation used as an antidiarrheal may lead to constipation. Therefore, it is advisable to begin with the granule formulation at a dose of 0.5 mg and gradually increase the dose while monitoring bowel movement frequency, stool consistency, and the severity of FI.

Although the maximum reimbursable dose under Japan's national health insurance is 2 mg/day, the guidelines from the National Institute for Health and Clinical Excellence (NICE) state that loperamide is a safe and dose-dependent medication, and the dose may be increased up to 16 mg/day until the desired stool consistency is achieved [1]. In the FI Guidelines [1], calcium polycarbophil is recommended with a grade of B, while loperamide hydrochloride is recommended with a grade of A.

If symptoms do not improve with these initial conservative measures, the patient should be referred to a specialized facility capable of performing advanced diagnostic testing and treatment.

1.5.3 Specialized Conservative Therapies (Fig. 64.2)

Pelvic Floor Muscle Training (PFMT)

Pelvic floor muscle training is a therapeutic approach aimed at strengthening the pelvic floor muscles, including the external anal sphincter and the levator ani, through repeated voluntary contractions. This method has been shown to improve both urinary and fecal incontinence. Although it remains unclear which subgroups of patients with FI benefit most from PFMT, it is generally indicated for individuals who are capable of understanding the training instructions and who possess sufficient motivation to continue the exercises at home.

It is important to note that simply instructing patients to "practice tightening the anus" is insufficient. Proper technique must be taught through direct examination and guidance to ensure effective engagement of the correct musculature. PFMT is a simple and low-cost intervention and when appropriately instructed has been reported to improve FI in 41–66% of cases [1]. In the FI Guidelines [1], PFMT is assigned a recommendation grade of C (meaning weak recommendation based on limited evidence without complete consensus).

Biofeedback Therapy (Fig. 64.4)
Biofeedback (BF) therapy involves the use of devices such as anal electromyography or anorectal manometry to provide patients with real-time visual feedback on pelvic floor muscle activity. This allows patients to perform pelvic floor muscle training more effectively by consciously adjusting their muscle contractions based on the feedback provided [15]. The primary goals of BF therapy in the treatment of FI are to enhance the strength and endurance of the pelvic floor muscles, including the external anal sphincter, and to normalize rectal sensation. As with PFMT, the specific patient populations most likely to benefit from BF therapy remain unclear. Therefore, BF therapy is best suited for

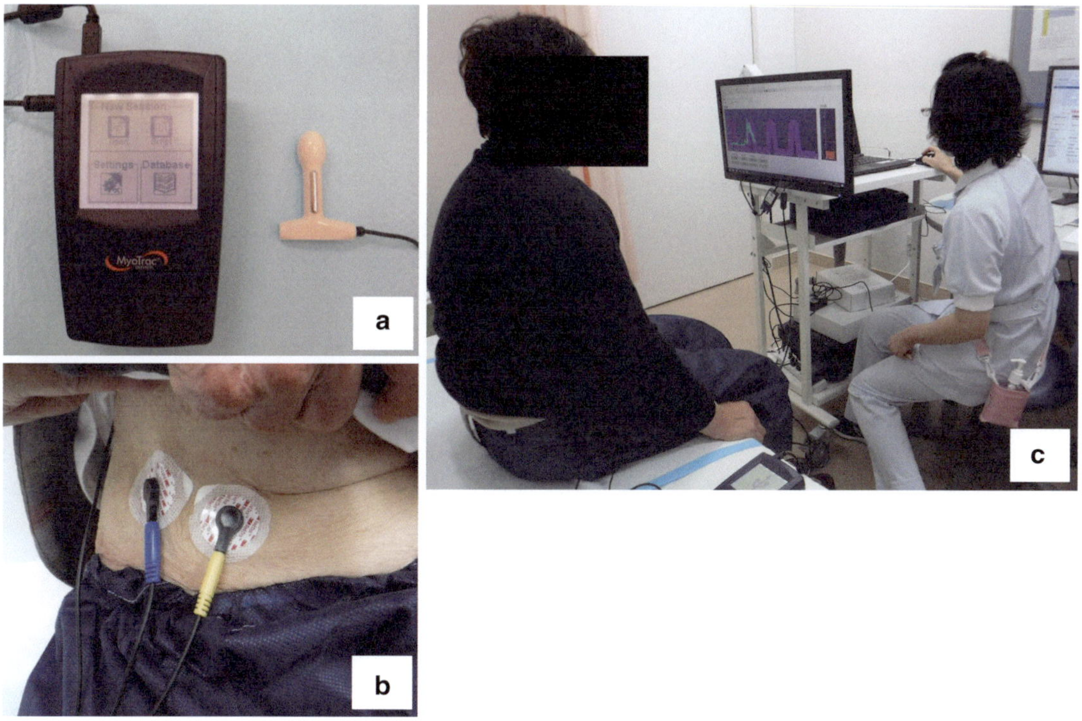

Fig. 64.4 Biofeedback therapy for fecal incontinence. (cited from Ref. [15]). (**a**) Anal electromyography (EMG) probe inserted into the anal canal to measure anal sphincter activity. (**b**) Surface EMG electrodes placed on the external oblique abdominal muscles to measure abdominal muscle activity (MyoTrac™ Infinity, MP Japan, Tokyo). (**c**) Patients visually monitor both anal sphincter contraction and abdominal muscle activity on a display and perform training under the guidance of a therapist

patients who can understand the training protocol and are motivated to continue pelvic floor exercises at home.

The reported efficacy of BF therapy for FI ranges from 70% to 80%. A meta-analysis of six randomized controlled trials (RCTs) [16] found that the odds ratio for the effectiveness of BF therapy compared to other treatments was 1.2 (95% CI: 0.7–2.1). The 2022 European guidelines [17] rated pelvic floor physiotherapy, including PFMT and BF therapy, as having a "moderate recommendation" despite the low level of evidence. In contrast, although BF therapy requires BF equipment, it can be effectively instructed and has no side effects. Therefore, the 2021 American College of Gastroenterology guidelines [18] strongly recommend BF therapy based on moderate-quality evidence, and the sixth edition of the International Consultation on Incontinence [3] assigns it a recommendation grade of A. In the FI Guidelines [1], BF therapy is assigned a recommendation grade of C.

Anal Insert Device for Fecal Incontinence

This therapy involves the insertion and placement of a specialized device into the rectum and anal canal to act as a plug, thereby preventing FI. However, patients with normal anorectal sensation often find the presence of the device uncomfortable and intolerable. Therefore, this method is considered more suitable for patients with diminished anorectal sensation, such as those with spinal cord injury or elderly individuals. In Japan, the Peristeen® Anal Plug (Coloplast, Tokyo) was previously available, but its production was discontinued in June 2023. As a result, there are currently no anal insert device for FI available for clinical use in Japan.

Transanal Irrigation (Fig. 64.5)

Transanal irrigation (TAI), also referred to as retrograde colonic irrigation, is a therapeutic method that involves regularly emptying the rectum and left colon via transanal infusion of water to prevent FI. It is also effective in managing refractory constipation. Due to the time and effort required for irrigation, this therapy is typically indicated for patients with refractory FI or constipation. It is commonly used in patients with spinal cord injury or pediatric patients with spina bifida, who often present with both FI and constipation. It is also beneficial for patients with low anterior resection syndrome (LARS), who frequently experience severe defecatory dysfunction.

The effectiveness of TAI is often assessed by its continuation rate, which has been reported to range from 50% to 80% [19]. In Japan, the Peristeen® Anal Irrigation System (Coloplast, Tokyo) was approved for insurance coverage in April 2018 but only for patients with refractory defecation disorders due to spinal cord injury, excluding those who had undergone rectal surgery. This exclusion was based on a clinical study involving 32 patients with refractory defecation disorders using a balloon catheter, in which rectal perforation occurred in three cases—two of whom had LARS and one who had undergone rectopexy for rectal prolapse [20].

To enable safe use of TAI in patients with a history of rectal surgery, including those with LARS, a cone catheter was developed and received regulatory approval in November 2020. The cone catheter lacks a balloon and is designed so that only the tip enters the rectum, thereby minimizing the risk of rectal injury from balloon inflation or catheter insertion. It is anticipated that TAI using the cone catheter will be approved for broader indications, including patients with LARS and those with refractory FI or constipation unrelated to spinal cord injury. In the FI Guidelines [1], TAI is assigned a recommendation grade of B.

1.5.4 Surgical Treatment (Fig. 64.3)

Surgical treatment should be considered when FI does not sufficiently improve with conservative

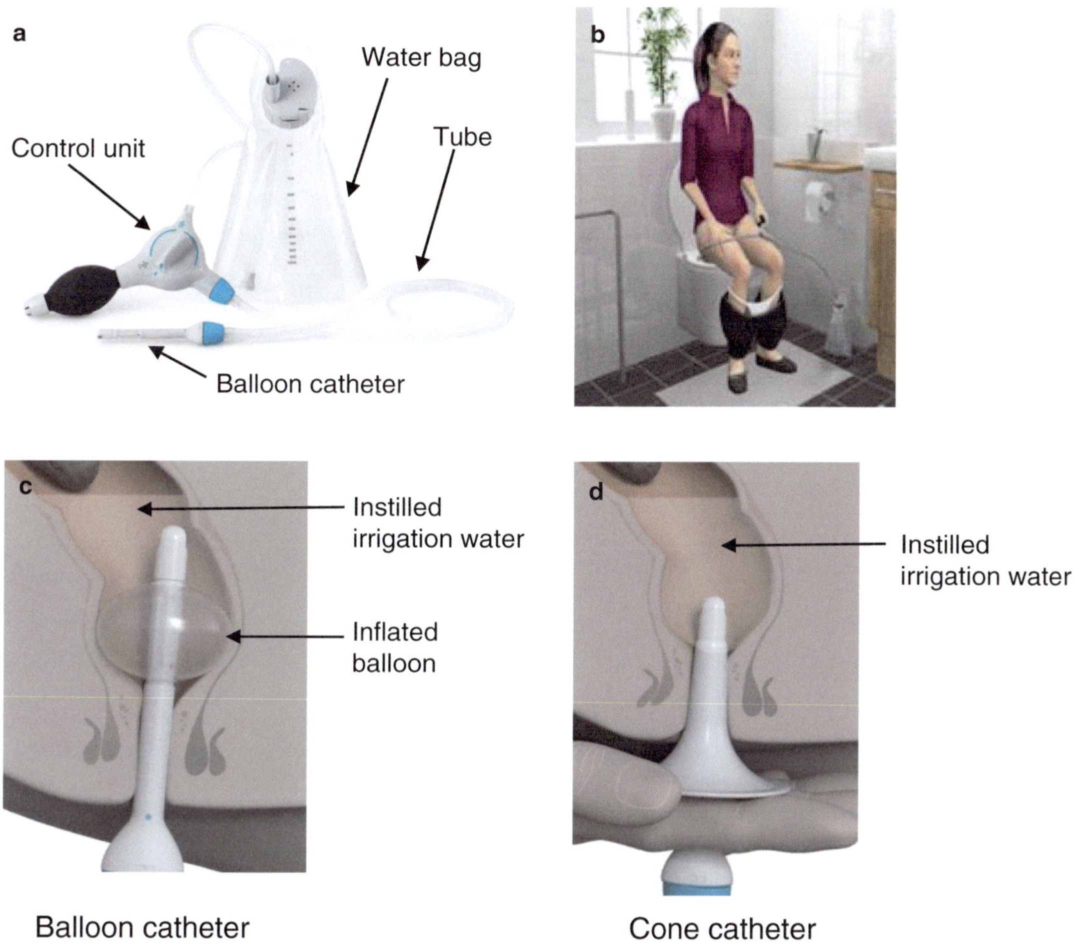

Fig. 64.5 Transanal irrigation (Images provided by Coloplast K.K.). (**a**) Peristeen® Transanal Irrigation Syste—Peristeen Plus (Coloplast, Tokyo). (**b**) Unlike traditional gravity-based systems that require suspending a water bag at height, this device uses a pump, allowing the irrigation bag to remain on the floor. (**c**) Balloon catheters prevent catheter dislodgement and leakage during irrigation by inflating the balloon. (**d**) Cone catheters, which lack a balloon, must be manually held in place during irrigation. However, only the tip enters the rectum, and there is no balloon-induced pressure, reducing the risk of rectal injury

therapy. In patients with severe spinal cord injury who have failed conservative treatment and for whom other surgical options are not appropriate, antegrade continence enema or stoma creation may be indicated.

In the absence of severe spinal cord injury, the first step is to evaluate for the presence of anal sphincter disruption using endoanal ultrasonography. If no disruption is detected, sacral neuromodulation is considered the first-line surgical option.

First-Line Surgical Procedures

Sacral Neuromodulation (Fig. 64.6)

Sacral neuromodulation (SNM) is a surgical treatment that improves FI by electrically stimulating the sacral nerves involved in defecation using an implantable neurostimulator. A key advantage of SNM is its selectivity—patients can undergo a test stimulation to determine its efficacy before permanent implantation. If the electrical stimulation is ineffective during the test period, the lead can be

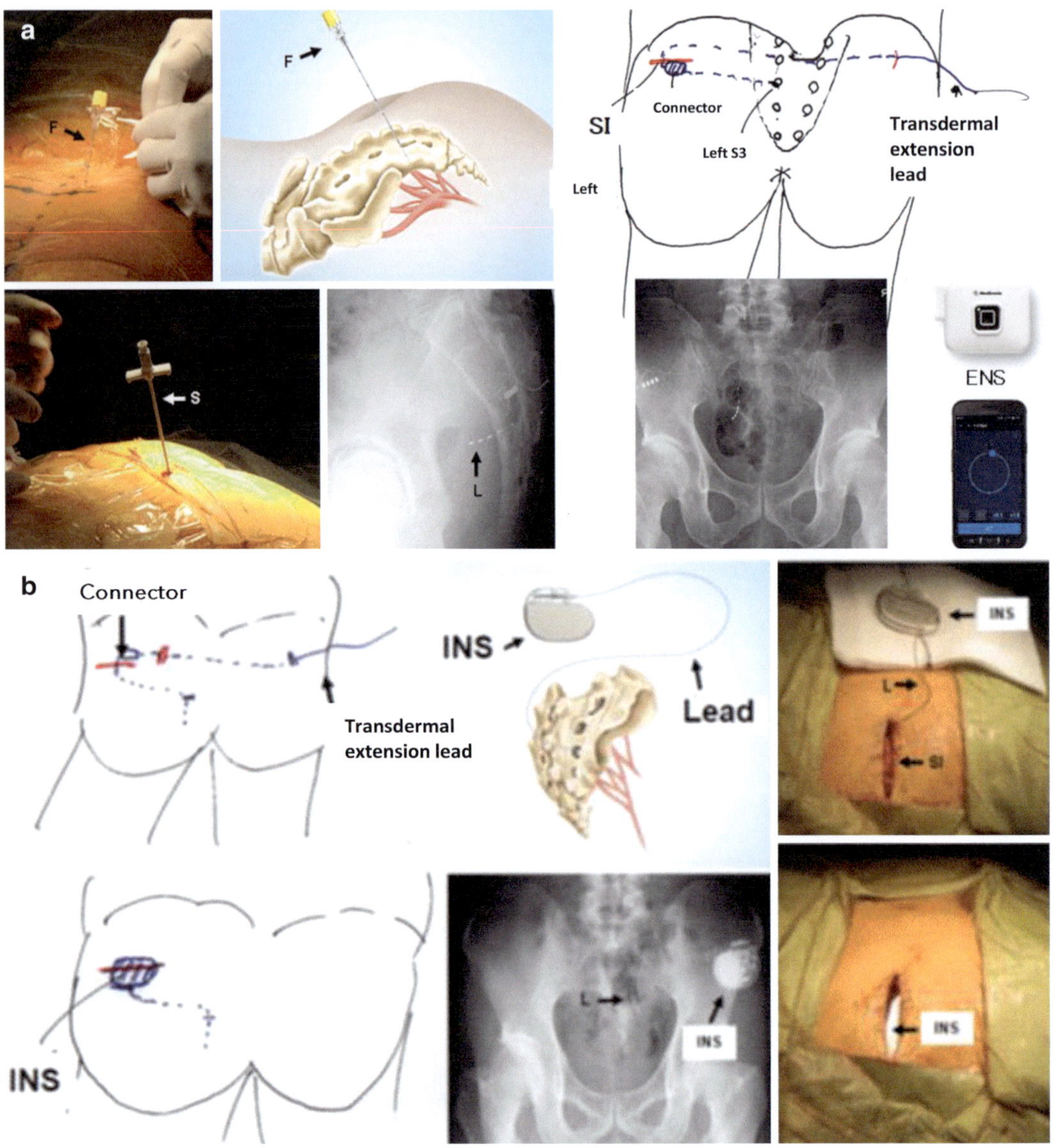

Fig. 64.6 Sacral neuromodulation (Some images provided by Medtronic Japan Co., Ltd.). (**a**) Stage 1: Test stimulation procedure. (**b**) Stage 2: Permanent implantation procedure. Abbreviations: F Foramen needle, S Lead introducer sheath, L Lead (electrical stimulation lead), SI Skin incision, S3 Third sacral foramen, ENS External nerve stimulator, INS Implantable nerve stimulator

removed, allowing the patient to return to their baseline condition. This reversibility, combined with its selectivity, makes SNM a minimally invasive and effective surgical option. Since Tanagho et al. first reported its use for urinary incontinence in 1982 and Matzel et al. extended its application to FI in 1995, approximately 350,000 patients worldwide had undergone SNM by April 2022. The intention-to-treat efficacy for FI is reported at 63% in short-term outcomes (≤1 year) and 54% in long-term outcomes (≥3 years). For urinary incontinence, efficacy rates range from 67% to 80%

[21]. In Japan, SNM was approved for insurance coverage in April 2014 for FI refractory to conservative therapy and in September 2017 for refractory overactive bladder. In the FI Guidelines [1], SNM is the only surgical treatment assigned a recommendation grade of A.

Previously, patients with implanted SNM devices were ineligible for MRI. However, since November 2022, the electrodes and neurostimulators used in SNM have been approved for conditional use with 1.5 T and 3.0 T whole-body MRI. Additionally, while earlier devices were nonrechargeable and required replacement every 5–7 years under local anesthesia, a rechargeable, MRI-compatible device was released in February 2023.

The mechanism of action of SNM is not fully understood. While it is established that the sacral nerves play a central role in continence via the pudendal nerve, which controls the urethral and anal sphincters, the therapeutic effects of SNM are now believed to involve not only direct muscle stimulation but also modulation of afferent sensory pathways in the spinal cord, autonomic regulation of colonic motility, and influence on supraspinal centers involved in micturition and defecation [21].

Anal Sphincteroplasty

If endoanal ultrasonography reveals a sphincter defect that is believed to be the cause of FI, either SNM or sphincteroplasty may be indicated. Anal sphincteroplasty has been shown to significantly improve FI in many patients, with approximately 80% achieving good continence at 1 year postoperatively. However, recurrence and deterioration are common, with success rates declining to around 50% at 5 years and as low as 6% at 10 years [22]. Therefore, when a sphincter defect is identified, the choice between SNM and sphincteroplasty should be made after a thorough discussion with the patient regarding the advantages and limitations of each approach. In the FI Guidelines [1], sphincteroplasty is assigned a recommendation grade of B.

Second-Line Surgical Procedures

If SNM and sphincteroplasty are ineffective or not indicated, second-line options include antegrade continence enema (ACE), graciloplasty, ventral rectopexy, and stoma creation. However, as of 2023, ACE, graciloplasty, and ventral rectopexy are performed at only a limited number of institutions in Japan.

Antegrade Continence Enema (ACE)

This procedure involves creating a cecostomy through which enemas are administered regularly to manage FI. In addition to open and laparoscopic approaches, minimally invasive cecostomy creation using colonoscopy has been reported. Compared to transanal irrigation, ACE requires less irrigation fluid and shorter administration time. However, it still involves surgery and may raise psychological concerns related to body image, similar to a stoma. In the FI Guidelines [1], ACE is assigned a recommendation grade of C.

Graciloplasty

This technique involves wrapping the gracilis muscle from the leg around the anal canal to augment sphincter function. While effective in experienced hands for severe FI, it is associated with a high rate of complications and reoperations. The procedure is technically demanding and requires significant training and case volume. Due to the widespread adoption of SNM, graciloplasty is now rarely performed worldwide. In the FI Guidelines [1], this procedure is assigned a recommendation grade of D (meaning very weak recommendation, reflecting disagreement among committee members).

Ventral Rectopexy

This procedure, performed via laparoscopy or laparotomy, involves incising the peritoneum on the right side of the rectum from the sacral promontory to the rectouterine (or rectovesical) pouch, dissecting the rectovaginal (or rectoprostatic) septum to the pelvic floor, and suturing a mesh to the ventral aspect of the lower rectum and the sacral promontory. First described by D'Hoore et al. in 2004, it was originally developed for rectal prolapse and is notable for preserving the autonomic nerves on the dorsal side of the rectum. It is indicated for FI caused by rectal intussusception or rectocele and is more commonly performed in women. However, concerns about long-term mesh-related complications have led to its exclusion from surgical treatment recommendations for FI in both the 2022 European guidelines [17] and the 2021 American College of Gastroenterology guidelines [18]. Although described in the Japanese FI Guidelines [1], it is not assigned a recommendation grade and is not considered a standard treatment.

Stoma

Stoma creation is generally considered a last resort for severe FI, but it should not be viewed as a treatment failure. If the psychological impact of altered body image can be accepted, it represents a straightforward and definitive solution. According to a survey of 69 patients with stomas created for FI [23], the median score for postoperative activity level was eight out of ten. Furthermore, 83% of respondents reported "little" or "no" restriction in daily life due to the stoma, indicating that quality of life was better poststoma than during severe FI. In the FI Guidelines [1], stoma creation is assigned a recommendation grade of B.

Experimental Surgical Therapies: Regenerative Medicine

Although still in the research phase, anal sphincter regenerative therapy involving the transplantation of cultivated autologous skeletal muscle cells into the external anal sphincter have shown promise in improving urge FI. Frudinger et al. [24] reported that in 39 patients with urge FI due to external anal sphincter dysfunction or rupture, injection of cultured cells derived from the pectoralis muscle into the external anal sphincter resulted in a ≥50% reduction in FI episodes in 31 patients (79.5%) after 1 year. These findings suggest promising future developments in regenerative medicine for FI.

2 Conclusion

This chapter has provided an overview of FI based on the *Clinical Guidelines for Fecal Incontinence 2017*. As awareness and clinical practice surrounding FI continue to expand, it is hoped that FI will no longer be regarded as a "silent affliction" but rather as a "common and treatable" symptom, gaining broader societal understanding and acceptance.

Take-Home Message

FI can be classified into passive and urge types based on symptoms, and the cause can often be estimated based on medical history and anorectal examination. After excluding organic causes such as colorectal cancer, inflammatory bowel disease, and rectal prolapse, initial management should be tailored to the symptom type, underlying cause, and severity—beginning with dietary, lifestyle, and bowel habit guidance, as well as pharmacotherapy. FI caused by diarrhea due to excessive or inappropriate laxative use can often be resolved by discontinuing or adjusting the medication. If symptoms do not sufficiently improve with initial treatment, referral to a specialized facility is recommended.

Competing Interests The author(s) has no competing interests to declare that are relevant to the content of this manuscript.

References

1. The Japan Society of Coloproctology. Practice guidelines for fecal incontinence, 2017 edition. Tokyo: Nankodo; 2017. (in Japanese)
2. Mimura T. Definition and epidemiology of fecal incontinence. Geka (Surgery). 2017;79:212–9. (in Japanese)
3. Bliss D, et al. Assessment and conservative management of faecal incontinence and quality of life in adults. In: Abrams P, et al., editors. Incontinence. 6th ed. ICUD-ICS; 2017. p. 1993–2085.
4. Mimura T, et al. Current situations of the management of fecal incontinence in Japanese institutions. J Jpn Soc Coloproctol. 2012;65:101–8. (in Japanese)
5. Mimura T. Types and characteristics of excretory disorders: fecal incontinence. In: Goto H, et al., editors.

Theory and practice of excretion rehabilitation. 2nd ed. Tokyo: Nakayama Shoten; 2022. p. 102–7. (in Japanese).
6. Mimura T. Fecal incontinence. In: Koike K, et al., editors. Latest treatments for gastrointestinal diseases 2019–2020. Tokyo: Nankodo; 2019. p. 92–7. (in Japanese).
7. Mimura T, et al. Fecal incontinence. In: 3rd, editor. Supplement to Japanese clinical medicine. Tokyo: Nihon Rinsho Sha; 2020. p. 413–9. (in Japanese).
8. Mimura T, et al. Anorectal function testing. Rinsho Kensa (Clinical Laboratory Testing). 2022;66:853–61. (in Japanese)
9. Mimura T. Characteristics and treatment of defecation disorders in the elderly. Rinsho Rounen Kango (Clinical Geriatric Nursing). 2018;25:2–13. (in Japanese).
10. Mimura T. Treatment algorithm for fecal incontinence. Mod Phys. 2017;37:68–73. (in Japanese).
11. Ogata H, et al. Validation study of the Japanese version of the Fecal incontinence quality of life scale. Color Dis. 2012;14:194–9.
12. Orkin BA, et al. The digital rectal examination scoring system (DRESS). Dis Colon Rectum. 2010;53:1656–60.
13. Mimura T. Treatment and care of defecation disorders based on symptoms: Fecal incontinence. In: Goto H, et al., editors. Theory and practice of excretion rehabilitation. 2nd ed. Tokyo: Nakayama Shoten; 2022. p. 464–72. (in Japanese).
14. Mimura T. Basics of bowel care (bowel habits and daily life). In: Goto H, et al., editors. Theory and practice of excretion rehabilitation. 2nd ed. Tokyo: Nakayama Shoten; 2022. p. 428–35. (in Japanese).
15. Honma Y, et al. Physiotherapy (pelvic floor muscle training, biofeedback therapy): defecation disorders. In: Goto H, et al., editors. Theory and practice of excretion rehabilitation. 2nd ed. Tokyo: Nakayama Shoten; 2022. p. 373–7. (in Japanese).
16. Enck P, et al. Biofeedback therapy in fecal incontinence and constipation. Neurogastroenterol Motil. 2009;21:1133–41.
17. Assmann SL, et al. Guideline for the diagnosis and treatment of faecal incontinence: AUEG/ESCP/ESNM/ESPCG collaboration. United European Gastroenterol J. 2022;10:251–86.
18. Wald A, et al. ACG clinical guidelines: management of benign anorectal disorders. Am J Gastroenterol. 2021;116:1987–2008.
19. Mimura T. Treatment and care of defecation disorders: transanal irrigation therapy. In: Goto H, et al., editors. Theory and practice of excretion rehabilitation. 2nd ed. Tokyo: Nakayama Shoten; 2022. p. 438–43. (in Japanese).
20. Mimura T, et al. Transanal irrigation for refractory disordered defecation: a prospective multicenter clinical study in Japan. J Jpn Soc Coloproctol. 2018;71:70–85. (in Japanese)
21. Mimura T. Sacral neuromodulation: principles and mechanisms of action. In: Goto H, et al., editors. Theory and practice of excretion rehabilitation. 2nd ed. Tokyo: Nakayama Shoten; 2022. p. 377–83. (in Japanese).
22. Glasgow SC, et al. Long-term outcomes of anal sphincter repair for fecal incontinence: a systematic review. Dis Colon Rectum. 2012;55:482–90.
23. Norton C, et al. Patients' views of a colostomy for fecal incontinence. Dis Colon Rectum. 2005;48:1062–9.
24. Frudinger A, et al. Skeletal muscle-derived cell implantation for the treatment of sphincter-related faecal incontinence. Stem Cell Res Ther. 2018;9:233–52.

Diagnosis and Treatment of DGBI of the Anorectum, Functional Anorectal Pain

65

Kotaro Maeda

Abstract

Functional anorectal pain is subdivided into three categories (levator ani syndrome, unspecified functional anorectal pain, proctalgia fugax) based on the duration of pain and the presence or absence of tenderness elicited by posterior traction of the puborectalis muscle after excluding organic diseases that may cause rectal pain. Levator ani syndrome presents chronic or recurrent rectal pain lasting 30 min or longer, which serves to distinguish it from the shorter pain episodes characteristic of proctalgia fugax. Levator ani syndrome involves tenderness elicited by posterior traction of the puborectalis muscle and serves to distinguish it from unspecified functional anorectal pain, which presents with similar symptoms but lacks this specific tenderness. Proctalgia fugax presents a sudden, severe rectal pain that lasts from a few seconds to several minutes (rarely up to 30 min) and resolves completely. Symptoms must have been present for at least 6 months, and all criteria must be met during the most recent 3 months in functional anorectal pain. Conservative treatment is usually performed for functional anal pain.

K. Maeda (✉)
Medical Cooperation Himawariseishinkai Oumeimai Hospital, Ome, Tokyo, Japan
e-mail: maeda@oumeimai.or.jp

Keywords

Functional anorectal pain · Levator ani syndrome · Unspecified functional anorectal pain · Proctalgia fugax · Anorectal pain

1 Functional Anorectal Pain

Functional anorectal pain is classified as one of *functional anorectal disorders* according to the internationally recognized Rome IV diagnostic criteria (Table 65.1) [1]. Based on the duration of pain and the presence or absence of tenderness, functional anorectal pain is further subdivided into the following categories: levator ani syndrome (F2a), unspecified functional anorectal pain (F2b), and proctalgia fugax (F2c) (Table 65.1). In clinical practice, these subtypes often exhibit overlapping features [2].

Table 65.1 Functional anorectal disorders (Rome IV Classification) [1]

F. Functional anorectal disorders
F1. Fecal incontinence
F2. Functional anorectal pain
F2a. Levator ani syndrome
F2b. Unspecified functional anorectal pain
F2c. Proctalgia fugax
F3. Functional defecation disorders

H. Kaneko et al. (eds.), *Disorders of Gut-Brain Interaction*,
https://doi.org/10.1007/978-981-95-6974-8_65

1.1 Levator Ani Syndrome

1.1.1 Concept and Definition

According to the Rome IV criteria, levator ani syndrome is characterized by a dull, vague pain or a sensation of pressure in the high rectum, which often worsens in the sitting position compared to standing or lying down. Physical examination may reveal spasm and tenderness of the levator ani muscle, vagina, or pelvic floor. Tenderness is often more pronounced on the left side than the right [1].

In Rome III, functional anorectal pain was classified into chronic and transient types. Levator ani syndrome was defined as a functional disorder characterized by chronic or recurrent anorectal pain lasting more than 20 min, with tenderness elicited by posterior traction of the puborectalis muscle during digital rectal examination. The pain was described as dull or as a sensation of urgency [3]. Historically, chronic anorectal pain has been referred to by various terms, including levator ani syndrome, levator spasm, puborectalis syndrome, piriformis syndrome, pelvic tension myalgia, levator syndrome, levator elevation syndrome, levator ani spasm syndrome, and spastic levator ani syndrome [3–5].

1.1.2 Epidemiology

The overall prevalence of anorectal pain from all causes is reported to be 11.6%, with levator ani syndrome accounting for 6.6% [6]. The prevalence is slightly higher in women (7.4%) than in men (5.7%). The age of onset ranges widely from 6 to 90 years, with a peak incidence between 30 and 60 years [6].

1.1.3 Etiology and Pathophysiology

Levator ani syndrome is thought to result from spasm of the pelvic floor muscles and elevated resting anal pressure [2]. Recent studies have reported that many individuals with dyssynergic defecation exhibit tenderness of the levator ani muscle. Improvement of dyssynergia through biofeedback therapy suggests that rectoanal dyssynergia may underlie the pathophysiology of levator ani syndrome (Table 65.2) [7]. In 2020, Zhang et al. demonstrated that patients with functional anorectal pain had lower peak amplitudes and prolonged latencies in rectal sensory-evoked potentials compared to healthy controls, suggesting that impaired afferent sensory perception in the anorectal region may contribute to the pathophysiology (Table 65.2) [8]. Additionally, these patients exhibited lower voluntary contraction pressures, increased maximum tolerable volume during rectal distension, and a correlation between anal resting pressure and peak sensory evoked potentials, indicating a possible link between anal pressure and afferent signaling pathways in patients with functional anorectal pain [8]. Other contributing factors may include peripheral inflammation, altered peripheral and central sensory processing, and psychosocial factors [9].

Table 65.2 Suggested pathophysiological mechanisms of functional anorectal pain

1. Dyssynergic defecation in the rectoanal region
Many patients with dyssynergic defecation exhibit tenderness of the levator ani muscle.
Dyssynergia improves with biofeedback therapy.
2. Reduced afferent sensory perception in the anorectal region
Latency of rectal sensory-evoked potentials is prolonged compared to healthy individuals.
Peak amplitude of rectal sensory-evoked potentials is lower than in healthy individuals.

1.1.4 Diagnostic Criteria

According to the Rome IV criteria, the diagnostic standards for levator ani syndrome require that all four items listed in Table 65.3 be fulfilled. Symptoms must have been present for at least 6 months, and all criteria must be met during the most recent 3 months [1].

Item 1 specifies that the pain must be chronic or recurrent in nature. Item 2 defines the duration of pain as lasting 30 min or longer, which serves to distinguish it from the shorter pain episodes characteristic of proctalgia fugax (F2c) as classified in Table 65.1. Item 3, which involves tenderness elicited by posterior traction of the puborectalis muscle, serves to distinguish levator ani syndrome from unspecified functional anorectal pain (F2b), which presents with similar

Table 65.3 Diagnostic criteria for levator ani syndrome [1]

All of the following criteria must be met:
Chronic or recurrent rectal pain
Pain lasting 30 min or longer
Tenderness of the puborectalis muscle upon posterior traction
Exclusion of other conditions that may cause rectal pain, such as the following:
Inflammatory bowel disease
Intramuscular abscess or anal fissure
Thrombosed hemorrhoids
Prostatitis
Coccydynia
Major structural abnormalities of the pelvic floor
Symptoms must have been present for at least 6 months, and all criteria must be met during the most recent 3 months.

Table 65.4 Diagnostic approach for functional anorectal pain

History taking:
Frequency, duration, and characteristics of pain
Presence of other symptoms or signs of inflammation
Physical examination:
1. Anorectal inspection and digital rectal examination
Assess for rectal pain and tenderness upon posterior traction of the puborectalis muscle
Exclude anorectal diseases such as hemorrhoids and prostatitis
Exclude rectal masses or inflammatory conditions
2. Abdominal examination
Assess for abdominal tenderness and peritoneal signs
Investigations:
Colonoscopy
Abdominal CT/MRI
Abdominal ultrasonography
For treatment selection: perform anorectal manometry and balloon expulsion test.

symptoms but lacks this specific tenderness (Table 65.1). Item 4 establishes the requirement to exclude organic diseases that may cause anorectal pain, such as inflammatory bowel disease, intramuscular abscesses, anal fissures, thrombosed hemorrhoids, prostatitis, coccydynia, or significant structural abnormalities of the pelvic floor.

1.1.5 Diagnosis and Differential Diagnosis

History Taking

A thorough history should confirm the presence of chronic or recurrent rectal pain lasting more than 30 min and persisting for over 6 months (Table 65.3). Inquiry should also include symptoms suggestive of inflammatory or anorectal diseases, such as diarrhea, hematochezia, anorectal masses, or pelvic organ prolapse.

Physical Examination

Anorectal inspection and digital rectal examination should assess for hemorrhoids, anal fissures, perianal abscesses, fistulas, and other anorectal conditions. Prostate examination may help diagnose prostatitis. Examination should also evaluate for structural abnormalities such as levator ani injury or hematoma (Table 65.4 and Fig. 65.1). Posterior traction of the puborectalis muscle should be performed to assess for tenderness, aiding in the differentiation between levator ani syndrome and unspecified functional anorectal pain (Tables 65.1, 65.3, and 65.4 and Fig. 65.1). Abdominal examination should consider ischemic or inflammatory bowel disease and assess for tenderness or peritoneal signs.

Imaging Studies

Colonoscopy, barium enema, abdominal and transanal ultrasonography, and abdominal/pelvic CT or MRI should be performed as needed to exclude organic pathology (Table 65.4 and Fig. 65.1).

1.1.6 Treatment

Various treatment modalities for levator ani syndrome are summarized in Table 65.5 [9–12]. According to a review by the American Academy of Family Physicians, sitz baths, fiber supplementation, and biofeedback therapy are recommended for functional anorectal pain [10].

A comparative study of three treatment modalities—galvanic electrical stimulation, levator ani massage with sitz baths, and biofeedback therapy with psychological counseling—showed

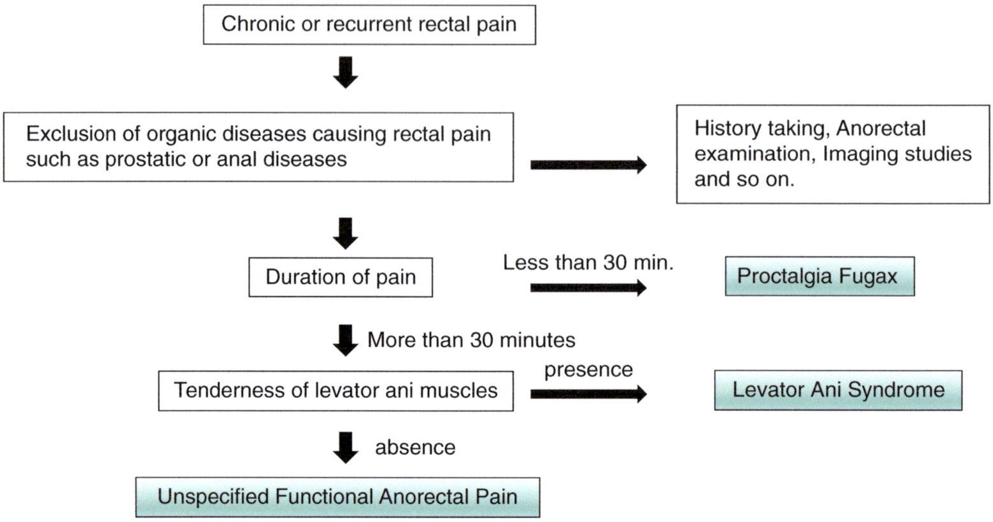

Fig. 65.1 Diagnostic flowchart for functional anorectal pain

Table 65.5 Treatment options for levator ani syndrome

Sitz baths
Fiber supplements
Biofeedback therapy
Sacral neuromodulation (SNM)
Galvanic electrical stimulation
Injections: Triamcinolone and botulinum toxin
Topical nitroglycerin
Muscle relaxants: Methocarbamol, diazepam, and cyclobenzaprine
Digital massage of the levator ani muscle

Table 65.6 Indicators for selecting treatment for functional anorectal pain

1. Biofeedback therapy
Patients with elevated anal resting pressure on anorectal manometry
Patients unable to expel the balloon during expulsion test
Patients with defecatory disorders
2. Sacral neuromodulation or galvanic electrical stimulation
Patients with normal anal resting pressure on anorectal manometry

that 87% of patients in the biofeedback group achieved pain remission, compared to 45% in the electrical stimulation group and 22% in the massage group. These improvements were sustained for up to 12 months [7].

A meta-analysis of 27 studies involving 1538 patients with functional anorectal pain found that triamcinolone injections, sacral neuromodulation (SNM), and biofeedback therapy were the most effective treatments. Galvanic stimulation, botulinum toxin injections, and topical nitroglycerin were less effective [11]. SNM and biofeedback therapy were most effective in reducing pain severity. Biofeedback therapy is the first-line treatment for patients with elevated anal resting pressure or defecatory disorders, while SNM or electrical stimulation may be considered for patients with normal resting pressure (Table 65.6). Although triamcinolone injections may improve symptoms, their analgesic effect is limited [11].

In principle, treatment should be tailored to the patient's symptoms using a multidisciplinary approach, including lifestyle modification, pharmacologic, behavioral, and physical therapies [9]. In clinical practice, some patients may continue to report severe symptoms despite various treatments, necessitating the use of analgesics. However, opioids should be avoided, and surgical interventions should be reserved as a last resort [4, 9].

1.2 Unspecified Functional Anorectal Pain

1.2.1 Concept and Definition

According to the Rome IV criteria, unspecified functional anorectal pain is defined as anorectal pain that presents with symptoms similar to levator ani syndrome but without tenderness elicited by posterior traction of the levator ani muscle [1].

1.2.2 Epidemiology

There are no epidemiological studies specifically focused on unspecified functional anorectal pain.

1.2.3 Etiology and Pathophysiology

The etiology and pathophysiology remain unclear.

1.2.4 Diagnostic Criteria

The diagnostic criteria for unspecified functional anorectal pain require that items 1, 2, and 4 in Table 65.3 be fulfilled. Symptoms must have been present for at least 6 months, and all three criteria must be met during the most recent 3 months. Notably, item 3, which involves tenderness of the puborectalis muscle upon posterior traction, is absent (Table 65.1 and Fig. 65.1) [1].

1.2.5 Diagnosis and Differential Diagnosis

The diagnostic and differential diagnostic approach is the same as that for levator ani syndrome (Fig. 65.1).

1.2.6 Treatment

Treatment options are outlined in Table 65.5. Unlike in levator ani syndrome, biofeedback therapy, which is effective for that condition, is not considered beneficial for unspecified functional anorectal pain [1, 2]. As shown in Table 65.6, anorectal manometry and balloon expulsion tests should be performed. If anal resting pressure is normal and balloon expulsion is successful, biofeedback therapy should not be employed. Instead, sacral neuromodulation (SNM) or galvanic electrical stimulation may be considered [11].

1.3 Proctalgia Fugax

1.3.1 Concept and Definition

Also referred to as transient rectal pain [5], proctalgia fugax is defined in the Rome IV criteria as a sudden, severe rectal pain that lasts from a few seconds to several minutes (rarely up to 30 min) and resolves completely [1]. In 90% of patients, the pain is localized to the rectum. The episodes are infrequent, with 51% of patients experiencing five or fewer episodes per year. The pain is described as cramping, gnawing, tingling, or stabbing and ranges from uncomfortable to unbearable. Approximately 50% of patients report that the pain interferes with daily activities or awakens them from sleep [1].

1.3.2 Epidemiology

The prevalence is estimated to be between 8% and 18%, with no significant sex differences [1]. Although rare, cases have been reported in preadolescent children, including a seven-year-old [1].

1.3.3 Etiology and Pathophysiology

The pathophysiology is not well understood, but abnormal smooth muscle contractions may be involved [1]. The triggers for pain episodes are also unclear [12], although episodes often occur following stress or anxiety [1]. In rare cases, congenital hypertrophy of the internal anal sphincter with elevated anal resting pressure has been reported [12].

1.3.4 Diagnostic Criteria

According to Rome IV, the diagnostic criteria for proctalgia fugax require that all four items listed in Table 65.7 be met. Symptoms must have been present for at least 6 months, and all criteria must be fulfilled during the most recent 3 months [1].

1.3.5 Diagnosis and Differential Diagnosis

After excluding organic diseases that may cause anorectal pain, diagnosis is based on the characteristic nature and duration of the pain (Fig. 65.1).

Table 65.7 Diagnostic criteria for proctalgia fugax [1]

All of the following criteria must be met:
1. Recurrent rectal pain not related to defecation
2. Pain lasting from a few seconds to several minutes (up to a maximum of 30 min)
3. No anorectal pain between episodes
4. Exclusion of other conditions that may cause rectal pain, such as the following:
Inflammatory bowel disease
Intramuscular abscess or anal fissure
Thrombosed hemorrhoids
Prostatitis
Coccydynia
Major structural abnormalities of the pelvic floor
Symptoms must have been present for at least 6 months, and all criteria must be met during the most recent 3 months.

1.3.6 Treatment

Because the pain episodes are brief, treatment is generally not practical. Patients should be reassured that the condition is benign and that no preventive treatment is currently available [1, 12]. However, in patients experiencing pain episodes lasting more than 20 min, inhaled *salbutamol* has been reported to be more effective than placebo [1, 12].

Take-Home Message

When diagnosing anorectal pain, especially in excluding organic causes, careful consideration is necessary. Anorectal examination should assess for conditions such as pelvic organ prolapse and prostatitis. However, findings may not be easily observed depending on the patient's position or degree of straining, so examination during straining may be helpful. Additionally, because the expression and degree of pain vary among individuals, it is necessary to consider the psychological background of the patient when making a diagnosis.

Competing Interests The author(s) has no competing interests to declare that are relevant to the content of this manuscript.

References

1. Rao SSC, et al. Anorectal disorders. Gastroenterology. 2016;150:1430–42.
2. Grimaud JC, et al. Manometric and radiologic investigations and biofeedback treatment of chronic idiopathic anal pain. Dis Colon Rectum. 1991;34:690–5.
3. Bharucha AE, et al. Functional anorectal disorders. Gastroenterology. 2006;130:1510–8.
4. Maeda K, et al. Levator ani syndrome. Sanka to Fujinka (Obstet Gynecol). 2013;80:897–900. (in Japanese)
5. Fukudo S, et al. ROME III Japanese edition. Kyowa Kikaku. 2008:400–13. (in Japanese)
6. Bharucha AE, et al. An update on anorectal disorders for gastroenterologists. Gastroenterology. 2014;146:37–45.
7. Chiarioni G, et al. Biofeedback is superior to electrogalvanic stimulation and massage for treatment of levator ani syndrome. Gastroenterology. 2010;138:1321–9.
8. Zhang Q, et al. Impaired anorectal afferents is a potential pathophysiological factor associated with functional pain. Front Neurol. 2020;11:577025.
9. Bharucha AE, et al. Anorectal and pelvic pain. Mayo Clin Proc. 2016;91:1471–86.
10. Cohee MW. Benign anorectal conditions: evaluation and management. Am Fam Physician. 2020;101:24–33.
11. Byrnes KG, et al. Optimal management of functional anorectal pain: a systematic review and network meta-analysis. Eur J Gastroenterol Hepatol. 2022;34:249–59.
12. Wald A, et al. ACG clinical guidelines: management of benign anorectal disorders. Am J Gastroenterol. 2021;116:1987–2008.

66 Diagnosis and Treatment of DGBI of the Anorectum, Functional Defecation Disorders, Dyssynergic Defecation

Tomoko Takahashi

Abstract

Normal defecation involves a coordinated response to rectal wall distension, leading to the urge to defecate and synchronized activation of abdominal pressure, pelvic floor relaxation, and anal sphincter relaxation. In contrast, functional defecation disorders are characterized by difficulty evacuating stool despite no morphological abnormalities, and one major cause is dyssynergic defecation. This condition results from impaired coordination between intraabdominal pressure, pelvic floor muscles, and anal sphincters during defecation. Symptoms include excessive straining, incomplete evacuation, and a sense of anorectal blockage.

Initial management for the patients who have these complications should include dietary modifications, bowel habit improvement, and appropriate laxative use.

Patients with persistent symptoms after using initial management may benefit from referral to specialized centers for advanced diagnostics and therapy.

Diagnosis requires specialized tests such as anorectal manometry, high-resolution manometry, surface electromyography, balloon expulsion test, and defecography. First-line treatment is a biofeedback therapy, which retrains muscle coordination and improves rectal sensation. Studies report a 70–80% success rate, with benefits lasting over 2 years.

Keywords

Functional defecation disorders · Dyssynergic defecation · Pelvic floor incoordination · Anismus · Obstructed defecation

1 Introduction

In normal defecation, the presence of an adequate volume of stool causes distension of the rectal wall. This distension stimulus is transmitted via the sacral nerves to the cerebral cortex, resulting in the sensation of the urge to defecate. Rectal distension also triggers the rectoanal excitatory reflex, leading to a transient contraction of the external anal sphincter. This is followed by the rectoanal inhibitory reflex, which causes relaxation of the proximal internal anal sphincter and allows for the descent of rectal contents for sampling. If the conditions are appropriate for defecation, the individual assumes a defecatory posture (seated on the toilet with forward trunk flexion), increases intraabdominal pressure through straining, and relaxes the puborectalis muscle and external anal sphincter, resulting in stool expulsion.

T. Takahashi (✉)
Kameda Medical Center, Chiba, Japan
e-mail: takahashi.tomoko@kameda.jp

H. Kaneko et al. (eds.), *Disorders of Gut-Brain Interaction*,
https://doi.org/10.1007/978-981-95-6974-8_66

In contrast, functional defecation disorders are defined as a form of constipation characterized by difficulty in defecation or a sensation of incomplete evacuation due to the inability to adequately and comfortably expel stool from the rectum, despite the absence of morphological abnormalities [1–3]. One of the primary causes is dyssynergic defecation [4].

2 Disease Concept

Dyssynergic defecation is defined as a lack of coordination among the anal and pelvic floor muscles and the abdominal musculature (intraabdominal pressure) during defecation. Specifically, it involves inadequate relaxation or paradoxical contraction of the anal and pelvic floor muscles or insufficient rectal propulsive force (abdominal pressure). This condition is also referred to as pelvic floor incoordination or anismus.

3 Symptoms

Symptoms may include excessive straining during defecation, a sensation of incomplete evacuation, a feeling of anorectal obstruction, and prolonged time required for defecation. However, these symptoms are not specific to dyssynergic defecation, and diagnostic testing is necessary for confirmation.

4 Epidemiology

The prevalence of dyssynergic defecation is not well established due to the requirement for specialized anorectal functional testing for diagnosis. It is estimated to be present in 20–81% of patients diagnosed with functional constipation [5–9], and it is reported to be more common in women [10].

5 Diagnostic Criteria and Evaluation

Immediate use of specialized diagnostic tests for functional defecation disorders is not recommended. Initial management should include conservative measures such as improving bowel habits, increasing dietary fiber intake, and discontinuing medications that may worsen constipation. If these measures are ineffective, osmotic or stimulant laxatives may be introduced. Diagnostic testing should be reserved for cases that remain refractory to these interventions [11].

The Rome IV criteria provide diagnostic standards for dyssynergic defecation (Table 66.1) [3]. Diagnostic evaluation includes anorectal manometry or anal surface electromyography (EMG), balloon expulsion test, defecography, or dynamic magnetic resonance imaging (dynamic MRI).

Table 66.1 Rome IV diagnostic criteria for dyssynergic defecation

The patient must satisfy diagnostic criteria for functional constipation and/or irritable bowel syndrome with constipation[a]
At least two abnormal findings from the following three tests:
(a) Abnormal balloon expulsion test
(b) Abnormal anorectal evacuation pattern with manometry or anal surface EMG
(c) Impaired rectal evacuation by imaging
Inappropriate contraction of the pelvic floor as measured with anal surface EMG or manometry with adequate propulsive forces during attempted defecation[b]

[a]Symptoms must have been present for at least 6 months, and all criteria must be met during the most recent 3 months

[b]This criterion is defined by age- and gender-appropriate normal values for the technique

6 Anorectal Manometry and Surface Electromyography

Under normal conditions, anal resting pressure exceeds rectal pressure at rest. During straining, the anal sphincter relaxes in coordination with an increase in rectal (abdominal) pressure, resulting in a decrease in anal pressure. In dyssynergic defecation, however, anal pressure may paradoxically increase or fail to change during attempted defecation. High-resolution anorectal manometry (HR-ARM) is particularly useful, as it allows simultaneous measurement of rectal and anal pressures.

Four patterns of rectoanal coordination have been identified using HR-ARM or EMG [12]:

1. Increased rectal pressure with paradoxical anal contraction
2. Inadequate rectal pressure with increased anal pressure
3. Increased rectal pressure with absent or incomplete anal relaxation
4. Inadequate rectal pressure with absent or incomplete anal relaxation

7 Defecography

Defecography involves the expulsion of simulated stool (a mixture of barium and flour) under fluoroscopy or MRI to assess for morphological or functional abnormalities. It is considered the gold standard for diagnosing obstructed defecation. It is also useful for differentiating functional defecation disorders from structural abnormalities such as rectocele or rectal intussusception.

In dyssynergic defecation, findings may include poor expulsion of simulated stool, absence of physiological perineal descent during straining, and paradoxical contraction of the puborectalis muscle (Fig. 66.1). Additionally, a lack of change in the anorectal angle is commonly observed rather than shaping of anorectal angle during straining [13]. Defecography performed in the seated position is considered more informative than MRI, although radiation exposure to the lower abdomen and reproductive organs is a limitation, particularly in younger patients.

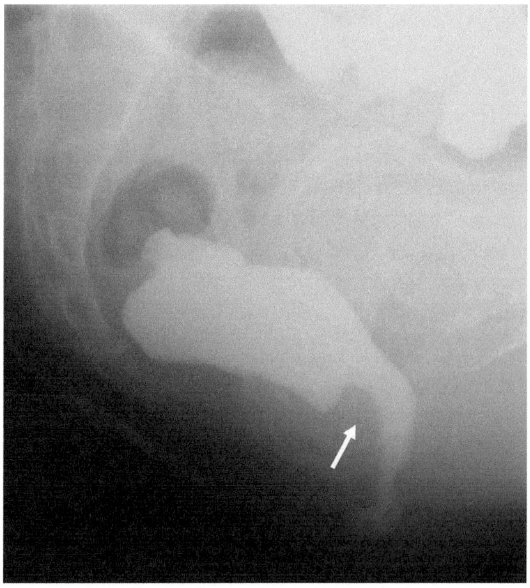

Fig. 66.1 Defecography image during straining in dyssynergic defecation. The arrow indicates paradoxical contraction of the puborectalis muscle, resulting in impaired expulsion of simulated stool

8 Balloon Expulsion Test

In this test, a balloon is inserted into the rectum of a seated patient and inflated with 50 mL of water. The patient is then asked to expel the balloon within 1–3 min. This test is a useful screening tool for functional defecation disorders, particularly for diagnosing pelvic floor incoordination [14].

9 Treatment

Biofeedback (BF) therapy is considered effective. BF therapy is defined as a technique or phenomenon that enables conscious regulation of internal physiological states by providing feedback of biological information that is normally unconscious. In dyssynergic defecation, the goal is to correct incoordination among rectal pressure (abdominal pressure), the puborectalis muscle, and the anal sphincter during straining, as well as to normalize rectal sensation. To correct dyssynergia, surface EMG or anorectal manometry is used. Sessions typically last 30–60 min and involve training in contraction and relaxation of the anal muscles and appropriate increases in abdominal pressure. These sessions are conducted twice weekly for a total of 5–10 sessions (Figs. 66.2 and 66.3). Normalization of rectal sensation is achieved by performing balloon expulsion exercises with varying volumes of water while undergoing corrective training for coordination disorders.

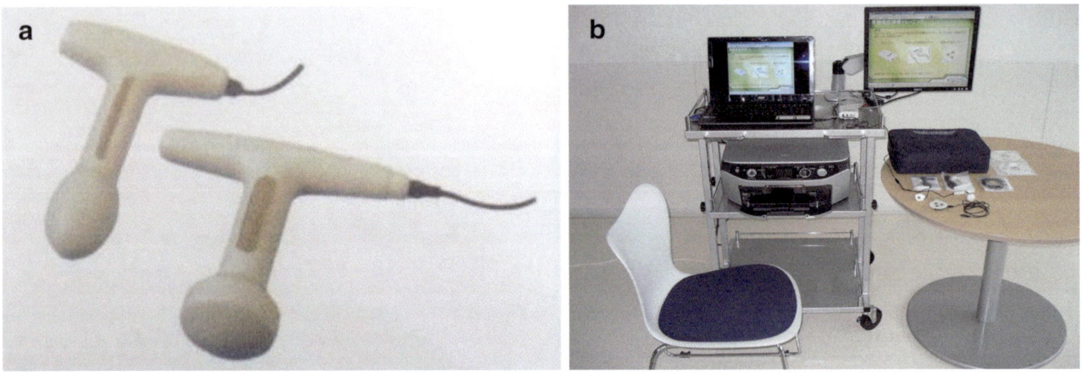

Fig. 66.2 Anorectal biofeedback equipment. Left, probe; right, full device setup

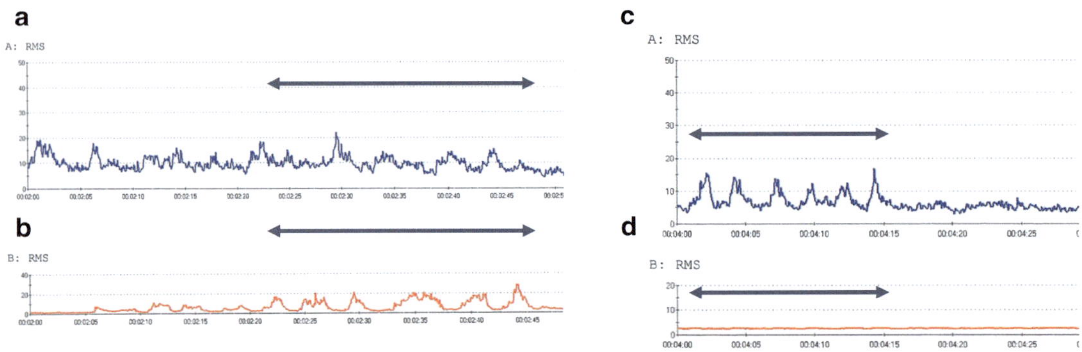

Fig. 66.3 Biofeedback therapy using surface electromyography of the anal region. (**a**) Anal EMG during the first training session, (**b**) Abdominal EMG during the first training session, (**c**) Anal EMG during the fifth training session, (**d**) Abdominal EMG during the fifth training session. Arrows indicate voluntary anal contractions instructed at a frequency of once per second. During the first session, the patient was unable to contract the anal muscles as instructed and exhibited excessive abdominal muscle contraction. By the fifth session, appropriate anal contractions were observed, and unnecessary abdominal contractions had resolved

10 Prognosis

Randomized controlled trials (RCTs) have reported success rates of 70–80% for biofeedback therapy [15], with effects lasting for more than 2 years after completion of the treatment course [16, 17].

Take-Home Message
Although the diagnostic tests and treatments described are available only at specialized centers, initial management—including dietary modification, improvement of bowel habits, and appropriate use of laxatives—is consistent with standard treatment for chronic constipation. Through careful attention to treatment response and patient-reported symptoms, clinicians can identify patients who may benefit from referral to specialized care.

Competing Interests The author(s) has no competing interests to declare that are relevant to the content of this manuscript.

References

1. Chatoor D, et al. Constipation and evacuation disorders. Best Pract Res Clin Gastroenterol. 2009;23:517–30.
2. Mimura T. Defecatory disorders (anorectal functional disorders). Diagnosis and Treatment. 2013;101:285–90. (in Japanese)
3. Rao SS, et al. Anorectal disorders. Gastroenterology. 2016;150:1430–42.
4. Classification of chronic constipation. Japanese Society of Gastroenterology, Chronic Constipation Diagnosis and Treatment Study Group (eds.). Clinical practice guidelines for chronic constipation 2017. Tokyo: Nankodo; 2017:3–5. (in Japanese).
5. Kuijpers HC. Application of the colorectal laboratory in diagnosis and treatment of functional constipation. Dis Colon Rectum. 1990;33–39
6. Wald A, et al. Contributions of evacuation proctography and anorectal manometry to evaluation of adults with constipation and defecatory difficulty. Dig Dis Sci. 1990;35:481–7.
7. Surrenti E, et al. Audit of constipation in a tertiary referral gastroenterology practice. Am J Gastroenterol. 1997;92:1471–5.
8. Rao S, et al. How useful are manometric tests of anorectal function in the management of defecation disorders? Am J Gastroenterol. 1997;92:469–75.
9. Nullens S, et al. Regional colon transit in patients with dyssynergic defecation or slow transit constipation. Gut. 2012;61:1132–9.
10. Rao SSC, et al. Dyssynergic defecation: demographics, symptoms, stool patterns, and quality of life. J Clin Gastroenterol. 2004;38:680–5.
11. Bharucha AE, et al. Anorectal disorders. In: Drossman DA, et al., editors. Rome IV functional gastrointestinal disorders: disorders of gut-brain interaction, vol. 2. Raleigh, NC: Rome Foundation; 2017.
12. Rao SS, et al. Diagnosis and treatment of dyssynergic defecation. J Neurogastroenterol Motil. 2016;22:423–35.
13. Wozniak MM, et al. Evacuation proctography. In: Santoro GA, editor. Pelvic floor disorders: a multidisciplinary textbook. 2nd ed. Springer; 2021. p. 133–62.
14. Minguez M, et al. Predictive value of the balloon expulsion test for excluding the diagnosis of pelvic floor dyssynergia in constipation. Gastroenterology. 2004;126:57–62.
15. Heymen S, et al. Randomized, controlled trial shows biofeedback to be superior to alternative treatments for patients with pelvic floor dyssynergia-type constipation. Dis Colon Rectum. 2007;50:428–41.
16. Lee HJ, et al. Long-term efficacy of biofeedback therapy in patients with dyssynergic defecation: results of a median 44-month follow-up. Neurogastroenterol Motil. 2015;27:787–95.
17. Rao SS, et al. Long-term efficacy of biofeedback therapy for dyssynergia: a randomized controlled trial. Am J Gastroenterol. 2010;105:890.

Diagnosis and Treatment of DGBI of the Anorectum, Functional Defecation Disorders, Evacuation Disorder

67

Toshiki Mimura

Abstract

Evacuation disorder (ED) is defined as the inability to adequately and comfortably evacuate stool from the rectum, even when the stool is soft. It presents symptoms such as difficulty in defecation and a sensation of incomplete evacuation. ED is classified into functional ED, such as pelvic floor incoordination, and structural ED, such as rectocele and rectal intussusception. ED is common, accounting for 41% of chronic constipation with a prevalence of approximately 1.4% in the general population in Japan.

Defecography is the most useful tool for diagnosing and distinguishing between functional and structural ED. However, rectocele and rectal intussusception are frequently observed on defecography even in asymptomatic individuals. Therefore, the presence of these findings in patients with defecatory symptoms does not necessarily indicate that they are the cause of the symptoms, and careful clinical correlation is required. Defecography is also valuable for accurately identifying patients with obsessive-compulsive defecation disorder who do not actually have constipation.

Treatment options include bowel habit training, laxatives, suppositories, and enemas, which may provide some benefit. However, biofeedback therapy is the most effective treatment for functional ED. For structural ED, surgical interventions, such as rectocele repair or ventral rectopexy, may be effective in carefully selected patients.

Keywords

Constipation · Evacuation disorder · Dyssynergic defecation · Pelvic floor incoordination · Inadequate defecatory propulsion · Rectocele · Rectal intussusception · Defecography · Balloon expulsion test · Biofeedback therapy

1 Introduction

Regarding chronic constipation, dietary and lifestyle guidance or pharmacologic therapy are often discussed for infrequent bowel movement-type constipation. However, there also exists difficult defecation-type constipation, characterized by straining and a sensation of incomplete evacuation. In some cases, biofeedback therapy or even surgery may be effective, depending on the underlying cause. This section focuses on evacu-

T. Mimura (✉)
Division of Gastroenterological, General and Transplant Surgery, Department of Surgery, Jichi Medical University, Shimotsuke, Japan
e-mail: mimurat@jichi.ac.jp

H. Kaneko et al. (eds.), *Disorders of Gut-Brain Interaction*,
https://doi.org/10.1007/978-981-95-6974-8_67

ation disorder, the primary pathophysiological mechanism underlying difficult defecation-type constipation.

1.1 Concept and Definition

Evacuation disorder is defined as a condition in which stool, even when soft, cannot be evacuated from the rectum in an adequate and comfortable manner [1–3]. Depending on whether the cause is functional or structural, evacuation disorders are classified into functional evacuation disorders and structural evacuation disorders (Table 67.1).

1.2 Epidemiology

There are no large-scale epidemiological studies specifically investigating evacuation disorders. However, in a study of 147 patients diagnosed with chronic constipation based on symptoms alone, colonic transit studies and defecography revealed that 51 patients (35%) had evacuation disorder alone, and 10 patients (7%) had combined slow transit constipation and evacuation disorder, resulting in a total prevalence of 41% for evacuation disorder [4]. According to the 2019 National Health and Nutrition Survey in Japan, the prevalence of self-reported constipation was 3.5%, suggesting that the prevalence of evacuation disorder in the general population is approximately 1.4%. Thus, evacuation disorder is not rare and represents a clinically important subtype of chronic constipation.

Table 67.1 Classification of evacuation disorders

Evacuation disorder	Functional evacuation disorder	Pelvic floor incoordination (=dyssynergic defecation) Inadequate defecatory propulsion Rectal hyposensitivity Rectal hypocontractility
	Structural evacuation disorder	Rectocele rectal intussusception sigmoidocele enterocele megarectum

1.3 Etiology and Pathophysiology

1.3.1 Functional Evacuation Disorder

Functional evacuation disorder is caused by functional abnormalities such as impaired pelvic floor muscle coordination or altered rectal sensation. The two main pathophysiological mechanisms are pelvic floor incoordination and inadequate defecatory propulsion [5].

Pelvic floor incoordination refers to a condition in which the levator ani muscle, including the puborectal muscle and external anal sphincter, fails to relax or paradoxically contracts during straining, when it should remain relaxed. This condition is also referred to as dyssynergic defecation. For a detailed discussion, see Chap. 66.

Dyssynergic Defecation

Inadequate defecatory propulsion is caused by insufficient increase in intraabdominal pressure during straining due to weakened abdominal muscles and is often related to aging or sarcopenia.

1.3.2 Structural Evacuation Disorder

Structural evacuation disorder is caused by anatomical abnormalities such as weakening of the rectovaginal septum or rectal support structures. Common causes include rectocele, rectal intussusception, sigmoidocele, enterocele, and megarectum, with rectocele and rectal intussusception being the most prevalent [1–3].

- Rectocele: A condition specific to women, in which the anterior rectal wall bulges into the vaginal cavity when intraabdominal pressure rises during straining due to weakening of the rectovaginal septum [6]. For details, see Chap. 68.
- Rectal intussusception: A condition in which the rectal wall, whose fixation has become impaired due to factors such as age-related tissue weakening, invaginates into the distal rectum during straining. This intussusception can

obstruct the passage of stool or cause the invaginated rectal mucosa to be misperceived as retained feces, resulting in symptoms such as difficulty in defecation and a sensation of incomplete evacuation. However, it is important to note that rectal intussusception is frequently observed on defecography even in asymptomatic individuals. Therefore, the presence of rectal intussusception on imaging in a patient reporting defecatory symptoms does not necessarily indicate that the intussusception is the cause of those symptoms, and careful clinical correlation is required.

1.4 Diagnosis and Examination

1.4.1 Symptoms

Common symptoms include difficulty in defecation, a sensation of incomplete evacuation, frequent bowel movements due to feeling of residual stool, and excessive straining. In rectocele, additional symptoms may include vaginal or perineal discomfort, bulging of the vaginal wall during straining, and vaginal digitation—manual pressure on the posterior vaginal wall or perineum to assist stool evacuation. In rectal intussusception, the intussuscepted rectal mucosa may be mistaken for feces, leading to a sensation of incomplete evacuation despite the absence of stool in the rectum—a so-called false urge to defecate. Furthermore, both rectocele and rectal intussusception may also cause passive fecal incontinence a few hours after defecation due to retained stool without being fully evacuated during defecation.

1.4.2 Digital Rectoanal Examination

In suspected pelvic floor incoordination, the patient is instructed to strain during digital rectoanal examination. Normally, the anus and perineum descend during straining, but in dyssynergia, paradoxical anal contraction may occur.

In rectocele, palpation of the anterior rectal wall may reveal generalized weakness of the rectovaginal septum or a localized defect. In addition, during straining, the posterior vaginal wall may prolapse through the vaginal introitus, which is why rectocele is classified as a type of pelvic organ prolapse.

1.4.3 Specialized Examinations

Functional evacuation disorders can be diagnosed using defecography, balloon expulsion test, and anal electromyography (EMG). Among these, defecography is considered the most useful [7] because it most accurately replicates actual defecation and can also diagnose structural abnormalities such as rectocele and rectal intussusception.

- *Defecography* evaluates perineal descent, anorectal angle, coordination of pelvic floor muscle and anal sphincter during simulated defecation, and presence and degree of rectocele or rectal intussusception. For details, see Chap. 62.

  In healthy individuals, perineal descent and anal opening occur during straining, and simulated stool is expelled completely within 30 s. In functional evacuation disorders, perineal descent may be absent or reversed, the anus may not open, and simulated stool is not expelled.

  In rectocele, the anterior rectal wall bulges toward the vagina beyond the expected virtual line of the original anterior rectal wall. Barium trapping—residual contrast in the rectocele after defecation—suggests that the rectocele is the cause of symptoms. If vaginal digitation eliminates the barium trapping and symptoms such as feeling of incomplete evacuation or vaginal discomfort, the rectocele is confirmed as clinically significant.

  In rectal intussusception, the proximal rectum is invaginated into the distal rectum (Fig. 67.1). The Oxford classification is used to grade severity based on the extent of prolapse. Grades III (the advanced portion reaching the upper anal canal) and IV (extending into the anal canal) are considered clinically significant. Grade V, in which the prolapse extends outside the anal canal, represents mucosal prolapse or complete rectal prolapse.
- Balloon expulsion test: A balloon is inserted into the rectum, inflated with water, and the

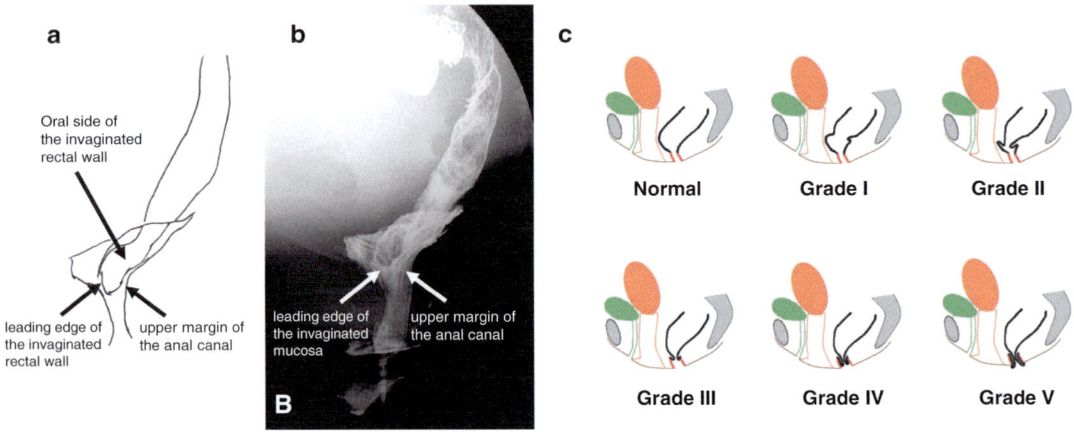

Fig. 67.1 Rectal Intussusception. (Cited from Ref. (3). (**a**) Schematic illustration of rectal intussusception. (**b**) Defecography image of rectal intussusception. The proximal rectum is prolapsing into the distal rectum, with the leading edge reaching the upper margin of the anal canal, consistent with *Grade III rectal intussusception*. (**c**) Oxford Classification of rectal intussusception. *Grade I*: High rectorectal intussusception. *Grade II*: Low rectorectal intussusception. *Grade III*: Rectoanal intussusception reaching the upper margin of the anal canal. *Grade IV*: Rectoanal intussusception entering the anal canal. *Grade V*: External prolapse of the rectum beyond the anal canal

patient is asked to expel it. Failure to expel within 1 min suggests functional evacuation disorder. This examination is simple and is used as a screening test for functional defecation disorder. For details, Chap. 63.

- *Anal electromyography (EMG)*: Electrodes are placed in the anus and on the abdominal wall to assess electrical activity of the anal sphincter and abdominal muscles during each of anal squeezing and straining. Abnormally increased anal sphincter activity during straining suggests pelvic floor incoordination. For details, see Chap. 61.
- *Anorectal manometry*: According to the Rome criteria, pelvic floor incoordination is diagnosed when, during straining, the anal pressure does not decrease by more than 20% from resting pressure. However, this criterion is based on the flawed assumption that anal pressure must decrease during defecation. In reality, defecation occurs when the rectal pressure, elevated by the defecation reflex and increased intraabdominal pressure during straining, exceeds the anal pressure, even if the anal pressure during straining is higher than that at rest. In fact, in healthy individuals without defecatory symptoms, anal pressure usually increases during straining. Grossi et al. [8] performed anorectal manometry in 85 asymptomatic individuals and found that according to the Rome criteria, 74 (87%) would be misdiagnosed with functional evacuation disorder. Due to this high false-positive rate, the authors concluded that "anorectal manometry is of limited accuracy for discriminating between healthy people and patients with functional evacuation disorder." Therefore, anorectal manometry is not appropriate for diagnosing pelvic floor incoordination.

  However, this test is useful for evaluating propulsive force. If the increase in rectal pressure during straining is less than 45 mmHg above baseline, the patient can be diagnosed with inadequate defecatory propulsion.

1.5 Differential Diagnosis

A key differential diagnosis for evacuation disorder is obsessive-compulsive defecation disorder, which is not a true form of constipation [1–3]. Obsessive-compulsive defecation disorder is a condition in which patients, driven by obsessive thoughts, report a persistent sensation of incomplete evacuation (*false urge to defecate*) and engage in excessive straining or frequent toilet visits, despite the absence of stool in the rectum. This condition is not caused by anorectal dysfunction but rather by psychological factors.

Therefore, conventional constipation treatments aimed at promoting stool evacuation are ineffective. Instead, management should focus on cognitive behavioral therapy and psychological or psychiatric interventions, with appropriate explanation of the condition to the patient.

In patients with obsessive-compulsive defecation disorder, defecography typically shows rapid and complete expulsion of the simulated stool without any finding of evacuation disorders, such as rectocele or rectal intussusception, and no residual simulated stool remains in the rectum. Despite these normal findings, these patients strongly complain of a sensation of incomplete evacuation. Thus, defecography is extremely valuable not only for distinguishing between functional and structural evacuation disorders but also for accurately identifying patients with obsessive-compulsive defecation disorder who do not actually have constipation.

1.6 Treatment

Treatment options include bowel habit training, laxatives, suppositories, and enemas, which may provide some benefit. However, biofeedback therapy is the most effective treatment for functional evacuation disorders.

In patients with rectocele or rectal intussusception, simply showing the defecography video and explaining the condition often leads to understanding and reassurance, and many patients do not request further treatment. For those who do, surgical intervention may be considered. However, even if structural abnormalities are corrected surgically, symptom improvement is not guaranteed. Therefore, careful patient selection and thorough preoperative counseling are essential.

1.6.1 Biofeedback Therapy

Biofeedback therapy is effective for functional evacuation disorders. The *Japanese Clinical Practice Guidelines for Chronic Constipation 2017* state: "Biofeedback therapy is effective for chronic constipation caused by functional evacuation disorder and is recommended (Strength of Recommendation: Weak, Evidence Level: A)." This therapy is primarily indicated for pelvic floor incoordination (dyssynergic defecation); for further details, refer to Chap. 66.

1.6.2 Rectocele Repair

While laxatives and biofeedback therapy may provide some benefit in patients with *rectocele*, the definitive treatment is surgical repair and reinforcement of the *rectovaginal septum*. The *Japanese Clinical Practice Guidelines for Chronic Constipation 2017* state: "Surgical treatment is effective and recommended when the cause of constipation is rectal prolapse, rectocele, or rectal intussusception (Strength of Recommendation: Weak, Evidence Level: B)." For further details on treatment of rectocele, see Chaps. 68 and 69.

1.6.3 Ventral Rectopexy

Ventral rectopexy is one of surgical procedures for rectal intussusception. In this technique, a mesh is sutured to the ventral aspect of the distal rectum and anchored to the sacral promontory to correct the prolapse. It is generally indicated for grade III or IV rectoanal intussusception according to the Oxford classification [9]. As a relatively new procedure, it is typically performed laparoscopically or robotically.

According to a systematic review by Grossi et al. [9] of 18 studies involving 1238 patients, the overall symptomatic improvement rate was 83% (95% CI: 74–91%), and the anatomical recurrence rate of rectal intussusception was low, at 2–7% during the mean follow-up period of 31 months (range: 12–72 months). The complication rate ranged from 5% to 15%, with most being minor, such as wound infections or urinary retention. The conversion rate from laparoscopic to open surgery was 2% (range: 0–8%). The incidence of mesh-related complications, the most concerning adverse event, was 0.5% (95% CI: 0–3.9%). However, when mesh-related complications do occur, they can be severe, which may explain the limited adoption of this procedure.

2 Conclusion

This chapter has outlined the major pathophysiological mechanisms, diagnostic approaches, and treatment strategies for *evacuation disorder*. When patients continue to report difficulty in defecation or a sensation of incomplete evacuation despite soft stools achieved through laxative therapy, further evaluation—particularly with *defecography*—is warranted to identify the underlying cause and guide appropriate treatment.

Take-Home Message

Evacuation disorder is defined as the inability to adequately and comfortably evacuate stool from the rectum, even when the stool is soft. It presents with symptoms such as difficult defecation and a sensation of incomplete evacuation. The condition is classified into functional evacuation disorders, such as pelvic floor incoordination, and structural evacuation disorders, such as rectocele and rectal intussusception. Defecography is the most useful diagnostic tool. Biofeedback therapy is effective for functional disorders, while surgical interventions, such as rectocele repair or ventral rectopexy, may be appropriate for structural disorders. However, surgical indications must be carefully considered on a case-by-case basis.

Competing Interests The author(s) has no competing interests to declare that are relevant to the content of this manuscript.

References

1. Mimura T. Evacuation disorder (anorectal functional disorder). Diagn Ther. 2013;101:285–90. (in Japanese)
2. Mimura T, et al. Diagnosis and treatment of chronic constipation. J Jpn Soc Coloproctol. 2019;72:583–99. (in Japanese)
3. Mimura T, et al. Diagnosis and treatment of evacuation disorder. Diagn Ther. 2022;110:85–92. (in Japanese)
4. Voderholzer WA, et al. Clinical response to dietary fiber treatment of chronic constipation. Am J Gastroenterol. 1997;92:95–8.
5. Mimura T, et al. Functional evacuation disorder. In: 3rd, editor. Supplement to Japanese clinical: gastrointestinal syndromes. Tokyo: Nihon Rinsho Sha; 2020. p. 383–90. (in Japanese).
6. Mimura T, et al. Rectocele. In: 3rd, editor. Supplement to Japanese clinical: gastrointestinal syndromes. Tokyo: Nihon Rinsho Sha; 2020. p. 377–82. (in Japanese).
7. Mimura T, et al. Functional examinations for chronic constipation. Gastroenterol Hepatol Intern Med. 2019;5:163–73. (in Japanese)
8. Grossi U, et al. Diagnostic accuracy study of anorectal manometry for diagnosis of dyssynergic defecation. Gut. 2016;65:447–55.
9. Grossi U, et al. Surgery for constipation: systematic review and practice recommendations. Results II: hitching procedures for the rectum (rectal suspension). Color Dis. 2017;19:37–48.

68 Diagnosis and Treatment of Anorectal Dysfunction Due to Organic Disease, Rectocele

Kotaro Maeda

Abstract

Rectocele is one of the structural causes of organic defecatory disorders. Rectocele is defined as the protrusion of the anterior rectal wall toward the posterior vaginal wall due to weakening of the rectovaginal septum. However, since many cases are asymptomatic, diagnosis is typically reserved for symptomatic individuals. The size of the rectocele can be assessed via defecography, with some reports defining rectocele as a protrusion measuring ≥3 cm in length or depth. In principle, asymptomatic rectocele does not require treatment. Intervention is indicated only in symptomatic cases. Conservative management includes guidance on bowel habits, administration of laxatives, and increased dietary fiber intake. Biofeedback therapy may also be selected. If symptoms do not improve sufficiently with these measures, surgical treatment may be considered. Various surgical methods are available. Transvaginal anterior levatorplasty has been reported to yield favorable and long-term outcomes among them.

Keywords

Rectocele · Organic defecatory disorder · Rectovaginal septum · Pelvic organ prolapse · Surgical treatment of rectocele · Anterior levatorplasty

1 Definition and Concept

Rectocele is one of the structural causes of organic defecatory disorders, in which stool cannot be effectively evacuated due to an anatomical abnormality of the anorectal region [1]. It is characterized by the protrusion of the anterior rectal wall into the posterior vaginal wall due to weakening of the rectovaginal septum [1, 2]. In Japan, the condition was initially referred to as "rectovaginal wall relaxation syndrome," but the term "rectocele" is now more commonly used. It is classified as a type of pelvic organ prolapse and is frequently associated with other forms of pelvic organ prolapse [3]. Although often asymptomatic [4], rectocele may require treatment when accompanied by symptoms such as difficult defecation, a sensation of incomplete evacuation, or constipation.

K. Maeda (✉)
Medical Corporation Himawariseishinnkai Oumeimai Hospital, Ome, Tokyo, Japan
e-mail: maeda@oumeimai.or.jp

H. Kaneko et al. (eds.), *Disorders of Gut-Brain Interaction*,
https://doi.org/10.1007/978-981-95-6974-8_68

2 Epidemiology

In Western countries, the prevalence of rectocele among women aged 50 years and older is reported to be 30–50%. However, no epidemiological data are currently available from Japan. One Western study reported that 12% of women aged 18–24 years without childbirth experience had rectoceles measuring ≥1 cm. According to Japanese reports, rectocele can occur across a wide age range (20–80 years), with peak incidence between 40 and 60 years.

3 Etiology and Pathophysiology

Weakening of the rectovaginal septum is attributed to overstretching during vaginal delivery or chronic straining due to difficult defecation, which may lead to tearing of the rectovaginal membrane [5]. Additional contributing factors include aging, obesity, weakening of pelvic support structures postmenopause, and neuropathy of the pelvic floor muscles.

Under normal conditions, straining increases intraabdominal pressure, which raises intrarectal pressure and facilitates stool expulsion toward the anus. In rectocele, however, the increased pressure is directed toward the weakened rectovaginal septum (i.e., the anterior rectal wall), causing stool to become trapped within the rectocele, leading to symptoms such as difficult defecation and a sensation of incomplete evacuation (Fig. 68.1). These symptoms may worsen in the standing position or in the evening, manifesting as a sensation of perineal pressure or perineal pain.

A characteristic finding in rectocele patients is manual assistance during defecation (digitation), in which the patient applies pressure to the posterior vaginal wall with a finger. This maneuver supports the weakened rectovaginal septum, redirecting pressure toward the anus and facilitating smoother defecation.

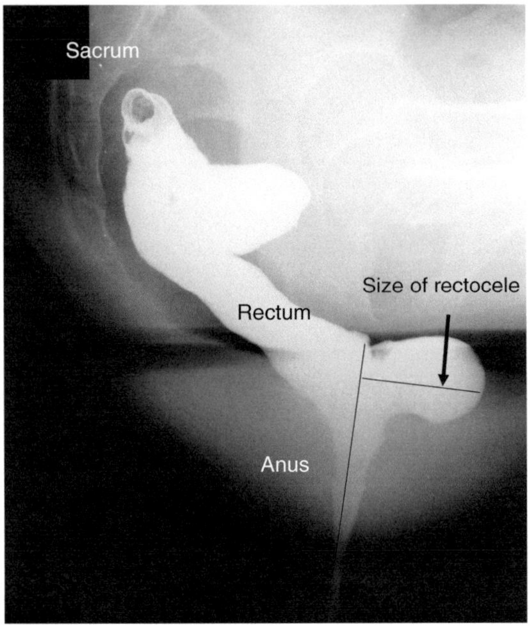

Fig. 68.1 Defecographic findings of rectocele

4 Diagnostic Criteria

Rectocele is defined as the protrusion of the anterior rectal wall toward the posterior vaginal wall. However, since many cases are asymptomatic, diagnosis is typically reserved for symptomatic individuals. The size of the rectocele can be assessed via defecography, with some reports defining rectocele as a protrusion measuring ≥3 cm in length or depth [6] (Fig. 68.1).

5 Diagnosis and Differential Diagnosis

Patients may present with symptoms such as difficult defecation, a sensation of incomplete evacuation, perineal pressure or discomfort, perineal pain, a feeling of perineal descent, or a vaginal mass. In such cases, rectocele should be suspected, and appropriate examinations should be conducted. Medical history should include inquiries about manual assistance during defecation, childbirth, and surgical history. Since fecal incontinence is reported in 40% and urinary incontinence in 21% of rectocele patients, these symptoms should also be assessed [3].

5.1 Physical Examination

Inspection and palpation of the rectum, vagina, and perineum, including bimanual examination, are essential. Straining maneuvers should always be performed during examination. Visual inspection may reveal posterior vaginal wall prolapse and coexisting conditions such as vaginal prolapse, uterine prolapse, cystocele, or rectal prolapse, as well as perineal descent [3]. During digital rectal examination, hooking a finger toward the vaginal side may help identify the rectocele (Fig. 68.2). Bimanual examination during straining should also assess for the presence of sigmoidoceles, enteroceles, or peritoneoceles between the vagina and rectum.

5.2 Imaging Studies

Defecography can confirm the presence and size of a rectocele during straining (Fig. 68.1) and assess for residual contrast material, rectal intussusception, or rectal prolapse during defecation. When contrast medium is applied to the vagina, defecography can also aid in diagnosing sigmoidoceles, enteroceles, and peritoneoceles [7]. Although CT and MRI can detect rectocele, dynamic MRI and 3D-CT allow for real-time evaluation and are useful for diagnosing coexisting pelvic organ prolapse.

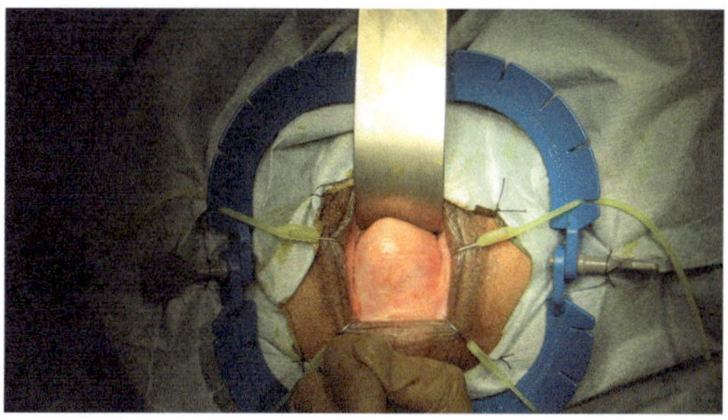

Fig. 68.2 Intraoperative findings of rectocele

6 Treatment

In principle, asymptomatic rectocele does not require treatment. Intervention is indicated only in symptomatic cases.

6.1 Conservative Treatment

Conservative management includes guidance on bowel habits (e.g., avoiding excessive straining), administration of laxatives, and increased dietary fiber intake. Biofeedback therapy may also be selected. If symptoms do not improve sufficiently with these measures, surgical treatment may be considered.

6.2 Surgical Treatment

6.2.1 Indications

Given that rectocele is a benign condition, surgical indications should be carefully evaluated in consultation with the patient. Surgery is generally indicated for large rectoceles (typically $\geq$5 cm), cases unresponsive to conservative treatment, patients with residual barium on post-defecation imaging, those requiring manual assistance during defecation, or those presenting with a vaginal mass [2, 3].

6.2.2 Surgical Techniques

Various surgical methods are available (see Table 68.1). The fundamental principle is to plicate, excise, or reinforce the weakened rectovaginal septum. Reinforcement may involve autologous tissue or mesh. Symptom improvement rates vary depending on surgical indication

Table 68.1 Surgical treatments for rectocele

1. *Transanal surgery*
Plication techniques: Block method, Sarles method, and Khubchandani method Resection technique: PPH (not suitable for large rectoceles)
2. *Transvaginal surgery*
Posterior colporrhaphy GYNEMESH (nonabsorbable polypropylene soft mesh)
3. *Reinforcement of the rectovaginal septum*
Transvaginal anterior keratoplasty
4. *Transabdominal fixation*
Rectovaginovesicopexy

and technique, but transvaginal anterior levatorplasty has been reported to yield favorable and long-term outcomes [3].

Take-Home Message

During evaluation of constipation and related symptoms, it is essential to examine the vagina to assess for rectocele and other forms of pelvic organ prolapse. Rectocele is often observed in women, even in asymptomatic cases. When determining treatment strategy, it is crucial to assess the degree of correlation between the rectocele and the patient's symptoms, considering the size of the rectocele and the response to conservative therapy.

Competing Interests The author(s) has no competing interests to declare that are relevant to the content of this manuscript.

References

1. Japanese Society of Stoma and Continence Rehabilitation. Glossary of terms for stoma and continence rehabilitation. 4th ed. Tokyo: Kanehara Publishing; 2020. (in Japanese).
2. Maeda K, et al. Rectocele. Mod Phys. 2017;37:83–5. (in Japanese).
3. Maeda K, et al. Outcomes of transvaginal anterior levatorplasty with posterior colporrhaphy for symptomatic rectocele. J Anus Rectum Colon. 2021;5:137–43.
4. Yoshioka H, et al. Physiological and anatomic assessment of patients with rectocele. Dis Colon Rectum. 1991;34:704–8.
5. Aiger F, et al. The rectogenital septum: morphology, function, and clinical relevance. Dis Colon Rectum. 2004;47:131–40.
6. Takao Y. Rectocele. In: Anazawa S, et al., editors. Continence rehabilitation. Tokyo: Nakayama Shoten; 2009. p. 140–2. (in Japanese).
7. Maeda K, et al. Transvaginal peritoneocele repair with anterior levatorplasty for patient with a rectocele and an enterocele. Surg Today. 2021;51:844–7.

Diagnosis and Treatment of Anorectal Dysfunction Due to Organic Disease, Rectal Prolapse

69

Hidetoshi Katsuno

Abstract

Rectal prolapse refers to a condition in which the rectum descends and may protrude through the anus. It is classified as either complete rectal prolapse, where the full thickness of the rectum is externally visible, or occult prolapse (rectal intussusception), which remains within the anal canal. Multiple pathophysiological mechanisms have been proposed, including sliding hernia, intussusception progression, and pelvic floor dysfunction. Diagnosis is based on clinical examination and may require imaging studies such as defecography for occult cases. Differential diagnosis from hemorrhoids and identification of coexisting pelvic organ prolapse are essential in preoperative assessment.

Surgical treatment is broadly categorized into perineal and abdominal approaches. Perineal techniques—such as the Gant-Miwa and Delorme procedures—are often chosen for elderly or high-risk patients due to their minimal invasiveness. Abdominal procedures, including laparoscopic or robot-assisted rectopexy, are associated with lower recurrence rates but require general anesthesia. Ventral rectopexy, in particular, preserves pelvic autonomic nerves and may reduce postoperative constipation.

The choice of surgical approach should be individualized based on patient condition and institutional capabilities. Comprehensive evaluation, including assessment for coexisting pelvic organ prolapse, is crucial for successful management.

Keywords

Rectal prolapse · Rectal intussusception · Rectopexy · Laparoscopic surgery

1 Definition and Etiology

Rectal prolapse is classified into two types: complete rectal prolapse, in which the rectum intussuscepts and protrudes externally through the anus, and occult rectal prolapse (rectal intussusception), in which the prolapse remains within the rectal lumen. Several theories have been proposed regarding its pathogenesis, including the sliding hernia theory, which posits that the anterior rectal wall invaginates into the anal canal from a deep cul-de-sac (Douglas pouch); the intussusception theory, which suggests progression from occult to complete prolapse; and the pelvic floor dysfunction theory, which attributes the condition to weakening of the pelvic floor muscles, anal sphincter, and supporting struc-

H. Katsuno (✉)
Department of Surgery, Fujita Health University Okazaki Medical Center, Okazaki, Japan
e-mail: katsuno@fujita-hu.ac.jp

H. Kaneko et al. (eds.), *Disorders of Gut-Brain Interaction*,
https://doi.org/10.1007/978-981-95-6974-8_69

Table 69.1 Anatomical features associated with rectal prolapse

No.	Feature
1.	Deep cul-de-sac (Douglas pouch or rectovesical pouch)
2.	Redundant sigmoid colon
3.	Elongated mesorectum
4.	Diastasis of the levator ani muscle
5.	Perineal descent
6.	Patulous anal sphincter
7.	Loss of support by the uterus and bladder

Table 69.2 Differential diagnosis between rectal prolapse and hemorrhoids

Feature	Rectal prolapse	Hemorrhoids
Visual inspection	Circumferential prolapse	Radial protrusions
Digital rectal examination	Flaccid rectal wall within the rectum and full-thickness prolapse	Engorged venous plexus
Anorectal manometry	Decreased pressure	Normal pressure

tures. However, no single theory fully explains the condition, and it is generally accepted that multiple factors contribute to its development. The anatomical features commonly observed in rectal prolapse are summarized in Table 69.1.

2 Diagnosis

Patients typically present with complaints of rectal protrusion and anal bleeding, necessitating differentiation from hemorrhoids. The distinguishing features of rectal prolapse and hemorrhoids are outlined in Table 69.2. Diagnosis is relatively straightforward when prolapse is observed during abdominal straining on the examination table. However, in many outpatient cases, prolapse is not evident during routine physical examination. In such instances, straining on a portable toilet can be helpful. If this is not feasible, patients may be asked to bring photographs of the prolapse taken during symptomatic episodes.

Rectal intussusception cannot be diagnosed through physical examination alone; defecography is a valuable diagnostic tool, though its availability is limited to specialized centers. Chronic rectal prolapse may be associated with mucosal edema or ulceration. In rare cases, a prolapsed rectal tumor may be the leading point of intussusception, making total colonoscopy essential preoperatively to exclude organic disease. Additionally, since rectal prolapse may coexist with other forms of pelvic organ prolapse—such as rectocele, vaginal prolapse, uterine prolapse, and cystocele—comprehensive preoperative evaluation is crucial [1]. The classification of rectal prolapse is illustrated in Fig. 69.1.

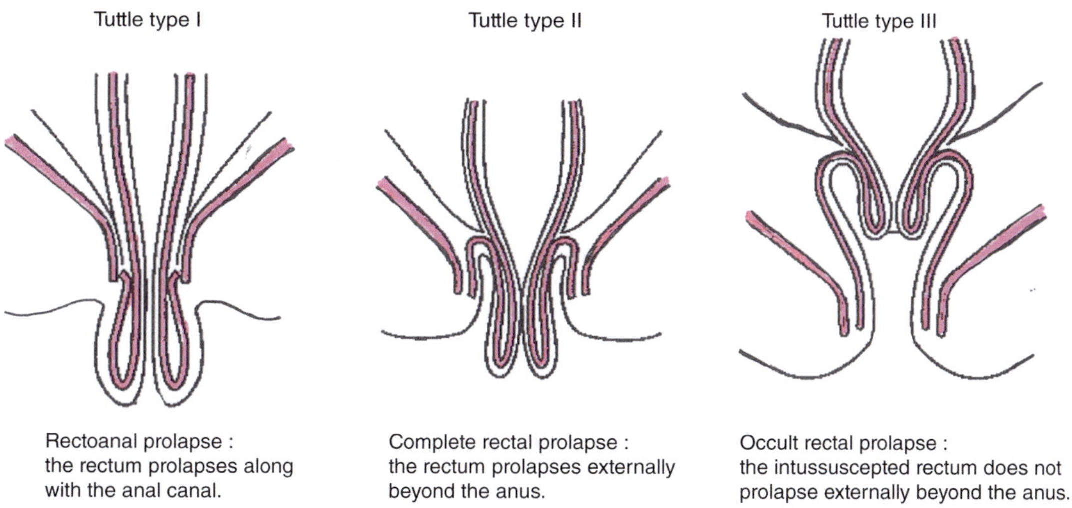

Fig. 69.1 Classification of rectal prolapse

3 Treatment

Surgical treatment for rectal prolapse is broadly categorized into perineal approaches and abdominal approaches (Table 69.3). Perineal procedures can be performed under spinal or local anesthesia and are associated with minimal systemic impact, making them widely used. However, they are associated with a high recurrence rate. In contrast, abdominal procedures—particularly laparoscopic surgery, which has been covered by insurance in Japan since 2012 [2]—are increasingly performed. Reports of robot-assisted surgery also exist [3], although this is not yet covered by insurance in Japan. Abdominal procedures require general anesthesia and are therefore limited to specialized centers, but they offer lower recurrence rates [4]. Below are representative techniques for each approach:

Table 69.3 Surgical treatments for rectal prolapse

Approach	Procedure
Perineal procedures	Gant-Miwa procedure Thiersch procedure Delorme procedure Altemeier procedure
Abdominal procedures	Rectopexy (open, laparoscopic, or robot-assisted approaches): Ripstein procedure Wells procedure Suture rectopexy + Resection Reropexy (Frykman-Goldberg procedure) Ventral rectopexy

3.1 Perineal Procedures

- *Gant-Miwa procedure*: The most commonly performed perineal surgery in Japan. This technique involves full-thickness ligation of the prolapsed rectal wall from the mucosal side, creating multiple mucosal nodules to plicate the bowel wall and reduce the prolapse. Due to its high recurrence rate when performed alone, it is often combined with the Thiersch procedure to reinforce the anal sphincter (Gant-Miwa + Thiersch). Care must be taken to avoid deep sutures that may perforate the bowel.
- *Thiersch procedure*: First described in 1891 by German surgeon Karl Thiersch, this technique involves circumferential placement of a *silver* wire (now commonly nylon, Teflon, or polyester tape) around the external anal sphincter to prevent prolapse. While it has a high recurrence and infection rate, it is suitable for high-risk patients due to its feasibility under local anesthesia.

- *Delorme procedure*: Introduced in 1900 by French military surgeon Edmond Delorme, this technique involves sleeve resection of the mucosa from the prolapsed segment, plication of the exposed muscular layer, and reanastomosis of the mucosal edges. It is widely used in Europe.
- *Altemeier procedure*: Reported in 1952 by American surgeon William Altemeier, this transanal approach involves full-thickness resection of the redundant rectosigmoid colon, followed by an anterior levatorplasty, and it is primarily used in Western countries. Whereas the Gant-Miwa + Thiersch and Delorme procedures are suitable for relatively short-segment prolapse (approximately 5 cm or less), the Altemeier procedure is indicated for longer-segment cases. Due to the risk of anastomotic leakage, a temporary diverting stoma may be created.

3.2 Abdominal Procedures

Abdominal rectopexy is associated with a lower recurrence rate than perineal procedures and is the first-line option for patients who can tolerate general anesthesia. The rectum is mobilized and suspended cranially and then fixed to the anterior sacral surface. Representative techniques include the following:

- *Ripstein procedure* uses Teflon mesh to wrap and fix the anterior rectal wall to the sacrum.
- *Wells procedure* employs Ivalon sponge to fix the posterior rectal wall.
- *Suture rectopexy* involves direct suturing of the rectal mesentery to the sacrum.
- *Ventral rectopexy*: A relatively new technique reported by D'Hoore et al. in 2004, in which the anterior rectal wall is fixed to the sacral promontory using mesh [5]. This approach preserves the autonomic nerves on the dorsal side of the rectum, resulting in a lower incidence of postoperative constipation.

A systematic review found that both perineal and abdominal procedures improve postoperative quality of life (QoL), with no significant differences between surgical techniques [6].

4 Conclusion

Abdominal procedures for rectal prolapse are associated with lower recurrence rates, and the number of *minimally invasive laparoscopic surgeries* is increasing. In practice, the choice of surgical technique depends on patient factors (e.g., age, general health) and institutional capabilities (e.g., availability of general anesthesia). It is essential to understand the characteristics of each procedure thoroughly.

Take-Home Message

- Preoperative evaluation should consider the possibility of *pelvic organ prolapse*, including rectocele, vaginal prolapse, uterine prolapse, and cystocele.
- In cases where diagnosis is challenging, referral to specialized centers capable of performing straining examinations or defecography should be considered.
- Perineal procedures, which can be performed under spinal or local anesthesia, are widely used due to their minimal systemic impact. Abdominal procedures require general anesthesia and are therefore performed only in specialized facilities. Compared to perineal procedures, abdominal procedures have a lower recurrence rate, and it is covered by insurance when performed laparoscopically.

Competing Interests The author(s) has no competing interests to declare that are relevant to the content of this manuscript.

References

1. Maeda K, et al. Pelvic organ prolapse. Modern Phys. 2017;37:75–7. (in Japanese).
2. Hanai K, et al. Selection of surgical procedures and techniques for laparoscopic rectopexy in complete rectal prolapse. Surgery. 2009;63:1697–702. (in Japanese).
3. Ayav A, et al. Robotic-assisted pelvic organ prolapse surgery. Surg Endosc. 2005;19:1200–3.
4. Koide Y, et al. Techniques and outcomes of rectopexy for rectal prolapse. J Japan Soc Coloproctol. 2012;65:840–6. (in Japanese).
5. D'Hoore A, et al. Long-term outcome of laparoscopic ventral rectopexy for total rectal prolapse. Br J Surg. 2004;91:1500–5.
6. Tou SBS, et al. Surgery for complete (full-thickness) rectal prolapse in adults. Cochrane Database Syst Rev. 2015;11:1–66.

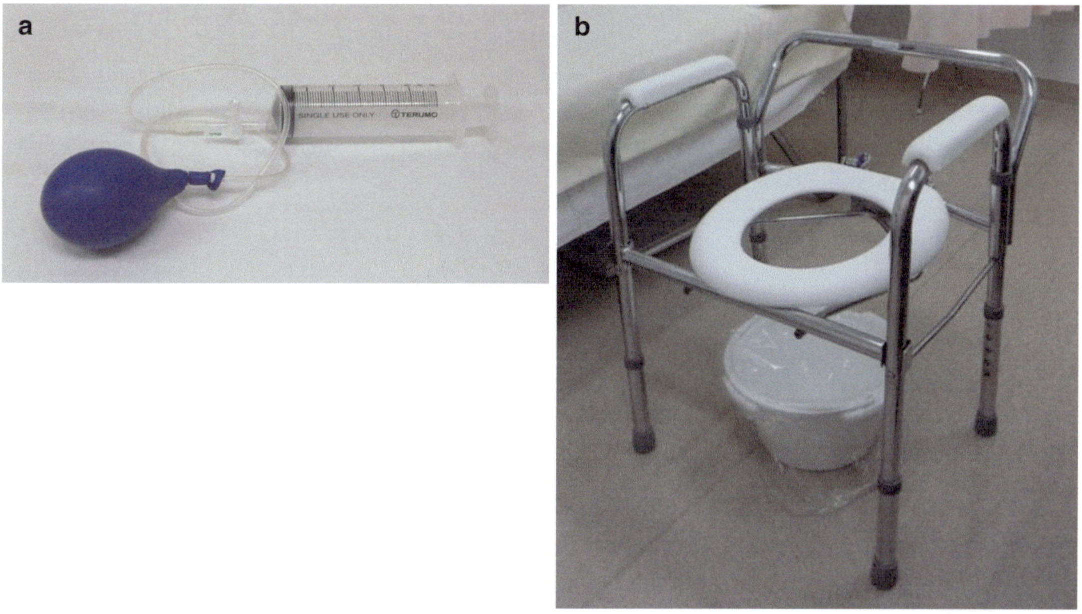

Fig. 70.1 Rectal balloon expulsion training. In the lateral decubitus position, a *rectal balloon* (**a**) is inserted into the patient's anus and inflated with 50 mL of air to ensure close contact with the lower rectal margin. Up-and-down anal movements are confirmed. The patient then sits on a *portable commode* (**b**) to perform balloon expulsion training. (**a**) Rectal balloon. (**b**) Portable commode used during rectal balloon expulsion training

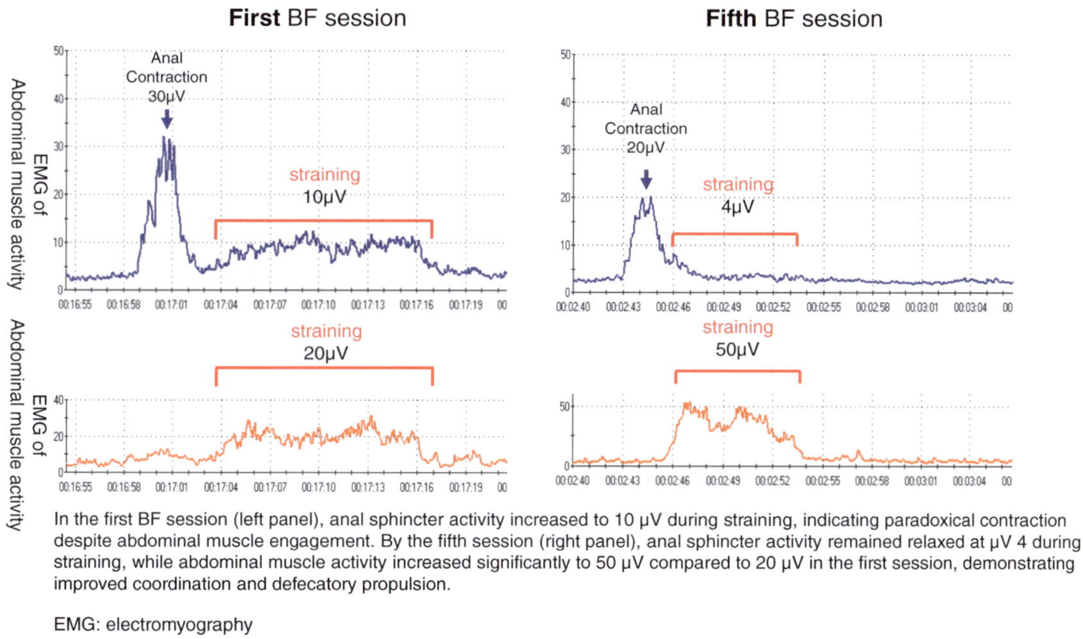

Fig. 70.2 Electromyographic tracings during biofeedback (BF) therapy for constipation. In the first BF session (left panel), anal sphincter activity increased to 10 μV during straining, indicating paradoxical contraction despite abdominal muscle engagement. By the fifth session (right panel), anal sphincter activity remained relaxed at 4 μV during straining, while abdominal muscle activity increased significantly to 50 μV compared to 20 μV in the first session, demonstrating improved coordination and defecatory propulsion. EMG electromyography

By the third session, abdominal activity during straining began to improve. By the fourth session, the patient could expel the balloon independently. By the fifth session, anal sphincter activity remained relaxed at 4 μV during straining, while abdominal muscle activity had markedly increased to 50 μV (Fig. 70.2b), compared to 20 μV in the first session. With improvement in both pelvic floor coordination and inadequate defecatory propulsion, the patient's symptoms were resolved, and BF therapy was concluded.

PEG LD laxative was continued at a dose of four sachets/day while elobixibat hydrate was discontinued. Enemas became unnecessary, and bowel movements stabilized at 1–2 times/day. Although stool consistency improved from BSFS types 5–6 to type 4, the feeling of evacuation difficulty remained absent.

4 Discussion

This patient had a functional defecation disorder due to pelvic floor incoordination and inadequate defecatory propulsion. Pelvic floor incoordination, also known as dyssynergic defecation, occurs when the pelvic floor muscles—including the puborectalis and external anal sphincter—fail to relax or paradoxically contract during straining, despite the need for relaxation to allow defecation. Inadequate defecatory propulsion results from insufficient abdominal muscle strength, leading to inadequate intraabdominal pressure during straining [1].

Defecography is a valuable diagnostic tool for functional evacuation disorders. It replicates actual defecation and can diagnose both functional and structural defecation disorders, such as rectocele and rectal intussusception. In healthy individuals, defecography shows perineal descent, anal canal opening during straining, with near-complete evacuation of simulated stool within 20–30 seconds. In contrast, functional defecation disorders show absent or paradoxical perineal movement during straining, the anal canal does not open, or even if it does, the stimulated stool is not completely evacuated.

In this case, the absence of perineal descent and incomplete evacuation despite anal canal opening confirmed the diagnosis of functional defecation disorder (pelvic floor incoordination).

BF therapy is an effective treatment for functional defecation disorders [2]. The goal of BF therapy for functional defecation disorders is to train patients to contract abdominal muscles effectively during straining while maintaining relaxation of the pelvic floor muscles and external anal sphincter. Patients with functional defecation disorders often fail to generate effective abdominal muscle contraction during straining and simultaneously contract the pelvic floor muscles and external anal sphincter; however, they are usually unwere of this condition. In BF therapy, anal EMG and abdominal muscle EMG are used to help patients become aware of their ana and abdominal muscle activity. The physical therapist guides the patients in adopting a forward-leaning posture during defecation and applying effective intraabdominal pressure during straining. Together, the patient and physical therapist work to improve pelvic floor incoordination.

In addition, rectal balloon expulsion training involves inflating a balloon placed in the rectum with 50 mL of air or water to simulate stool. Patients are trained to maintain relaxation of the pelvic floor muscles and voluntarily expel the balloon [3].

The reported efficacy of BF therapy for functional defecation disorders is approximately 70–80% [2]. A meta-analysis of four RCTs by Enck et al. showed that BF therapy was significantly more effective than other treatments for constipation due to pelvic floor incoordination, with an odds ratio of 3.7 (95% CI: 2.1–6.3) [4]. Combined anal EMG and balloon training has also been shown to significantly improve symptoms and quality of life [5]. In Japan, the 2017 Clinical Practice Guidelines for Chronic Constipation recommend BF therapy for functional defecation disorders with evidence level A and recommendation grade 2 [6]. Despite its evidence level A, the recommendation grade remains low due to the limited number of facilities capable of performing BF therapy in Japan. It is hoped that, in the future, defecography and BF therapy will became more widely available in Japan, increasing the number of centers able to treat patients like the present case.

Take-Home Message

The feeling of evacuation difficulty is a characteristic symptom of defecation disorder-type constipation. It may result from IBS-C with hard stool or defecation disorders even when stools are soft. Defecation disorders should be evaluated using defecography to distinguish between functional and structural causes. When functional (pelvic floor incoordination or inadequate propulsion), biofeedback therapy is indicated. If a patient reports evacuation difficulty, stool consistency should be assessed, and referral to a facility capable of performing defecography should be considered if symptoms persist despite soft stools.

Competing Interests The author(s) has no competing interests to declare that are relevant to the content of this manuscript.

References

1. Mimura T, et al. Diagnosis and treatment of defecation disorders. Diagn Ther. 2022;110:85–92. (in Japanese).
2. Homma Y, et al. Physical therapy (pelvic floor muscle training, biofeedback therapy) for defecation disorders. In: Theory and practice of continence rehabilitation. 2nd ed. Tokyo: Nakayama Shoten; 2022. p. 373–7. (in Japanese).
3. Mimura T. Effectiveness of biofeedback therapy using rectal balloon expulsion training for constipation with pelvic floor incoordination. Biofeedback Res. 2011;38:43–50. (in Japanese).
4. Enck P, et al. Biofeedback therapy in fecal incontinence and constipation. Neurogastroenterol Motil. 2009;21:1133–41.
5. Mimura T, et al. Effectiveness of biofeedback therapy using anal EMG and rectal balloon expulsion training for constipation with pelvic floor incoordination. Biofeedback Res. 2012;39:23–31. (in Japanese).
6. Research Group on Diagnosis and Treatment of Chronic Constipation, affiliated with the Japanese Society of Gastroenterology. CQ5-10: is biofeedback therapy effective for chronic constipation? In: Guidelines for the management of chronic constipation 2017. Tokyo: Nankodo; 2017. p. 82–4. (in Japanese).

Case Discussion, Feeling of Incomplete Defecation

71

Yuko Homma and Toshiki Mimura

Abstract

A 51-year-old woman presented with a one-year history of feeling of incomplete defecation and vaginal bulging during defecation. She did not experience evacuation difficulty but relieved the residual stool sensation by repeatedly straining while pressing the vaginal bulge with her finger to evacuate stool trapped in the rectocele. Digital rectal examination revealed a large, deep rectocele on the anterior rectal wall. Defecography showed a 2.1 cm rectocele with trapping of pseudo-stool at the end of straining. Vaginal digitation effectively assisted complete evacuation and resolved the residual feeling. The patient underwent anterior levatorplasty via a transperineal approach. Seven months after surgery, defecography confirmed disappearance of the rectocele, complete evacuation of pseudo-stool, and resolution of symptoms.

The feeling of incomplete defecation is a common symptom of defecation disorders, classified as structural or functional and diagnosed by defecography. Structural defecation disorders, including rectocele and rectal intussusception, may require surgical treatment; however, the degree of symptom improvement varies. Therefore, it is necessary to carefully evaluate the extent to which structural changes contribute to symptom manifestation. It is important to provide thorough explanations tailored to each patient's condition so that patients can ultimately select and decide on their treatment options.

Keywords

Feeling of incomplete defecation · Defecation disorder · Rectocele · Structural defecation disorder · Defecography

1 Introduction

Feeling of incomplete defecation is defined as the sensation that stool remains in the rectum after defecation. This symptom often arises when stool is not fully evacuated from the rectum. However, in some cases, this sensation occurs despite complete evacuation, a condition referred to as obsessive-compulsive defecation neurosis, characterized by a false urge to defecate without any physical retention of stool [1].

This symptom is commonly observed in defecation disorders, even when stool is soft. Defecation disorders are classified into the following [2]:

Y. Homma (✉) · T. Mimura
Department of Surgery, Division of Gastroenterological, General and Transplant Surgery, Jichi Medical University, Shimotsuke, Japan
e-mail: y.homma@jichi.ac.jp

H. Kaneko et al. (eds.), *Disorders of Gut-Brain Interaction*,
https://doi.org/10.1007/978-981-95-6974-8_71

- Structural defecation disorder: rectocele, rectal intussusception, etc.
- Functional defecation disorder: pelvic floor incoordination and inadequate defecatory propulsion

Defecography is a valuable diagnostic tool for distinguishing between these conditions and for differentiating them from obsessive-compulsive defecation neurosis.

2 Case Presentation (Structural Defecation Disorder: Rectocele)

- *Patient*: A 51-year-old female
- *Chief complaints*: Feeling of incomplete defecation and vaginal bulging during defecation
- *Medical history*: Unremarkable
- *Present illness*: The patient had experienced a sensation of incomplete defecation and vaginal bulging during defecation for 4 years. She underwent two transanal rectocele repair surgeries at another hospital three and 2 years ago, respectively. Although symptoms initially improved, they recurred 1 year ago, prompting her visit to our department. While taking laxatives, her stool was soft (BSFS type 5), and the defecation frequency was moderately increased at 4–5 times per day. Although she did not experience evacuation difficulty during defecation, she felt an incomplete evacuation at the end of defecation. To relieve this feeling, she repeatedly applied pressure to the posterior vaginal wall with a finger inserted into the vagina while straining, thereby facilitating the evacuation of stool trapped in the rectocele.
- *Anorectal examination*: Perianal sensation was normal. No stool was palpable in the rectum. A large, deep rectocele was detected on the anterior rectal wall. Anal resting tone was slightly elevated, with normal squeeze pressure. No rectocele prolapse was observed from the vaginal introitus during straining in the lateral position.

3 Clinical Course

Despite two prior rectocele repair surgeries, a large rectocele was still palpable, and the symptoms such as feeling of incomplete defecation were also characteristic of rectocele. Therefore, defecography was performed to evaluate the rectocele.

3.1 Defecographic Findings

During straining, the anterior rectal wall bulged toward the vaginal side, forming a 2.1-cm-deep rectocele (Fig. 71.1a). Although the simulated stool was completely expelled by the end of straining, a portion remained trapped within the rectocele (Fig. 71.1b), correlating with the patient's sensation of incomplete evacuation. When the patient applied pressure to the vaginal bulge during straining—mimicking her usual defecation behavior—the trapped stool was fully expelled, and the sensation of incomplete evacuation disappeared.

3.2 Preoperative Diagnosis

Since vaginal digitation was effective both in daily life and during defecography, the rectocele was deemed to have high pathological significance. The patient was informed that surgical correction has an approximately 80% success rate in such cases. After discussing the benefits and risks, she opted for surgery of rectocele repair.

3.3 Treatment Course

An anterior levatorplasty was performed via a perineal approach. The rectovaginal septum was dissected between the vagina and rectum, and the puborectalis muscle was sutured to reinforce the septum. The patient was discharged on postoperative day 6 without complications. Postoperatively, the sensation of incomplete evacuation resolved, and vaginal digitation was no longer necessary.

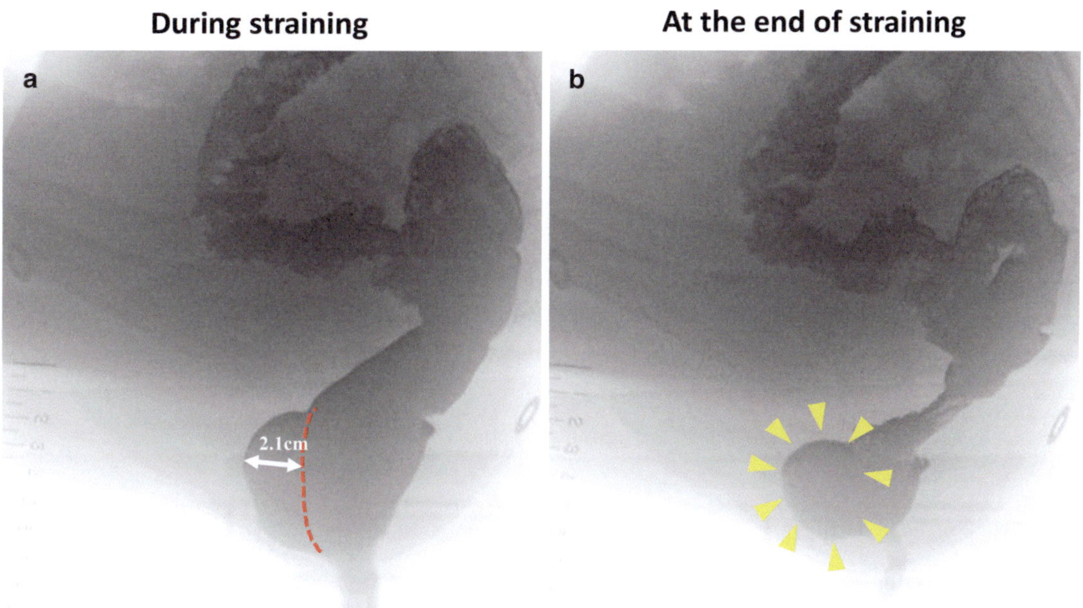

Fig. 71.1 Preoperative defecography. (**a**) During straining, a 2.1 cm bulge (dotted line) was observed in the anterior rectal wall, consistent with a diagnosis of rectocele. (**b**) At the end of straining, a portion of the simulated stool remained trapped within the rectocele (trapping; arrowhead), and the patient reported a sensation of incomplete evacuation

3.4 Postoperative Defecography (Seven Months Later)

Except for a small residual bulge at the most cranial site, the rectocele had resolved (Fig. 71.2a). Simulated stool was almost completely expelled without trapping (Fig. 71.2b), and the patient no longer reported a sensation of incomplete evacuation.

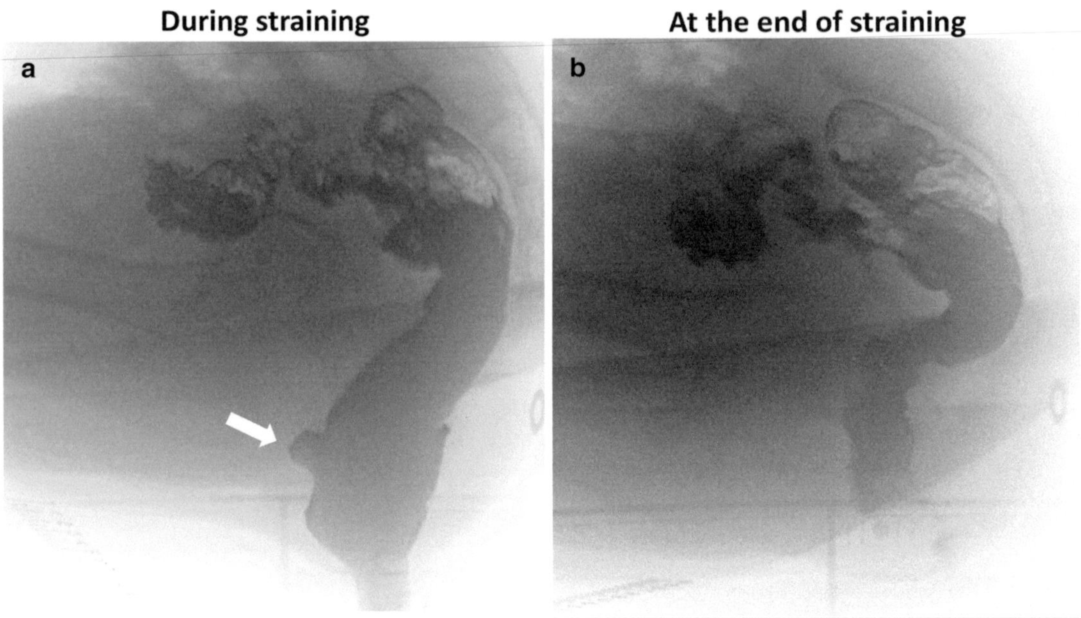

Fig. 71.2 Defecography at 7 months postoperatively. (**a**) During straining, the rectocele had resolved except for a small residual bulge at the most cranial site (white arrow). (**b**) At the end of straining, the small bulge observed in (**a**) had disappeared, no trapping was seen, and the simulated stool was almost completely expelled. The patient no longer reported a sensation of incomplete evacuation

4 Discussion

The feeling of incomplete defecation is a common symptom in defecation disorders. Defecography is a highly useful diagnostic tool that simulates actual defecation and helps identify both structural (e.g., rectocele, rectal intussusception) and functional (e.g., pelvic floor incoordination) defecation disorders. It also available for determining the appropriateness of surgical intervention.

Rectocele is a structural defecation disorder unique to women, caused by weakening of the rectovaginal septum [2]. During straining, increased intraabdominal pressure causes the anterior rectal wall to bulge into the vaginal cavity. In addition to aging and childbirth, chronic straining due to defecation difficulties caused by pelvic floor muscle coordination disorders is considered to be a cause of rectovaginal septum weakness. In normal individuals, the vector of the fecal expulsion force generated by an increase in intrarectal pressure during defecation is directed toward the anus, enabling the expulsion of stool. In rectocele, distension of the anterior wall of the rectum causes the vector of the fecal expulsion force to disperse toward the vagina, resulting in insufficient fecal expulsion force and causing a sensation of incomplete evacuation. Even when the rectum is emptied, trapping of stool within the rectocele can cause a persistent sensation of incomplete evacuation. On the other hand, many individuals with rectocele remain asymptomatic, indicating that rectocele is not always the cause of incomplete evacuation or a target for treatment. This highlights the difficulty in determining appropriate management.

Rectocele can be identified by digital rectal examination, particularly when abnormal laxity or a hernia-like defect is palpated in the rectovaginal septum. On defecography, rectocele is diagnosed when the anterior rectal wall bulges beyond the expected anatomical line toward the vagina during straining.

Regarding the pathological significance of rectocele, defecography is useful. First, regarding the size of rectocele, Shorvon et al. performed defecography on 21 asymptomatic nulliparous women and found rectocele in 17 cases (83%), of which 16 were less than 2 cm in size and only 1 case exceeded 2 cm [3]. In other words, rectocele measuring 2 cm or less is considered to have little pathological significance. Additionally, after the expulsion of pseudostool, residual pseudostool remains within the rectocele (trapping) and the patient reports a sensation of incomplete evacuation, the rectocele is considered to have significant pathological significance as the cause of the sensation of incomplete evacuation. Furthermore, if the patient is asked to perform vaginal digitation and both the trapping of pseudostool and the sensation of incomplete evacuation resolve, the rectocele is deemed to have extremely high pathological significance as the cause of the sensation of incomplete evacuation.

The fundamental treatment for rectocele is surgical treatment aimed at reinforcing the rectovaginal septum. As previously described, defecographic findings are valuable in assessing the clinical relevance of a rectocele. Accordingly, we routinely refer to these findings when discussing surgical indications with patients at our institution. Specifically, the following three defecographic findings are considered predictive factors for symptom improvement after surgery: (1) a large rectocele (≥2 cm), (2) positive pseudostool trapping, and (3) effective digital assistance during defecation. The success rate of surgery improves as the number of criteria increases (the success rate is 50% with 0 criteria, 60% with 1 criterion, 70% with 2 criteria, and 80% with 3 criteria). Surgery is offered only to patients who understand and accept the predicted success rate. Therefore, some patients may decline surgery even with an 80% success rate, while others may opt for surgery even with a 50% success rate. In this case, the patient met all three criteria and experienced complete symptom resolution postoperatively.

Surgical approaches include transanal, transvaginal, perineal, and transabdominal routes, each with multiple techniques. Each surgical procedure has its advantages and disadvantages, and surgical outcomes are reported differently depending on the indication, follow-up period, and definition of success. Therefore, the choice of procedure is determined by the institutional expertise and surgeon preference and other factors [2]. At our institution, anterior levatorplasty or defect-specific repair via the perineal approach is preferred.

A systematic review by Grossi et al. [4] found no significant differences in outcomes among surgical techniques. Overall symptom improvement was 73% (95% CI: 67–78%), but improvement rates for specific symptoms were lower: excessive straining (38%), incomplete evacuation (44%), and vaginal digitation (43%).

Defecography is not only useful for determining surgical indications but also for explaining the condition to patients. In some patients, defecography helps them understand that their feeling of incomplete evacuation or evacuation difficulty is caused by a rectocele. Once they also understand why vaginal digitation is effective, many feel reassured by this explanation and choose not to undergo surgery. Because rectocele is a benign, nonlife-threatening condition, it is essential that treatment decisions for rectocele causing incomplete evacuation are ultimately made by the patients themselves, supported by thorough, individualized explanations tailored to their specific condition.

Take-Home Message

The feeling of incomplete defecation is a common symptom of defecation disorders, which are classified as structural or functional. It is diagnosed by defecography. Structural defecation disorders include rectocele and rectal intussusception, for which surgical treatment is the fundamental approach. However, because the degree of symptom improvement after surgery varies, it is necessary to carefully evaluate the extent to which structural changes contribute to symptom manifestation. It is important to provide thorough explanations tailored to each patient's condition so that patients can ultimately select and decide on their treatment options.

Competing Interests The author(s) has no competing interests to declare that are relevant to the content of this manuscript.

References

1. Mimura T, et al. Diagnosis and treatment of chronic constipation. J Japan Soc Coloproctol. 2019;72:583–99. (in Japanese).
2. Mimura T, et al. Rectocele (gastrointestinal syndrome IV). Japanese J Clin Med. 2020;12:377–82. (in Japanese).
3. Shorvon PJ, et al. Defecography in normal volunteers: results and implications. Gut. 1989;30:1737–49.
4. Grossi U, et al. Surgery for constipation: systematic review and practice recommendations; results IV: recto-vaginal reinforcement procedures. Color Dis. 2017;19:73–91.

72 Case Discussion, Functional Anal Pain

Shota Takano

Abstract

Pain localized to the rectum or anus that cannot be differentiated through diagnostic testing or pathological examination is classified as functional anorectal pain. While no standardized treatment has been established, various therapeutic approaches have been reported, including electrical stimulation and pharmacotherapy.

Keywords

Functional anorectal pain · Pelvic floor muscles · Hypertonicity · Hypersensitivity · Tibial nerve stimulation · Transanal electrical stimulation · Biofeedback therapy · Spinal cord stimulation therapy

1 Introduction

Pain localized to the rectum or anus that cannot be differentiated through diagnostic testing or pathological examination is classified as functional anorectal pain. Although the precise etiology remains unclear, proposed contributing factors include spasms of pelvic floor muscles such as the internal anal sphincter and puborectalis muscle, psychological factors such as stress, rectal intussusception, posterior pelvic compartment prolapse, and pelvic nerve dysfunction. While no standardized treatment has been established, various therapeutic approaches have been reported, including electrical stimulation and pharmacotherapy [1].

2 Case Presentation

Patient: A 45-year-old male
Chief Complaint: Anal pain
Medical History: None
Family History: Unremarkable
Allergies: None reported
Smoking History: Nonsmoker
Alcohol use: Occasional social drinking
Present illness: The patient reported longstanding anorectal pain exacerbated by prolonged sitting. Recently, pain has also occurred in the standing position. The pain does not worsen during defecation.

3 Clinical Course

To exclude organic diseases such as inflammatory bowel disease (IBD), colorectal cancer, anal stenosis, rectal prolapse, rectocele, fistula, and anal fissure, the patient underwent digital rectal

S. Takano (✉)
Department of Functional Anorectal Disorder, Coloproctology Center, Takano Hospital, Kumamoto, Japan
e-mail: micw@takano-hospital.jp

H. Kaneko et al. (eds.), *Disorders of Gut-Brain Interaction*,
https://doi.org/10.1007/978-981-95-6974-8_72

examination, anoscopy, transanal ultrasonography, and sigmoidoscopy. No abnormalities were detected.

[Anorectal Manometry]

- Resting pressure: 134 mmHg
- Voluntary squeeze pressure: 302 mmHg

[Anal Electrical Sensory Testing]

- Lower anal canal: 1.0 mA
- Upper anal canal: 1.6 mA

[Rectal Sensory Balloon Distension Test]

- First sensation threshold: 10 mL
- Urge to defecate threshold: 30 mL
- Maximum tolerable volume: 80 mL

These findings suggested mild hypertonicity of the anal sphincter and hypersensitivity of the anal canal and rectum. A diagnosis of functional anorectal pain was made. Treatment was initiated with tibial nerve stimulation and oral pregabalin. After 1.5 months with insufficient response, therapy was transitioned to transanal electrical stimulation, biofeedback therapy, and oral duloxetine. Although pain was slightly alleviated, the effect remained inadequate (Face Pain Scale score: 4), prompting the initiation of spinal cord stimulation therapy.

In the first stage, a stimulation electrode was inserted into the epidural space between the L3 and L4 vertebrae and advanced cranially, with the electrode positioned between Th9 and L2. Following a one-week trial stimulation period with positive response, the second stage involved implantation of the permanent pulse generator. Pain subsequently improved, and the patient continues to receive regular follow-up for device management (Fig. 72.1).

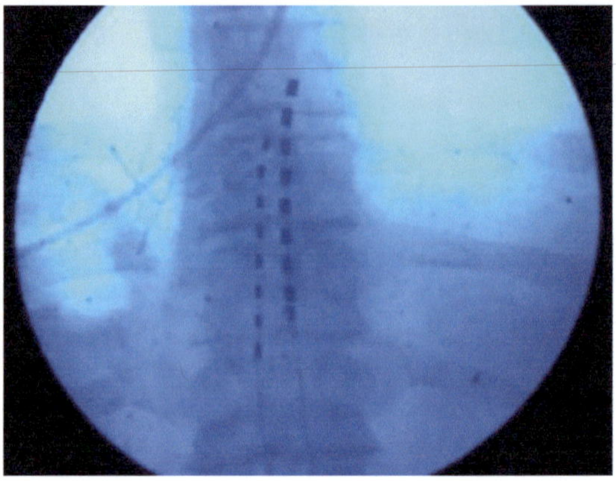

Fig. 72.1 Implantation of the permanent pulse generator

4 Discussion

The etiology of functional anorectal pain remains unclear. Potential contributing factors include spasms of pelvic floor muscles such as the internal anal sphincter and puborectalis muscle, psychological stress, rectal intussusception, posterior pelvic compartment prolapse, and pelvic nerve dysfunction. Due to the uncertain pathophysiology, no definitive treatment has been established. However, several therapeutic modalities have been reported:

- *Pharmacotherapy* includes antispasmodics such as diazepam, pregabalin, tricyclic antidepressants, and tramadol-based agents [2].
- *Biofeedback therapy* involves insertion of an anal electromyography probe or anal manometry catheter, allowing patients to visually monitor physiological changes and perform targeted training.
- *Electrical stimulation therapy* includes tibial nerve stimulation and transanal electrical

stimulation using low-frequency currents administered in multiple sessions [3].

- *Spinal cord stimulation therapy* involves insertion of stimulation electrodes into the epidural space and subcutaneous implantation of a pulse generator for continuous stimulation. This therapy is covered by insurance and is practiced in Japan.
- *Nerve block injections*: Targeting the pudendal nerve, sacral nerves, inferior hypogastric plexus, and ganglion impar has been reported.
- *Myotomy*: Indicated when the internal anal sphincter measures ≥3.5 mm in thickness. In cases of levator ani spasm syndrome, the puborectalis muscle is incised.
- *Other therapies* include puborectalis muscle massage, thermotherapy, botulinum toxin injections, and warm water enemas.

Take-Home Message

It is not uncommon for patients with anorectal pain to have comorbid psychiatric conditions, often expressing dissatisfaction or anxiety regarding treatment efficacy. While various treatment options have been described, the level of evidence supporting each is variable. Nonetheless, it is essential for clinicians to be familiar with a broad range of therapeutic strategies to provide individualized care and offer appropriate treatment options to patients.

Competing Interests The author(s) has no competing interests to declare that are relevant to the content of this manuscript.

References

1. Simrén M, et al. Update on Rome IV Criteria for Colorectal Disorders: Implications for Clinical Practice. Curr Gastroenterol Rep. 2017;19:15.
2. Atkin GK, et al. Patient Characteristics and Treatment Outcome in Functional Anorectal Pain. Dis Colon Rectum. 2011;54(7):870–5.
3. Takano S, et al. Bilateral posterior tibial nerve stimulation for functional anorectal pain-short term outcome. Int J Colorectal Dis. 2016;31(5):1053–4.

Case Discussion, Fecal Incontinence

73

Tatsuya Abe

Abstract

This chapter focuses on the clinical evaluation and management of passive fecal incontinence (FI), illustrated through a case involving a 70-year-old female presenting with postdefecation soiling. Diagnostic assessment revealed reduced resting anal pressure and thinning of the internal anal sphincter, consistent with internal anal sphincter dysfunction. Despite preserved voluntary squeeze pressure, the patient exhibited symptoms characteristic of passive FI. Conservative treatment with calcium polycarbophil, a bulking agent, effectively reduced leakage by improving stool consistency. Internal anal sphincter dysfunction is a common etiology of passive FI, particularly in older adults, and may result from aging, obstetric trauma, or fibrosis. This chapter discusses the pathophysiology, diagnostic approach—including anorectal manometry and endoanal ultrasonography—and therapeutic strategies for FI. Emphasis is placed on the importance of stool consistency in symptom control and the role of pharmacologic agents as first-line therapy. The chapter also highlights the need for differential diagnosis, particularly in distinguishing overflow incontinence due to chronic constipation. While conservative management is often sufficient, surgical options may be considered in refractory cases. Overall, this chapter underscores the value of individualized, symptom-based treatment in improving patient outcomes and quality of life.

Keywords

Anorectal manometry · Bristol Stool Form Scale · Calcium polycarbophil · Daikenchuto · Internal anal sphincter · Loperamide hydrochloride · Maximum resting pressure · Passive fecal incontinence

1 Introduction

Fecal incontinence is defined as "symptoms of involuntary or uncontrolled loss of feces from the anus" [1]. It is classified into three types: passive fecal incontinence, in which stool leaks without the patient's awareness or urge to defecate; urge fecal incontinence, in which the patient experiences an urge to defecate but is unable to reach the toilet in time; and mixed fecal incontinence, which presents with features of both types [1]. The primary risk factors for fecal incontinence include decreased contractile strength of the internal and external anal sphincters, alterations in rectal sensation or compli-

T. Abe (✉)
Department of Proctology, Kunimoto Hospital, Anorectal Surgery, Asahikawa, Japan
e-mail: t-abe@cf6.so-net.ne.jp

H. Kaneko et al. (eds.), *Disorders of Gut-Brain Interaction*,
https://doi.org/10.1007/978-981-95-6974-8_73

Table 73.1 Wexner score (Cleveland Clinic Fecal Incontinence Score)

Symptom	Never (0)	<1/ month (1)	<1/ week (2)	<1/ day (3)	≥1/ day (4)
Solid stool leakage	⓪	1	2	3	4
Liquid stool leakage	0	1	2	③	4
Gas leakage	0	1	2	③	4
Wears pad	0	1	2	3	④
Lifestyle alteration	0	1	②	3	4

The total score is calculated by summing the points for each item. A score of 0 indicates normal continence, while a score of 20 represents the most severe incontinence. (Adapted from Reference [1]

○: Score of the presented case

ance, abnormal stool consistency, and central or peripheral nervous system disorders [2]. In general, the severity of fecal incontinence is considered to increase in the order of gas leakage, liquid stool leakage, and solid stool leakage. The Wexner score (Table 73.1), which accounts for the frequency of incontinence and its impact on daily life, is a simple and widely used tool for assessing severity [1].

If the leakage is minimal—such as slight soiling of underwear—treatment may not be necessary. However, when symptoms negatively affect physical or mental health or daily activities (e.g., noticeable odor, need to carry a change of clothes, perianal dermatitis, social withdrawal), some form of treatment is warranted [2].

2 Case Presentation (Passive Fecal Incontinence)

Patient: A 70-year-old female

Chief complaint: Soiling of underwear after defecation

Medical history: Hypertension since age 60

Obstetric history: Two vaginal deliveries

Present illness: The patient had long experienced a sensation of anal dampness. Over the past six months, she noticed increasing frequency of underwear soiling several hours after defecation, prompting her to seek medical attention.

Physical examination: No significant findings

Bowel habits: Several soft stools per day and no use of laxatives

Wexner score: 12 (Table 73.1)

3 Clinical Course

Anorectal examination revealed a scar at the left posterior aspect of the vaginal introitus, likely from an episiotomy. Digital rectal examination showed reduced resting anal tone, while voluntary contraction produced strong pressure on the examining finger. Proctoscopy revealed small amounts of yellowish soft stool and mucus in the rectum.

Anorectal manometry showed a maximum resting pressure of 17 mmHg (institutional reference range: 40–100 mmHg) and a maximum voluntary squeeze pressure of 146 mmHg (reference: 80–200 mmHg). Endoanal ultrasonography did not reveal any clear disruption of the internal or external anal sphincters, but the internal anal sphincter was thin, measuring less than 1 mm (reference: ≥2 mm) (Fig. 73.1).

Based on these findings, the patient was diagnosed with passive fecal incontinence due to internal anal sphincter dysfunction. As there was no leakage of solid stool, it was hypothesized that firming the stool consistency could reduce incontinence. Administration of calcium polycarbophil (0.5 g, three times daily) was initiated and proved effective.

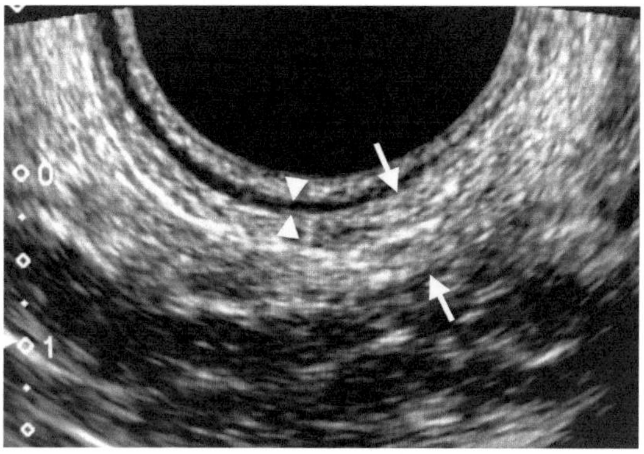

Fig. 73.1 Endoanal ultrasonographic image. No disruption is observed in the internal anal sphincter (arrowhead) or external anal sphincter (arrow); however, the internal anal sphincter is thinned to less than 1 mm in thickness

4 Discussion

The most common cause of fecal incontinence is internal anal sphincter dysfunction [3]. Fibrosis or thinning of the internal anal sphincter leads to decreased resting anal pressure, resulting in passive fecal incontinence. This condition is typically mild and more prevalent among older adults. Because no sphincter disruption is observed, it was previously classified as idiopathic fecal incontinence [4]. Patients often report symptoms such as "a sensation of anal dampness" or "soiling of underwear some time after defecation" (postdefecation passive fecal incontinence).

The anal sphincters may be damaged by anorectal surgery, childbirth, trauma, rectal prolapse, or aging. Injury to the internal anal sphincter reduces resting pressure and predisposes to passive fecal incontinence, whereas damage to the external anal sphincter reduces voluntary squeeze pressure and predisposes to urge fecal incontinence [2]. Even with normal sphincter function, patients with rectal hypersensitivity or chronic diarrhea may experience urge fecal incontinence. Conversely, patients with reduced rectal sensation may have impaired evacuation, leading to leakage of retained stool or overflow fecal incontinence [4].

As fecal incontinence is a benign condition and not life-threatening, conservative treatments such as pharmacotherapy and pelvic floor muscle training are generally the first-line approaches [1]. Bowel dysfunctions such as diarrhea and constipation are frequently associated with fecal incontinence. In general, the higher the stool water content and frequency of defecation, the greater the risk of incontinence. Therefore, for fecal incontinence associated with soft or loose stools, initial treatment should aim to firm the stool using bulking agents (e.g., dietary fiber, thickening agents) or antidiarrheal medications [5].

The dosage of these agents should be adjusted to achieve a stool consistency corresponding to types 3 (slightly firm) or 4 (normal) on the Bristol Stool Form Scale [1]. Calcium polycarbophil, a treatment for irritable bowel syndrome (IBS), exhibits high water absorption and gel formation under neutral conditions in the small and large intestines [6]. It retains water in the gastrointestinal tract and modulates intestinal transit, making it effective for both diarrhea-predominant and constipation-predominant IBS. Due to its bulking properties, calcium polycarbophil is frequently used in specialized centers in Japan for the treatment of fecal incontinence [3, 6]. If stool consistency remains insufficiently firm, low-dose loperamide hydrochloride may be added [1].

In contrast, for fecal incontinence due to reduced rectal sensation or defecation disorders, regular rectal evacuation using suppositories or enemas may be effective [5]. In children with fecal impaction or encopresis (overflow fecal incontinence), polyethylene glycol (macrogol 4000) is recommended [5]. Daikenchuto, a traditional Japanese herbal medicine, has been reported to be effective in elderly patients with fecal incontinence due to impaired evacuation [7]. Several observational studies have shown that daikenchuto improves rectal sensation and evacuation in patients with constipation [7].

Pelvic floor muscle exercises and biofeedback therapy may also be effective for fecal incontinence [1]. In the present case, internal anal sphincter function was impaired, while the maximum voluntary squeeze pressure—an indicator of external anal sphincter function—was within normal limits. The external anal sphincter and other pelvic floor muscles are innervated by the somatic nervous system, whereas the internal anal sphincter is autonomically innervated. Therefore, it remains unclear whether voluntary contraction training can improve internal anal sphincter function [2].

Take-Home Message

- Mild fecal incontinence often responds well to pharmacotherapy and can be managed effectively in general clinical settings.
- In cases of overflow fecal incontinence, where loose stool leaks from the rectum, antidiarrheal agents may be mistakenly prescribed.
- In patients with underlying chronic constipation, digital rectal examination or imaging should be performed to assess for fecal impaction.
- If conservative treatment fails or in severe cases, surgical interventions such as sphincteroplasty or sacral neuromodulation should be considered.

Competing Interests The author(s) has no competing interests to declare that are relevant to the content of this manuscript.

References

1. The Japan Society of Coloproctology. Clinical practice guidelines for fecal incontinence in Japan, vol. 2024. 2nd ed. Tokyo: Nankodo; 2024. p. 2–78. (in Japanese)
2. Abe T, et al. Diagnosis and treatment of fecal incontinence. Medicina. 2016;53:1428–31. (in Japanese)
3. Mimura T, et al. Current situation of the management of fecal incontinence in Japanese institutions: diagnosis and treatment. J Jpn Soc Coloproctol. 2012;65:101–8. (in Japanese)
4. Abe T. Diagnosis and treatment of fecal incontinence. In: Clinical approach to constipation for all physicians. Tokyo: Yodosha; 2022. p. 143–9. (in Japanese).
5. Abe T. Overview of pharmacotherapy. In: Continence rehabilitation: theory and practice. 2nd ed. Tokyo: Nakayama Shoten; 2022. p. 446–50. (in Japanese).
6. Abe T, et al. Calcium polycarbophil in the management of fecal incontinence. Br J Med Med Res. 2016;12:1–7.
7. Abe T, et al. Clinical efficacy of Japanese herbal medicine daikenchuto in the management of fecal incontinence: a single-center, observational study. J Anus Rectum Colon. 2019;3:160–6.

Topics, Low Anterior Resection Syndrome (LARS) 74

Keiji Koda

Abstract

Low anterior resection syndrome (LARS) occurs in approximately 80% of patients after sphincter-preserving surgery for low rectal cancer, causing defecatory dysfunction and social difficulties. Its pathogenesis remains unclear. This article discusses two major factors: impaired neorectal motility due to disruption of autonomic nerves to the proximal colon and anal dysfunction from nerve injury to the remaining rectum and internal anal sphincter. Additionally, the rectosigmoid brake, a colonic region involved in continence and potentially affected by rectal cancer surgery, may contribute to LARS. Its role warrants further investigation.

Keywords

Low anterior resection syndrome (LARS) · Altered colonic motility · Denervated neorectum · Rectosigmoid brake · Colonic transit time · Anal sphincter dysfunction

K. Koda (✉)
Surgery Unit, Coloproctology Center Takano Hospital, Kumamoto, Japan

Low anterior resection syndrome (LARS) refers to a condition characterized by defecatory dysfunction following sphincter-preserving operations (SPO) for rectal cancer, which results in significant psychological and social consequences for patients. It has been reported to occur in approximately 80% of cases [1]. Due to the variety of defecatory symptoms involved, LARS has recently been defined as a syndrome that leads to a decline in patients' quality of life and social functioning [2]. The etiology is multifactorial, but it is believed that intraoperative damage to multiple components responsible for normal defecatory physiology results in functional impairment [3]. This section focuses on one of the contributing factors to LARS: altered colonic motility following surgical manipulation and its relationship to postoperative defecatory dysfunction.

1 Neural Innervation of the Left Colon Used as a Rectal Substitute in SPO and Surgical Impact

In sphincter-preserving operations (SPO) for rectal cancer, including low anterior resection, the affected rectum is partially or nearly completely resected depending on tumor location. Reconstruction is typically performed using the left colon as a substitute for the resected rectum. The extrinsic innervation of the left colon includes

H. Kaneko et al. (eds.), *Disorders of Gut-Brain Interaction*,
https://doi.org/10.1007/978-981-95-6974-8_74

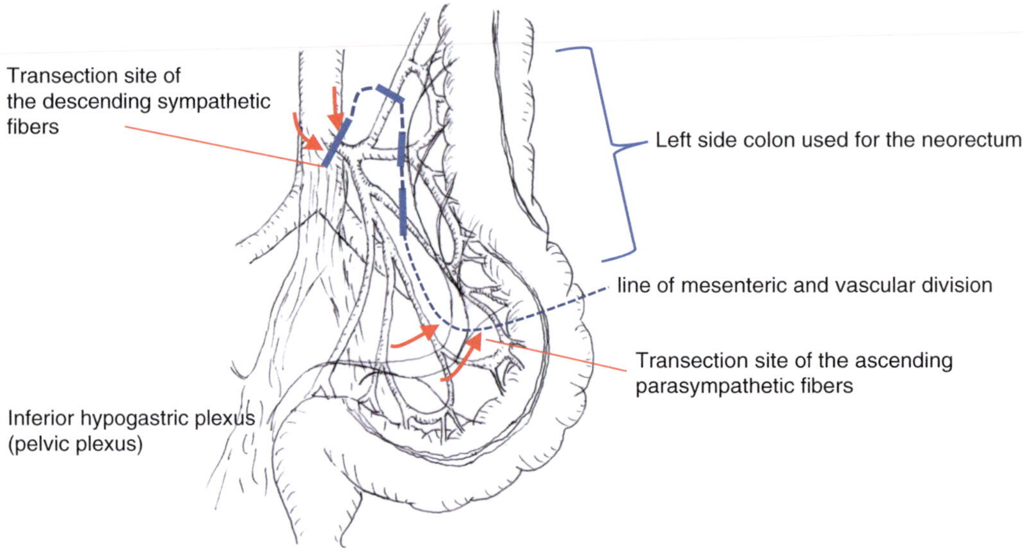

Fig. 74.1 Denervation of the neorectum due to intraoperative manipulation. Both the ascending parasympathetic fibers from the pelvic plexus and the descending sympathetic fibers near the inferior mesenteric artery (IMA) are severed

parasympathetic fibers ascending from the pelvic plexus through the mesentery and sympathetic fibers descending along the inferior mesenteric artery (IMA), which innervate the descending colon, sigmoid colon, and rectum [4]. During lymphadenectomy in rectal cancer surgery, if the IMA is resected at its root or preserved at its root and then resected after branching of the superior rectal artery (SRA), the sympathetic fibers running along these arteries are severed. Additionally, mesenteric dissection proximal to the tumor may disrupt parasympathetic fibers ascending from the pelvic plexus. Consequently, the remaining left colon used for reconstruction becomes a denervated neorectum, lacking both sympathetic and parasympathetic innervations (Fig. 74.1). The length of this denervated neorectum varies depending on whether the IMA is ligated at its root or more distally at the SRA [5].

2 Neural Innervation of the Residual Rectum After Low Anterior Resection

The lower rectum and anal canal receive innervation from fibers of the inferior hypogastric plexus (pelvic plexus), which enter the rectal wall at approximately the 2 o'clock and 10 o'clock positions, about 8 cm from the anal verge, near the superior aspect of the prostate [6]. In low rectal cancer surgery, these nerves may be damaged or severed. Although the exact impact of this on anal and lower rectal function and its contribution to LARS remains unclear, it may explain why sphincter dysfunction can occur postoperatively even in the absence of direct manipulation of the anal sphincter [3].

3 Gastrointestinal Motility and LARS

3.1 Hyperactivity of the Colon and External Denervation

As described above, SPO procedures significantly alter the neural innervation of the left colon and residual rectum, potentially leading to postoperative motility patterns that differ markedly from preoperative physiology. Keane et al. reported that both antegrade and retrograde colonic reflexes observed postprandially in the left colon are reduced in patients with LARS compared to those without, suggesting this as a contributing factor [7]. Mochiki et al. found that the gastrocolic reflex, measured using a barostat proximal to the anastomosis after low anterior resection, was more pronounced in patients with severe LARS symptoms, indicating that an exaggerated postprandial gastrocolic reflex may be a causative factor [8]. Similarly, Emmertsen et al., who developed the LARS score, reported that excessive neorectal motility after meals was more common in patients with severe LARS, suggesting that neural damage may play a more significant role than anatomical changes in the development of LARS [9].

In animal studies, we observed that colonic segments with surgically severed extrinsic nerves exhibited approximately 150% increased motility, even when blood flow was preserved [10]. Other studies have reported similar findings, with denervation leading to a 130% increase in colonic motility, potentially contributing to LARS [11]. The increased motility of the denervated neorectum using the denervated colon may be one of the causes of LARS.

In human studies, pressure sensors placed in the colon during scheduled endoscopy one year after sphincter-preserving surgery for rectal cancer revealed spastic, disorganized waves in the neorectum. Among 49 patients with such findings, 12 (24%) reported severe urgency and 18 (37%) reported moderate urgency. In contrast, among 88 patients without disorganized motility during the one-hour observation period, only 6 (7%) and 28 (32%) reported severe and moderate urgency, respectively. These findings suggest that disorganized and excessive neorectal motility may contribute to LARS in humans.

Furthermore, when the IMA is preserved and the SRA is ligated, the length of the denervated neorectum is theoretically shorter than when the IMA is ligated at its root. In such cases, the frequency of neorectal spasms is reportedly lower [5].

A recent study using radioisotopes to measure colonic transit time found that patients with high LARS scores had shorter colonic transit times than those with fewer symptoms, suggesting that hypermotility may influence LARS development [12].

3.2 Role of the Rectosigmoid Brake

Recent advances in high-resolution colon manometry, which uses sensors spaced every 1–2 cm instead of the older 3–4 channel systems, have provided new insights. The existence of the sphincter of O'Beirne, proposed in the nineteenth century and located approximately 10–17 cm from the anal verge, has been revisited. Chen et al. observed that contractions and relaxations in the rectosigmoid region in response to large peristaltic waves corresponded with anal sphincter activity, supporting the functional significance of the sphincter of O'Beirne [13].

In patients with severe constipation, relaxation in this region was absent until bisacodyl was administered, which then induced relaxation and strong peristalsis, leading to defecation [14]. Lin et al. reported that patients with fecal incontinence exhibited fewer postprandial retrograde and antegrade waves in the rectosigmoid region. Furthermore, sacral neuromodulation (SNM) has been shown to significantly enhance retrograde peristaltic waves originating from the rectosigmoid region. This mechanism, known as the rectosigmoid brake [15], plays a critical role in preventing the inflow of colonic contents into the rectum. It has been reported that the involvement of the rectosigmoid brake is not only essential in the pathophysiology of fecal incontinence but also represents one of the mechanisms by which SNM exerts its therapeutic effect [16].

In rectal cancer surgery, the rectosigmoid region responsible for this brake is often resected. The extent to which this contributes to LARS remains unclear, but disruption of the rectosigmoid brake mechanism may be related to the fecal incontinence observed in LARS.

High-resolution manometry studies in LARS patients have shown that, after bisacodyl administration, short-cycle antegrade peristalsis was more frequent in patients with LARS than in patients without LARS and correlated with LARS scores. Additionally, large peristaltic waves from the right to left colon, typically seen in healthy individuals, were less frequent in LARS patients [17].

4 Conclusion

The pathogenesis of LARS involves both postoperative anal dysfunction and impaired function of the neorectum, indicating that multiple factors contribute to symptom development. Although research into neorectal motility remains ongoing, elucidating these mechanisms is expected to provide valuable insights for symptom management.

Take-Home Message
While defecatory dysfunction following sphincter-preserving surgery for rectal cancer has been recognized since the 1980s, it was only after 2010 that LARS gained attention in major medical journals. The field remains relatively young. SPO procedures often involve severing extrinsic nerves, potentially impairing autonomic reflexes and intestinal function essential for normal defecation. Future surgical approaches should aim to preserve function while maintaining oncologic efficacy, and therapeutic strategies to compensate for impaired anal and neorectal function should continue to be explored.

Competing Interests The author(s) has no competing interests to declare that are relevant to the content of this manuscript.

References

1. Martellucci J. Low anterior resection syndrome: a treatment algorithm. Dis Colon Rectum. 2016;59:79–82.
2. Keane C, et al. International consensus definition of low anterior resection syndrome. Dis Colon Rectum. 2020;63(3):274–84.
3. Koda K, et al. Ethology and management of low anterior resection syndrome based on the normal defecation mechanism. Surg Today. 2019;49(19):803–8.
4. Netter FH. The Netter collection of medical illustrations. USA: Novartis; 1997.
5. Koda K, et al. Denervation of the neorectum as a potential cause of defecatory disorder following low anterior resection for rectal cancer. Dis Colon Rectum. 2005;48(2):210–7.
6. Ishiyama G, et al. Nerves supplying the internal anal sphincter: an immunohistochemical study using donated elderly cadavers. Surg Radiol Anat. 2014;36(10):1033–42.
7. Keane C, et al. Altered colonic motility is associated with low anterior resection syndrome. Colorect Dis. 2021;23(2):415–23.
8. Mochiki E, et al. Barostat examination of proximal site of the anastomosis in patients with rectal cancer after low anterior resection. World J Surg. 2001;25(11):1377–81.
9. Emmertsen KJ, et al. A hyperreactive postprandial response in the neorectum - the clue to low anterior resection syndrome after total mesorectal excision surgery? Colorect Dis. 2013;15(10):e599–606.
10. Shimizu K, et al. Induction and recovery of colonic motility/ decfecatory disorders after extrinsic denervation of the colon and rectum in rats. Surgery. 2006;139(3):395–406.
11. Lee WY, et al. Surgical autonomic denervation results in altered colonic motility: an explana-

tion for low anterior resection syndrome? Surgery. 2008;143(6):778–83.
12. Ng KS, et al. Colonic transit in patients after anterior resection: prospective comparative study using single-photon emission CT/CT scintigraphy. Br J Surg. 2020;107(5):567–79.
13. Chen JH, et al. The sphincter of O'Beirne—Part 1: high-resolution manometry evidence of a functional sphincter. Dig Dis Sci. 2021;66(10):3516–28.
14. Chen JH, et al. The sphincter of O'Beirne—Part 2: report of a case of chronic constipation with autonomous dyssynergia. Dig Dis Sci. 2021;66(10):3529–41.
15. Lin AY, et al. The "rectosigmoid brake": review of an emerging neuromodulation target for colorectal functional disorders. Clin Exp Pharmacol Physiol. 2017;44(7):719–28.
16. Lin AY, et al. Faecal incontinence is associated with an impaired rectosigmoid brake and improved by sacral neuromodulation. Colorect Dis. 2022;24(12):1556–66.
17. Asnong A, et al. Exploring the pathophysiology of LARS after low anterior resection for rectal cancer with high-resolution colon manometry. Neurogastroenterol Motil. 2022;34(11):e14432.

75 Topics, Pediatric Functional Disorders of Intestinal Tract: Pediatric Chronic Functional Constipation

Miwako Nakano

Abstract

Constipation is a common symptom. Surveys using the Rome III criteria found constipation in at least 10–20% of children in Japan. The children who visit the doctor primarily complaining of constipation may have more than moderate levels of chronic constipation and a gradual decline in rectal sensitivity, which may be unnoticed by them or their families. Since they are suffering from various symptoms, it is better to start medication immediately rather than wasting time with general guidance on lifestyle and diet. It is effective to introduce lifestyle guidance once medication has alleviated symptoms to a certain extent and the patient feels more comfortable. The goal of treatment is to achieve a "nonconstipated state," defined as having bowel movements at least three times per week that are easy and complete, without a sensation of incomplete evacuation. Fecal impaction. If present, it must be removed. After disimpaction or in cases without impaction, a combination of oral and transrectal treatments is used to maintain a "nonconstipated state." Sometimes it takes months or years to achieve nonconstipated state without pharmacological treatment. So it is important that every caregivers around the child understand the knowledge of constipation and body.

Mild constipation children should be treated by improvement of lifestyle.

Keywords

Pediatric chronic functional constipation · Fecal impaction and disimpaction · Overflow incontinence · Osmotic laxatives · Transrectal therapy · Lifestyles guidance for constipation · Defecation diary

M. Nakano (✉)
Yoshikawa Kids Clinic, Tokyo, Japan

Suzuki Children's Clinic, Urawa, Japan
e-mail: info@yoshikawa-kids.com

Functional gastrointestinal disorders (FGIDs) in children, as in adults, can manifest with diverse symptoms throughout the gastrointestinal tract—from the esophagus to the anus—and their severity may improve or worsen with growth. This section focuses on one such condition: chronic functional constipation in children.

The Japanese Society of Pediatric Gastroenterology, Hepatology and Nutrition and the Japanese Pediatric Gastrointestinal Motility Society jointly established a guideline committee, which published the first edition of the Clinical Practice Guidelines for Pediatric Chronic Functional Constipation in 2013 [1]. The committee primarily consisted of pediatric gastroenterologists and pediatric surgeons, and a revision committee was launched in 2023. New Guidelines were published in 2025.

H. Kaneko et al. (eds.), *Disorders of Gut-Brain Interaction*,
https://doi.org/10.1007/978-981-95-6974-8_75

1 Definition of Constipation in Children

According to the guidelines, constipation is defined as "a condition in which bowel movements are delayed or difficult," and constipation syndrome is defined as "a condition in which symptoms due to constipation are present and require diagnosis or treatment." Although this definition may appear vague and difficult to apply clinically, it is important because the condition is often not self-reported. In children, symptoms are typically recognized by caregivers, and constipation often goes unnoticed until it becomes severe. Children may not complain of symptoms, and those who have experienced constipation since infancy may consider it normal and not recognize it as distressing. Early detection is difficult unless caregivers are attentive.

2 Epidemiology of Chronic Constipation in Children

The prevalence of constipation in children varies widely depending on the study. As a common condition, its reported frequency is influenced by how constipation is defined, as well as by racial, cultural, and social factors.

A review cited in the guidelines reports a prevalence ranging from 0.7% to 29.6% internationally. In Japan, the 2016 National Livelihood Survey by the Ministry of Health, Laboure and Welfare reported symptomatic prevalence rates of 0.58% in boys and 0.66% in girls aged 0–9 years and 0.46% in boys and 1.45% in girls aged 10–19 years [2].

Surveys based on defecation frequency among elementary school children report constipation rates ranging from 5.7% to 18.5% [1]. An Internet-based survey using the Rome III criteria found constipation in 18% of children aged 0–3 years, 16–20% of elementary school children, and 20% of high school students [3]. These findings suggest that the actual prevalence of constipation is significantly higher than that indicated by symptomatic reporting alone.

While constipation is generally more common in girls, more severe cases are often observed in boys, particularly during early childhood.

3 Pathophysiology of Chronic Functional Constipation in Children

In adults, chronic functional constipation often presents as infrequent defecation with normal colonic transit time. In contrast, most pediatric cases involve stool retention at the anorectal level, resembling difficult defecation-type constipation in adults. Because diagnostic testing used in adults is often impractical in children, colonic transit time is not well established but is presumed to be normal in most cases.

Constipation in children is thought to result from immature defecatory coordination. It frequently begins around the time of weaning, when stools become more formed, although it can also start earlier during the period of loose stools. As stool accumulates, it becomes harder and larger, making defecation more difficult. Persistent fecal impaction leads to chronic rectal distension, reduced rectal sensitivity, and further stool accumulation, creating a vicious cycle of constipation (Fig. 75.1). For young children, the pain associated with difficult defecation can be a source of significant fear. Even when they feel the urge to defecate, they may voluntarily contract the external anal sphincter to retain stool, leading to stool withholding behavior. This further exacerbates constipation, reinforcing both physiological and psychological cycles of chronicity. Although defecatory coordination may improve with growth and maturation, the timing varies greatly among individuals. If rectal dysfunction progresses faster than developmental improvement, constipation may persist into adulthood. Colonic motility and defecation are regulated by the autonomic nervous system, making stress a significant factor. Environmental influences such as home, daycare, or school settings, as well as the child's sensitivity to pain, fear, and anxiety, can affect the course of constipation.

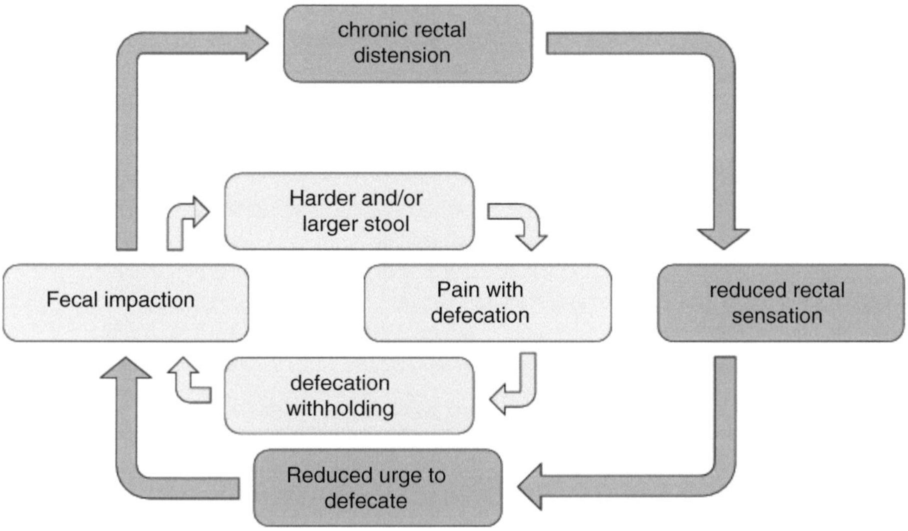

Fig. 75.1 Vicious cycle of constipation. ○: Physiological vicious cycle at the rectal level, ●: Psychological vicious cycle

4 Diagnosis and Symptoms of Constipation

The diagnostic and treatment flow is illustrated in Fig. 75.2. Diagnosis is based on medical history, including developmental history, symptoms, and physical examination. Underlying diseases, comorbidities, and medication effects must also be considered. Abdominal palpation often reveals fecal masses, although they may be difficult to detect if the stool is soft. Abdominal bloating may not be apparent if the child can pass gas. Fecal impaction can be confirmed by digital rectal examination, but if consent is not obtained, suprapubic ultrasound or plain abdominal X-ray may be useful. If the child resists examination, it should not be forced. In advanced cases, contrast enema may be performed, sometimes serving both diagnostic and therapeutic purposes. If organic diseases such as Hirschsprung's disease or low-type anorectal malformations are suspected, referral to a specialized center is recommended.

Treatment is indicated when stool retention is accompanied by any of the following symptoms. The guidelines use the Rome IVcriteria as a diagnostic reference (Table 75.1) [4].

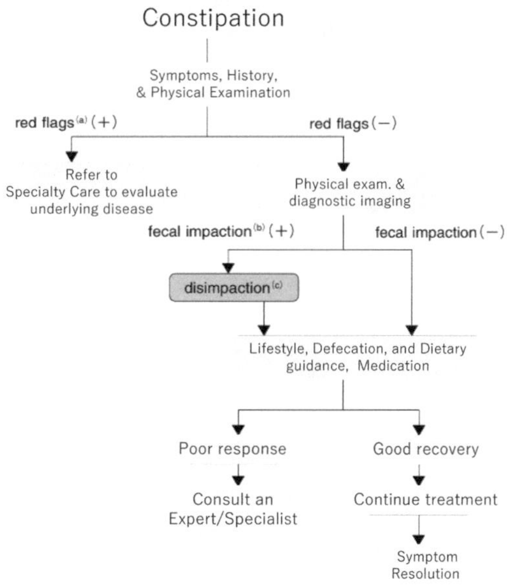

Fig. 75.2 Diagnostic and treatment flowchart for constipation [1] (partially modified by the author)

Not all symptoms are present in every case, and children often visit clinic complaining only the most prominent symptoms. Careful history-taking often reveals multiple symptoms previously unrecognized as related to constipation.

Table 75.1 Diagnostic criteria for functional constipation (Rome IV)

Must include ***one month of at least two*** *of the following in infants up to 4 years of age:*
1. Two or fewer defecations per week
2. History of excessive stool retention
3. History of painful or hard bowel movements
4. History of large diameter stools
5. Presence of a large fecal mass in the rectum
In toilet trained children, the following additional criteria may be used:
6. At least one episode/week of incontinence after the acquisition of toileting skills
7. History of large diameter stools which may obstruct the toilet

4.1 Defecation Frequency and Stool Consistency

The diagnostic criteria include defecation fewer than twice per week or no bowel movement for more than five consecutive days. However, some children may pass small amounts of stool frequently and be mistakenly considered to have normal bowel habits. Others may appear to have daily bowel movements but still retain large amounts of stool. Therefore, frequency alone is not a reliable indicator. Stool consistency is assessed using the Bristol Stool Form Scale (BS), as in adults. However, young children may perceive normal stools as "hard," so the key is whether the stool is easy for the child to pass. Even soft stools that are very large or thick, or that clog the toilet, should be considered indicative of constipation. These stools are often malodorous.

4.2 Symptoms of Difficult Defecation

Repeated straining, visible stool at the anus that cannot be expelled, and severe pain during defecation are signs of fecal impaction. As a result of withholding the urge to defecate, the interval between the initial sensation of defecation and actual bowel movement may extend to several hours or even one to two days. Although this behavior and associated pain may become less noticeable with age, they often persist. Toilet training can trigger or worsen stool withholding behavior. Some children may urinate in the toilet but insist on defecating in a diaper, causing distress for caregivers. Toilet refusal may persist into school age and even be misinterpreted as a developmental disorder.

4.3 Bleeding

Rectal bleeding may occur due to congestion from fecal impaction or anal fissures caused by hard stools. Rectal prolapse is also often associated with constipation.

4.4 Fecal Incontinence

Overflow incontinence is a symptom of fecal impaction. While some children may pass large stool columns, most experience soiling of underwear with small amounts of BS type 1 stool or loose stool, often without awareness. In severe cases, incontinence may occur during sleep or continuously. Significant leakage can cause perianal skin irritation and erosion.

4.5 Bowel Obstruction Symptoms Due to Fecal Impaction

Symptoms include discomfort, nausea/vomiting, abdominal bloating, abdominal pain, decreased appetite, and worsening picky eating. Persistent urge to defecate may lead to irritability, restlessness, and reduced concentration. Urinary symptoms such as increased frequency, enuresis, and nocturnal enuresis may also occur and in severe cases urinary retention. Many children visiting emergency departments with abdominal pain are found to have constipation. True acute constipation is rare; most cases represent acute exacerbations of chronic constipation. Therefore, follow-up after initial treatment at emergency OPD is essential.

5 Treatment of Constipation

Any child suffering from constipation is a candidate for treatment, and strict adherence to diagnostic criteria is not necessary. The goal of treatment is to achieve a "nonconstipated state," defined as having bowel movements at least three times per week that are easy and complete, without a sensation of incomplete evacuation.

5.1 Explanation

Before initiating treatment, it is essential to explain the pathophysiology of constipation and the child's current condition to both the child and the caregivers. This helps ensure understanding and cooperation with the treatment plan.

5.2 Disimpaction

The first step is to assess for fecal impaction. If present, it must be removed.

The standard approach is transrectal, using manual disimpaction, glycerin enemas, or colonic irrigation, which may take several days. In severe cases, hospitalization and sedation may be required for transrectal disimpaction. Once partial disimpaction is achieved, oral medications can be started.

If impaction is mild and transrectal methods are difficult (especially in older children), oral laxatives may be used. Caregivers should be informed of the possible symptoms, temporary worsening and associated risks during initial treatment.

5.3 Maintenance Therapy

If there is no fecal impaction, or fecal retention is present in the rectum but rectal distension is mild, maintenance therapy can be started. In cases of treatment difficulty or poor response, early referral to a specialist or experienced facility is recommended.

5.3.1 Lifestyle, Defecation, and Dietary Guidance

In mild cases not meeting diagnostic criteria, lifestyle modifications should be attempted first [5]. If no improvement is seen after about one month—or if caregivers have already tried such measures—pharmacologic treatment should be initiated. Once symptoms improve with medication, lifestyle and dietary guidance can be more effectively introduced.

Some children may resist changes due to strong preferences or environmental limitations, so care should be taken not to overburden caregivers or enforce changes rigidly.

Lifestyle Guidance

Create a supportive environment for defecation (e.g., accessible toilets), reduce excessive stress, and promote a regular, relaxed daily routine to support autonomic nerve system regulation. Adequate sleep and early rising are especially important. While no specific exercise is proven to aid defecation, moderate physical activity is encouraged.

Dietary Guidance

A regular, nutritionally balanced diet is essential. Breakfast is particularly important for improving constipation. Adequate fiber intake and reducing picky eating are recommended. However, eating small amounts or having a picky diet may be related to personality, and improvement may require time and growth. Rather than forcing disliked foods, it is better to focus on enjoyable meals and increasing overall intake. Misconceptions about diet are common among caregivers, so consultation with a dietitian may be helpful.

Defecation Guidance

Avoiding stool withholding is critical for both prevention and treatment. In young children, persuasion and coercion are ineffective; instead, stool consistency should first be improved with medication. If the child can use the toilet, encouraging regular toileting at set times may be effective. This applies to maintenance therapy as well.

Establishing a habit of sitting on the toilet at regular times, regardless of urge, can gradually lead to successful defecation. Toilet sessions should not be too long and should be stopped if the child resists. Morning defecation is not essential; any time when the child feels relaxed is acceptable.

Defecation Diary

Even in children who appear to have no issues, keeping a defecation diary for about a week once or twice a year can help to detect latent constipation and facilitate early treatment. When used as part of treatment, the diary serves as a behavioral therapy tool and should be recommended to all patients, though not forced if the burden on caregiver is excessive. It typically includes records of treatment, defecation times, stool consistency and volume, and relevant life events.

5.3.2 Pharmacologic Maintenance Therapy

After disimpaction or in cases without impaction, a combination of oral and transrectal treatments is used to maintain a "nonconstipated state."

5.4 Oral Medications

Osmotic laxatives These are the first-line agents. In mild cases, sugar-based laxatives such as lactulose, oligosaccharides, or malt extract may be effective, especially in children under one year. Magnesium oxide, a saline laxative, is widely used despite national health insurance system stating it is not indicated for children under five. It is effective across all ages, typically dosed at 0.2–1.5 g/day in 1–3 divided doses. If high doses are needed, switching agents or adding enemas may be preferable. Although hypermagnesemia is a concern, it is generally not problematic in children without underlying conditions, and routine serum magnesium monitoring is not commonly performed.

Polyethylene glycol (PEG) is increasingly used and is recommended in Western guidelines. Its efficacy and safety have been confirmed in Japan, and it is approved for use in children aged two years and older by national insurance system.

Stimulant Laxatives Sodium picosulfate is used as a rescue medication when osmotic laxatives fail to maintain a "nonconstipated state." Due to its palatability, it is sometimes used daily. However, it may cause abdominal pain and urgency, making it less suitable for children attending school or daycare. Senna-based agents, including herbal formulations, are generally not recommended for children, though they may be used from around age 10.

5.4.1 Other Agents

Epithelial function modulators and bile acid transporter inhibitors are rarely used in children but may be considered around puberty. Prokinetics, nonsenna herbal medicines, and probiotics may be helpful in some cases but are generally considered adjunctive. In children with high intestinal sensitivity, calcium polycarbophil may be used.

Because treatment is often long term, medication choice should consider palatability and compatibility with the child's lifestyle. Individual responses vary, and there is no need to insist on the use of stimulant or osmotic laxatives.

5.4.2 Transrectal Therapy

If oral medications fail to maintain a "nonconstipated state," if stool is too loose for oral agents, or if oral medications do not produce predictable urges—interfering with school or daycare—enemas or suppositories may be used alone or in combination. Although past traumatic experiences with enemas may cause resistance, proper explanation and instruction can help both child and caregiver understand their role in preventing fecal impaction. When used appropriately, their effectiveness is clear and sustainable.

6 Prognosis

Constipation has a high recurrence rate. Even when symptoms improve, the underlying pathophysiology may persist. Some children maintain good bowel habits with growth and can discontinue treatment. On the other hand, if mild constipation persists, it may recur immediately and also recurrence in adulthood. It is important to confirm that a "nonconstipated state" is maintained during gradual medication tapering and after discontinuation. Establishing healthy rectal and colonic function during childhood lays the foundation for adult gastrointestinal health. Therefore, constipation should be treated more proactively.

Take-Home Message
Constipation is a common symptom, but children who visit the doctor primarily complaining of constipation may have chronic constipation and a gradual decline in rectal sensitivity, which may be unnoticed by them or their families. In other words, it is often a "disease." Since they are suffering, it is better to start medication immediately rather than wasting time with general guidance on lifestyle and diet. It is effective to introduce lifestyle guidance once medication has alleviated symptoms to a certain extent and the patient feels more comfortable.

Treatment should be viewed not as a cure but as a supportive strategy—maintaining rectal and colonic health while awaiting physical and psychological maturation. Misconceptions about childhood defecation and constipation are common, even among healthcare providers. Greater awareness and early intervention, including public education on healthy bowel habits, are essential.

Competing Interests The author(s) has no competing interests to declare that are relevant to the content of this manuscript.

References

1. Japanese Society for Pediatric Gastroenterology, Hepatology and Nutrition; Japanese Pediatric Gastrointestinal Motility Society. Clinical practice guidelines for pediatric chronic functional constipation. Tokyo: Shindan to Chiryo Sha; 2025. (in Japanese).
2. Ministry of Health, Labour and Welfare. 2016 National Livelihood Survey. (in Japanese).
3. Japan Toilet Research Institute (NPO). Toilet Lab Survey. https://www.toilet.or.jp/activitiess/?id=research.
4. Douglas A. Drossman: functional gastrointestinal disorders: history, pathophysiology, clinical features, and Rome IV. Special issue of *Gastroenterology*; May 2016.
5. Nakano M. Special feature: Scientific perspectives on pediatric constipation—"How to provide lifestyle and defecation guidance". Shonika Shinryo. 2020;51:757–63. (in Japanese).

Part X

Practical Treatment

Practical Treatment, the Science of "Illness Begins in the Mind"

76

Toshikatsu Okumura

Abstract

In Japan, there is a traditional proverb: "Illness begins in the mind." Indeed, it is a common experiential understanding that one's mental state can influence physical health. For instance, stress is known to trigger or exacerbate irritable bowel syndrome (IBS). While the concept that "illness begins in the mind" is widely recognized, the underlying mechanisms remain largely unexplored. In the present chapter, possible mechanisms are shown to clarify the concept. Knowledge regarding the relationship between the central nervous system (CNS) and gastrointestinal functions such as gastrointestinal motility, visceral sensation, and intestinal barrier function is increasing. For over 35 years, our research group has consistently investigated CNS regulation of gastrointestinal function. For instance, neuropeptide orexin acts centrally in the brain to improve gastrointestinal motility, visceral sensation, and intestinal barrier function. In turn, decrease in orexin signaling in the brain may induce gastrointestinal dysmotility, visceral hypersensitivity, and leaky gut. These features are characteristic of the clinical presentation of IBS. Thus, impaired orexin function may provide a unifying explanation for the multifaceted pathophysiology of IBS. In this context, IBS ("illness") may arise from reduced central orexin signaling ("mind"), supporting the concept that "illness begins in the mind."

Keywords

Irritable bowel syndrome · Brain · Orexin · Visceral hypersensitivity · Leaky gut

1 Introduction

In Japan, there is a traditional proverb: "Illness begins in the mind." Indeed, it is a common experiential understanding that one's mental state can influence physical health. It is well established that psychological stress can induce peptic ulcers, a phenomenon supported by investigations conducted following major disasters such as the Great Hanshin-Awaji Earthquake (1995) and the Great East Japan Earthquake (2011) [1, 2]. Stress is also known to trigger or exacerbate irritable bowel syndrome (IBS), a type of functional gastrointestinal disorder (FGID) [3]. Furthermore, stress has been reported to worsen organic gastrointestinal diseases such as inflammatory bowel disease (IBD) [4].

Although IBS is frequently observed in the general population (nonpatient IBS), what distin-

T. Okumura (✉)
Asahikawa Medical University, Asahikawa, Japan
e-mail: okumurat@asahikawa-med.ac.jp

H. Kaneko et al. (eds.), *Disorders of Gut-Brain Interaction*,
https://doi.org/10.1007/978-981-95-6974-8_76

guishes those who seek medical care (patient IBS)? Previous studies have shown that individuals with patient IBS tend to seek medical attention not only due to the severity of gastrointestinal symptoms but also due to psychological distress and health-related anxiety [5]. In other words, patient IBS may be viewed as a manifestation of health anxiety ("mind") expressed through healthcare-seeking behavior ("illness"). While the concept that "illness begins in the mind" is widely recognized, the underlying mechanisms remain largely unexplored.

2 The Nervous System and Immune Regulation

To scientifically understand the proverb "illness begins in the mind," it is essential to elucidate the mechanisms by which the nervous system ("mind") regulates or disrupts immune function ("illness"). The following summarizes current research findings on neuroimmune regulation.

2.1 Sympathetic Nervous System and Immune Modulation

The sympathetic nervous system plays a role in immune regulation [6]. β_2-Adrenergic receptors, which are receptors for catecholamines—the physiologically active substances of the sympathetic nervous system—are expressed on the surface of lymphocytes. Stimulation of these receptors suppresses lymphocyte egress from lymph nodes, thereby maintaining homeostasis of lymphocyte dynamics. Cross-talk between β_2-adrenergic receptors and chemokine receptors has also been demonstrated, indicating a mechanism by which neural signals are translated into immune responses.

This regulation of lymphocyte dynamics by the sympathetic nervous system via β_2-adrenergic receptors may be involved in the pathophysiology of inflammatory diseases. In mouse models of multiple sclerosis and allergic dermatitis, administration of β_2-adrenergic receptor agonists suppressed disease progression, whereas mice lacking β_2-adrenergic receptor expression exhibited exacerbated disease. These findings suggest that β_2-adrenergic receptor signaling exerts anti-inflammatory effects and that sympathetic nervous system regulation of lymphocyte dynamics may influence the pathogenesis of inflammatory diseases—implying that such diseases ("illness") are modulated by the sympathetic nervous system ("mind").

2.2 Parasympathetic Nervous System and Immune Modulation

In 2000, Tracy and colleagues proposed the concept of the *vagal cholinergic antiinflammatory pathway* in *Nature* [7]. This concept posits that stimulation of the efferent vagus nerve (cholinergic pathway) exerts systemic antiinflammatory effects. Subsequent studies identified the splenic branch of the vagus nerve as a critical efferent pathway. Vagal stimulation activates $\alpha7$ nicotinic acetylcholine receptors ($\alpha7$nAChR) on macrophages in the spleen, suppressing the production of inflammatory cytokines such as TNF-α, thereby reducing systemic inflammation [8].

This demonstrates a mechanism by which the parasympathetic nervous system ("mind") regulates inflammation ("illness"). More recently, in 2020, Professor Kanai's group at Keio University reported in *Nature* that gastrointestinal signals are transmitted via the hepatic branch of the vagus nerve to the central nervous system, where they are integrated and relayed back through the efferent vagus nerve to regulate intestinal T regulatory cells (Tregs), thereby modulating intestinal inflammation [9]. Research on parasympathetic immune regulation and its relevance to disease is rapidly advancing.

Moreover, therapeutic strategies for several diseases leveraging vagus nerve inflammation control are being investigated. Recent reports indicate that vagus nerve stimulation has improved disease states in conditions such as rheumatoid arthritis and Crohn's disease, a type of inflammatory bowel disease [10–12].

3 Central Nervous System Regulation of Gastrointestinal Function: The Role of the Gut-Brain Axis in IBS Pathophysiology

While research on autonomic nervous system-mediated immune regulation is accumulating, knowledge regarding the relationship between the central nervous system (CNS) and visceral function remains limited. For over 35 years, our group has consistently investigated CNS regulation of gastrointestinal function. Recently, we have focused on comprehensive analyses of central mechanisms governing visceral perception and intestinal permeability.

The importance of understanding the *gut-brain axis* is emphasized in the Rome IV criteria, revised in 2016 [13]. Clarifying the mechanisms of visceral hypersensitivity and leaky gut—key pathophysiological features of IBS influenced by the Gut-Brain Axis—and developing novel therapies based on these insights is a rational approach. The following section discusses our research on orexin, a neuropeptide, and its role in central regulation of gastrointestinal function and IBS pathophysiology.

3.1 What Is Orexin?

Orexin is a neuropeptide identified in 1998 by Sakurai et al. during a search for novel bioactive substances using orphan G protein-coupled receptors [14]. Orexin is uniquely produced exclusively in neurons of the lateral hypothalamus, a region known as the feeding center. Intracerebroventricular administration of synthetic orexin in rats increased food intake, leading to the initial hypothesis that orexin promotes feeding behavior.

Subsequent studies revealed that orexin neurons project widely throughout the brain and influence various neural pathways. Orexin plays a critical role in maintaining wakefulness, and narcolepsy has been linked to orexin system dysfunction. Orexin receptor antagonists are now clinically used as hypnotics [15]. Our group has been at the forefront of research demonstrating that orexin acts centrally to enhance gastrointestinal function. This section outlines our findings on the physiological and pathophysiological significance of orexin in the brain-gut axis.

3.2 Orexin and Gastric Acid Secretion and Gastrointestinal Motility

Intracerebroventricular administration of orexin-A in rats dose-dependently increased gastric acid secretion [16]. This effect was not replicated by intraperitoneal administration of orexin-A or intracerebroventricular administration of orexin-B, indicating that orexin-A acts centrally to stimulate gastric acid secretion. Structure-activity relationship studies further revealed that the two disulfide bonds in orexin-A are essential for this effect [17]. The orexin-induced increase in gastric acid secretion was completely blocked by atropine pretreatment or surgical vagotomy, indicating vagus nerve dependency. Regarding the brain sites involved in orexin's action, the following have been identified: the origin of the vagus nerve, which controls the stomach, is located in the dorsal nucleus of vagus nerve; direct axonal projections from orexin-containing cells in the lateral hypothalamus are found in the dorsal nucleus of vagus nerve; and the dorsal nucleus of vagus nerve is excited by orexin. It is thought that orexin activated-specific receptors on neurons in the dorsal nucleus of the vagus nerve, thereby inducing vagus nerve excitation.

Moreover, the gastric acid secretion induced by intravenous 2-deoxy-D-glucose (2-DG) was blocked by the orexin-1 receptor (OX_1R) antagonist SB334867, confirming the involvement of endogenous central orexin in gastric acid regulation [18]. Furthermore, it was clarified that this pathway is the result of orexin binding to OX1R. These findings suggest that orexin neurons in the lateral hypothalamus stimulate OX1R-expressing neurons in the DMV, leading to vagal activation and enhanced gastric acid secretion.

Additionally, orexin centrally enhances gastric and colonic motility, and this effect, like gastric acid secretion, is vagus nerve-dependent [19, 20].

3.3 Orexin and Visceral Sensory Modulation

Visceral hypersensitivity refers to an increased sensitivity to sensations arising from the gastrointestinal tract. In 1973, Ritchie et al. demonstrated that patients with irritable bowel syndrome (IBS) exhibit a lower pain threshold in response to rectal distension [21], suggesting a mechanism for the abdominal pain commonly observed in IBS. This concept has since become well established and is now considered a principal mechanism underlying abdominal pain in patients with functional gastrointestinal disorders (FGIDs) such as IBS.

Our research has investigated the effects of orexin on visceral perception. We found that orexin acts centrally to attenuate visceral sensitivity [22]. This orexin-induced visceral analgesia involves downstream signaling pathways including dopamine, opioids, adenosine, and cannabinoids. Additionally, other neuropeptides such as ghrelin and oxytocin also exert central visceral analgesic effects. Ghrelin appears to utilize the orexinergic system to mediate its effects, while orexinergic neurons may act upstream of oxytocin in modulating visceral sensation [23].

3.4 Central Nervous Regulation in Intestinal Barrier Function

Disruption of the intestinal barrier, or leaky gut, has been implicated not only in gastrointestinal disorders such as IBS but also in systemic diseases including Alzheimer's disease [24]. Leaky gut has been observed in all IBS subtypes—diarrhea-predominant, constipation-predominant, and mixed-type. While peripheral mechanisms regulating intestinal barrier function have been extensively studied, the role of the central nervous system (CNS) has remained unclear.

Using a rat model of leaky gut, we demonstrated that central signaling via orexin, ghrelin, and oxytocin improves intestinal barrier function [25–27]. This rapid, neurally mediated regulation of the gut barrier is particularly relevant for understanding the pathophysiology of stress-related gastrointestinal disorders such as IBS. Orexinergic neurons in the lateral hypothalamus activate the vagus nerve, which in turn improves leaky gut via the vagal cholinergic pathway. These findings highlight the role of the CNS, through autonomic pathways such as the vagus nerve, in regulating intestinal barrier integrity.

IBS is frequently comorbid with psychological disturbances such as depression and anxiety. Both intestinal barrier dysfunction and psychological symptoms may originate from central nervous system dysregulation, providing a unified explanation for the deep involvement of the brain in the pathophysiology of IBS.

3.5 Orexin and IBS

Based on our findings, we propose that in healthy individuals, normal orexin signaling maintains gastrointestinal motility and visceral sensory function, including normal pain thresholds in response to rectal distension. A reduction in orexin signaling may lead to gastrointestinal dysmotility, visceral hypersensitivity, and leaky gut. Moreover, orexin has been reported to enhance appetite, regulate sleep-wake cycles, and exert antidepressant effects. Therefore, diminished orexin signaling may also contribute to sleep disturbances, anorexia, and depressive symptoms.

These features—gastrointestinal dysmotility, visceral hypersensitivity, leaky gut, sleep disturbances, anorexia, and depression—are characteristic of the clinical presentation of IBS. Thus, impaired orexin function may provide a unifying explanation for the multifaceted pathophysiology of IBS. In this context, IBS ("illness") may arise from reduced central orexin signaling ("mind"), supporting the concept that "illness begins in the mind" (Fig. 76.1).

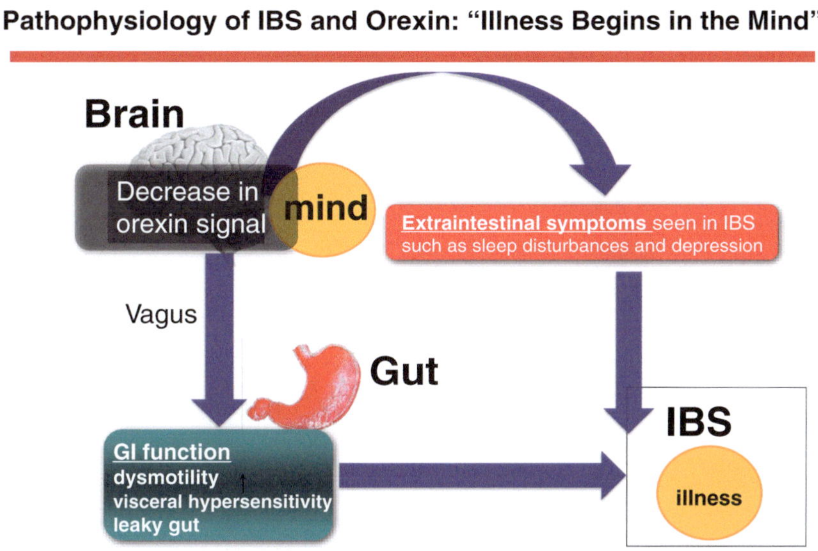

Fig. 76.1 Pathophysiology of IBS and Orexin: "Illness Begins in the Mind". A decrease in central orexin signaling ("mind") activates the vagus nerve, leading to the development of key IBS pathophysiological features: gastrointestinal dysmotility, visceral hypersensitivity, and leaky gut ("illness"). This reduction in orexin signaling also contributes to extraintestinal symptoms commonly seen in IBS, such as sleep disturbances and depression, providing a unified explanation for the disorder

4 Clinical Implications of "Illness Begins in the Mind"

These findings suggest that even in animal models, modulation of brain function (e.g., via intracerebroventricular administration of orexin) can influence the pathophysiology of IBS. Such insights should be translated into clinical practice. In treating FGIDs such as IBS, where patients present with prominent symptoms like *abdominal pain, constipation*, and *diarrhea*, treatment strategies often focus on controlling gastrointestinal symptoms. This typically involves medications that act directly on the gut.

However, many patients do not achieve sufficient symptom relief with these approaches. Considering the concept that "illness begins in the mind," therapeutic strategies targeting the "mind"—such as anxiolytics and antidepressants that act on the CNS—may be necessary. Importantly, effective modulation of the "mind" also requires a strong patient-physician relationship.

IBS is known to have a high placebo response rate. Harnessing this effect requires a therapeutic alliance built on trust and communication. The placebo effect is mediated by central nervous mechanisms, and reassurance—such as explaining that IBS is not life-threatening and that improvement is achievable—can help regulate the "mind."

It is particularly important to explain the *gut-brain axis* and why abdominal symptoms may occur despite normal test results. Without such understanding, some patients may engage in "doctor shopping," believing that something has been missed.

Demonstrating that "illness begins in the mind" applies to IBS opens new avenues for treatment development. Elucidating the mechanisms behind this concept holds great promise for managing a wide range of diseases.

Take-Home Message

Patients with functional gastrointestinal disorders (FGIDs) such as irritable bowel syndrome (IBS) often present with prominent gastrointestinal symptoms, including abdominal pain, constipation, and diarrhea. Consequently, treatment strategies tend to focus primarily on controlling these gastrointestinal manifestations. In such cases, therapeutic approaches typically involve medications that act directly on the gastrointestinal tract to regulate its function.

However, when these pharmacological interventions fail to achieve satisfactory symptom relief, it becomes necessary to consider the concept that "illness begins in the mind." This perspective underscores the importance of treatment strategies aimed at modulating the mind, which may include interventions targeting the central nervous system, such as anxiolytics or antidepressants.

Competing Interests The author(s) has no competing interests to declare that are relevant to the content of this manuscript.

References

1. Aoyama N, et al. Peptic ulcers after the Hanshin-Awaji earthquake: increased incidence of bleeding gastric ulcers. Am J Gastroenterol. 1998;93(3):311–6.
2. Kanno T, et al. Peptic ulcers after the Great East Japan earthquake and tsunami: possible existence of psychosocial stress ulcers in humans. J Gastroenterol. 2013;48(4):483–90.
3. Fukudo S, et al. Evidence-based clinical practice guidelines for irritable bowel syndrome 2020. J Gastroenterol. 2021;56(3):193–217.
4. Araki M, et al. Psychologic stress and disease activity in patients with inflammatory bowel disease: a multicenter cross-sectional study. PLoS One. 2020;15(5):e0233365.
5. Levy RL, et al. Psychosocial aspects of the functional gastrointestinal disorders. Gastroenterology. 2006;130(5):1447–58.
6. Nakai A, et al. Adrenergic control of lymphocyte trafficking and adaptive immune responses. Neurochem Int. 2019;130:104320.
7. Borovikova LV, et al. Vagus nerve stimulation attenuates the systemic inflammatory response to endotoxin. Nature. 2000;405(6785):458–62.
8. Huston JM, et al. Splenectomy inactivates the cholinergic anti-inflammatory pathway during lethal endotoxemia and polymicrobial sepsis. J Exp Med. 2006;203(7):1623–8.
9. Teratani T, et al. The liver-brain-gut neural arc maintains the Treg cell niche in the gut. Nature. 2020;585(7826):591–6.
10. Koopman FA, et al. Vagus nerve stimulation inhibits cytokine production and attenuates disease severity in rheumatoid arthritis. Proc Natl Acad Sci USA. 2016;113(29):8284–9.
11. Genovese MC, et al. Safety and efficacy of neurostimulation with a miniaturised vagus nerve stimulation device in patients with multidrug-refractory rheumatoid arthritis: a two-stage multicentre, randomised pilot study. Lancet Rheumatol. 2020;2(9):e527–38.
12. Sinniger V, et al. A 12-month pilot study outcomes of vagus nerve stimulation in Crohn's disease. Neurogastroenterol Motil. 2020;32(1):e13911.
13. Drossman DA, Hasler WL. Rome IV—functional GI disorders: disorders of gut-brain interaction. Gastroenterology. 2016;150(6):1257–61.
14. Sakurai T, et al. Orexins and orexin receptors: a family of hypothalamic neuropeptides and G protein-coupled receptors that regulate feeding behavior. Cell. 1998;92(4):573–85.
15. Bassetti CLA, et al. Narcolepsy—clinical spectrum, aetiopathophysiology, diagnosis and treatment. Nat Rev Neurol. 2019;15(9):519–39.
16. Takahashi N, et al. Stimulation of gastric acid secretion by centrally administered orexin-A in conscious rats. Biochem Biophys Res Commun. 1999;254(3):623–7.
17. Okumura T, et al. Requirement of intact disulfide bonds in orexin-A-induced stimulation of gastric acid secretion that is mediated by OX1 receptor activation. Biochem Biophys Res Commun. 2001;280(4):976–81.
18. Yamada H, et al. A selective orexin-1 receptor antagonist, SB334867, blocks 2-DG-induced gastric acid secretion in rats. Neurosci Lett. 2005;376(2):137–42.
19. Nozu T, Okumura T. Endogenous orexin-A in the brain mediates 2-deoxy-D-glucose-induced stimulation of gastric motility in freely moving conscious rats. J Gastroenterol. 2012;47(4):404–11.
20. Nozu T, Okumura T. Central orexin-A increases colonic motility in conscious rats. Neurosci Lett. 2011;498(2):143–6.
21. Ritchie J. Pain from distension of the pelvic colon by inflating a balloon in the irritable colon syndrome. Gut. 1973;14(2):125–32.
22. Okumura T, Nozu T. Antinociceptive action against colonic distension by brain orexin in conscious rats. Brain Res. 2015;1598:12–7.
23. Okumura T, Nozu T. Central regulatory mechanisms of visceral sensation in response to colonic distension with special reference to brain orexin. Neuropeptides. 2021;86:102129.

24. Camilleri M. Leaky gut: mechanisms, measurement and clinical implications in humans. Gut. 2019;68(8):1516–26.
25. Okumura T, Nozu T. Brain orexin improves intestinal barrier function via the vagal cholinergic pathway. Neurosci Lett. 2020;714:134592.
26. Ishioh M, et al. Ghrelin acts in the brain to block colonic hyperpermeability in response to lipopolysaccharide through the vagus nerve. Neuropharmacology. 2020;173:108116.
27. Okumura T, Nozu T. Oxytocin acts centrally in the brain to improve leaky gut through the vagus nerve and a cannabinoid signaling in rats. Physiol Behav. 2022;254:113914.

77 Practical Treatment, Explore Issues with Psychosomatic Medicine Treatment

Hiroshi Kaneko

Abstract

Functional gastrointestinal disorders (FGIDs), such as irritable bowel syndrome (IBS), are characterized by chronic digestive symptoms without identifiable structural abnormalities. Effective diagnosis and treatment require a psychosomatic perspective, which recognizes the complex interaction between the gut, brain, and psychological factors. A purely biomedical approach often fails to capture the full clinical picture. The biopsychosocial model, central to psychosomatic medicine, provides a comprehensive framework for understanding symptom development, influenced by stress, emotional regulation, past trauma, and behavioral responses. Cognitive behavioral therapy (CBT) exemplifies this approach by addressing maladaptive thoughts and behaviors that perpetuate symptoms. Evidence supports CBT's role in reducing symptom severity and psychological distress. However, successful FGID management extends beyond CBT alone—it involves careful patient-doctor communication, validation of the patient's experience, and integration of psychological, behavioral, and medical care. Psychosomatic assessment is essential for identifying factors such as anxiety, depression, somatization, and coping styles, which can guide individualized treatment. Ultimately, a psychosomatic approach enhances diagnostic accuracy, therapeutic relationships, and long-term outcomes for FGID patients.

Keywords

Functional gastrointestinal disorders (FGIDs) · Psychosomatic medicine · Biopsychosocial model · Cognitive behavioral therapy (CBT) · Gut-brain axis · Patient-doctor communication · Somatization · Stress and emotion regulation · Individualized treatment · Autogenic training

H. Kaneko (✉)
Division of Internal Medicine, Hoshigaoka Maternity Hospital, Nagoya, Japan
e-mail: hkaneko@fujita-hu.ac.jp

1 Definition of Psychosomatic Disorders

Psychosomatic disorders are defined as "physical diseases in which psychosocial factors are closely involved in the onset and course, and in which organic or functional abnormalities are recognized. However, physical symptoms associated with other psychiatric disorders, such as neurosis or depression, are excluded" (Japanese Society of Psychosomatic Medicine, 1991) (in Japanese).

Conditions such as irritable bowel syndrome (IBS), migraine, and hypertension are considered

H. Kaneko et al. (eds.), *Disorders of Gut-Brain Interaction*,
https://doi.org/10.1007/978-981-95-6974-8_77

psychosomatic disorders when psychosocial factors significantly influence the manifestation, persistence, or improvement of symptoms. Thus, the term "psychosomatic disorder" refers not to a specific disease entity but to a pathological condition. When documenting a diagnosis in the medical record, it is appropriate to specify, for example, "irritable bowel syndrome (psychosomatic disorder)." Representative physical diseases that are better conceptualized as psychosomatic disorders depending on the clinical context are listed in Table 77.1.

The Diagnostic and Statistical Manual of Mental Disorders (DSM), developed by the American Psychiatric Association, was revised in 2013 with the release of DSM-5 (the most recent version being DSM-5-TR, published in March 2022). Although the term "psychosomatic disorder" is not used in the DSM, the chapter on *Somatic Symptom and Related Disorders* includes a category titled *Psychological Factors Affecting Other Medical Conditions* (Table 77.2). According to the DSM-5, common clinical examples include asthma exacerbated by anxiety, denial of the need for treatment for acute chest pain, and insulin manipulation in diabetes for the purpose of weight loss. Adverse effects may range from acute and immediate medical consequences (e.g., Takotsubo cardiomyopathy) to chronic and long-term outcomes (e.g., hypertension induced by chronic occupational stress). Affected medical conditions include those with well-defined pathophysiology (e.g., diabetes, cancer, coronary artery disease), functional syndromes (e.g., migraine, irritable bowel syndrome (IBS), fibromyalgia), and idiopathic medical symptoms (e.g., pain, fatigue, dizziness).

In the International Classification of Diseases, tenth Revision (ICD-10)—with ICD-11 officially adopted by the World Health Organization in January 2022 and currently being prepared for implementation in Japan—the concept corresponding to psychosomatic disorders is found under *Behavioral Syndromes Associated with Physiological Disturbances and Physical Factors* (F5). This includes categories such as eating disorders (F50), sexual dysfunction (F52), and *Psychological and Behavioral Factors Associated with Disorders or Diseases Classified Elsewhere* (F54). Examples of conditions categorized under F54 include asthma, dermatitis and eczema, gastric ulcer, ulcerative colitis, and urticaria. Additionally, within the category of *Neurotic, Stress-Related, and Somatoform Disorders* (F4), the subcategory *Somatoform Autonomic Dysfunction* (F45.3) corresponds to what has traditionally been referred to in Japan as "autonomic imbalance."

Table 77.1 Physical diseases that are better understood as psychosomatic disorders

System	Representative conditions
Respiratory system	Bronchial asthma, hyperventilation syndrome, psychogenic cough, laryngeal spasm, and chronic obstructive pulmonary disease (COPD)
Cardiovascular system	Essential hypertension, essential hypotension, orthostatic hypotension, coronary artery disease (angina pectoris, myocardial infarction), and certain arrhythmias
Gastrointestinal system	*Irritable bowel syndrome (IBS), functional dyspepsia (FD),* gastric and duodenal ulcers, acute gastric mucosal lesions, ulcerative colitis, biliary dyskinesia, chronic pancreatitis, chronic hepatitis, aerophagia, *psychogenic vomiting, diffuse esophageal spasm, and esophageal achalasia*
Endocrine/ metabolic system	Eating disorders (anorexia nervosa, bulimia nervosa), hyperthyroidism, diabetes mellitus, psychogenic polydipsia, deprivation dwarfism, simple obesity, and pseudo-Bartter syndrome
Neuromuscular system	Tension-type headache, migraine, chronic pain, spasmodic torticollis, writer's cramp, blepharospasm, and trigeminal neuralgia
Other conditions	Rheumatoid arthritis, fibromyalgia, low back pain, hyperhidrosis, alopecia areata, chronic urticaria, atopic dermatitis, menopausal syndrome, temporomandibular joint disorder, glossodynia, and stomatitis

Table 77.2 DSM-5 criteria corresponding to psychosomatic disorders

Psychological factors affecting other medical conditions
Diagnostic code: 316 (F54)
A. A medical symptom or condition (other than a mental disorder) is present.
B. Psychological or behavioral factors adversely affect the medical condition in at least one of the following ways:
1. The psychological factors have influenced the course of the medical condition, as evidenced by a close temporal association between the psychological factors and the onset, exacerbation, or delayed recovery of the medical condition.
2. The psychological factors interfere with the treatment of the medical condition (e.g., poor adherence to prescribed medical regimens).
3. The psychological factors constitute additional well-established health risks for the individual.
4. The psychological factors influence the underlying pathophysiology, triggering or exacerbating symptoms, or necessitating medical attention.
C. The psychological and behavioral factors in Criterion B are not better explained by another mental disorder (e.g., panic disorder, major depressive disorder, posttraumatic stress disorder).
Specify current severity:
Mild: Increases medical risk (e.g., inconsistent adherence in the treatment of hypertension).
Moderate: Worsens the underlying medical condition (e.g., anxiety exacerbating asthma).
Severe: Results in hospitalization or emergency room visits.
Extreme: Results in severe, life-threatening consequences (e.g., ignoring symptoms of a myocardial infarction)

2 Classification of Psychosomatic Disorders

Based on accumulated clinical experience, psychosomatic disorders can be classified into the following three categories:

2.1 Group I: Psychosocial Stress as a Trigger or Exacerbating Factor

This group includes cases in which psychosocial stress acts as a precipitating or aggravating factor in the development of physical illness. Examples include major life events (e.g., entering school, starting a job, relocating, bereavement) and daily life stressors (e.g., interpersonal conflicts, academic or occupational burdens) that precede the onset or recurrence of disease. Additionally, psychological states such as anxiety, depression, and anger may influence symptom severity.

2.2 Group II: Psychological Burden in Chronic Illness

This group encompasses chronic diseases such as bronchial asthma, rheumatoid arthritis, and malignancies, which tend to follow a prolonged and relapsing course. These conditions often lack a clear prognosis and impose significant physical, psychological, and financial burdens. The added psychosocial distress may lead to the development of anxiety and depression.

2.3 Group III: Psychosocial Factors Interfering with Treatment and Disease Management

In this group, psychosocial factors hinder appropriate treatment or disease management, thereby adversely affecting the clinical course. Patients may exhibit strong distrust toward medical care or demonstrate behaviors that obstruct therapeutic interventions.

3 Assessment Items in Psychosomatic Disorders

3.1 Cross-Sectional Perspective

It is important to assess how psychosocial factors are currently influencing the course of the physical illness. For example, stress related to interpersonal relationships at school or work may correlate with the frequency and severity of abdominal pain (e.g., as recorded in a bowel movement diary). Similarly, job promotions or transfers may be associated with the intensity of headaches (e.g., documented in a headache diary). The use of self-monitoring tools such as symptom diaries can facilitate this evaluation.

3.2 Longitudinal Perspective

In the diagnosis and treatment of psychosomatic disorders, it is essential to organize the clinical narrative along a temporal axis. This includes evaluating the patient's condition prior to symptom onset—referred to as "predisposing factors"—which may, in some cases, involve traits established during early childhood. It also involves identifying "precipitating factors," such as significant life events occurring around the time of symptom emergence, including school entry, employment, marriage, or accidents. Furthermore, attention must be given to "perpetuating factors" that hinder symptom resolution or improvement, such as maladjustment to academic or occupational demands, burdens associated with new living environments, or complications related to insurance or compensation claims. Structuring the clinical assessment in this chronological manner facilitates a more comprehensive understanding of the disorder and informs the development of an effective treatment strategy.

3.3 Life Events and Daily Stressors

It is essential to assess the presence or absence of life events and daily stressors, as outlined in Table 77.3, on an individual basis. In addition to conventional stressors, attention must also be directed toward emerging societal stressors associated with recent social changes. These include demographic shifts such as population aging and the decline in the working-age population, the widespread use of social networking services (SNS) and online gaming; diversification in work styles, employment while undergoing treatment for illnesses such as cancer, and the transition to remote work, online education, and virtual meetings prompted by the COVID-19 pandemic. These evolving phenomena represent new sources of stress that must be considered in clinical evaluation.

3.4 Biopsychosocial Model

The biopsychosocial model, proposed by Engel GL, provides a framework for understanding disease and illness behavior (e.g., seeking medical attention for minor symptoms). This model aligns with the principles of psychosomatic medicine, which emphasize a holistic understanding of the patient that integrates both physical and psychological dimensions. Evaluation items based on this model are summarized in Table 77.4.

3.5 Personality Traits and Behavioral Patterns in Psychosomatic Patients

Patients with psychosomatic disorders often exhibit personality traits or behavioral tendencies that predispose them to somatization of stress. Common patterns include the following:

(i) Perfectionism and obsessive traits: Individuals who feel compelled to do everything precisely or who ruminate excessively.
(ii) Overadaptation: Individuals who suppress their emotions, avoid expressing their thoughts, and strive to meet others' expectations. Although they may appear to have no interpersonal issues, they often harbor inter-

Table 77.3 Life cycle, developmental tasks, and potential psychosocial stressors

1. *Childhood*
Infancy and early childhood: basic trust (sense of security) and basic life habits (autonomy)
Relationship with mother—lack of affection or physical contact and anxiety about being abandoned
Family atmosphere—parental conflict, separation, divorce, illness, death, relationship with in-laws, etc.
Discipline—overly strict (overly controlling), inconsistent, neglectful, and abuse
Relationship with siblings—birth of younger siblings, conflict over parents, being an only child, etc.
School age: foundation of social adaptability (competence)
Home life—relationship with parents, absence of mother, absence of father, overly strict discipline, parental (marital) relationship, gaming addiction, poverty, etc.
School life—relationships with friends and teachers, academic performance, bullying, etc.
2. *Adolescence and Young Adulthood: Establishment of Ego Identity and Sexual Identity (Autonomy)*
Home life—individuation from parents (conflict between dependence and independence), etc.
School life—relationships with friends (including the opposite sex) and teachers, academic performance, issues related to advancement, entrance exam failure, club activities, etc.
Social life—romantic relationships, marriage, employment, etc.
3. *Adulthood and Middle Age: Intimacy and "Nurturing and Care".*
Home life—marriage, relationship with spouse, infertility, childbirth and parenting, parental roles, children's education, children's independence, changes in relationships with parents, housing conditions, job transfers, dual-income households, etc.
Social life—employment, job content and suitability, competition for promotion, job transfers, promotions, relationships with supervisors, colleagues and subordinates, work environment, overwork, balancing work with childcare, caregiving or medical treatment, commuting time, job changes, bankruptcy, unemployment, relationships with people in the community, remote work, online meetings, etc.
4. *Early Old Age (Regressive Phase, Menopause) and Old Age: Sense of Integrity and "Wisdom".*
Home life—children's independence, changes in relationships with children, illness or death of spouse, illness or death of close relatives, elder-to-elder caregiving, divorce, etc.
Social life—retirement, financial insecurity, loss of social roles, loss of life purpose, reemployment, relationships with people in the community, etc.

Table 77.4 Patient evaluation grid

Domain	Current	Around onset	Early childhood
Biological (physical)	Physical symptoms and findings Physical examination finding Medications in use Abnormal test results	Initial symptoms Changes in physical condition Changes in medications used	History of physical illness Family history of physical and mental illness
Psychological	Physical and psychological complaints Psychological state Expectations for treatment	Changes in psychological state Changes in mood and behavior Psychological testing Requests for psychological support	Personality development Defense mechanisms and interpersonal responses Past psychiatric history
Social factors	Cohabiting Individuals Occupation Social stress Physical environment	Changes in Economic status Occupational changes Changes in living environment Changes in physical environment	Parental occupational history Early life interpersonal relationships

Adapted from Leigh et al. [1]. Also cited in Textbook of Internal Medicine, ninth ed. Nakayama Shoten; 2019:88. (in Japanese)

Table 77.5 Characteristics of alexithymia

1. Poor capacity for fantasy and imagination
2. Inability to verbalize internal conflicts
3. Restricted experience and expression of emotions
4. Tendency to use actions rather than words to express emotions or avoid conflict
5. Difficulty in communicating with interviewers or clinicians
6. Tendency to describe trivial details endlessly rather than expressing emotions
7. Thought content is more focused on external events than on internal fantasies or emotions

nal dissatisfaction, anger, or self-loathing, leading to stress accumulation.

(iii) Alexithymia: A personality trait proposed by Sifneos PE to explain the symptoms of psychosomatic disorders. Its characteristics are listed in Table 77.5. Alexithymia may also be observed in other psychiatric disorders. Patients with psychosomatic disorders often have diminished awareness of bodily sensations, a condition referred to as alexisomia.

(iv) Type A behavior pattern: Characterized by (1) aggressiveness, (2) ambition, (3) competitiveness, and (4) a constant sense of time urgency. Although traditionally considered a risk factor for coronary artery disease, this association has been subject to debate in recent years.

3.6 Differential Diagnosis of Psychiatric Disorders

It is well known that patients with depression often first present to internal medicine clinics. Many psychiatric disorders manifest primarily with physical symptoms (e.g., headache, nausea, insomnia). In such cases, psychosocial factors may contribute to symptom onset, necessitating careful differentiation from psychiatric disorders. Disorders requiring differential diagnosis are listed in Table 77.6.

Additionally, neurodevelopmental disorders may cause abnormal bodily sensations, leading to physical complaints. It is important to consider developmental disorders in the evaluation of psychosomatic conditions. For example, comorbid attention deficits have been reported in patients with IBS. However, due to concerns about overdiagnosis, such considerations should be limited to cases where there is significant impact on academic or occupational functioning and should be approached with caution.

Table 77.6 Representative psychiatric disorders requiring differential diagnosis from psychosomatic disorders

Mood disorders: major depressive disorder
Anxiety disorders: panic disorder, social anxiety disorder, posttraumatic stress disorder (PTSD), acute stress disorder, generalized anxiety disorder, obsessive-compulsive disorder (OCD)
Somatoform disorders
Borderline personality disorder
Schizophrenia
Malingering and factitious disorder
Behavioral problems and habits
Neurodevelopmental disorders

4 Etiology and Pathophysiology of Psychosomatic Disorders

Understanding the etiology and pathophysiology of psychosomatic disorders requires an integrated perspective that considers both psychosocial factors (e.g., stress) and biological mechanisms. The following subsections outline key theoretical and physiological frameworks:

4.1 Stress Theory

Biologically, stress refers to a state of internal disequilibrium caused by various external stimuli (stressors). Physical or environmental stressors—such as cold exposure or physical restraint—can induce a triad of physiological responses: (1) gastric and duodenal ulcers, (2) thymic atrophy, and (3) adrenal cortex hypertrophy. Hans Selye demonstrated that similar responses occur in reaction to psychological stressors as well. These nonspecific responses, regardless of the type of stressor, represent the body's defense mechanisms and are considered essential for maintaining adaptation.

Selye termed this response the general adaptation syndrome, which is commonly known as the stress theory. It is conceptualized in three stages: the alarm reaction, the stage of resistance, and the stage of exhaustion.

4.2 Emotional Information Processing

Emotions—such as anger, fear, joy, and sadness—are transient and intense affective states triggered by specific stimuli. Biologically, emotions are responses to the fulfillment, frustration, or threat to innate needs essential for individual or species survival. In individuals with alexithymia, it is hypothesized that there is either a disruption in the verbalization of emotional experiences or a fundamental impairment in emotional processing itself. Some studies suggest that these impairments may be due to disrupted communication between the right and left cerebral hemispheres or between the limbic system and the cerebral cortex.

4.3 Hypothalamic-Pituitary-Adrenal (HPA) Axis

When the body is exposed to stress, the paraventricular nucleus of the hypothalamus secretes corticotropin-releasing factor (CRF), which is transported via the hypophyseal portal system to the anterior pituitary gland. This stimulates the release of adrenocorticotropic hormone (ACTH), which in turn promotes the secretion of cortisol from the adrenal cortex. This cascade constitutes the hypothalamic-pituitary-adrenal (HPA) axis, a critical physiological response system essential for survival, often accompanied by activation of the autonomic nervous system.

Animal studies have shown that HPA axis reactivity is heightened by early-life stressors such as maternal separation or inadequate parental care during the lactation period. Furthermore, recent research has highlighted the role of the gut microbiota in modulating HPA axis responsiveness. The stability and regulation of the HPA axis are increasingly understood to be influenced by the composition and activity of the gut microbiota.

5 Diagnosis of Psychosomatic Disorders Based on Etiology and Pathophysiology

The diagnosis of psychosomatic disorders involves a combination of (1) exclusionary diagnosis, which rules out organic diseases and psychiatric disorders, and (2) positive diagnosis, which identifies the relationship between symptoms and psychosocial factors (i.e., the mind-body interaction).

5.1 Exclusionary Diagnosis

The exclusion of organic disease should be conducted by general internists or primary care physicians. For example, in cases of chronic abdominal pain and altered bowel habits, clinicians should assess for signs of colorectal cancer or inflammatory bowel disease through medical interviews, physical examinations, and basic laboratory tests such as blood work and fecal occult blood testing. If red flag symptoms suggestive of serious pathology are present, referral to a specialist (e.g., gastroenterologist) for advanced diagnostics such as colonoscopy is warranted.

If a psychiatric disorder is suspected, referral to a psychiatrist is appropriate. In cases where the patient is resistant to psychiatric consultation, it may be helpful to propose comanagement initially.

5.2 Positive Diagnosis

Although psychosomatic disorders are characterized by a close relationship between physical symptoms and psychosocial factors, patients are not always aware of this connection and may even deny it. Therefore, the initial consultation should emphasize active listening and a thorough clinical interview to establish a strong patient-physician relationship. This approach can help patients recognize the mind-body connection, facilitating both diagnosis and treatment planning.

5.3 Psychological Testing

Psychological assessments may include personality inventories, intelligence tests, and instruments that evaluate coping strategies and quality of life (QoL). These tools serve as adjuncts to diagnosis. Given potential patient resistance, clinicians should explain the purpose of testing and administer it only when appropriate. No single test can capture the entirety of a patient's personality or condition; therefore, it is necessary to select a test battery that combines various psychological tests according to the purpose. This typically includes both self-report questionnaires and projective tests to provide complementary insights.

The Hospital Anxiety and Depression Scale (HADS) is a widely used, copyright-free questionnaire that is simple to administer and frequently employed in clinical research.

5.4 Psychophysiological Testing

These tests assess central nervous system function (e.g., electroencephalography, brain imaging) and autonomic nervous system function at the organ level. Examples include orthostatic testing, pupillometry, electrogastrography, digital photoplethysmography, and heart rate variability analysis. Polysomnography (PSG), which monitors sleep and respiratory patterns, is essential for diagnosing sleep-related breathing disorders.

Evaluating psychosomatic disorders from both psychodynamic and physiological perspectives is useful for identifying treatment-resistant cases and selecting appropriate therapies. Visualizing pathophysiological processes can also enhance patient understanding and engagement. Brain imaging techniques such as SPECT, PET, fMRI, and near-infrared spectroscopy (NIRS) are expected to become increasingly accessible in general clinical practice.

6 Treatment of Psychosomatic Disorders

Key psychosomatic treatment modalities are summarized in Table 77.7. Among psychotherapeutic approaches, autogenic training (AT), transactional analysis, behavioral therapy, and cognitive therapy are commonly employed in psychosomatic medicine.

6.1 Autogenic Training (AT)

AT is a self-hypnosis technique developed with a focus on the health-promoting effects of entering a hypnotic state. Its core mechanism is self-induced relaxation. Although early hypnosis emphasized the concept of "sleep," its effects may have been confused with those of increased

Table 77.7 Major psychosomatic therapeutic modalities

1. Physical therapy provided by general internal medicine or clinical specialties
2. Lifestyle guidance
3 Psychotherapy through interviews (counseling)
4. Pharmacotherapy (e.g., psychotropic medications, Kampo medicine)
5. Environmental adjustment
6. Autogenic training and progressive muscle relaxation
7. Psychoanalytic therapy: transactional analysis
8. Behavioral therapy: biofeedback therapy
9. Cognitive therapy
10. Family therapy
11. Sandplay therapy
12. Bibliotherapy
13. Music therapy
14. Group therapy
15. Fasting therapy
16. Eastern therapies: Morita therapy, Naikan therapy, acupuncture and moxibustion, yoga therapy, Zen-based therapy, qigong
17. Gestalt therapy
18. Others

Adapted from: Textbook of Internal Medicine, ninth ed. Nakayama Shoten; 2019:88. (in Japanese)

suggestibility, decreased level of consciousness, and relaxation. AT evolved independently and has become a widely accepted treatment in psychosomatic medicine.

The standard AT practice (Table 77.8) consists of a background formula and six standard formulas, which are silently repeated to induce specific physical sensations, such as heaviness and warmth in the arms. Additional techniques include organ-specific formulas, volitional training formulas targeting behavioral change, and advanced practices such as meditative exercises and autonomic neutralization.

If functional gastrointestinal disorders (FGIDs) could be explained solely by sympathetic overactivation due to stress, then any relaxation technique that activates the parasympathetic nervous system should be effective. However, there is currently insufficient evidence supporting the efficacy of AT for functional dyspepsia (FD), and few studies demonstrate its effectiveness for IBS. High-quality randomized controlled trials (RCTs) are needed.

Some clinicians provide books or videos to encourage patients to practice AT independently. However, for AT to be effective, it is essential to enhance motivation through psychoeducation, provide guided sessions initially, and encourage repeated practice with self-monitoring. Importantly, the "autogenic" in AT refers to "self-generating," not to be confused with "autonomic" as in the autonomic nervous system. The term indicates, first, a psychophysiological perspective that promotes autonomous processes of self-normalization, and second, a methodological meaning that involves promoting self-normalization functions independently. In other words, it implies "transitioning to a state of autonomy that brings about self-normalization through one's own efforts." It is important to intervene in a manner that leverages the characteristics of AT based on an accurate understanding of its concept and usefulness.

Table 77.8 Standard formulas for autogenic training

Formula type	Training content	Formula statement
Background formula	Relaxation training	"I am calm and relaxed."
Formula 1	Heaviness in limbs	"My arms and legs feel heavy."
Formula 2	Warmth in limbs	"My arms and legs feel warm."
Formula 3	Cardiac regulation	"My heart beats calmly and regularly."
Formula 4	Respiratory regulation	"My breathing is calm and easy."
Formula 5	Abdominal warmth	"My abdomen feels warm."
Formula 6	Forehead cooling	"My forehead feels pleasantly cool."

Adapted from Kaneko et al. [2]

6.2 Cognitive Behavioral Therapy (CBT)

CBT is a series of therapeutic techniques that focus on thoughts and cognitions related to the onset, maintenance, and exacerbation of symptoms and guide individuals toward appropriate actions to improve or control symptoms. It is characterized by targeting factors that contribute to the maintenance or exacerbation of symptoms to achieve symptom control. In CBT, after assessing how symptoms are maintained or exacerbated by specific situations, cognitive processes, emotions, physical sensations, and behaviors, interventions are tailored to address each of these elements (Fig. 77.1).

CBT has demonstrated some efficacy for IBS, with growing evidence supporting its use. However, studies on its effectiveness for FD are limited, and reports of CBT use for FGIDs in Japan remain scarce. Barriers include limited access to trained providers and delivery systems. Nevertheless, CBT is generally more acceptable to gastroenterologists and psychosomatic physicians than hypnosis, suggesting potential for broader adoption.

In Japan, CBT is covered by health insurance for depression, and familiarity with its principles is beneficial.

Recent studies have explored the cost-effectiveness of Internet-based CBT for IBS. However, some reports question its long-term efficacy, warranting cautious interpretation. While CBT focuses on modifying maladaptive

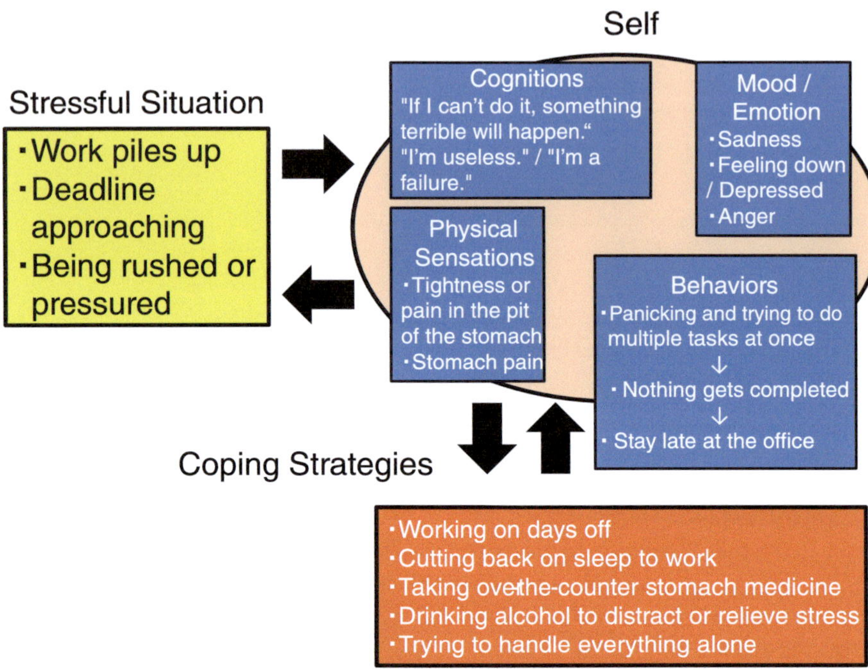

Fig. 77.1 Example of cognitive behavioral therapy (CBT) assessment. In this case, within a stressful environment, pessimistic cognition (e.g., "If I can't do it, something terrible will happen.") arises, leading to negative emotions (such as sadness, depression, and anger), and the emergence of stress-related physical symptoms (e.g., stomach pain). At the same time, ineffective behaviors (such as panicking and trying to do multiple tasks at once) occur. The coping strategy used—cutting back on sleep to work—is ad hoc and ineffective and instead contributes to symptom exacerbation. By creating a worksheet like this and filling it out together with the patient, a shared understanding of the factors maintaining or worsening the symptoms can be developed, leading to various practical interventions. It is also used as homework, allowing the patient to complete it at home to deepen their understanding

thoughts and behaviors that perpetuate symptoms (Fig. 77.1), it does not directly address the underlying psychophysiological mechanisms. Therefore, after achieving initial symptom control, further interventions targeting these mechanisms may be necessary.

Emerging forms of CBT abandons the idea of correcting thoughts and cognition, focusing instead on distancing oneself from them and not reacting to them, and to a greater or lesser extent, it contains elements of mindfulness.

This concept, rooted in Zen meditation and integrated into American psychotherapy, was emphasized when it was actively introduced into CBT. It corresponds to the attitude of observing without reacting to what arises in one's mind and body. Such practices lead to a reduction in symptoms as a result of no longer being swayed by symptoms or anxiety. While these efforts are still in their early stages, promising results have been obtained for FGID, and further development is anticipated in the future.

7 Practical Considerations for Treatment Selection Including Psychosomatic Approaches

The most recent editions of the clinical practice guidelines for FD and IBS are the second revisions. Notably, the treatment algorithm for IBS places greater emphasis on psychosomatic considerations compared to that for FD. A treatment flowchart for FD that incorporates psychosomatic perspectives is presented in Fig. 77.2.

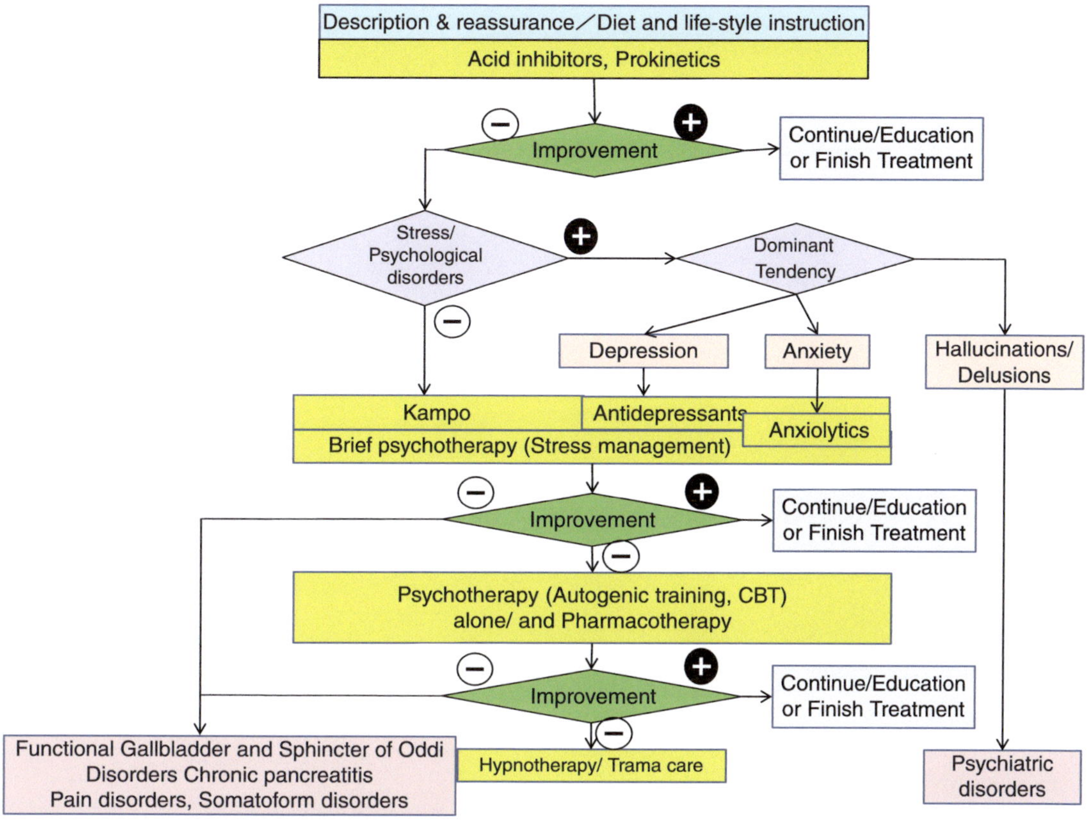

Fig. 77.2 Treatment flowchart for functional dyspepsia including psychosomatic approaches

In some cases, hallucinations or delusions—such as olfactory reference syndrome (e.g., "I must be bothering others with my smell")—may be present. For treatment-resistant cases, clinicians should consider functional disorders of the biliary or pancreatic systems, which may present with symptoms similar to FD. Additionally, some patients may require treatment from the perspective of somatic symptom disorder or chronic pain.

8 Conclusion

Many chronic functional disorders, including functional gastrointestinal disorders (FGIDs), remain poorly understood in terms of pathophysiology at the current level of medical science. In many cases, multiple pathological mechanisms are intricately intertwined, making it difficult to apply a linear, cause-and-effect model of medical care. As a result, patient satisfaction is not always achieved through conventional biomedical approaches alone.

There is a growing call for holistic medicine, personalized care, and patient-centered approaches. A treatment structure that integrates both cross-sectional and longitudinal perspectives—grounded in a strong patient-physician relationship—is essential. However, this area remains insufficiently supported by current health insurance systems.

The economic burden of FGIDs, along with their impact on social productivity and societal loss, is becoming a concern comparable to that of depression. In clinical practice, the challenge lies in how to deliver high-quality care in a limited time frame to patients with moderate to severe symptoms who do not respond to standard pharmacotherapy targeting the gastrointestinal tract.

To meet this challenge, it is essential to perform accurate diagnosis and implement evidence-based pharmacological and nonpharmacological therapies. When symptoms or their impact on daily life do not improve, healthcare providers must work collaboratively with patients to construct a pathophysiological model of symptom generation and continue treatment longitudinally.

Take-Home Message

- The foundation of care lies in accurate diagnosis and the appropriate application of evidence-based treatments.
- In refractory cases, clinicians must be prepared to take on the responsibility of providing care that not only addresses symptoms but also enhances the patient's social functioning and sense of purpose.
- A solid grounding in psychosomatic medicine—its knowledge, attitudes, and practices—is required.

Competing Interests The author(s) has no competing interests to declare that are relevant to the content of this manuscript.

References

1. Leigh H, et al. The patient evaluation grid: a systematic approach to comprehensive care. Gen Hosp Psychiatry. 1980;2(3).
2. Kaneko H, et al. Expected developments in the treatment of functional dyspepsia: a psychosomatic approach. Nihon Shokakibyo Gakkai Zasshi. 2016;113:947–58. (in Japanese).

Further Reading

Komaki M, et al., eds. Guidelines for the diagnosis and treatment of psychosomatic disorders. Kyowa Kikaku; 2006. (in Japanese).

Kaneko H. General internal medicine—Psychosomatic disorders. In: Nangaku M, Ban S, eds. Textbook of internal medicine, 9th ed., Vol. 1. Nakayama Shoten; 2020. pp. 86–92. (in Japanese).

Kubo C, ed. Standard textbook of psychosomatic medicine, 3rd ed. Igaku Shoin; 2009. (in Japanese).

Terminology Committee of the Japanese Society of Psychosomatic Medicine & Academic Training Committee of the Japanese Society of Psychosomatic Internal Medicine, eds. Dictionary of psychosomatic medicine terms, 3rd ed. Miwa Shoten; 2020. (e-book, in Japanese).

The Japanese Society of Gastroenterology, ed. Clinical practice guidelines for functional gastrointestinal disorders 2021—Functional Dyspepsia (FD), 2nd rev. Nankodo; 2021. (in Japanese).

The Japanese Society of Gastroenterology, ed. Clinical practice guidelines for functional gastrointestinal disorders 2020—Irritable Bowel Syndrome (IBS), 2nd rev. Nankodo; 2020. (in Japanese).

Kaneko H. Functional dyspepsia. In: Nakai Y, et al., eds. Psychosomatic internal medicine—From diagnosis to treatment. Asakura Shoten; 2022. pp. 173–7. (in Japanese).

78 Practical Treatment, Physical Findings in the Abdomen, Physical Findings: Inspection, Auscultation, Percussion, Palpation

Takeshi Mizukami

Abstract

Abdominal physical examination remains crucial in diagnosing functional gastrointestinal disorders (FGIDs). It provides real-time insights into patient conditions, including responses to positional and respiratory changes that imaging cannot replicate. Furthermore, it offers unique diagnostic clues for FGIDs like intestinal motility disorders and visceral hypersensitivity through inspection, auscultation, percussion, and palpation. This chapter details a comprehensive abdominal examination, covering preparation and the systematic order of inspection, auscultation, percussion, and palpation. It also discusses findings that contribute to the examination of FGIDs, such as abdominal morphology, distension (e.g., ascites, Mesenterium commune), postoperative scars, vascular signs indicative of hepatic dysfunction, intestinal motility patterns, vascular lesions, liver size, intestinal gas distribution, peritoneal irritation, unique colonic anatomies in Japanese patients, inflammation, organ characteristics, fecal masses, and key tenderness points.

T. Mizukami (✉)
Department of Endoscopy Center, NHO Kurihama Medical and Addiction Center,
Yokosuka, Japan
e-mail: mi-zukami@violin.ocn.ne.jp

Keywords

Abdominal physical examination · FGIDs · Visceral hypersensitivity · Auscultation · Percussion · Palpation

1 Introduction

In the diagnosis of functional disorders, the complete exclusion of organic disease is a fundamental prerequisite. Although the evaluation of physical findings is a cornerstone of clinical practice, recent trends—particularly in the field of gastroenterology—have increasingly prioritized imaging studies over physical examination. Even in standard medical textbooks, the sections dedicated to "abdominal physical examination techniques" have been gradually reduced.

Computed tomography (CT) scans provide clear visualization of intraabdominal masses, inflammation, and ascites and allow for the observation of gas and fecal retention sites. Ultrasonography and magnetic resonance imaging (MRI) can depict fine details within the biliary and pancreatic ducts. Although endoscopy is invasive, it enables comprehensive evaluation of the entire gastrointestinal tract. Given the speed and diagnostic accuracy of these modalities, the decline in abdominal physical examination may be, to some extent, unavoidable.

H. Kaneko et al. (eds.), *Disorders of Gut-Brain Interaction*,
https://doi.org/10.1007/978-981-95-6974-8_78

However, abdominal examination allows for real-time observation of the patient's symptoms, including the effects of positional changes and respiratory variation—factors that imaging cannot replicate. In the clinical setting, clues to diagnosing FGIDs such as intestinal motility disorders and visceral hypersensitivity can currently only be obtained through surface-level inspection, auscultation, percussion, and palpation. Moreover, the act of physical examination itself enhances communication with the patient and can be effectively utilized in the management of FGIDs.

This section outlines the techniques for obtaining physical findings during abdominal examination, including traditional methods. It also explains the pathophysiology of FGIDs in conjunction with representative abdominal X-rays, CT colonography, and endoscopic images.

2 Preparation Before Examination

Prior to the examination, the physician should inform the patient about the methods and content of the physical assessment. It is essential to ensure patient privacy and avoid inducing embarrassment. In shared hospital rooms, curtains should be drawn, and a towel should be placed over the knees of female patients wearing skirts. When examining patients of the opposite sex, a nurse of the same sex as the patient should be present.

For procedures such as liver palpation, approaching from the patient's right side is advantageous. To prevent transmission of infection, skin irritation, or discomfort from cold hands or instruments, hand hygiene must be performed before examining each patient. Fingernails should be trimmed, and both hands and the stethoscope should be warmed prior to palpation.

3 Order of Examination

Abdominal examination consists of four components: inspection, auscultation, percussion, and palpation. These should be performed in order of increasing invasiveness: inspection → auscultation → percussion → palpation. The abdomen is divided into nine regions for systematic evaluation (see Fig. 78.1).

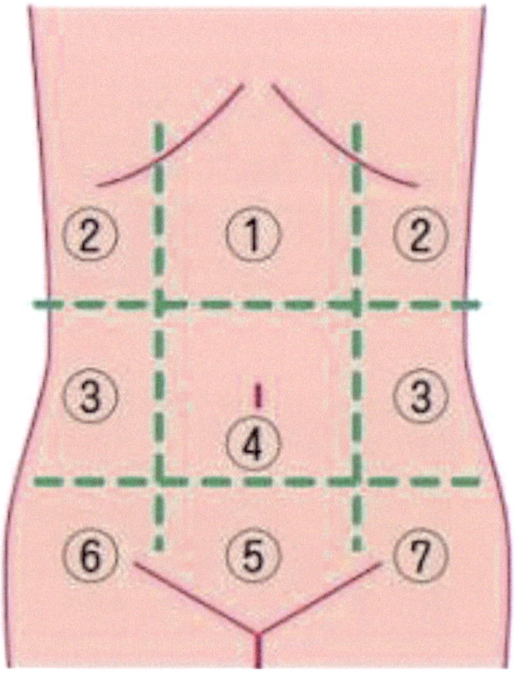

Fig. 78.1 Abdominal regions. ① Epigastric region, ② hypochondriac region, ③ flank region, ④ umbilical region, ⑤ lower abdominal region, ⑥ ileocecal region right iliac fossa), ⑦ left lower quadrant

4 Inspection

Preparation: Expose the abdomen down to the suprapubic region and extend the knees.

4.1 Abdominal Wall

Positional changes and respiratory instructions may be given as needed.

4.1.1 Morphology

1. *Distension*: Observe changes in the standing (anterior and lateral views) and supine positions, noting respiratory variation and abdominal muscle tension.
   - Bilateral dorsal protrusion in the supine position suggests ascites.
   - *Abdominal distension in the standing position may suggest Mesenterium commune* (Fig. 78.2) *or postural effects* [1].

     In cases of *Mesenterium commune*, the entire colon descends into the pelvic cavity when standing. Additionally, *postural or respiratory influences* may cause hepatic ptosis, leading to complaints of *abdominal bloating*. In both conditions, the symptoms typically resolve when the patient assumes a *supine position*.
2. *Postoperative scars*: Postoperative adhesions can affect FGIDs, including constipation.

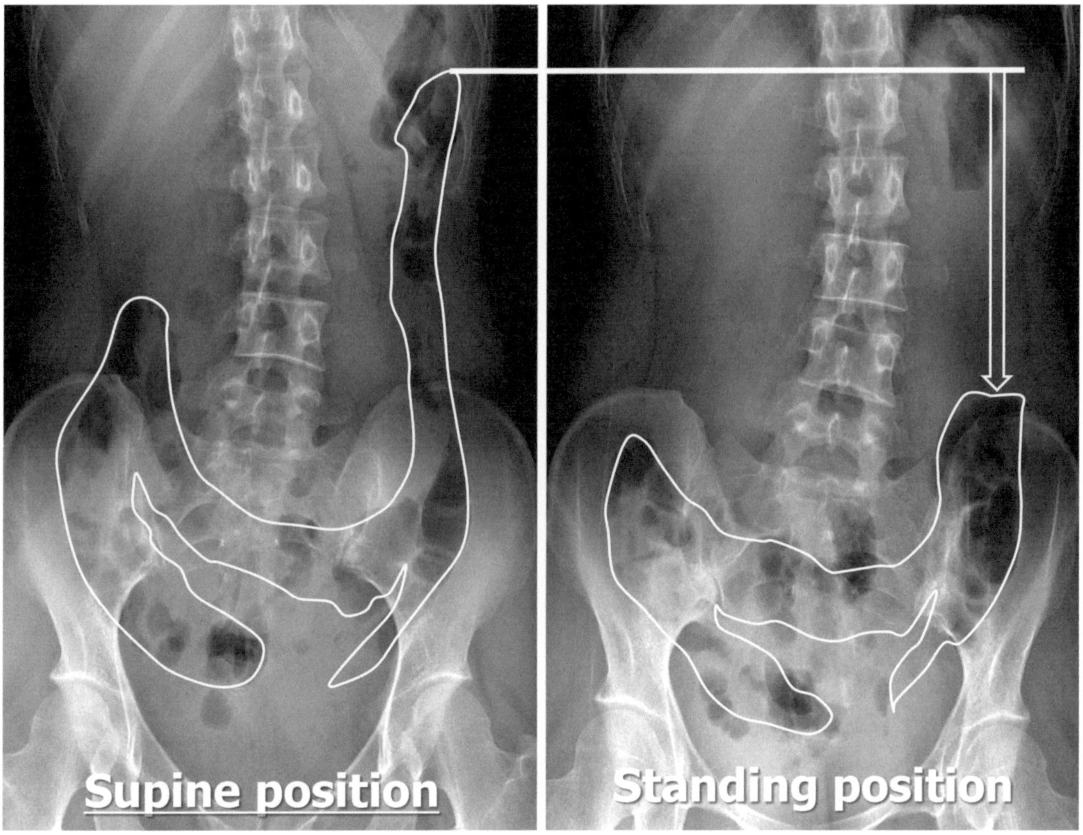

Fig. 78.2 Abdominal X-ray in complete mesocolon. The entire colon descends into the pelvic cavity in the standing position

- *Gastrectomy*: Confirm the size of the surgical scar and inquire about the extent of resection.
  →Consider dumping syndrome or blind loop syndrome.
- *Postpancreatectomy*: May result in indigestion due to pancreatic enzyme deficiency.
- *Cholecystectomy*: May cause disruption of bowel rhythm or bile acid diarrhea.
- *Colorectal or appendectomy*: Inquire about the resected area.
  → Terminal ileum resection may lead to bile acid diarrhea.
- *Postgynecologic surgery*: Pelvic adhesions may cause difficult defecation.

3. *Venous engorgement and spider angiomas*:
   - Suggestive of hepatic dysfunction.
   - May be associated with excessive alcohol intake or diarrhea induced by lactulose.
4. *Striae distensae and umbilical contour*:
   - Indicate subcutaneous fat thickness.
   - May reflect significant weight fluctuations or endocrine disorders.
   - Also observed in patients with excessive food intake or dietary restriction leading to normal-transit constipation.
5. *Umbilical and Inguinal hernias* (Fig. 78.3):
   - The colon may herniate into the inguinal canal, potentially contributing to difficult defecation.
6. *Subcutaneous masses*:
   - Become more prominent with abdominal muscle contraction.
   - Respiratory movement:
     – Anterior-posterior movement suggests abdominal wall origin.
     – Vertical movement suggests intraabdominal origin.

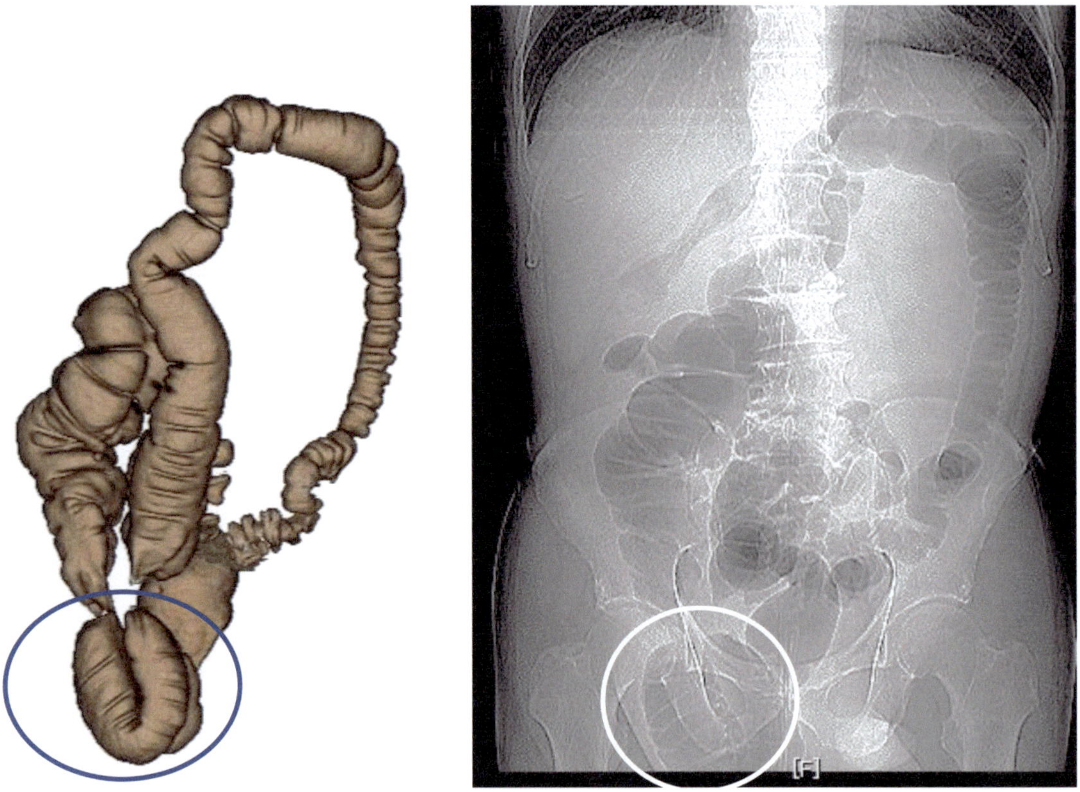

Fig. 78.3 CT colonography. Abnormal configuration with the ascending colon descending and herniating into the inguinal canal. Also visible on abdominal X-ray

– Lack of movement suggests retroperitoneal origin.

7. *Courvoisier's sign*:
   - Painless enlargement of the gallbladder
   - → Suggestive of cholangiocarcinoma or ampullary carcinoma.
8. *Grey-Turner's sign (flank ecchymosis) and Cullen's sign (periumbilical ecchymosis)*:
   → Indicate hemorrhagic extravasation, as seen in severe pancreatitis.

4.1.2 Rigidity of the Rectus Abdominis (e.g., Parkinson's Disease)

May suggest decreased activities of daily living (ADL).

1. *Respiration*
   - *Tachypnea with shallow breathing*: Suggests peritoneal irritation.
     →Pain exacerbated by deep breathing (e.g., hepatic abscess, Fitz-Hugh-Curtis syndrome).
   - *Deep and rapid breathing*:
     →Kussmaul respiration, indicative of diabetic ketoacidosis.

5 Auscultation: Evaluation of Intestinal Function and Exclusion of Vascular Lesions

1. *Vascular bruits*: Auscultate along arterial pathways (see Fig. 78.4).

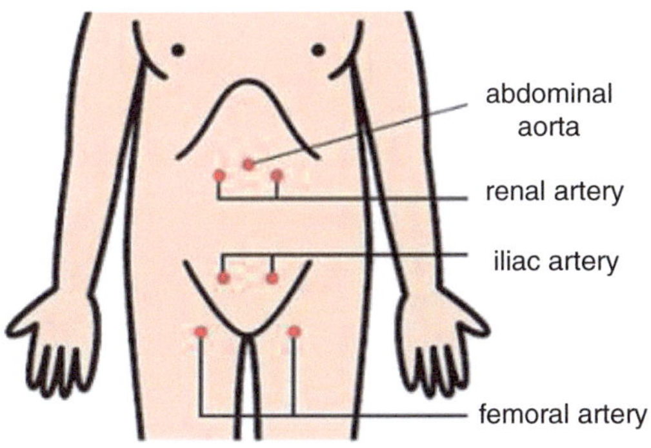

Fig. 78.4 Auscultation sites for vascular bruits

→May indicate abdominal aortic aneurysm, valvular heart disease, or vasculitis.

2. *Bowel sounds*:
   Bowel sounds reflect intestinal motility, which is influenced by food intake and psychological stress.
   - *Typically*:
     – *Normal*: low-pitched, 4–12 sounds/min.
     – *Postprandial*: high-pitched, >12 sounds/min.
     – *Decreased*: often seen in constipation.
     – *Absent*: concerning for ileus or peritonitis.
     – *Hyperactive*: associated with diarrhea or early mechanical obstruction.

5.1 Pathological Findings

- Absence of bowel sounds for >5 minutes → Suggests functional ileus or peritonitis.
- Persistent hyperactive, high-pitched sounds (>12/min) → Suggests diarrhea or mechanical ileus.
- "Metallic sounds" in bowel obstruction result from friction between luminal contents and mucosa.

5.2 Physiological Findings

(a) *Postprandial intestinal motility*:
   1. Gastric contents remain for 2–4 hours, with mixing movements.
      →Swallowed air may remain in the stomach and occasionally produce loud sounds with movement.
   2. Gastric emptying into the small intestine triggers peristalsis lasting 3–8 hours.
      →Even asymptomatic individuals exhibit peristalsis during digestion.
   3. The colon functions in 6–7 cm segments with:
      (i) *Mixing contractions* (nonpropulsive).
      (ii) *Propulsive contractions*, including giant migrating contractions (GMCs), especially postawakening or post-

prandially, as part of the *gastrocolic reflex*.

→ These occur 1–2 times/day, moving feces from the right to the left colon, temporarily halting at the rectosigmoid junction.

→ Mixing sounds are weak and rarely auscultated; propulsive contractions produce strong bowel sounds and often coincide with an urgent need to defecate.

→ In *irritable bowel syndrome (IBS)*, heightened sensitivity to bile acids may prolong postprandial colonic hypermotility [2].

(b) *Stress-related intestinal motility*:

→ In IBS, psychological stress enhances and prolongs intestinal motility [3, 4].

1. Gastric emptying is similar in healthy individuals and IBS patients [5].

→ Except in aerophagia, gastric bubble sounds are not stress-sensitive.

2. Small intestinal dysmotility is reported under stress [6]. In IBS with abdominal bloating, small bowel transit time is shortened [7].

→ Hyperactive bowel sounds may be auscultated in such cases.

→ Aerophagia or small intestinal bacterial overgrowth (SIBO) may also cause increased bowel sounds.

3. Colonic motility, assessed via smooth muscle electromyography, identifies three primary patterns: segmental contractions, propulsive contractions, and GMCs.
   - In diarrhea-predominant IBS, postprandial GMCs and segmental contractions in the sigmoid colon are often absent.
   - In constipation-predominant IBS, both segmental and propulsive contractions are typically preserved.

The author has reported that during unsedated colonoscopy, peristalsis was frequently observed in diarrhea-predominant IBS (Fig. 78.5), while segmental contractions were observed in some cases of constipation-predominant IBS (Fig. 78.6), which disappeared upon relaxation [8].

During endoscopic examination in diarrhea-predominant IBS, borborygmi are often audible. On auscultation, strong peristaltic sounds may be heard, particularly in response to patient anxiety or tension.

In constipation-predominant IBS, segmental contractions are typically silent, and bowel sounds are generally absent.

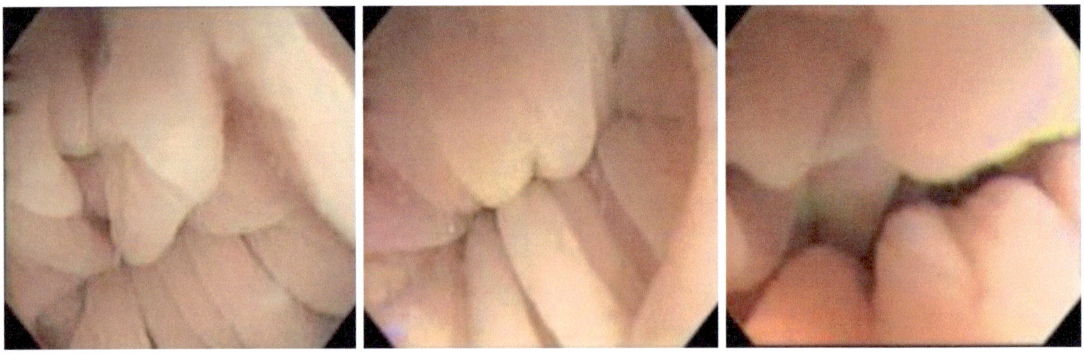

Fig. 78.5 Strong peristalsis in diarrhea-predominant IBS

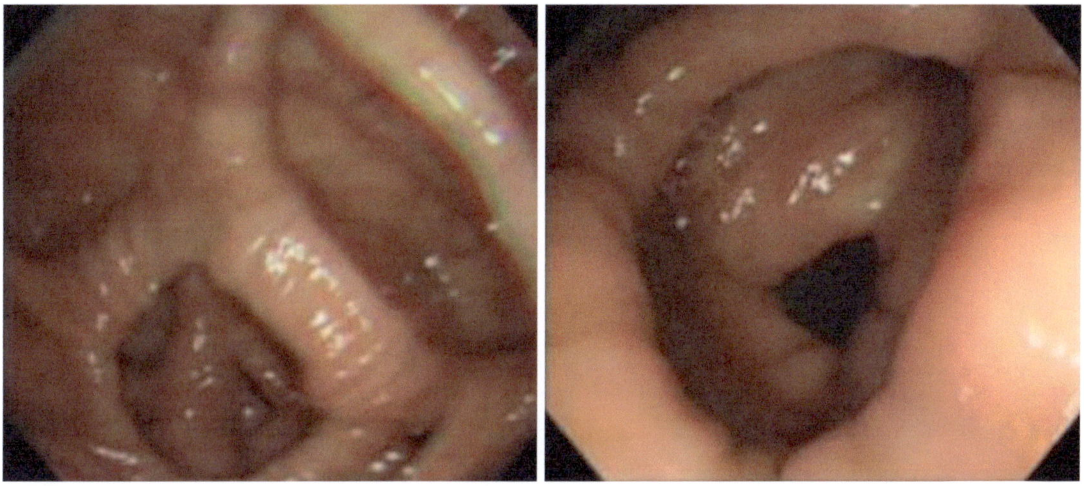

Fig. 78.6 Segmental contractions in constipation-predominant IBS

6 Percussion

Percussion provides information on liver size, gas presence, and distribution and may indicate peritoneal irritation or inflammation.

1. *Liver evaluation*:
   - Percuss the right costal margin to estimate liver protrusion (Fig. 78.7).
   - Place a stethoscope over the epigastrium and stroke the right costal margin to assess sound transmission.

     → Some patients may perceive liver descent or enlargement as vague abdominal discomfort.
2. *Pain induced by percussion*:

   → Suggests peritoneal irradiation sign.
   - Right costal margin: cholecystitis, cholangitis, hepatic abscess, and hepatomegaly.
   - Costovertebral angle: ureteral or renal calculi.
   - Back: pancreatitis and renal calculi.
3. *Gas presence and distribution*:
   - Normal intestinal gas volume: ~200 mL [9]; may be absent (Fig. 78.8).
   - Types of intestinal gas:
     - Swallowed air: nitrogen and oxygen.
     - Fermentation: hydrogen and methane.
     - Acid-base reaction: carbon dioxide (rapidly absorbed from the gastric mucosa)

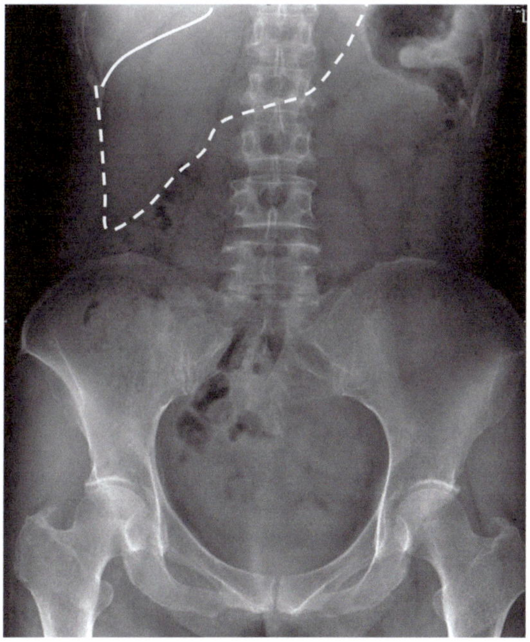

Fig. 78.7 Hepatic ptosis. The liver descends approximately two vertebral bodies below the costal margin

     → Aerophagia and fermentation-derived gases are most clinically relevant.
4. *Stomach bubble*:
   - Results from air swallowed during meals or aerophagia (Fig. 78.9).
   - Postprandial CO_2 produced by neutralization of gastric acid may also contribute.

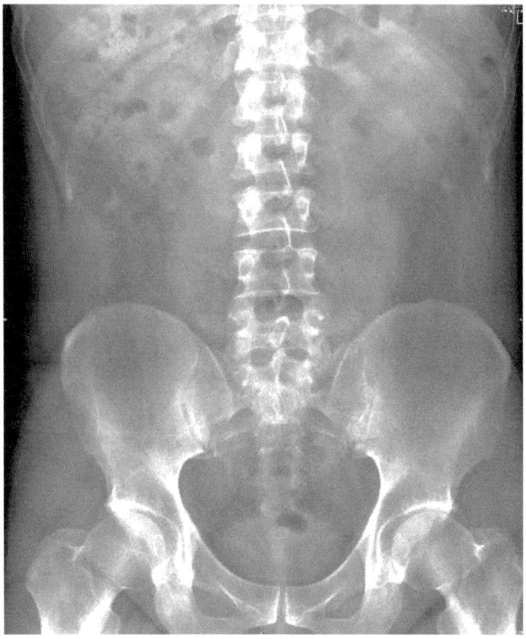

Fig. 78.8 Case with minimal intestinal gas

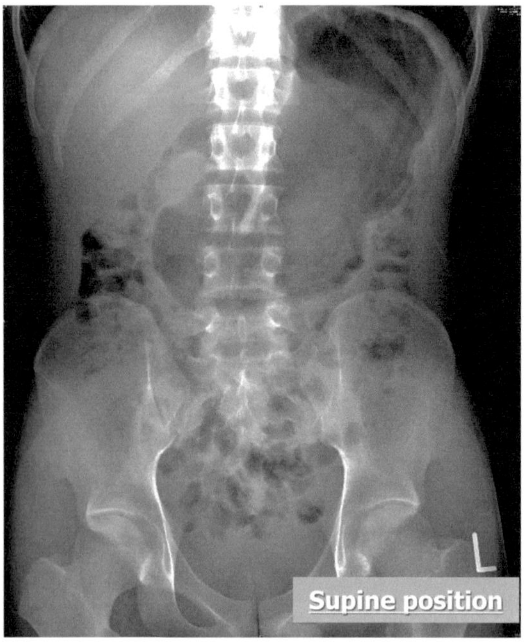

Fig. 78.9 Large gastric bubble in a patient with aerophagia

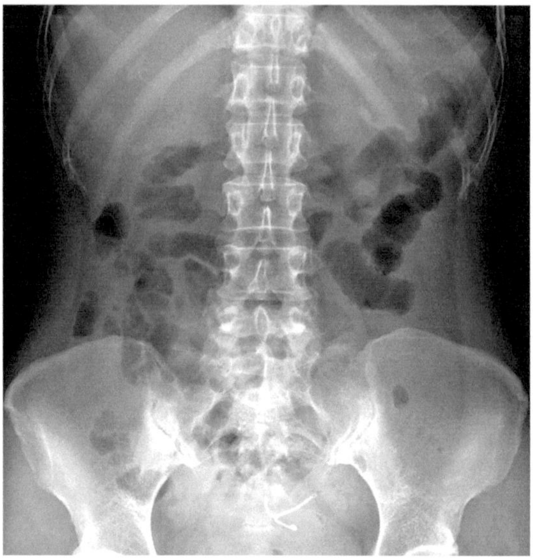

Fig. 78.10 Exocrine pancreatic insufficiency responding to pancrelipase therapy

→ Produces low-pitched tympany in the epigastrium.

5. *Small intestinal gas*:
   - Normally minimal due to rapid transit.
   - Present in indigestion, *SIBO*, or excessive aerophagia.
     - Pancreatic exocrine secretion insufficiency, such as chronic pancreatitis (Fig. 78.10).
     - Gastrinoma with impaired enzyme activation.
     - Alcoholism with accelerated transit time (Fig. 78.11)

       → Tympany around the umbilicus; epigastric gas helps differentiate small bowel origin.
6. *Colonic gas*:
   - From gastric/small bowel transit or *constipation*.

     → Low-pitched tympany over colonic regions.
   - Transverse and sigmoid colon accumulate gas in supine position.
   - In constipation, gas is mainly colonic; coexisting small bowel gas suggests additional pathology.

     → Textbook colonic anatomy [10] (Fig. 78.12) is rare in Japanese patients. Variants include the following:

- Descending colon running centrally (Fig. 78.13a).
- Entire colon in the pelvis (Fig. 78.13b).
- Redundant colon throughout the abdomen (Figure 78.13c)
  → Especially common in constipation-predominant IBS [8].
  → Consider unexpected colonic positioning during examination.

– Large tympany around the umbilicus → sigmoid volvulus (Fig. 78.14).
– Tympany over liver → chilaiditi syndrome (Fig. 78.15): colonic interposition between the liver and diaphragm.

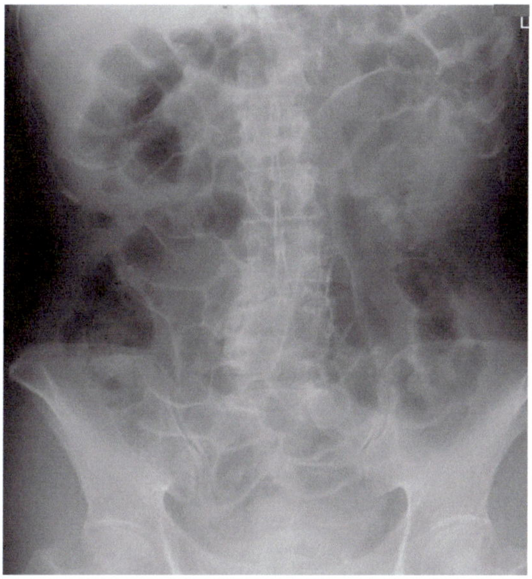

Fig. 78.11 Small intestinal gas in a heavy alcohol consumer

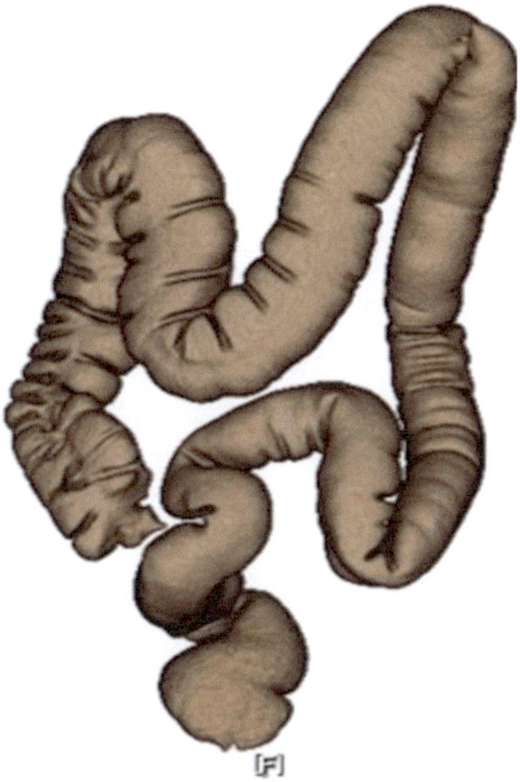

Fig. 78.12 Textbook colonic anatomy. The ascending and descending colon are retroperitoneally fixed [10]

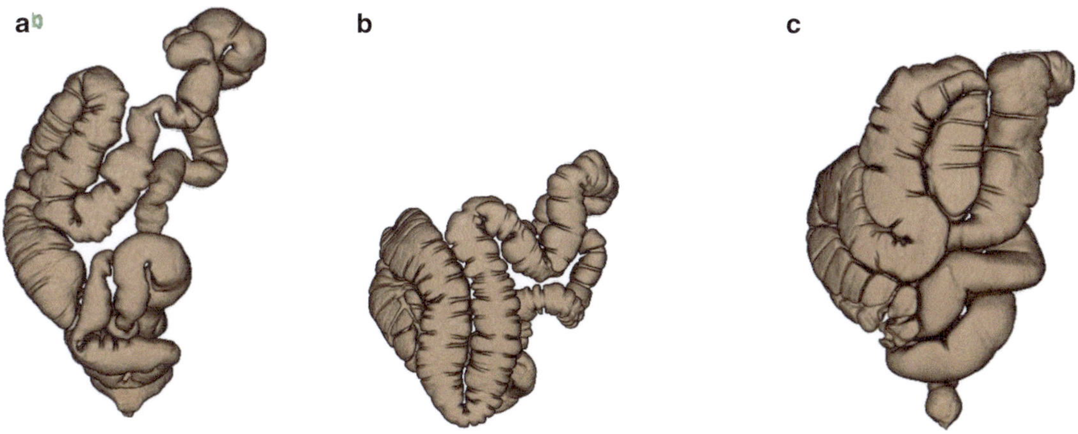

Fig. 78.13 Examples of colonic morphological variants. (**a**) Descending colon runs centrally, (**b**) entire colon located in the pelvic cavity, (**c**) redundant colon distributed throughout the abdominal cavity

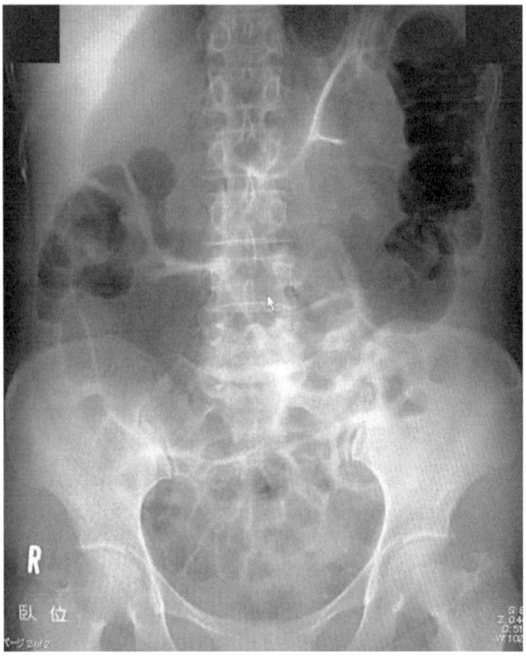

Fig. 78.14 Sigmoid volvulus. "Coffee bean sign" observed on abdominal X-ray

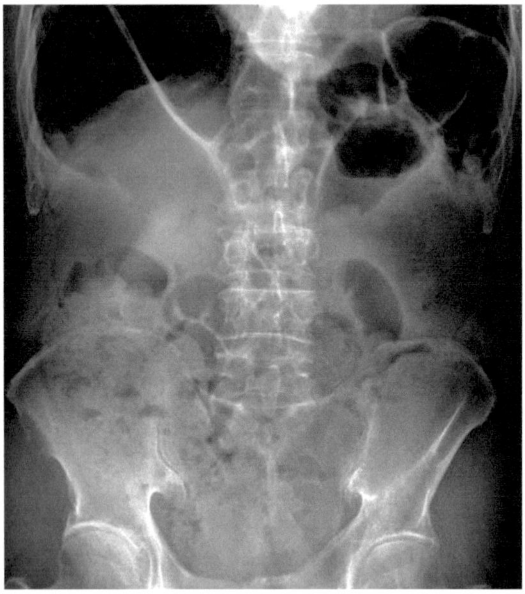

Fig. 78.15 Chilaiditi syndrome. Interposition of the colon between the liver and right diaphragm

7 Palpation

Tender point allows estimation of intraabdominal inflammation, organ size, consistency, and surface characteristics. Only structures firmer than surrounding soft tissue are detectable. In luminal organs, content volume and consistency can be assessed.

Ensure trimmed nails and warm hands. Gently compress the abdominal wall to assess intraabdominal conditions. Obesity, thick abdominal muscles, or strong muscle tension complicates evaluation. Gradual pressure synchronized with respiration may reduce resistance.

- *Liver*: Evaluate for hepatomegaly and surface irregularities.
- *Kidneys, gynecologic organs, intraabdominal arteries*:
  Large ovarian cysts, uterus myoma, and *arterial aneurysms* may be palpable.
  Care must be taken not to mistake the *iliac artery* for *fecal masses* during palpation.
- *Tenderness points* (Fig. 78.16): Peritoneal irritation signs and referred pain, mainly used for diagnosing intraabdominal inflammation (including traditional signs).
  1. *Murphy's sign*: Pain halts inspiration when pressing under right costal margin → Acute cholecystitis.
  2. *McBurney's, Lanz's, and Monroe's points* → Appendicitis.
  3. *Rosenstein's sign*: Increased pain in left lateral decubitus compared to supine position when pressing right periumbilical area → peritonitis or acute appendicitis.
  4. *Rovsing's sign*: Pressing left lower abdomen increases pain in right lower quadrant → peritonitis.
  5. *Blumberg sign:* Press vertically on the abdominal wall with the hand and release suddenly to feel a sharp pain

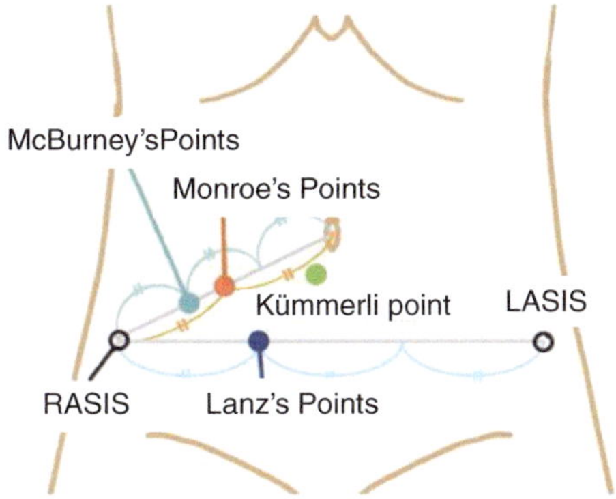

Fig. 78.16 Tenderness points

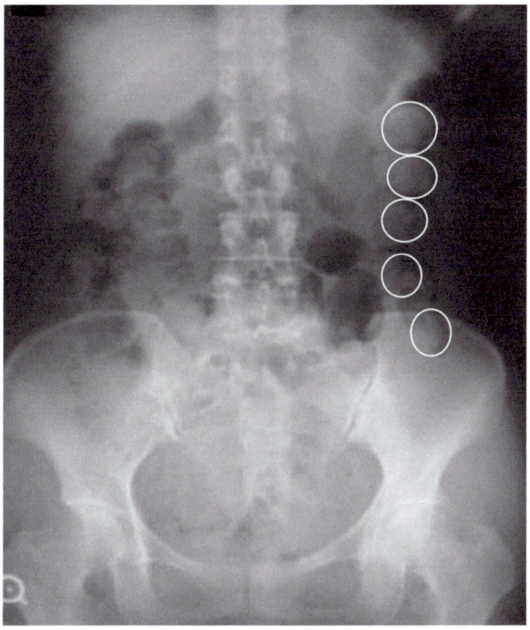

Fig. 78.17 Retained formed stool in the descending colon

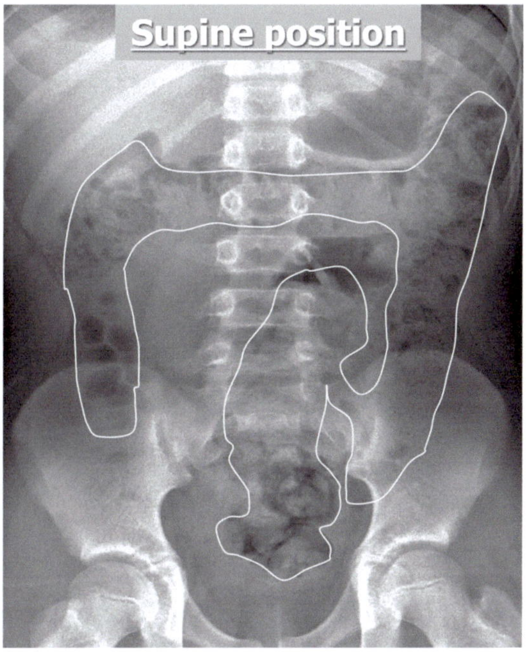

Fig. 78.18 Hard fecal mass in the rectum. Indicative of rectal constipation with absent defecatory urge

called "Rebound tenderness." → peritonitis.

6. Boas' point: Left side of T10–T12 → gastric ulcer.
7. Boas' *gallbladder point*: Right side of T9–T10 → biliary disease.

Estimation of stool form and volume in the colon: Fecal palpation is only possible when feces are firmer than surrounding tissue, typically in the descending colon or beyond. Japanese colonic anatomy varies; colon may not be present at expected sites [8]. After complete defecation, left colon may be empty.

- Feces palpable in descending colon post-defecation → incomplete evacuation (Fig. 78.17).
- Feces in rectum without urge → Rectal hyposensitivity (so-called rectal constipation) (Fig. 78.18).

Stress-related visceral hypersensitivity: Stress lowers sensory thresholds in IBS [11], even with normal motility [6]. → Abdominal pain on palpation in the absence of organic disease may indicate hypersensitivity.

8 Conclusion

This chapter has presented the methods of abdominal physical examination in conjunction with the pathophysiology of functional gastrointestinal disorders (FGIDs) and representative clinical imaging. When considering the patient's condition, time constraints, and healthcare costs, physical examination should be utilized as a complementary tool alongside imaging studies.

Take-Home Message

- Physical findings offer a wealth of real-time information.
- They are invaluable not only for supplementing imaging diagnostics but also for verifying symptoms as they are described by the patient during the clinical encounter.
- The integration of physical examination into routine practice enhances diagnostic accuracy and strengthens the physician-patient relationship, particularly in the management of FGIDs.

Competing Interests The author(s) has no competing interests to declare that are relevant to the content of this manuscript.

References

1. Barba E, et al. Visible abdominal distension in functional gut disorders: objective evaluation. Neurogastroenterol Motil. 2023;35:e14466.
2. Narducci F, et al. Colonic motility and gastric emptying in patients with irritable bowel syndrome. Effect of pretreatment with octylonium bromide. Dig Dis Sci. 1986;31:241–6.
3. Almy TP, et al. Alterations in colonic function in man under stress; experimental production of sigmoid spasm in healthy persons. Gastroenterology. 1949;12:425–36.
4. Fukudo S, et al. Brain-gut response to stress and cholinergic stimulation in irritable bowel syndrome. A preliminary study. J Clin Gastroenterol. 1993;17:133–41.
5. Nielsen OH, et al. Gastric emptying rate and small bowel transit time in patients with irritable bowel syndrome determined with 99mTc-labeled pellets and scintigraphy. Dig Dis Sci. 1986;31:1287–91.
6. Mayer EA, et al. Role of visceral afferent mechanisms in functional bowel disorders. Gastroenterology. 1990;99:1688–704.
7. Hebden JM, et al. Abnormalities of GI transit in bloated irritable bowel syndrome: effect of bran on transit and symptoms. Am J Gastroenterol. 2002;97:2315–20.
8. Mizukami T, et al. Colonic dysmotility and morphological abnormality frequently detected in Japanese patients with irritable bowel syndrome. Intest Res. 2017;15:236–43.
9. Zar S, et al. Review article: bloating in functional bowel disorders. Aliment Pharmacol Ther. 2002;16:1867–76.
10. Mizukami T, et al. Development and application of water immersion method in colonoscopy. J Jpn Soc Gastroenterol Endosc. 2023;65:19–28. (in Japanese)
11. Drossman DA, et al. Alterations of brain activity associated with resolution of emotional distress and pain in a case of severe irritable bowel syndrome. Gastroenterology. 2003;124:754–61.

Further Readings

Chronic Constipation Diagnosis and Treatment Study Group. Clinical practice guidelines for chronic constipation 2017. Tokyo: Nankodo; 2017. (in Japanese).

Japanese Society of Gastroenterology. Clinical practice guidelines for functional gastrointestinal disorders 2020. Tokyo: Nankodo; 2020. (in Japanese).

79 Practical Treatment, Physical Findings in the Abdomen, Digital Rectal Examination

Noriaki Manabe

Abstract

Digital rectal examination (DRE) is a crucial physical examination technique that contributes significantly to diagnosis, particularly in functional gastrointestinal disorders where organic diseases must be excluded. It serves as an important screening tool for anorectal functional disorders. DRE allows assessment of anal sphincter function, tone, sensation, presence and consistency of stool, and the need for disimpaction. It also aids in excluding rectal and prostatic tumors. Absolute contraindication for DRE is lack of patient consent, while relative contraindications include recent anal surgery, anal stricture, or severe anal pain. The procedure involves visual inspection of the perianal area, followed by palpation of the distal rectum and anal canal with a lubricated finger. Key steps include assessing sphincter tone at rest and during voluntary contraction and relaxation and evaluating the rectal wall for abnormalities. While DRE's reliability in assessing anal sphincter function in fecal incontinence patients has shown conflicting results, recent scoring systems like DRESS score demonstrate good correlation with anorectal manometry. DRE is a reliable bedside tool for evaluating dyssynergic defecation and screening patients who require further physiological testing like anorectal manometry. Complications are rare and typically mild, such as discomfort or abrasions, which can be minimized with proper lubrication and patient instruction. DRE is a valuable skill for evaluating anorectal function and screening patients for more specialized tests in cases of fecal incontinence or chronic constipation, though adequate training is essential for proficiency.

Keywords

Digital rectal examination · Anorectal function · Fecal incontinence · Chronic constipation · Dyssynergic defecation

1 Introduction

In general internal medicine outpatient settings, physical examination is reported to contribute approximately 5–15% to diagnostic accuracy. Therefore, conducting a thorough physical examination is of paramount importance. Digital rectal examination (DRE) should be performed not only in patients presenting with hematochezia but also in broader clinical contexts. However, due to embarrassment experienced by both phy-

N. Manabe (✉)
Division of Endoscopy and Ultrasonography, Department of Clinical Laboratory Medicine, Kawasaki Medical School, Okayama, Japan
e-mail: n_manabe@med.kawasaki-m.ac.jp

H. Kaneko et al. (eds.), *Disorders of Gut-Brain Interaction*,
https://doi.org/10.1007/978-981-95-6974-8_79

sicians and patients, this examination is often omitted. It is thus essential to explain its necessity to patients in advance. In particular, when examining female patients, the presence of a same-gender nurse is mandatory.

In the diagnosis of functional gastrointestinal disorders (FGIDs), it is essential not only to exclude organic diseases but also to screen for functional disorders of the anorectal region. DRE plays a significant role in this context. Specifically, DRE is a critical component of the physical examination, involving visual inspection of the perianal skin, palpation of the distal rectum and anal canal, and, when appropriate, fecal occult blood testing using stool adhered to the examination glove. These steps greatly contribute to determining subsequent diagnostic and therapeutic strategies.

2 Indications for Digital Rectal Examination

DRE allows for the assessment of anal sphincter function, tone, and sensation, the presence and characteristics of stool, the effectiveness of laxatives, and the necessity for manual disimpaction [1]. It is also a valuable technique for excluding rectal tumors and, in male patients, prostatic neoplasms.

3 Contraindications to Digital Rectal Examination

The absolute contraindication to DRE is the absence of patient consent. Relative contraindications include recent anorectal surgery, anal stenosis, and severe anal pain. However, in cases of significant anal pain, the examination may be performed under local anesthesia with the patient's consent [2].

4 Relevant Anatomy for Digital Rectal Examination

The rectum begins at the rectosigmoid junction and is distinguished from the colon by the absence of taeniae coli (Fig. 79.1). The anal canal begins at the anorectal junction and is demarcated by the anorectal ring, located at the superior attachment of the puborectalis muscle. In adults, the anal canal typically measures 3–5 cm in length and terminates at the anal verge, where the anal canal epithelium transitions to perianal skin.

The anal canal is divided by the dentate line. The region 6–12 mm above the dentate line consists of transitional epithelium—columnar, cuboidal, and stratified squamous—and is referred to as the cloacogenic zone. This area contains diffuse autonomic nerve fibers. Below the dentate line to the anal verge, the epithelium is stratified squamous without skin appendages such as hair follicles, sebaceous glands, or sweat glands and is termed the anoderm. This region is richly innervated by somatic nerve fibers, which explains why most painful anal disorders originate in the lower anal canal [3].

The internal anal sphincter, composed of smooth muscle, maintains tonic contraction to allow for continence. The external anal sphincter, composed of skeletal muscle, is under voluntary control and contracts in response to the sensation of defecation, thereby delaying bowel movements.

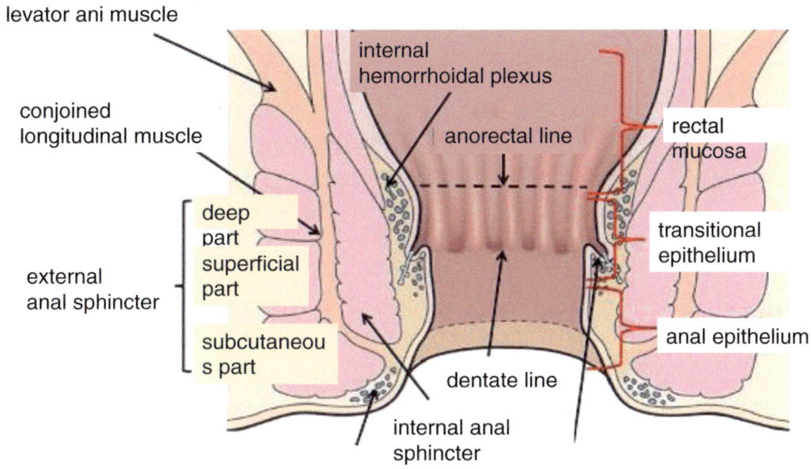

Fig. 79.1 Anatomy related to digital rectal examination. Anatomical structures relevant to performing a digital rectal examination

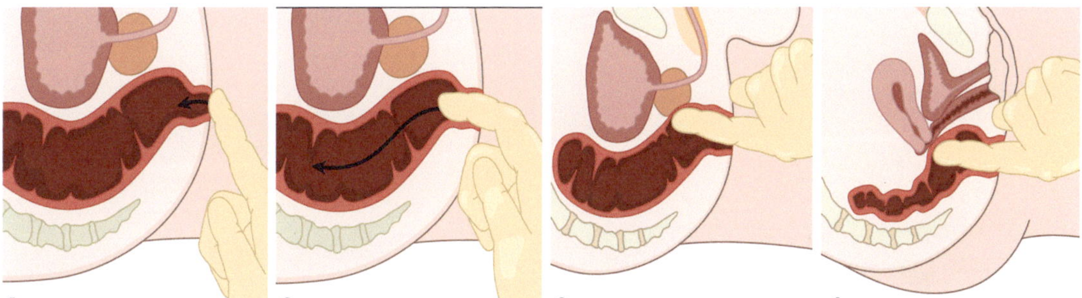

1 2 3 4

1. Insert the tip of the gloved index finger into the anus

2. Introduce your finger to follow the curve of the sacrum

3 and 4. Rotate the finger anteriorly to palpate the anterolateral and lateral walls and the prostate or cervix.

(Reproduced with permission from Elsevier)

Fig. 79.2 Procedure for digital rectal examination. Steps of the digital rectal examination procedure. (Adapted from Ref. [4])

5 Procedure for Digital Rectal Examination [4] (Fig. 79.2)

DRE can be performed in various positions, including standing, knee-chest, and prone positions. The left lateral position is the most commonly used. In postoperative patients or those unable to maintain this position, the choice of position should consider both physician preference and patient capability.

Before beginning the examination, the examiner should wear two gloves on the dominant hand and one glove on the nondominant hand. The examination begins with inspection of the perineal area. The buttocks are gently separated to observe the perianal region for external lesions. For example, in patients with severe anal pain, the presence of anal fissures or thrombosed external hemorrhoids may obviate the need for DRE.

If rectal prolapse is suspected based on symptoms, the patient should be asked to strain, allowing direct observation of prolapsed hemorrhoids or rectal mucosa.

Next, the examiner prepares for palpation of the anal canal and rectum. Lubricant is applied to the index finger of the dominant hand and to the patient's anus. The patient is instructed to exhale to relax the anal sphincter. The examiner gently inserts the index finger into the anal canal, advancing into the rectum while minimizing discomfort. A slight tightening may be felt at the anorectal ring.

Once inside the rectum, the examiner rotates the finger circumferentially to palpate the rectal wall thoroughly, ensuring no small lesions are missed. The finger is then withdrawn to the anal canal, and the patient is instructed to contract the anus and then strain as if defecating. This allows assessment of sphincter tone and detection of nodules, irregularities, or tenderness.

In male patients, the prostate should be palpated by rotating the finger anteriorly, assessing its size, shape, consistency, and the presence of nodules or tenderness.

Before removing the finger, the patient is asked to strain again and then relax the sphincter. The examiner pulls out the finger and checks the gloves for blood and, if there is any fecal matter, checks its characteristics. If bleeding is suspected but not visible, a fecal occult blood test may be performed using the stool on the glove.

6 Clinical Utility of Digital Rectal Examination

Several studies have evaluated the accuracy of DRE in patients with fecal incontinence. Some report a strong correlation between DRE findings and anal sphincter parameters at rest and during contraction [5], while others report poor correlation [6]. Recently, the Digital Rectal Examination Scoring System (DRESS), which uses a 0–5 scale, has been developed and shows good correlation with anorectal manometry results [7] (Table 79.1).

Table 79.1 Digital rectal examination scoring system (DRESS)

Resting score	
0	No anal tone at all; anus is completely open
1	Extremely low tone
2	Slightly low tone
3	Normal tone
4	Slightly high tone
5	Extremely high tone
Contraction score	
0	No contraction at all
1	Mild contraction
2	Considerable contraction but weaker than normal
3	Normal contraction
4	Strong contraction
5	Extremely strong contraction, causing pain to the examining finger

This table is reproduced from a paper by Orkin et al. [7]

Comparative studies between DRE and ultrasonography for assessing sphincter defects show good correlation when defects are large (150–270°), but poor correlation when defects are small (<90°) [8]. Coura et al. reported a sensitivity of 90% but a specificity of only 28%, indicating limited diagnostic accuracy [9].

These discrepancies may be due to factors such as examiner finger size, technique, experience, and patient cooperation, all of which can affect results and lead to interexaminer variability. Therefore, DRE is considered to have limited reliability in evaluating anal sphincter function in patients with fecal incontinence. However, recent studies suggest that when performed by well-trained examiners, DRE correlates more closely with other modalities [10].

In contrast, a prospective study comparing DRE and anorectal manometry in patients with rectal sphincter dyssynergia reported excellent results: sensitivity 75%, specificity 87%, and positive predictive value 97% [11]. Similar findings have been confirmed in other studies. Additionally, DRE findings show moderate correlation with imaging-based diagnoses of rectocele [12].

These findings support the use of DRE as a reliable bedside tool for evaluating rectal sphincter dyssynergia and for screening patients who may require further physiological testing such as anorectal manometry.

7 Complications

Complications associated with DRE are generally rare and mild. The most common issues include patient discomfort and minor abrasions around the anus, which can be prevented with adequate lubrication. Patients who are extremely tense may experience pain due to anal sphincter contraction. In such cases, instructing the patient to exhale deeply and, if necessary, using a lubricant containing local anesthetic can help alleviate discomfort [13].

8 Conclusion

DRE is not only useful for diagnosing defecatory disorders but also serves as a screening tool to identify patients who may require advanced diagnostic procedures such as anorectal manometry. As a primary bedside assessment of anorectal function, DRE is a valuable technique. A normal DRE can effectively exclude many anorectal functional disorders. Conversely, if further evaluation is deemed necessary based on DRE findings, both further examination for organic disease using anoscopy and functional assessments such as anorectal manometry should be performed.

In the United States, despite clinical training, many residents lack proficiency in DRE, particularly in assessing anal sphincter tone in patients with fecal incontinence—a situation that has raised concerns [14]. This issue is similarly observed in Japan. Recent studies have demonstrated that DRE can provide evaluations comparable to anorectal manometry and have highlighted its clinical utility. At the same time, these studies emphasize the need for proper training to master the technique.

Take-Home Message
DRE is a useful bedside examination for patients with fecal incontinence or chronic constipation, as it not only evaluates anorectal function but also screens patients who require further examination such as anorectal manometry.

Competing Interests The author(s) has no competing interests to declare that are relevant to the content of this manuscript.

References

1. Royal College of Nursing. Digital rectal examination and manual removal of faeces: guidance for nurses. 3rd ed. London: RCN; 2003.
2. Muris JW, et al. The diagnostic value of rectal examination. Fam Pract. 1993;10:34–7.
3. Barleben A, et al. Anorectal anatomy and physiology. Surg Clin North Am. 2010;90:1–15.
4. Steggall MJ. Digital rectal examination. Nurs Stand. 2008;22:46–8.
5. Hallan RI, et al. Comparison of digital and manometric assessment of anal-sphincter function. Br J Surg. 1989;76:973–5.
6. Hill J, et al. History and examination in the assessment of patients with idiopathic fecal incontinence. Dis Colon Rectum. 1994;37:473–7.
7. Orkin BA, et al. The digital rectal examination scoring system (DRESS). Dis Colon Rectum. 2010;53:1656–60.
8. Dobben AC, et al. Anal inspection and digital rectal examination compared to anorectal physiology tests and endoanal ultrasonography in evaluating fecal incontinence. Int J Color Dis. 2007;22:783–90.
9. Coura MM, et al. Is digital rectal exam reliable in grading anal sphincter defects? Arq Gastroenterol. 2016;53:240–5.
10. Evans P, et al. Validating the inter-rater reliability of an anorectal assessment tool. Gastrointest Nurs. 2015;13:42–6.
11. Tantiphlachiva K, et al. Digital rectal examination is a useful tool for identifying patients with dyssynergia. Clin Gastroenterol Hepatol. 2010;8:955–60.
12. Rachaneni S, et al. Digital rectal examination in the evaluation of rectovaginal septal defects. Int Urogynecol J. 2017;28:1401–5.
13. Talley NJ. How to do and interpret a rectal examination in gastroenterology. Am J Gastroenterol. 2008;103:820–2.
14. Attaluri A, et al. Trainee vs expert assessment of digital rectal examination (DRE) for anorectal dysfunction: does experience matter? A prospective study. Am J Gastroenterol. 2009;104:S484–500.

Practical Treatment, Treatment of Intractable Abdominal Pain

80

Tsukasa Nozu

Abstract

In Japan, physicians may overlook functional disorders in patients without detectable abnormalities, despite functional abdominal pain being a common human experience. Among functional gastrointestinal disorders (FGIDs), centrally mediated abdominal pain syndrome (CAPS) is notably difficult to manage and significantly impairs quality of life. CAPS is characterized by chronic abdominal pain unrelated to meals or defecation and lacks peripheral autonomic signs despite severe pain. It frequently coexists with psychiatric conditions and often leads to doctor shopping and unnecessary procedures.

The pathophysiology suggests a central origin, involving central sensitization following peripheral nerve injury, diminished visceral sensitivity to physiological stimuli, and dysfunction of descending pain modulation systems. CAPS patients may also have impaired pelvic nerve function. Differential diagnoses include anterior cutaneous nerve entrapment syndrome (ACNES), abdominal epilepsy, and abdominal migraine. Management requires a multidisciplinary approach, including psychiatric support, education about CAPS, realistic goal-setting, and use of antidepressants or psychological therapies. Early recognition and appropriate intervention are essential to avoid worsening symptoms and dependency on narcotics. Internists and gastroenterologists play a critical role in identifying and managing CAPS to improve patient outcomes.

Keywords

Centrally mediated abdominal pain syndrome · Central sensitization · Neuropathic pain · Doctor shopping · Patient-physician relationship

In Japan, where endoscopic examinations are widely available, physicians may fall into the pattern of not recognizing patients without detectable abnormalities as having a legitimate illness. However, functional abdominal pain is a universal human experience. Therefore, when evaluating patients with abdominal pain, it is essential to consider functional gastrointestinal disorders (FGIDs) alongside organic diseases.

T. Nozu (✉)
Asahikawa Medical University, Asahikawa, Japan
e-mail: tnozu@asahikawa-med.ac.jp

H. Kaneko et al. (eds.), *Disorders of Gut-Brain Interaction*,
https://doi.org/10.1007/978-981-95-6974-8_80

Patients with FGIDs who are dissatisfied with their medical care often experience heightened anxiety, leading to doctor shopping, which in turn exacerbates their abdominal pain. Repeated consultations across multiple institutions may result in the development of refractory abdominal pain [1]. Among FGIDs, centrally mediated abdominal pain syndrome (CAPS) is one of the most challenging conditions to manage and significantly impairs patients' quality of life (QoL). This section focuses on CAPS as a representative disorder of refractory abdominal pain.

1 Definition

CAPS is the only FGID defined by the Rome IV criteria that is not classified based on a specific gastrointestinal organ responsible for the functional abnormality [2]. The Rome IV diagnostic criteria for CAPS are presented in Table 80.1 [2]. Abdominal pain in CAPS is typically unrelated to peripheral organ events such as meals, defecation, or menstruation.

Table 80.1 Diagnostic criteria[a] for centrally mediated abdominal pain syndrome (CAPS)[b]

Must include all of the following:
Continuous or nearly continuous abdominal pain
No or only occasional relationship of pain with physiological events (e.g., eating, defecation, or menses)[c]
Pain limits some aspect of daily functioning
The pain is not feigned
Pain is not explained by another structural or functional gastrointestinal disorder or other medical condition

[a]Criteria fulfilled for the last three months with symptom onset at least six months before diagnosis
[b]CAPS is typically associated with psychiatric comorbidity, but there is no specific profile that can be used for diagnosis
[c]Some degree of gastrointestinal dysfunction may be present
[d]Daily function could include impairments in work, intimacy, social/leisure, family life, and caregiving for self or others

2 Epidemiology

Community-based studies in Western countries report a prevalence of 0.5–2.2% in the general population [3]. CAPS is more common in women, with a peak onset in the 35–40 age range [3]. It is frequently associated with psychiatric comorbidities such as depression and anxiety disorders, increased visits to medical institutions, repeated endoscopic procedures, and a higher incidence of abdominal and pelvic surgeries. Patients often engage in doctor shopping, experience severely impaired QOL, and are frequently referred to tertiary care centers [1, 4].

3 Diagnosis

The first step is to exclude organic diseases. Diagnosis is then made by comparing the patient's symptoms to the Rome IV criteria (Table 80.1) [2]. Patients often describe their pain in terms such as "a burning sensation in the intestines" or "as if being gouged with a knife," and most are unable to localize the pain precisely. When the physician suggests a psychological component, patients may become irritable or deny the association. Loss experiences such as the death of a family member or miscarriage and life stressors are often implicated in the onset or exacerbation of symptoms. A notable feature is the lack of autonomic responses (e.g., sweating, tachycardia) despite reports of severe pain.

4 Pathophysiology

4.1 Neuropathic Pain

The frequent efficacy of low-dose tricyclic antidepressants (TCAs) in CAPS suggests a neuropathic mechanism. This type of pain is thought to involve visceral hypersensitivity at both peripheral and central levels. CAPS has little association with abdominal pain and events such as eating or defecation, and it is unlikely that pain is caused by stimulation of the intestines and increased firing of peripheral sensory nerves. Instead, abnormalities at the central level such as central visceral hypersensitivity are suspected.

4.2 Establishment of Central Visceral Hypersensitivity

When peripheral sensory nerves transmitting visceral sensations are damaged, sustained neural input to the central nervous system (spinal cord and brain) occurs. This persistent input induces a phenomenon known as central sensitization, leading to hypersensitivity. Although healing mechanisms eventually eliminate the neural input, the sensitization may persist, resulting in chronic central hypersensitivity. In this state, patients may continue to perceive pain even in the absence of sensory nerve stimulation from the intestine, leading to CAPS. Repeated abdominal surgeries are common in CAPS patients, and in some cases, surgery can cause nerve damage, and other factors such as pregnancy, childbirth, infections, and medications can also lead to similar nerve disorders.

4.3 Visceral Sensory Function in CAPS

Our group has evaluated human visceral sensory function using a barostat device. This method involves inflating a balloon in the rectum to determine the pressure threshold at which pain is perceived. In patients with irritable bowel syndrome (IBS), rectal pain thresholds are typically reduced, indicating visceral hypersensitivity [5]. In contrast, CAPS patients show no difference in pain thresholds compared to healthy controls, suggesting the absence of visceral hypersensitivity [5]. These findings indicate that while intestinal distension stimulates peripheral sensory nerve activity and is perceived as pain, this response remains within the normal physiological range. Therefore, the concept of CAPS as a disorder originating from central mechanisms is not contradicted by these results.

Next, instead of using strong distension stimuli that elicit pain, a physiological level of distension—one that does not induce pain in healthy individuals—was applied. The intensity of the sensation experienced during this distension was measured using a Visual Analogue Scale (VAS). The results showed that patients with IBS reported higher sensory intensity, whereas patients with CAPS reported lower intensity compared to healthy controls [5]. This suggests that in CAPS, there is sensory hyposensitivity to physiological distension stimuli. What do these findings imply?

Physiological stimuli in the rectum—such as the presence of stool or gas—are transmitted via the sacral parasympathetic nerves (pelvic nerves). Therefore, it is plausible that pelvic nerve dysfunction may be present in CAPS. If the pelvic nerves are damaged for any reason, sustained neural input to the spinal cord may occur, leading to central sensitization. At the same time, due to the nerve injury, peripheral nerve function is diminished, resulting in reduced responsiveness to physiological stimuli in the intestines.

This interpretation may provide a coherent explanation for the pathophysiology of CAPS.

4.4 Descending Pain Modulation

Afferent pain signals from the gastrointestinal tract are modulated by descending pain inhibitory pathways, which involve noradrenergic and serotonergic systems originating in the brainstem. These systems regulate neuronal excitability at the spinal dorsal horn, suppressing excessive central input. Dysfunction of this inhibitory system has been implicated in CAPS. Reduced central serotonergic signaling is also observed in psychiatric disorders such as depression, which aligns with the high comorbidity of CAPS with psychiatric conditions.

5 Differential Diagnosis

Differential diagnoses include malignancies of the gastrointestinal or genitourinary systems, inflammatory bowel disease, pelvic peritonitis, and acute intermittent porphyria. These conditions can generally be excluded through imaging, blood chemistry, and microbiological testing.

Abdominal pain may also originate from the abdominal wall rather than intraabdominal organs. Anterior cutaneous nerve entrapment syndrome (ACNES) accounts for 15–30% of abdominal wall pain cases [6] and is frequently misdiagnosed as CAPS or other FGIDs [7]. The anterior cutaneous branches of spinal nerves bend at 90° as they pass through the rectus abdominis muscle to reach the skin. In ACNES, these nerves are compressed at this point, causing pain. The causes include obesity, tight-fitting clothing, increased intraabdominal pressure, pregnancy, and increased estrogen and progesterone levels due to oral contraceptives, which result in swelling of the tissues surrounding the nerves and pressure on the nerves. However, the cause is unknown in many cases.

Symptoms include chronic pain at the lateral edge of the rectus abdominis, with a highly localized tender point (<2 cm in diameter). Abnormal skin sensations (hyperesthesia or hypoesthesia) may be present around the tender point. Pain worsens with abdominal wall tension and improves in the supine position but is exacerbated by standing, movement, or coughing. Local anesthetic injection at the tender point typically relieves the pain. Blood tests and imaging are usually unremarkable.

Other rare conditions that cause chronic abdominal pain without abnormalities on standard tests include abdominal epilepsy (a form of epilepsy with abdominal pain and EEG abnormalities) and abdominal migraine (recurrent midline abdominal pain with nausea and vomiting but no headache). These conditions must also be differentiated from CAPS.

6 Treatment

It is often difficult for general internists or gastroenterologists to manage CAPS independently. Psychiatric intervention is essential, but referral to psychiatry may be challenging. Establishing a strong patient-physician relationship and helping the patient understand the need for psychiatric treatment to alleviate abdominal pain is crucial. Simply stating that no abnormalities were found on tests is insufficient. Repeated explanations of the pathophysiology of CAPS help patients understand their condition and mark the first step toward treatment.

Patients who are not satisfied with their care may engage in doctor shopping or visit emergency departments at night, where they may be inappropriately prescribed narcotic analgesics, leading to dependency. To manage pain effectively, it is advisable to involve psychiatrists as part of the treatment team. Even after referral, continued involvement by the internist or gastroenterologist helps maintain patient trust.

When initiating treatment, it is important to clarify therapeutic goals. Many chronic pain patients expect complete pain relief, but striving for perfection may worsen or prolong symptoms. The goal should be to reduce abdominal pain to a level that does not interfere with daily life. Pharmacologic options include TCAs, serotonin-norepinephrine reuptake inhibitors (SNRIs), and selective serotonin reuptake inhibitors (SSRIs). Cognitive behavioral therapy and hypnotherapy may also be beneficial.

7 Conclusion

Abdominal pain is a key symptom in gastrointestinal disorders, but it more often results from functional abnormalities than from organic disease [3]. Therefore, internists and gastroenterologists must take FGIDs seriously to fulfill their professional responsibilities. CAPS significantly impairs QoL. To prevent the development of severe CAPS cases, the role of internists and gastroenterologists is important.

Take-Home Message

- CAPS is characterized by chronic abdominal pain that shows minimal correlation with gastrointestinal function.
- Central sensitization is thought to play a key role in its pathophysiology.
- CAPS is frequently accompanied by psychiatric comorbidities, including depression and anxiety.
- Many patients suffer from significant impairment in QoL and often engage in repeated doctor shopping.
- Building a strong patient-physician relationship is essential, and physicians treating abdominal pain must be familiar with the concept of CAPS.

Competing Interests The author(s) has no competing interests to declare that are relevant to the content of this manuscript.

References

1. Nozu T. Clinical analysis of Functional Gastrointestinal Disorders (FGIDs). J Fellow Jpn Soc Intern Med. 2001;13:713–8. (in Japanese).
2. Keefer L, et al. Centrally mediated disorders of gastrointestinal pain. Gastroenterology. 2016;150:1408–19.
3. Drossman DA, et al. U.S. householder survey of functional gastrointestinal disorders: prevalence, sociodemography, and health impact. Dig Dis Sci. 1993;38:1569–80.
4. Nozu T, et al. Inadequate health care-seeking behavior of Japanese patients with functional gastrointestinal disorders: a preliminary survey. J Gastroenterol. 2002;37:231–2.
5. Nozu T, et al. Altered rectal sensory response induced by balloon distention in patients with functional abdominal pain syndrome. Biopsychosoc Med. 2009;3:13.
6. Srinivasan R, et al. Chronic abdominal wall pain: a frequently overlooked problem. Practical approach to diagnosis and management. Am J Gastroenterol. 2002;97:824–30.
7. van Assen T, et al. Chronic abdominal wall pain misdiagnosed as functional abdominal pain. J Am Board Fam Med. 2013;26:738–44.

81 Practical Treatment, Forefront of Kampo Treatment

Hiroshi Takeda

Abstract

Kampo medicine, a traditional Japanese herbal system, is increasingly demonstrating its efficacy for functional gastrointestinal disorders (FGIDs) through randomized controlled trials (RCTs), complementing its classic use based on patient pattern (*sho*) diagnosis. This review synthesizes current clinical evidence and mechanisms of key Kampo formulas. For functional dyspepsia, *Rikkunshito* is the first-line treatment, proven to enhance ghrelin signaling and improve gastric motility. In cases of PPI-refractory GERD, Hangeshashinto offers significant therapeutic benefit. For irritable bowel syndrome (IBS), treatments are tailored to subtypes: Keishikashakuyakuto for mixed-type, Ninjinto for diarrhea-predominant, and Daikenchuto for constipation with bloating. Furthermore, Daikenchuto is effective for postoperative ileus and functional constipation by promoting intestinal motility and blood flow. Unlike single-target Western pharmaceuticals, these multicomponent medicines modulate integrated regulatory systems via prokinetic, anti-inflammatory, and psychotropic actions. This evidence confirms that Kampo medicine provides a valuable, multitarget therapeutic strategy for the complex pathophysiology of FGIDs, offering effective options where conventional treatments are limited.

Keywords

Kampo medicine · Functional gastrointestinal disorders (FGIDs) · Functional dyspepsia (FD) · Irritable bowel syndrome (IBS) · Gastroesophageal reflux disease (GERD) · Ghrelin · *Sho* (patient pattern)

1 Introduction

Traditionally, Kampo medicine has been prescribed based on the concept of *sho* (証, patient pattern). However, in recent years, its efficacy has increasingly been demonstrated through randomized controlled trials (RCTs) independent of *sho*-based diagnosis. This trend includes a growing body of research supporting the effectiveness of Kampo formulations in the treatment of functional gastrointestinal disorders (FGIDs).

To begin, a brief overview of the fundamental Kampo diagnostic framework of *yin-yang* and *kyo-jitsu* (deficiency-excess) is warranted [1]. A state of robust physical resistance to disease is classified as *jitsu* (excess), while a weakened

H. Takeda (✉)
Gastroenterology, Caress Memorial Hospital, Sapporo, Japan

Faculty of Pharmaceutical Sciences, Hokkaido University, Sapporo, Japan
e-mail: h_takeda@pharm.hokudai.ac.jp

H. Kaneko et al. (eds.), *Disorders of Gut-Brain Interaction*,
https://doi.org/10.1007/978-981-95-6974-8_81

state is termed *kyo* (deficiency). Patients are categorized into *Jitsu-sho* (excess pattern), *chukan-sho* (intermediate pattern), or *kyo-sho* (deficiency pattern). Additionally, a hypermetabolic state with systemic or localized heat is considered *yang*, whereas a hypometabolic, cold state is considered *yin*. Based on the combination of these axes, patients are classified into four categories, *yang*-excess, *yang*-deficiency, *yin*-excess, and *yin*-deficiency, which serve as guides for prescription selection.

In some cases, abdominal findings guide the choice of Kampo formula. Examples include the following:

- *Epigastric stiffness and discomfort (shinka-hiko)*: Pain or discomfort upon palpation of the epigastric region, indicating suitability for formulas such as Ninjinto or Shasinto -based formulas.
- *Splashing sounds in the stomach (ibushinsui-on)*: Audible water sounds upon light percussion of the epigastrium, suggesting the use of Ninjito.
- *Fullness and discomfort in the hypochondrium (kyokaku-kuman)*: Resistance under the costal margin, indicating the use of formulas containing Saiko (e.g., Shosaikoto).

2 Use of Kampo Medicine in Functional Gastrointestinal Disorders and Clinical Evidence

2.1 Esophageal Disorders

In patients with gastroesophageal reflux disease (GERD) who do not respond to proton pump inhibitor (PPI) therapy—so-called PPI-refractory GERD—are demonstrated approximately 40–50% in nonerosive gastroesophageal reflux disease (NERD). In such cases, clinicians often attempt modifications in PPI dosage or administration methods. Additionally, Kampo medicine, prokinetic agents, antacids, and mucosal protective agents are frequently used in combination.

RCTs involving PPI-refractory GERD patients have demonstrated that coadministration of Rikkunshito or Hangeshashinto yields therapeutic effects comparable to doubling the PPI dose [2]. In pediatric GERD, *Rikkunshito* has been reported to reduce esophageal acid exposure time and enhance esophageal clearance [3]. These findings suggest that combining Rikkunshito or Hangeshashinto with PPI therapy may be a promising treatment strategy for PPI-refractory GERD [4].

The Japanese GERD clinical practice guidelines also address this approach. In response to the clinical question, "Are there agents that provide additional benefit when combined with acid-suppressive therapy such as PPIs, including prokinetics and Kampo medicine?," the guidelines state: "Symptom improvement can be achieved by combining Kampo medicine with PPI therapy" [2].

2.2 Functional Dyspepsia (FD)

There is a growing consensus regarding the appropriate use of Kampo medicine in the treatment of functional dyspepsia (FD) [3, 4] (see Fig. 81.1) [5]. For postprandial distress syndrome (PDS), *Rikkunshito* is considered the first-line treatment. Depending on specific subjective and objective findings, Hangeshashinto, Bukuryoin, or Ninjinto may be selected. If these are ineffective, Kososan or Heisan, which possess anxiolytic and antidepressant properties, may be considered.

For epigastric pain syndrome (EPS), Anchusan is the first-line treatment. Depending on the clinical presentation, Hangeshashinto-, Bukuryoin-, Ninjinto-, Orento-, or Saiko-based formulas (Daisaikoto, Saikokeishito, Shigyakusan) may be used. If these are ineffective, Kososan or Heiisan may be considered.

Rikkunshito is the most widely used Kampo formula for FD in Japan. It is particularly effective in patients presenting with postprandial fullness or early satiety, especially when accompanied by anorexia. It is broadly applicable across the spectrum from intermediate to deficiency pat-

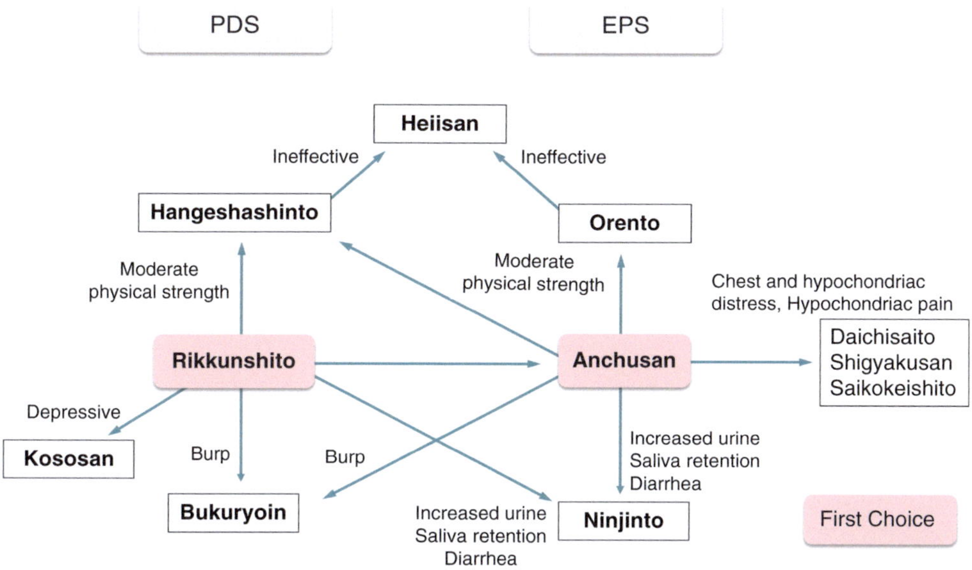

Fig. 81.1 Kampo treatment for functional dyspepsia (FD). (Adapted from Reference [5])

terns but is especially suitable for patients with classic deficiency symptoms such as fatigue, difficulty waking in the morning, postprandial drowsiness, and general malaise. While abdominal findings such as epigastric stiffness and splashing sounds are often used as targets, *Rikkunshito* can also be prescribed based solely on symptoms.

Hangeshashinto is the most important alternative to *Rikkunshito*. It is best suited for patients with moderate or greater constitution (intermediate pattern) and is not recommended for extremely thin individuals. It is typically indicated for epigastric discomfort and fullness, with or without accompanying symptoms such as borborygmi or diarrhea.

Bukuryoin is effective in patients with frequent belching that provides symptomatic relief. It is used in cases with more excess characteristics than *Rikkunshito*, but more deficiency than Hangeshashint*o*, and is also guided by findings such as epigastric stiffness and splashing sounds.

Ninjinto is considered when cold sensitivity is more pronounced than in cases treated with Rikkunshito. If the aforementioned formulas are ineffective, Heiisan or Kososan may be tried. These contain "*qi*-regulating" herbs and are expected to have anxiolytic and antidepressant effects.

For EPS, Anchusan is the first-line treatment, particularly in cases with epigastric pain and heartburn. It is used in deficiency-type patients. One of its components, Engosaku, contains alkaloids believed to exert potent analgesic effects.

Recent RCTs have increasingly demonstrated the efficacy of Rikkunshito in FD [3, 4, 6]. The first RCT by Tatsuta et al. (1993) compared Rikkunshito with gefarnate in 42 FD patients and found improvements in gastric emptying and dyspeptic symptoms after seven days of treatment. Harasawa et al. (1998) conducted a multicenter RCT in patients with dysmotility-type FD and demonstrated significant improvement in upper abdominal symptoms. Notably, Rikkunshito was particularly effective in improving anorexia, suggesting a unique mechanism of action distinct from other prokinetic agents. Suzuki et al. (2014) conducted a placebo-controlled RCT in 247 FD patients and reported significant improvement in epigastric pain and a trend toward improvement in postprandial fullness after eight weeks of Rikkunshito treatment. Post hoc analysis revealed that Rikkunshito was especially effective in *H. pylori*-negative patients with low plasma ghrelin levels. Tominaga et al. (2018) conducted a multicenter, placebo-controlled RCT (DREAM Study) and demonstrated that *Rikkunshito* significantly improved dyspeptic symptoms and quality of life (QoL).

Based on these RCT findings, the Japanese Society of Gastroenterology's FD clinical practice guidelines state the following in response to the clinical question, "Are Kampo medicines useful for FD?": "Rikkunshito is useful and recommended for use (evidence level A). Other Kampo medicines may be useful and are suggested for use (evidence level B)" [6].

2.3 Irritable Bowel Syndrome (IBS)

Kampo medicine is frequently employed in the treatment of irritable bowel syndrome (IBS). Initially, the selection of Kampo formulas is based on the patient's *sho* (pattern diagnosis), a practice known as *zui-sho* therapy (pattern-based treatment). A brief overview is provided here, with further details available in other chapters [4, 7] (Fig. 81.2).

- Keishikashakuyakuto (for deficiency to intermediate patterns) is the first-line treatment for mixed-type IBS. It is indicated in cases presenting with abdominal bloating, abdominal pain, and alternating diarrhea and constipation accompanied by tenesmus.
- Saikokeishito (for deficiency to intermediate patterns) is used when the patient exhibits relatively weak abdominal tone, with hypochondriac discomfort and tension of the rectus abdominis muscle.
- Shigyakusan (for intermediate to excess patterns) is appropriate for patients with psychological symptoms such as anxiety, insomnia, irritability, or depression.
- Shokenchuto (for deficiency patterns) is a modified version of Keishikashakuyakuto with the addition of maltose syrup (koi), often used in patients with significantly reduced vitality or in pediatric cases.
- Ninjinto (for deficiency patterns) is the first-line treatment for diarrhea-predominant IBS. It is indicated in patients with symptoms of *qi* deficiency, such as cold extremities, anorexia, and general fatigue.

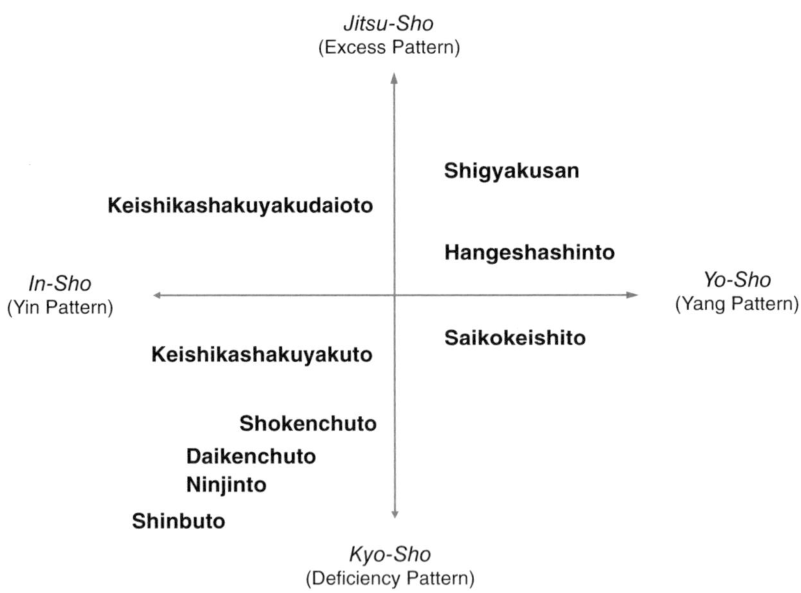

Fig. 81.2 Selection of Kampo medicines in irritable bowel syndrome (IBS). (Adapted from Ref. [7])

- Shinbuto (for deficiency patterns) is suitable for chronic watery diarrhea without abdominal pain, particularly when accompanied by general fatigue, cold limbs, dizziness, and palpitations.
- Hangeshashinto (for intermediate to deficiency patterns) is used in cases with epigastric fullness and borborygmi.
- Keishikashakuyakudaioto (for intermediate to deficiency patterns) is the first-line treatment for constipation-predominant IBS, especially when accompanied by spasmodic abdominal pain and abdominal bloating.
- Daikenchuto (for deficiency patterns) is used in cases with severe abdominal bloating due to gas, loud borborygmi, and intense abdominal pain. Although generally used for constipation-predominant IBS, it may also be effective in diarrhea-predominant cases.

In the treatment of IBS, pattern-based Kampo therapy is believed to enhance efficacy. However, Keishikashakuyakuto has demonstrated high effectiveness in IBS—particularly the alternating type—even without Kampo-specific diagnostic criteria, and some clinical evidence supports its use [4, 8].

For example, Sasaki et al. (1998) conducted an RCT comparing low-dose Keishikashakuyakuto with placebo in IBS patients and reported significant improvement in abdominal pain in diarrhea-predominant cases. Mizuno et al. (1985) conducted an RCT comparing Keishikashakuyakuto with mepenzolate bromide in IBS patients and found that the overall improvement rate was significantly higher in the Kampo group. Symptoms such as abnormal bowel movements, abdominal pain, flatulence, and abdominal bloating were significantly improved compared to the control group.

Additionally, Takeda et al. (2010) reported that Daikenchuto was effective in constipation-predominant IBS with abdominal bloating.

In summary:

- For mixed-type IBS: Keishikashakuyakuto.
- For diarrhea-predominant IBS: Ninjinto.
- For constipation-predominant IBS: Keishikashakuyakudaioto.
- For constipation-predominant IBS with abdominal bloating: Daikenchuto.

These formulas may be considered first-line treatments regardless of pattern diagnosis. However, if these treatments are ineffective, a reassessment of the patient's *sho* is warranted to guide further therapy.

The Japanese Society of Gastroenterology's IBS clinical practice guidelines address the clinical question, "Are Kampo medicines useful for IBS?" with the statement: "Some Kampo medicines are useful for IBS and are suggested for use (evidence level C)" [8].

2.4 Functional Constipation

The first-line Kampo medicine for the treatment of functional constipation is DaioKanzoto [4, 9] (Fig. 81.3) [10]. For hard, pellet-like stools in frail individuals or the elderly, Junchoto or Mashiningan is recommended. In cases of constipation-predominant irritable bowel syndrome (IBS), Keishikashakuyakudaioto is the preferred formula. All of these Kampo formulas contain Daio (Rhei Rhizoma), which exerts laxative effects primarily through its active components, sennosides A and B.

However, the pharmacological actions of *Daio* extend beyond its laxative properties. It is also known to possess antiinflammatory, psychotropic, and circulatory-enhancing effects, and thus its use is not limited solely to promoting bowel movements.

If these treatments are ineffective, formulas containing magnesium sulfate (e.g., Jokito series), which function similarly to saline laxatives, or Bofutsushosan may be considered.

Among Kampo formulas that do not contain Daio, Shokenchuto and Daikenchuto are notable. The former is used for constipation in frail pediatric patients, while the latter is indicated in cases with abdominal bloating due to intestinal gas accumulation.

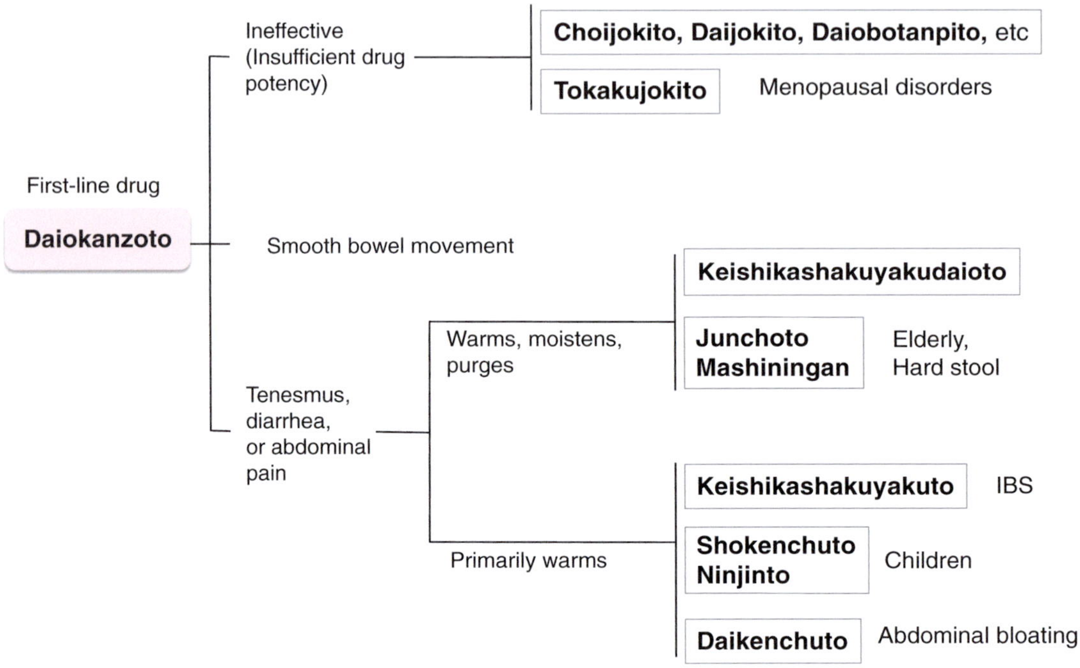

Fig. 81.3 Kampo treatment chart for constipation. (Adapted from Ref. [10]). IBS irritable bowel syndrome

Although stimulant and saline laxatives have been used for centuries, they generally lack robust clinical evidence. In contrast, Daikenchuto has been shown to be effective in the prevention and treatment of postoperative ileus.

Interestingly, Mashiningan and Junchoto have been reported in animal studies to promote defecation by increasing intestinal water secretion via activation of the CFTR (cystic fibrosis transmembrane conductance regulator) chloride channel, a mechanism similar to that of linaclotide [9].

2.5 Functional Diarrhea

From the perspective of Kampo medicine, diarrhea is classified into two types based on the *yin-yang* paradigm: *yin*-type diarrhea (chronic diarrhea) and *yang*-type diarrhea (acute infectious diarrhea). For yin-type diarrhea, formulas containing ingredients such as ginseng (Ninjin), dried ginger (Kankyo), aconite (Bushi), and atractylodes (Jutsu) are typically used. In contrast, formulas for yang-type diarrhea often include rhubarb (Daio), Coptis (Oren), and Peony (Shakuyaku) [4].

In clinical practice, Kampo medicine is more commonly used for chronic diarrhea. Chronic watery diarrhea is frequently observed in constitutionally weak individuals. In such cases, Shinbuto is considered the first-line treatment. It is particularly effective in patients who experience diarrhea triggered by cold exposure and is even more suitable when accompanied by dizziness, profound fatigue, and general debilitation.

If Shinbuto proves ineffective and the patient also presents with anorexia or postprandial fullness, Ninjinto should be considered. This formula contains dried ginger, which helps alleviate cold symptoms. If this is insufficient, aconite (Bushi) may be added to enhance the warming effect.

When neither of these formulas is effective, a combination of Shinbuto and Ninjinto may be used. This combination approximates the classical formula Bukuryo Shigyakuto, which is not available as a standardized extract but may offer therapeutic benefit.

In cases of diarrhea accompanied by epigastric stiffness (*shinka-hiko*) and abdominal rumbling, Hangeshashinto is indicated. Notably, Hangeshashinto has been shown in RCTs to be effective in treating delayed-onset diarrhea caused by irinotecan, a topoisomerase I inhibitor used in chemotherapy [11].

3 Mechanisms of Action of Major Kampo Medicines

Kampo medicines are composed of multiple crude drugs (herbal ingredients), each of which contains numerous bioactive compounds. As a result, it is generally difficult to explain the clinical effects of Kampo formulas solely through conventional pharmacological mechanisms. However, for several Kampo medicines, pharmacological actions underlying their clinical efficacy have been elucidated.

3.1 Rikkunshito

Rikkunshito is a representative Kampo formula used in patients with deficiency patterns. It consists of eight herbal ingredients: atractylodes (Sojutsu), ginseng (Ninjin), pinellia (Hange), poria (Bukuryo), jujube (Taiso), citrus peel (Chinpi), licorice (Kanzo), and fresh ginger (Shokyo). It is indicated for symptoms such as anorexia, general fatigue, epigastric discomfort or bloating, and splashing sounds in the epigastrium. Clinical indications include gastritis, gastric atony, gastroptosis with indigestion, and anorexia [3, 4]. Traditionally, Rikkunshito has been thought to exert its effects by improving gastric emptying and gastric adaptive relaxation. Our research has shown that several flavonoids contained in Chinpi, one of its components, antagonize serotonin 2B and 2C receptors, thereby promoting ghrelin secretion and enhancing appetite [12, 13]. Subsequent studies have demonstrated that these compounds act on multiple targets in both the gastrointestinal tract and central nervous system, thereby amplifying ghrelin signaling (Table 81.1 and Fig. 81.4) [13, 14]. In humans, Rikkunshito has been shown to increase plasma acyl-ghrelin levels, providing scientific validation of its pharmacological effects.

Table 81.1 Effects of Rikkunshito on ghrelin signaling

Mechanism	Target molecules/actions	Main active compounds Detected in human plasma
Increase in plasma ghrelin levels		
Promotion of ghrelin secretion	5-HT_{2B} receptor antagonism (peripheral)	HMF, hesperetin, nobiletin, and naringin (from Chinpi)
	5-HT_{2C} receptor antagonism (central)	Isoliquiritigenin, glycycoumarin (from Licorice), and hesperetin (from Chinpi)
	α2-Adrenergic receptor antagonism (peripheral)	Glycycoumarin (from licorice) and 8-shogaol[a] (from ginger)
	Type 1 CRF receptor antagonism (central)	Glycyrrhetinic acid, glycycoumarin (from licorice), nobiletin (from Chinpi)
Inhibition of ghrelin degradation	CES and BuChE inhibition (peripheral)	Pachymic acid (from Poria), glycycoumarin (from Licorice), 8-shogaol[a], and 8-gingerol[a] (from ginger)
Reversal of ghrelin resistance		
	Enhancement of GHSR1a activity (central and peripheral)	Atractylodin (from atractylodes)
	PDE3 inhibition (central)	HMF, nobiletin (from Chinpi), isoliquiritigenin (from Licorice)

Adapted from Reference [13]

HMF 3,3′,4′,5,6,7,8-heptamethoxyflavone; *CES* carboxylesterase; *BuChE* butyrylcholinesterase; *GHSR1a* growth hormone secretagogue receptor 1a; *PDE3* phosphodiesterase

[a]These compounds are detected in plasma only in conjugated forms

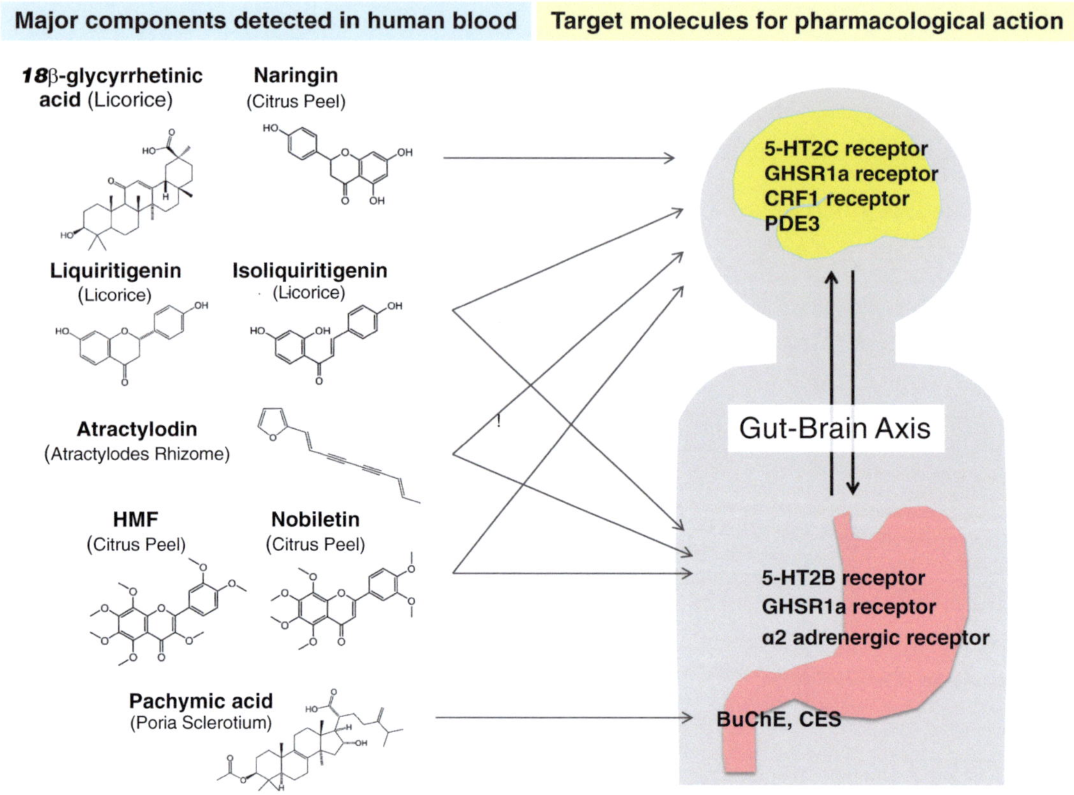

Fig. 81.4 Rikkunshito and its components act on the gut-brain axis. (Adapted from Reference [13]). HMF 3,3′,4′,5,6,7,8-heptamethoxyflavone; GHSR1a growth hormone secretagogue receptor 1a; CRF1 corticotropin-releasing factor receptor-1; PDE3 phosphodiesterase; BuChE butyrylcholinesterase; CES carboxylesterase

3.2 Hangeshashinto

Hangeshashinto comprises seven herbal ingredients: *Pinellia* (Hange), *Scutellaria* (Ogon), *Coptis* (Oren), ginseng (Ninjin), dried ginger (Kankyo), jujube (Taiso), and licorice (Kanzo). It is used in the treatment of functional dyspepsia (FD) and functional diarrhea. In oncology, it is also used for oral mucositis and irinotecan-induced cytotoxic diarrhea.

Its mechanism of action includes the suppression of excessive prostaglandin E_2 (PGE_2) production. In irinotecan-induced diarrhea, baicalin, a component of *Scutellaria*, inhibits β-glucuronidase, thereby preventing the deconjugation of the active metabolite SN-38 by gut microbiota. Additionally, berberine, an alkaloid in *Coptis*, exhibits central nervous system depressant, antispasmodic, and antidiarrheal effects, while saponin in ginseng have antistress properties [11].

3.3 Daikenchuto

Daikenchuto is a tonic formula composed of ginseng (Ninjin), Japanese pepper (Sansho), dried ginger (Kankyo), and maltose syrup (Koi). It is indicated for patients with abdominal coldness, pain, and bloating. Daikenchuto promotes small and large intestinal motility and increases intestinal blood flow, making it widely used for the treatment and prevention of postoperative ileus and constipation with abdominal bloating.

Its mechanism of action has been increasingly clarified. Daikenchuto enhances gastrointestinal motility from the pylorus to the small intestine during fasting, although high doses may suppress

① ↑ serotonin release from intestinal mucosal EC cells → ↑ gastrointestinal motility
② ↑ motilin release from intestinal mucosal endocrine cells → ↑ gastrointestinal motility
③ ↑ adrenomedullin release from intestinal mucosal epithelial cells → ↑ gastrointestinal blood flow
④ ↑ CGRP, substance P release from enteric neurons → ↑ gastrointestinal motility and blood flow

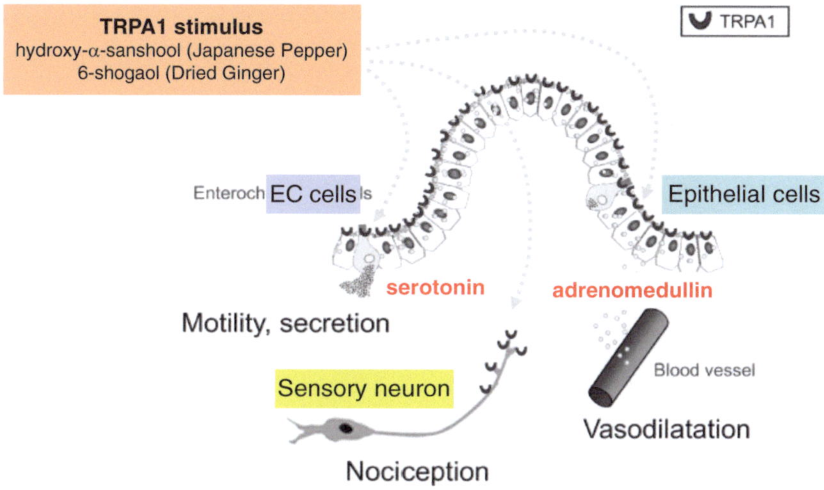

Fig. 81.5 Gastrointestinal motility-enhancing and blood flow-increasing effects of Daikenchuto. (Adapted from Reference [14]). EC enterochromaffin; CGRP calcitonin gene-related peptide; TRPA1 transient receptor potential A1)

motility. In the colon, it induces contractions both during fasting and postprandially. The contractile effect is mediated by hydroxy-sanshool, a component of Sansho, which stimulates cholinergic neurons by promoting acetylcholine release from the myenteric nervous plexus, leading to smooth muscle contraction.

Additionally, 6-shogaol, a compound in dried ginger, activates transient receptor potential ankyrin 1 (TRPA1) channels in the intestinal epithelium, promoting the release of adrenomedullin, which stimulates the calcitonin gene-related peptide (CGRP) receptors, thereby increasing intestinal blood flow (Fig. 81.5).

3.4 Keishikashakuyakuto

Keishikashakuyakuto consists of cinnamon bark (Keihi), peony root (Shakuyaku), jujube (Taiso), fresh ginger (Shokyo), and licorice (Kanzo). It is used in patients with reduced vitality who present with abdominal bloating, abdominal pain, and tenesmus associated with diarrhea or constipation. It is also used in cases of difficult defecation despite the urge to defecate, postlaxative abdominal pain, and postoperative bowel dysfunction.

Although its composition is identical to that of Keishito, Keishikashakuyakuto contains double the amount of Shakuyaku, resulting in significantly different pharmacological effects. Its antidiarrheal effect is attributed to the suppression of accelerated small intestinal transit, primarily mediated by paeoniflorin, a major component of Shakuyaku [1, 4].

4 Conclusion

Functional gastrointestinal disorders (FGIDs) are characterized by unclear etiologies and pathophysiologies. It is unlikely that a single functional abnormality is responsible for these conditions. Therefore, therapeutic agents that act on the body's regulatory systems as a whole are desirable. Western pharmaceuticals are often developed to target specific molecular pathways, which may explain their limited efficacy in FGIDs.

Kampo medicines, being multicomponent systems, have historically posed challenges for clinical trials and pharmacological elucidation within the framework of Western medicine. However, with the advancement of well-designed clinical studies and the introduction of novel research methodologies, our understanding of the clinical impact and mechanisms of Kampo medicines in FGIDs is gradually improving.

Continued progress in this field will depend on the efforts of clinicians and researchers in Japan, where high-quality Kampo medicines are routinely available under national health insurance.

Take-Home Message

In general patients with functional gastrointestinal disorders (FGIDs), several strategies can enhance satisfaction with Kampo therapy. One important approach is to clearly communicate the basic and clinical evidence supporting the treatment, thereby helping patients understand and accept the rationale for using Kampo medicine. It is also beneficial to inform patients in advance that therapeutic effects may take one to two months to become apparent. Furthermore, evaluating treatment efficacy after approximately two months and confirming the patient's willingness to continue therapy can help clarify the treatment plan and support adherence.

Competing Interests The author(s) has no competing interests to declare that are relevant to the content of this manuscript.

References

1. Japan Society for Oriental Medicine, Academic Education Committee. Textbook of Kampo medicine for specialists. Tokyo: Nankodo; 2010. (in Japanese).
2. Japanese Society of Gastroenterology. Clinical practice guidelines for Gastroesophageal Reflux Disease (GERD) 2021, 3rd Revised Edition. Tokyo: Nankodo; 2021. (in Japanese).
3. Takeda H. Rikkunshito and upper gastrointestinal disorders. Curr Ther. 2018;28:81–6. (in Japanese)
4. Takeda H. Functional gastrointestinal disorders and Kampo therapy. Clin Gastroenterol. 2015;30:257–62. (in Japanese).
5. Ishiwata M, et al. Chiryo (Therapy). 2009;91:1726–31. (in Japanese).
6. Japanese Society of Gastroenterology. Clinical practice guidelines for functional gastrointestinal disorders 2021— – Functional Dyspepsia (FD), 2nd Revised Edition. Tokyo: Nankodo; 2021. (in Japanese).
7. Shimada Y, et al. Clin Gastroenterol. 2000;3:66–71. (in Japanese).
8. Japanese Society of Gastroenterology. Clinical practice guidelines for Functional gastrointestinal Disorders 2020—irritable bowel syndrome (IBS), 2nd Revised Edition. Tokyo: Nankodo; 2020. (in Japanese).
9. Kono T. The role of Kampo medicine in chronic constipation. J Japan Soc Coloproctol. 2019;72:615–20. (in Japanese).
10. Akiba T. Sogo Rinsho (General Clinical Medicine). 2010;51:435–6. (in Japanese).
11. Mori K. Mechanism of irinotecan-induced Diarrhea and the effect of Hangeshashinto. Yakkyoku (Pharmacy). 2011;62:3509–13. (in Japanese).
12. Takeda H, et al. Rikkunshito, an herbal medicine, suppresses cisplatin-induced anorexia in rats via 5-HT2 receptor antagonism. Gastroenterology. 2008;134:2004–13.
13. Takeda H, et al. Scientific elucidation of the mechanism of action of Kampo medicine: Rikkunshito. Clin Gastroenterol. 2018;33:1349–56. (in Japanese).
14. Kono T, et al. Complementary and synergistic therapeutic effects of compounds found in Kampo medicine: analysis of daikenchuto. Front Pharmacol. 2015;6:159.

Further Readings

Tatsuta M, Iishi H. Effect of treatment with Liu-Jun-Zi-Tang (TJ-43) on gastric emptying and gastrointestinal symptoms in dyspeptic patients. Aliment Pharmacol Ther. 1993;7:459–62.

Harasawa S, et al. A multicenter, double-blind, post-marketing clinical trial of Rikkunshito for dysmotility-like dyspepsia. Igaku no Ayumi (Progress in Medicine). 1998;187:1207–29. (in Japanese).

Suzuki H, et al. Rikkunshito Study Group. Randomized clinical trial: rikkunshito in the treatment of functional dyspepsia—a multicenter, double-blind, randomized, placebo-controlled study. Neurogastroenterol Motil. 2014;26:950–61.

Tominaga K, et al. Rikkunshito simultaneously improves dyspepsia correlated with anxiety in patients with functional dyspepsia: a randomized clinical trial (the DREAM study). Neurogastroenterol Motil. 2018;

Sasaki D, et al. Clinical efficacy of Keishikashakuyakuto in irritable bowel syndrome. Rinsho Kenkyu (Clinical and Research). 1998;75:1136–52. (in Japanese).

Mizuno S, et al. Therapeutic effects of Keishikasha kuyakuto extract in irritable bowel syndrome. Shindan Chiryo (Diagnosis and Treatment). 1985;73:1143–52. (in Japanese).

Takeda H, et al. Kampo in gastroenterology. Jpn J Orient Psychosom Med. 2010;25:37–41. (in Japanese).

Practical Treatment, Practice of Family Medicine

82

Akira Uehara

Abstract

Most patients with functional gastrointestinal disorders (FGIDs/DGBI), who often engage in healthcare-seeking behaviors such as doctor shopping, typically visit family physicians first. Therefore, family physicians thoroughly understand the FGID/DGBI pathophysiology and consistently apply appropriate diagnostic and therapeutic strategies. To accurately assess their condition, it is essential to conduct a thorough history-taking focused on symptom characteristics, along with inquiries into past medical and family history, followed by a detailed physical examination. When necessary, additional diagnostic evaluations such as blood tests, urinalysis, radiography, ultrasonography, CT scans, and gastrointestinal endoscopy should be considered. When diagnosing FGIDs/DGBI, the first step in treatment is to clearly and thoroughly explain the condition to the patient. Initiating pharmacotherapy without this explanation often results in suboptimal outcomes. Since stress is a common trigger, it is also important to emphasize lifestyle modifications and stress management. These efforts are crucial in preventing doctor shopping and ensuring patient satisfaction. Pharmacotherapy should follow established clinical practice guidelines for each condition. Kampo medicine can also be effective in the treatment of FGIDs. If pharmacotherapy proves ineffective, psychological factors may be significant. In such instances, psychological counseling by a clinical psychologist or referral to a psychiatrist should be considered. In summary, building and maintaining a strong patient-physician relationship is vitally important.

Keywords

Family medicine · Healthcare-seeking behavior · Kampo medicine · Qi deficiency · Qi stagnation · Strong patient-physician relationship · Holistic medicine

1 Introduction

A considerable number of patients visit family physicians with chief complaints such as abdominal pain or constipation. To accurately assess their condition, it is essential to conduct a thorough history-taking focused on symptom characteristics, along with inquiries into past medical and family history, followed by a precise physical examination. When necessary, additional diagnostic evaluations such as blood tests, urinalysis, radiography, ultrasonography, CT scans, and gastrointestinal endoscopy should be considered. If

A. Uehara (✉)
Uehara Clinic, Sapporo, Japan
e-mail: akira-uehara@uehara-clinic.com

H. Kaneko et al. (eds.), *Disorders of Gut-Brain Interaction*,
https://doi.org/10.1007/978-981-95-6974-8_82

no organic disease is identified through this comprehensive assessment, a diagnosis of functional gastrointestinal disorder (FGID/DGBI: disorders of gut-brain interaction) is made, and appropriate treatment is initiated.

In reviewing cases of patients who presented with "stomach pain," the final diagnoses varied widely. While gastrointestinal diseases were most common, other diagnoses included abdominal aortic aneurysm dissection, myocardial infarction, pulmonary embolism, acute appendicitis, herpes zoster, pregnancy, and anxiety neurosis. These spanned internal medicine, surgery, dermatology, obstetrics and gynecology, and psychiatry. Accurately differentiating among these and promptly referring patients to appropriate specialists is both a challenge and a rewarding aspect of family medicine. Continuous professional development is essential for family physicians.

2 Instructive Case Report

The following cases provide valuable insights into the diagnosis and management of FGIDs.

2.1 Case 1

A 26-year-old man presented on November 21 with epigastric pain and nausea. At his request, upper gastrointestinal endoscopy was performed on November 25, revealing no abnormalities. Given his concurrent constipation, he was diagnosed with irritable bowel syndrome (IBS) and prescribed a standard treatment for two weeks. However, he returned on December 26 with persistent nausea and abdominal pain. Blood tests revealed anemia (hemoglobin 9.5 g/dL), prompting suspicion of inflammatory bowel disease such as Crohn's disease. Colonoscopy was performed on January 11 of the following year, revealing a tumor nearly obstructing the lumen of the ascending colon (Fig. 82.1). Biopsy confirmed adenocarcinoma. He was referred to a nearby general hospital for semiurgent surgery. Despite no family history of colorectal cancer, this was a case of sporadic, advanced colorectal cancer in a young adult. Retrospectively, his chief complaints of epigastric pain and nausea were likely due to subileus caused by the tumor. This case highlights the diagnostic challenges in FGIDs.

2.2 Case 2

A 26-year-old female midwife presented with sudden onset of heartburn and epigastric burning two days prior. Although upper endoscopy was recommended, she requested medication first, suspecting GERD. She was prescribed vonoprazan. As symptoms persisted, she returned the next day and consented to endoscopy. As shown

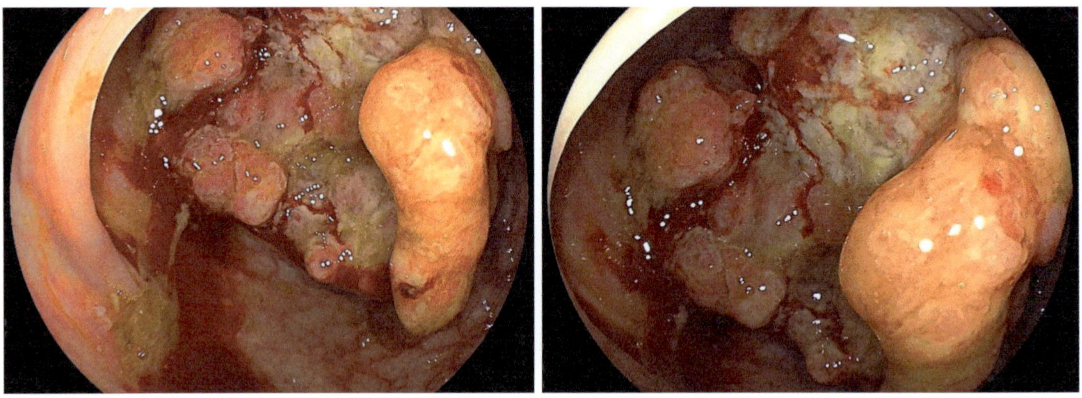

Fig. 82.1 Case 1. A cancerous lesion occupying nearly the entire lumen of the ascending colon beyond the hepatic flexure was observed

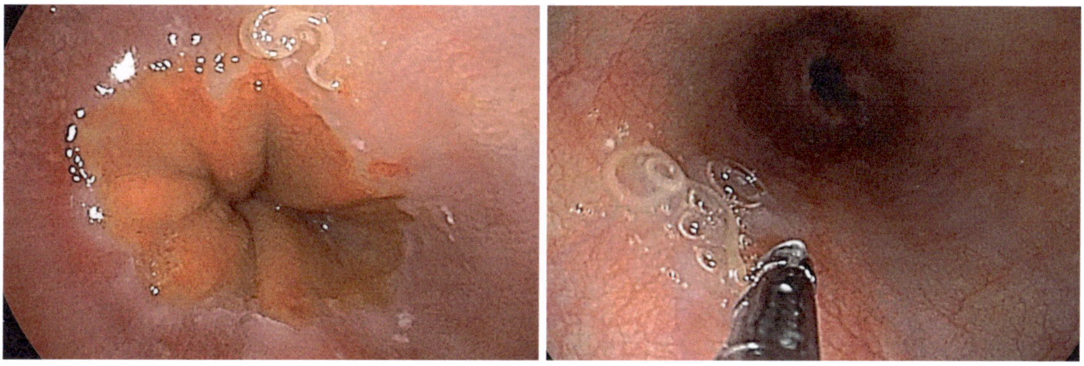

Fig. 82.2 Case 2. An Anisakis larva was embedded at the esophagogastric junction and was removed using biopsy forceps

in Fig. 82.2, an Anisakis larva was embedded at the lower esophagus and was removed with biopsy forceps, leading to immediate symptom resolution. Although her symptoms suggested GERD or functional dyspepsia (FD), the actual diagnosis was esophageal anisakiasis. Esophageal anisakiasis differs from gastric anisakiasis in that symptoms may include heartburn or epigastric burning rather than abdominal pain [1].

3 Healthcare-Seeking Behavior in FGID Patients

Nozu et al. analyzed the healthcare-seeking behavior of 3784 new patients at the Department of General Medicine, Hokkaido University Hospital. Patients were divided into 2 groups—63 diagnosed with FGIDs and 3721 with other conditions—and their healthcare-seeking behaviors were compared [2]. As shown in Table 82.1, 89% of FGID patients had visited other medical institutions prior to their current consultation, yet only 21% brought referral letters. In contrast, among patients with other conditions, only 22% had prior consultations, and 67% of those brought referral letters. These findings suggest that FGID patients are more likely to engage in "doctor shopping," indicating dissatisfaction with their family physicians. Nozu et al. attribute this to a lack of enthusiasm for FGID diagnosis and treatment among both family physicians and gastroenterologists, leading to inappropriate management and increased patient anxiety and dissatisfaction. To prevent such outcomes, family physicians must deepen their understanding of FGIDs and provide individualized, accurate care.

Table 82.1 Healthcare-seeking behavior of patients with functional gastrointestinal disorders [2]

	Patients with FGIDs	Patients with other diseases
	No. of patients (%)	
Seeing other physician(s) before for the same illness episode	56/63 (89%)	811/3721 (22%)
Changing physicians with professional referral	12/56 (21%)	542/811 (67%)
Changing physicians without professional referral	44/56 (79%)	269/811 (33%)

FGIDs Functional gastrointestinal disorders

4 Practical Management

When diagnosing FGIDs/DGBI, the first step in treatment is to clearly and thoroughly explain the condition to the patient. Initiating pharmacotherapy without this explanation often results in suboptimal outcomes. Educational booklets provided by pharmaceutical companies (e.g., on FD or diarrhea-predominant IBS) can be helpful in enhancing patient understanding. Since stress is a common trigger, it is also important to emphasize lifestyle modifications and stress management. These efforts are crucial in preventing doctor shopping and ensuring patient satisfaction.

Pharmacotherapy should follow established clinical practice guidelines for each condition. Kampo medicine is often effective in FGID treatment. As a Kampo specialist, the author actively incorporates Kampo therapy in clinical practice. *Rikkunshito* is frequently used for FD, *Keishikashakuyakuto* for IBS, *Keishikashakuyakudaioto* for constipation-predominant IBS, and *Hangeshashinto* for diarrhea-predominant IBS.

In cases where pharmacotherapy is ineffective, psychological factors may be significant. In such instances, psychological counseling by a clinical psychologist or referral to a psychiatrist is considered.

5 Innovations in Kampo Therapy for Functional Dyspepsia

Through active use of Kampo medicine, new insights have been gained regarding its application in FD. The latest treatment flowchart for FD from the Japanese Society of Gastroenterology (Fig. 82.3) includes *Rikkunshito* alongside acid-suppressive agents and prokinetics (e.g., acotiamide) as first-line therapy [3]. This revision reflects the growing body of basic and clinical evidence supporting *Rikkunshito*. However, in clinical practice, some patients do not respond as expected.

Upon investigation, it was noted that many of these patients exhibited enhanced retrograde peristalsis in the gastric antrum during endoscopy. In such cases, *Rikkunshito* was ineffective, whereas formulas with smooth muscle relaxant properties, such as *Bukuryoin* or *Daisaikoto*, were highly effective. Thus, *Rikkunshito* is suitable for patients with gastric hypomotility and smooth muscle relaxation, while *Bukuryoin* or *Daisaikoto* is more appropriate for those with antral hypertonicity. In Kampo terms, the former corresponds to a "Qi deficiency" type and the latter to a "Qi stagnation" type. This subclassification allows for more precise treatment [4]. Differentiation is based on endoscopic findings such as retrograde peristalsis from the pylorus to the antrum, belching with minimal insufflation, and bile reflux into the stomach, which indicate a "Qi stagnation" type. Diagnostic criteria for Qi deficiency and Qi stagnation are also used to support subclassification [5].

6 Conclusion

Patients with FGIDs often exhibit healthcare-seeking behaviors such as doctor shopping, underscoring the critical role of family physicians. To prevent adverse outcomes, family physicians must thoroughly understand FGID pathophysiology and consistently apply appropriate diagnostic and therapeutic strategies. When necessary, referral to clinical psychologists or psychiatrists should not be delayed.

Take-Home Message
Professor Masayoshi Namiki, the founding chair of the Third Department of Internal Medicine at Asahikawa Medical University and the author's mentor, emphasized the importance of holistic care with the words:"Do not treat the disease alone—treat the whole patient who has the disease," and "If you perform gastrointestinal endoscopy, you must also perform a psychological endoscopy." These teachings underscore the value of a strong patient-physician relationship and the essence of holistic medicine. For family physicians managing FGIDs/DGBI, there is no greater clinical pearl.

Competing Interests The author(s) has no competing interests to declare that are relevant to the content of this manuscript.

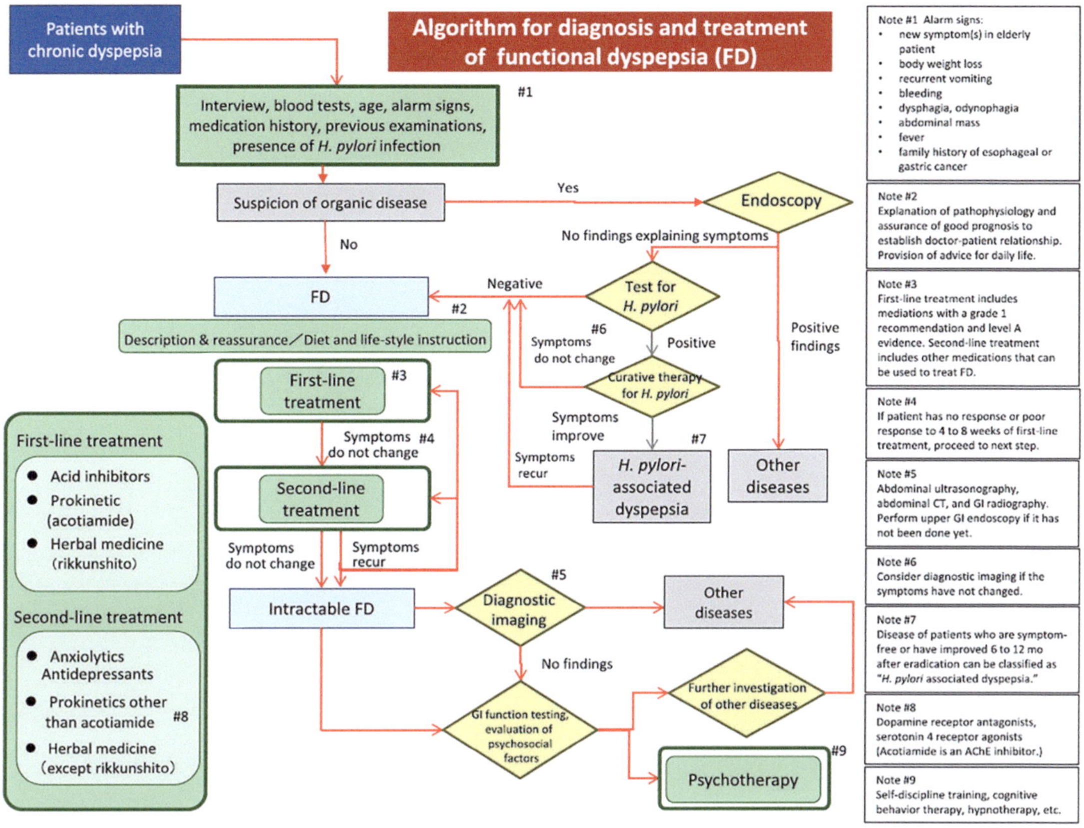

Fig. 82.3 Diagnostic and treatment flowchart for functional dyspepsia from the Japanese Society of Gastroenterology [3]

References

1. Uehara A, Okumura T. Esophageal anisakiasis mimicking gastroesophageal reflux disease. Am J Gastroenterol. 2017;112:532.
2. Nozu T, et al. Inadequate health care-seeking behavior of Japanese patients with functional gastrointestinal disorders: a preliminary survey. J Gastroenterol. 2002;37:231–2.
3. Miwa H, et al. Evidence-based clinical practice guidelines for functional dyspepsia 2021. J Gastroenterol. 2022;57:47–61.
4. Fukutomi T. Clinical commentary on 123 Kampo prescriptions—teachings of Dr. Iwao Yamamoto. Edited by Yamamoto Y. Tokyo: Medical Yukon; 2016. (in Japanese).
5. Terasawa K. Learning Japanese-Chinese medicine from case studies. 3rd ed. Tokyo: Igaku Shoin; 2012. (in Japanese).

83 Case Discussion, Esophagus

Osamu Tsuchida

Abstract

Symptoms such as chest pain, dysphagia, nausea and vomiting, loss of appetite, and aspiration into trachea are frequently encountered in clinical practice. It is essential to consider esophageal functional abnormalities in the differential diagnosis. We have proposed diagnostic algorithm for esophageal motility disorders using upper gastrointestinal video fluoroscopy and esophageal manometry. Following of exclusion diagnosis of organic lesions, GERD or FGIDs, psychological disorders, we actively diagnose esophageal motility disorders and treat patient with medication or psychosomatic intervention. Case 1 is a 39-year-old male with non-cardiac chet pain. He was diagnosed hypercontractile esophagus with esophageal manometry. He was treated medications of calcium channel blockers and nitroglycerin; symptoms subsequent improved. Case 2 is an 80-year-old male with Parkinson's disease, dysphagia, and loss of appetite. He was diagnosed achalasia (type III) with upper GI video fluoroscopy and esophageal manometry. Although initial treatment with medications led to improvement, the condition relapsed due to stress related to a natural disaster. Psychosomatic intervention contributed to subsequent recovery. Video fluoroscopy is a valuable screening tool that can be performed at any facility equipped with radiographic equipment. When abnormalities are detected, referral to a facility equipped with esophageal manometry is recommended to facilitate appropriate treatment. Broader adoption of this diagnostic approach in general clinical practice is strongly encouraged.

Keywords

Esophageal motility disorders · Non-cardiac chest pain · Upper GI video fluoroscopy · Esophageal manometry · Achalasia · Hypercontractile esophagus · Psychosomatic intervention

1 Diagnostic Methods for Esophageal Functional Abnormalities

Symptoms arising from esophageal functional abnormalities are diverse and may include chest pain, dysphagia, a sensation of food sticking, nausea and vomiting, heartburn, aspiration, and coughing. Patients experiencing these symptoms often consult departments such as cardiology, otolaryngology, pulmonology, or gastroenterol-

O. Tsuchida (✉)
Division of Psychosomatic Medicine, Functional Gastrointestinal Disorders, Saiseikai Iizuka-kaho Hospital, Iizuka, Japan
e-mail: tsuchida@iizuka-kaho.jp

H. Kaneko et al. (eds.), *Disorders of Gut-Brain Interaction*,
https://doi.org/10.1007/978-981-95-6974-8_83

ogy. However, even after undergoing examinations in these specialties, no organic lesions are frequently identified. Consequently, patients may be referred to psychiatry or psychosomatic medicine under the suspicion of psychogenic causes, where they are often given vague diagnoses such as anxiety disorders or depression and are prescribed psychotropic medications without clear therapeutic direction. This frequently leads to prolonged symptoms and repeated visits to multiple medical institutions, which is highly unfortunate for the patient.

One of the major reasons for the failure to accurately diagnose esophageal functional abnormalities is the limited availability and lack of widespread use of esophageal manometry equipment. Additionally, there is a general lack of awareness among physicians regarding the existence and clinical significance of esophageal functional abnormalities.

In response to this situation, our institution was among the first to introduce esophageal manometry equipment. To facilitate its effective use, we implemented upper gastrointestinal (GI) video fluoroscopy using barium as a screening method. When symptoms suggestive of esophageal functional abnormalities are present, as described above, we first perform standard imaging studies to exclude organic lesions. We then actively pursue a diagnosis of esophageal motility disorders using a proposed diagnostic algorithm [1]. Figure 83.1 illustrates this diagnostic algorithm. Among these, upper GI video fluoroscopy can be performed at any facility equipped with X-ray fluoroscopy. However, only a limited number of studies have been published in this field [2, 3]. Furthermore, standard examination methods and diagnostic criteria for video fluoroscopy remain ambiguous and lack objectivity [4].

To address this, our institution has standardized the upper GI video fluoroscopy procedure by establishing reference values for esophageal diameter and transit time based on healthy individuals. We proposed and reported diagnostic criteria consisting of eight items [5]. This method involves observing the esophagus in real time while the patient ingests barium, as used in gastric fluoroscopy. It provides a wealth of information from the images and offers a significant psychosomatic therapeutic benefit by allowing patients to view the video directly.

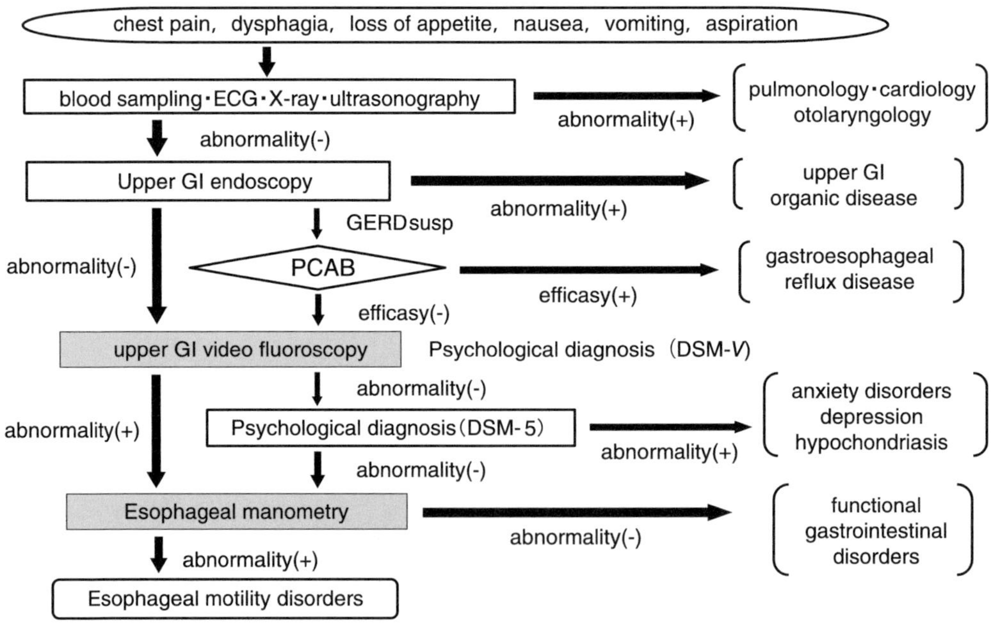

Fig. 83.1 Diagnostic algorithm for esophageal functional abnormalities. *PCAB* potassium-competitive acid blocker

Table 83.1 Diagnostic criteria for upper gastrointestinal video fluoroscopy

	(−) Normal	(+) Mild abnormality	(++) Severe abnormality
(1) Barium ingestion	Complete ingestion within test time	Partial ingestion within test time	Unable to ingest
(2) Swallowing from oral cavity to esophagus	No abnormality	Retention in piriform sinus or asymmetry	Aspiration into trachea
(3) Esophageal dilation	< 3.0 cm	3.0–4.0 cm	≥ 4.0 cm
(4) Barium retention in esophagus	No retention ≥10 s	Retention ≥10 s	Formation of fluid level
(5) Esophageal spasm	No spastic changes	Spastic changes present	Retrograde peristalsis present
(6) Gastroesophageal reflux	No reflux	Mild reflux	Severe reflux
(7) Gastric hypomotility	Continuous gastric motility	Intermittent gastric motility	No gastric motility
(8) Duodenal outflow	Outflow beyond ligament of Treitz	–	No outflow

Modified from Tsuchida [1]

Table 83.1 presents the diagnostic criteria. Each of the eight items is evaluated on a three-point scale: (−) indicates normal, while (+) and (++) are considered abnormal. Criterion (1) assesses the presence of eating disorders or cognitive decline, (2) evaluates swallowing function, (3) and (4) assess esophageal transit disorders, and (5) evaluates esophageal motility disorders. If abnormalities are observed in criteria (3) through (5), esophageal motility disorder is suspected, and esophageal manometry is performed for definitive diagnosis. The diagnosis of esophageal motility disorders follows the Chicago Classification version 4.0, proposed in 2020 [6].

Criterion (6) evaluates gastroesophageal reflux disease (GERD). If GERD is suspected, a challenge test using proton pump inhibitors (PPIs) or potassium-competitive acid blockers (PCABs) is conducted. Criterion (7) assesses gastric motility, and if hypomotility is suspected, prokinetic agents are considered. Criterion (8) evaluates duodenal transit, which is particularly useful for screening conditions such as superior mesenteric artery (SMA) syndrome.

Note: The following section presents two case studies of esophageal motility disorders diagnosed and treated according to this algorithm.

2 Case Presentation 1: Hypercontractile Esophagus

Patient: A 39-year-old male

Chief complaint: Chest pain

History of present illness: The patient experienced health deterioration due to workplace stress, which triggered the onset of chest pain in July. He visited a medical facility on July 25. Upper GI endoscopy revealed no organic lesions. Due to persistent chest pain, he was unable to continue working and took a leave of absence. He visited our hospital on August 3 for further examination.

Medical history: Appendectomy at age 8

Family history: Unremarkable

Social history: No alcohol use, positive smoking history, and no known allergies

Physical examination:

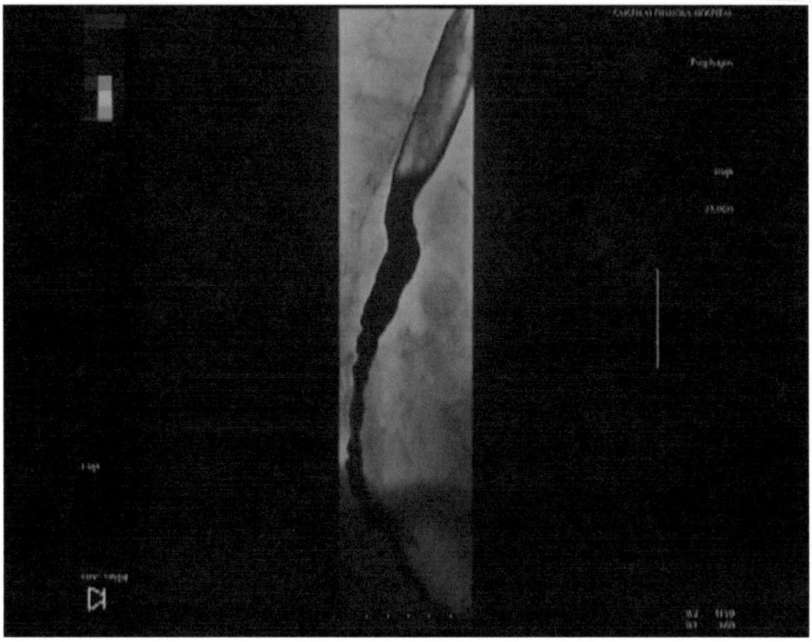

Fig. 83.2 Upper gastrointestinal video fluoroscopy in Case 1 (corkscrew-like esophageal spasm observed)

- Chest: Regular heart sounds
- Abdomen: Flat, soft, nontender, and normal bowel sounds

Diagnostic Course Blood tests, electrocardiogram, and chest CT showed no abnormalities. A PCAB challenge test was conducted under suspicion of GERD, but chest pain persisted. Suspecting esophageal motility disorder, upper GI video fluoroscopy was performed (Fig. 83.2), revealing a corkscrew-like esophageal spasm throughout the esophagus. The video was shown to the patient, and esophageal motility disorder was explained. Esophageal manometry was then performed (Fig. 83.3). Integrated relaxation pressure (IRP) and distal latency (DL) were within normal limits, but the mean distal contractile integral (DCI) was 7181.4 mmHg·s·cm, with four out of ten swallows exceeding 8000. Based on the Chicago Classification version 3.0 [7], the diagnosis was hypercontractile esophagus (Jackhammer esophagus).

Diagnosis

- # Hypercontractile esophagus (Jackhammer esophagus)

Treatment Course The patient was treated with oral calcium channel blockers (diltiazem) and sublingual nitroglycerin spray for chest pain.

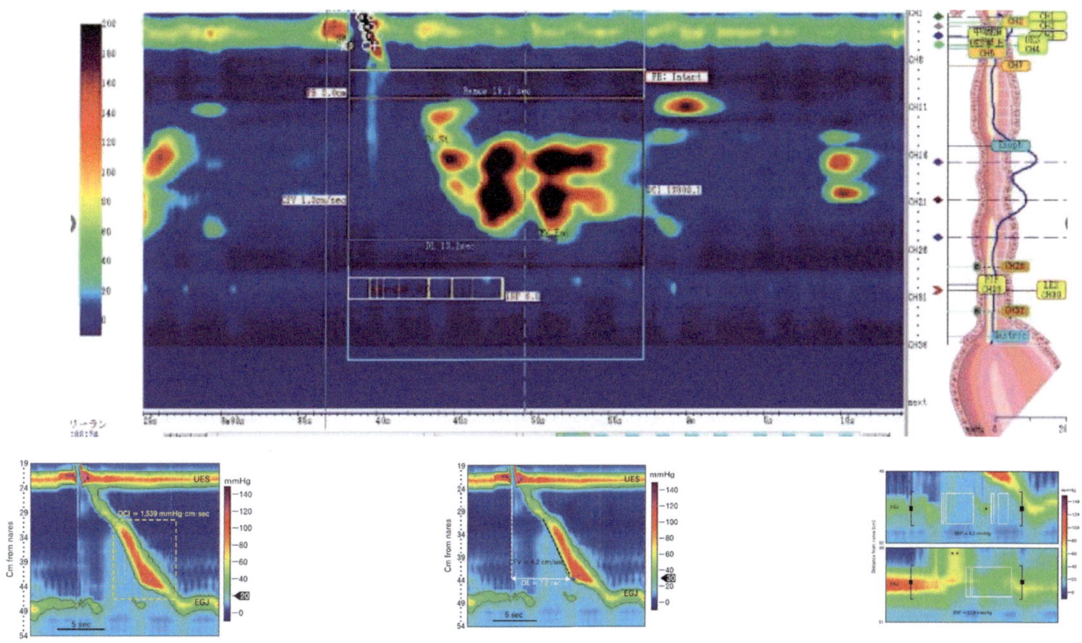

DCI(distal contractile integral)
(mmHg/s/cm)
(Normal range : <8000)

DL(distal latency) (sec)
Normal range: >4.5 sec)

IRP(Integrated relaxation pressure)
(Normal range: ≤15mmHg)

Fig. 83.3 Esophageal manometry in Case 1 (elevated DCI = 7181.4 mmHg·s·cm; 4 out of 10 swallows exceeded DCI 8000, consistent with hypercontractile esophagus)

Symptoms gradually improved. Autogenic training was introduced to address stress, resulting in complete resolution of chest pain and improved quality of life. The patient returned to work two months later. Four months after initiating treatment, follow-up esophageal manometry showed a DCI of 2688 mmHg·s·cm, with no swallows exceeding 8000, indicating normalization. Diltiazem therapy was continued, and the patient remains under outpatient follow-up.

3 Discussion

Chest pain without cardiac abnormalities is collectively referred to as non-cardiac chest pain (NCCP), accounting for approximately 70% of all chest pain cases. NCCP is common, with reported prevalence rates of approximately 25% in Western countries and 19% in Asia (China) [8]. A study using the Chicago Classification version 3.0 found that among NCCP patients, GERD was the most frequent cause (35%), followed by esophageal motility disorders (31%) [9]. Thus, esophageal motility disorders are not rare in patients with chest pain and should be considered in approximately 20% of cases.

Medications used to treat esophageal motility disorders include nitrates and calcium channel blockers, which are also used for angina pectoris. Since the esophagus, like coronary arteries, is composed of smooth muscle, these agents exert a smooth muscle-relaxing effect. It is important to note that when these drugs are used diagnostically for angina, their effectiveness in esophageal motility disorders may lead to misdiagnosis if not carefully considered.

Nonpharmacological treatments for NCCP include hypnotherapy and relaxation techniques. One study reported that hypnotherapy was effective in 80% of patients compared to 23% in the control group [10]. In this case, autogenic training incorporating hypnotherapeutic principles yielded favorable outcomes.

4 Case Presentation 2: Achalasia

Patient: An 80-year-old male

Chief complaints: Dysphagia and loss of appetite

History of present illness: Diagnosed with Parkinson's disease five years ago and has been receiving treatment in our neurology department. Dysphagia began three years ago and gradually worsened, leading to decreased appetite and weight loss. He visited our department in March.

Past medical history: Parkinson's disease diagnosed at age 75 (under treatment)

Social history: No alcohol or tobacco use, no known allergies

Physical Examination:

- Height, 160 cm, and weight, 48 kg
- Neurological findings: Resting tremor of the fingers (+) and brachybasia (+)
- Chest/abdomen: No abnormal findings

Diagnostic Course Upper GI endoscopy was performed to exclude organic lesions causes of dysphagia, but no abnormalities were found. Upper GI video fluoroscopy revealed esophageal dilation (maximum diameter 3.2 cm) and barium retention, raising suspicion of achalasia. Esophageal manometry confirmed the diagnosis with an IRP of 31.8 mmHg and a shortened DL of 3.5 s, consistent with type III achalasia (Table 83.2).

Table 83.2 Diagnostic criteria for esophageal motility disorders

≪Disorders of EGJ outflow: IRP ≧15.0 mmHg≫
Achalasia I: 100% Failed peristalsis
Achalasia II: 100% Failed peristalsis with PEP ≧20% swallows
Achalasia III: ≧20% Premature contraction (DL<4.5 s)
EGJOO (EGJ outflow obstruction):
≪Disorders of peristalsis: IRP < 15.0 mmHg≫
Absent contractility: 100% Failed Peristalsis
Distal esophageal spasm: ≧20% (DL<4.5 s)
Hypercontractile esophagus: ≧20% (DCI>8000 mmHg・ s・ cm)
Ineffective esophageal motility: >70% ineffective or ≧50% failed swallows

Partially adapted and translated from the Chicago Classification Version 4.0

Diagnosis

- #1 Achalasia type III
- #2 Parkinson's disease

5 Treatment Course

Achalasia type III is considered a condition in which esophageal spasm coexists with achalasia. In this case, both pathologies were thought to contribute to the patient's dysphagia. For treatment, a long-acting nitrate patch and a short-acting nitrate spray were administered as needed. The patient experienced marked symptomatic improvement, with increased appetite and weight gain to 50 kg.

However, in July of the following year, a heavy rain disaster caused a landslide on the mountain property owned by the patient, resulting in damage to neighboring homes and leading

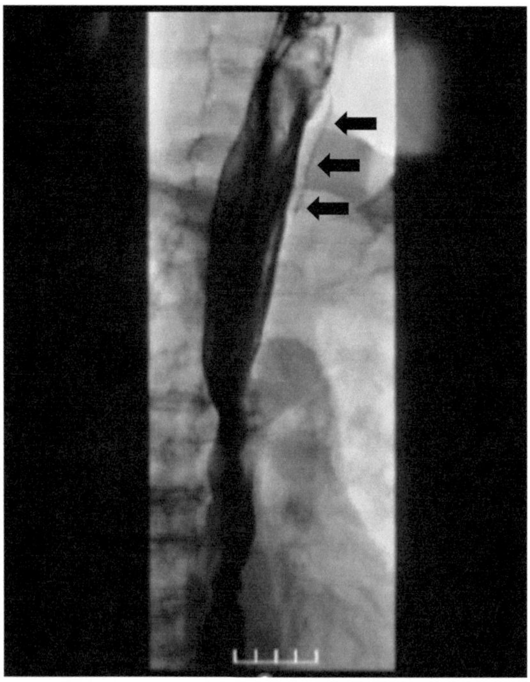

Fig. 83.4 Video fluoroscopy during recurrence in Case 2 (arrow indicates aspiration into the bronchial tree)

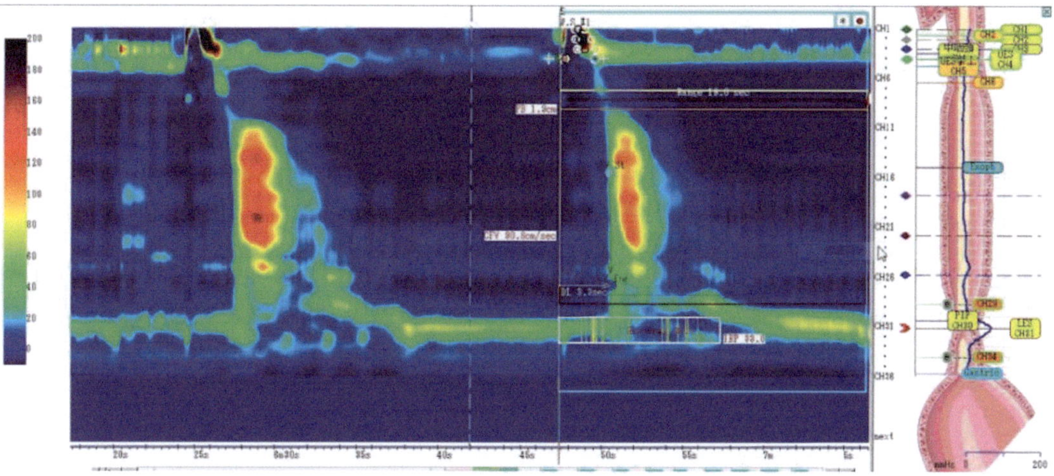

LES baseline pressure=51.0 mmHg (normal range: 15~45mmHg)
IRP=32.8 mmHg (normal range: ≤15mmHg)
DL=3.5 seconds (normal range: >4.5 sec, 70% of swallows less than 4.5 sec)
DCI=2877 mmHg·s·cm (normal range: <8000)

Fig. 83.5 Esophageal manometry during recurrence in Case 2 (IRP = 32.8 mmHg, mildly elevated; DL = 3.5 s, shortened)

to a legal compensation dispute. This event triggered a gradual recurrence of dysphagia and appetite loss. In August, upper GI video fluoroscopy revealed worsening achalasia (maximum esophageal diameter: 3.5 cm) and aspiration into the bronchial tree (Fig. 83.4). Esophageal manometry showed a slight increase in IRP to 32.8 mmHg (Fig. 83.5).

The patient expressed significant emotional distress, stating he was unable to sleep due to anxiety over the compensation issue. We responded with empathetic listening. Subsequently, a resolution was proposed by the insurance company, which alleviated the patient's anxiety. This coincided with an improvement in dysphagia.

One year later, follow-up video fluoroscopy showed improvement in achalasia (maximum esophageal diameter: 2.5 cm) and no evidence of aspiration, confirming clinical improvement. The patient continues to do well and remains under treatment for Parkinson's disease.

6 Discussion

This case involved a patient with Parkinson's disease who developed achalasia in the context of preexisting dysphagia. Although initial treatment led to improvement, the condition relapsed due to stress related to a natural disaster. Psychosomatic intervention contributed to subsequent recovery. Notably, the patient did not initially disclose the compensation dispute; it was only through repeated empathetic listening that this critical psychosocial factor emerged. This case underscores the importance of a patient-centered approach grounded in acceptance and empathy.

Achalasia has long been recognized as a psychosomatic disorder associated with stress. One study reported that 34% of 47 patients with achalasia had experienced emotional stress prior to disease onset [11]. In this case, the recurrence of achalasia was linked to disaster-related stress, and improvement was achieved through psychosomatic treatment. The ability to objectively monitor the disease course using video fluoroscopy and esophageal manometry adds further value to this case.

Take-Home Message

Symptoms such as chest pain, dysphagia, nausea and vomiting, and appetite loss are frequently encountered in clinical practice. It is essential to consider esophageal functional abnormalities in the differential diagnosis. Video fluoroscopy is a valuable screening tool that can be performed at any facility equipped with radiographic equipment and should be actively utilized. When abnormalities are detected, referral to a facility equipped with esophageal manometry is recommended to facilitate appropriate treatment. Broader adoption of this diagnostic approach in general clinical practice is strongly encouraged.

Competing Interests The author(s) has no competing interests to declare that are relevant to the content of this manuscript.

References

1. Tsuchida O. Diagnostic methods for esophageal functional abnormalities. Jpn Med J. 2009;4453:59–64. (in Japanese)
2. Hanning C, et al. Esophageal motility disorders. Radiology. 2007;47:123–36.
3. Brusori S, et al. Role of videofluorography in the study of esophageal motility disorders. Radiol Med. 2001;101:125–32.
4. Cedric GB, et al. Esophageal disease and testing. Taylor & Francis; 2005. p. 1–52.
5. Tsuchida O. Chest pain—the esophagus was the cause. Yuhisha; 2011. (in Japanese)
6. Rena Y, et al. Esophageal motility disorders on high-resolution manometry: Chicago classification version 4.0. Neurogastroenterol Motil. 2021;33:e14058.
7. Kahrilas PJ, et al. The Chicago classification of esophageal motility disorders, v3.0. Neurogastroenterol Motil. 2015;27:160–74.
8. Fass R, et al. Non-cardiac chest pain. J Clin Gastroenterol. 2008;42:636–46.
9. Juan GC, et al. Factors predictive of gastroesophageal reflux disease and esophageal cardiac chest pain. J Gastroenterol Hepatol. 2018;53:643–9.
10. Jones H, et al. Treatment of non-cardiac chest pain: a controlled trial of hypnotherapy. Gut. 2006;55:1403–8.
11. Cardi M, et al. Cardial achalasia and emotional stress: consideration on 47 clinical cases. Minerva Med. 1984;75:405–8.

Case Discussions, Gastroduodenal Lesions on DGBI

84

Hirokuni Okumi

Abstract

Functional dyspepsia (FD) is a common functional gastrointestinal disorder characterized by chronic upper abdominal discomfort in the absence of identifiable organic disease. In clinical practice, FD is frequently associated with comorbidities, including psychiatric disorders, other functional gastrointestinal disorders (FGIDs) such as irritable bowel syndrome (IBS) and gastroesophageal reflux disease (GERD), and other functional somatic syndromes (FSS) such as functional headache. These comorbid conditions can complicate both diagnosis and management. Additionally, FD shares overlapping symptoms with *Helicobacter pylori*-associated dyspepsia (HpD), posing a challenge for accurate differential diagnosis. This article presents clinical cases illustrating common patterns of FD: (1) FD with comorbid mental disorders, (2) FD with coexisting FGIDs, (3) FD with comorbid FSS, and (4) differential diagnosis between FD and HpD.

H. Okumi (✉)
Okumi Clinic, Ihoukai Medical Association, PsychoSomatic Medicine, Gastroenterology, Japanese Traditional (Kampo) Medicine, Osaka, Japan
e-mail: okuhiro@ihoukai.jp

Keywords

Functional dyspepsia · Comorbidity · Depression · Anxiety · Irritable bowel syndrome · Gastroesophageal reflux disorder · Functional somatic syndromes · *Helicobacter pylori*-associated dyspepsia

1 Case Presentation 1: Postprandial Distress Syndrome and Epigastric Pain Syndrome with Coexisting Psychiatric Disorders

Functional abnormalities of the upper abdomen presenting with epigastric discomfort and epigastric pain were historically referred to as "neurogenic gastritis" or "gastric atony," though these terms lacked clear definitions. Since the 1980s, the term *nonulcer dyspepsia* became standardized, and the condition was classified into subtypes—reflux type, gastritis type, and ulcer type—primarily characterized by heartburn, abdominal bloating, and epigastric pain. However, in the 1990s, the reflux type was reclassified as *gastroesophageal reflux disease (GERD)*. Following the Rome III criteria, the condition characterized by postprandial bloating and epigastric pain was established as *functional dyspepsia (FD)* (see Chap. 77).

H. Kaneko et al. (eds.), *Disorders of Gut-Brain Interaction*,
https://doi.org/10.1007/978-981-95-6974-8_84

1.1 Case Summary

- *Patient*: A 48-year-old female, homemaker
- *Chief complaints*: Loss of appetite, abdominal bloating, and stomach pain
- *History of present illness*: The patient had a history of recurrent epigastric to right hypochondrial pain. Since January of the previous year, she experienced persistent epigastric discomfort and pain following dinner. Over-the-counter medications were ineffective. After visiting a local clinic, she was referred to the gastroenterology department of a general hospital. No gross abnormalities were found, including on esophagogastroduodenoscopy (EGD). In January of the current year, she was referred to the psychosomatic medicine outpatient clinic.
- *Medical history*: Panic disorder
- *Psychosocial background*: Eldest daughter of three siblings, born to a father in the construction industry and a homemaker mother. Raised by a doting father and a somewhat overbearing mother. After graduating from high school and working part-time, she married at the age of 25, against her parents' wishes, to a husband from an old-established family. However, she divorced at age 30 due to the overinvolvement of her in-laws. She later remarried and currently leads a stable life aside from her gastrointestinal symptoms.

1.2 Examination Findings

- *Hospital Anxiety and Depression Scale (HADS)*: Anxiety 8 and depression 3
- *Gastrointestinal Symptom Rating Scale (GSRS)*: Abdominal pain 6, heartburn 6, reflux 6, nausea 6, abdominal bloating 6, and constipation 3

1.3 Clinical Course

Psychosocial factors such as overprotective parenting, traumatic experiences with her in-laws, and a premorbid personality characterized by excessive compliance were considered predisposing factors. Initially, *Rikkunshito* (a traditional Japanese herbal medicine) was prescribed. Due to her anxiety tendencies, *ethyl loflazepate* was added from the outset. Brief psychotherapy was also initiated. After six weeks, her abdominal discomfort stabilized except during episodes of overeating, though abdominal pain persisted. On day 90, a proton pump inhibitor (PPI) was added, resulting in partial symptom relief. Due to continued intermittent abdominal pain and bloating, the herbal prescription was changed to *Anchusan* on day 135, which led to marked improvement. The patient has since maintained a favorable clinical course.

1.4 Discussion

Postprandial distress syndrome (PDS), characterized by postprandial abdominal bloating and early satiety, and *epigastric pain syndrome (EPS)*, characterized by epigastric pain and burning unrelated to meals, are distinct subtypes of FD (1). However, overlap between the two is not uncommon (2). According to the Japanese Society of Gastroenterology's FD guidelines, evidence-based pharmacologic treatments include acid-suppressive agents such as proton pump inhibitors and H_2-receptor antagonists, as well as *acotiamide* and *Rikkunshito*. Additionally, commonly used agents include gastrointestinal prokinetics such as *mosapride* and *itopride*, and Japanese traditional medicines like *Anchusan*. In clinical practice, treatment should be tailored flexibly based on symptom presentation.

In this case, comorbid anxiety disorders such as panic disorder were present, and anxiolytics were introduced early in the treatment course. Such psychiatric comorbidities are frequently observed in patients with *functional gastrointestinal disorders (FGIDs)*. Therefore, when FGIDs are suspected, it is advisable to assess not only gastrointestinal symptoms but also the degree of anxiety and depression. The HADS, used in this case, is a simple and effective tool for evaluating psychiatric symptoms in general internal medicine settings.

2 Case Presentation 2: Functional Dyspepsia with Coexisting Other Functional Gastrointestinal Disorders

Within the spectrum of *functional gastrointestinal disorders (FGIDs)*, it is well recognized that *irritable bowel syndrome (IBS)* and *functional dyspepsia (FD)* frequently coexist. Similarly, comorbidity with *gastroesophageal reflux disease (GERD)* is also not uncommon.

2.1 Case Summary

- *Patient*: A 35-year-old female, office worker
- *Chief complaints*: Alternating diarrhea and constipation, early satiety, and intermittent chest discomfort
- *History of present illness*: Beginning around June two years prior, the patient began experiencing frequent episodes of diarrhea upon commuting to work. Subsequently, she developed alternating patterns of constipation and diarrhea. During this period, she also began experiencing intermittent sensations of chest tightness. Postprandial abdominal bloating became prominent, leading to reduced food intake. After visiting a local clinic, she was referred to the internal medicine and gastroenterology departments of a general hospital. Despite thorough evaluation, including endoscopy, no organic abnormalities were identified. Due to persistent symptoms, she was referred to the psychosomatic medicine outpatient clinic.
- *Past medical history*: Migraine
- *Physical examination*: Abdomen was flat and soft. Tympanic sounds were noted from the epigastrium and right hypochondrium to the ileocecal region. Bowel sounds were hyperactive.
- *Gastrointestinal Symptom Rating Scale (GSRS)*: Abdominal bloating 6, heartburn 5, and early satiety 4
- *Izumo scale*: Heartburn 0/1/0, abdominal pain 2/1/3, stomach heaviness 4/4/4, constipation 4/3/3, and diarrhea 4/3/1
- *Frequency Scale for the Symptoms of GERD (FSSG)*: Acid reflux 7/28 and dysmotility 15/28

2.2 Psychosocial Background

The patient is the eldest of three siblings, born to a civil servant father and a homemaker mother. She was raised in a harmonious family environment and attended an integrated elementary through high school program before enrolling in a law faculty at university. After graduation, she began working at an apparel company, but due to frequent stress from customer service, she changed jobs at age 30 and joined a textile company. Although interpersonal relationships at the new workplace were favorable, she was appointed as the lead for a new business project two years ago, which significantly increased her workload. It was during this period that her abdominal symptoms began to manifest.

2.3 Clinical Course

This case demonstrated the coexistence of FD, IBS, and GERD, all within the FGID spectrum. Notably, FD and GERD were not initially reported as chief complaints. However, detailed history-taking and self-administered symptom assessments revealed the presence of early satiety and chest discomfort, leading to the diagnosis of each respective condition. For GERD, an upper gastrointestinal endoscopy was performed, and the patient was diagnosed with *nonerosive reflux disease (NERD)*.

Pharmacological treatment was initiated based on both evidence and Kampo (Japanese Traditional Medicine) diagnostic principles. *Rikkunshito* was prescribed for FD. For IBS, *calcium polycarbophil* and probiotics were administered. For NERD, *lansoprazole* was prescribed.

A thorough psychosocial interview was conducted to assess environmental factors, including workload and interpersonal dynamics at the workplace. Based on these findings, coordination with the employer was undertaken to arrange a leave of absence and a phased return-to-work plan. Following these interventions, all symptoms gradually improved, and the patient was able to return to work on day 100 after the initial consultation.

2.4 Discussion

In FGIDs, overlapping disease concepts are common. However, patients with multiple symptoms often do not report all of them during the initial consultation. Therefore, self-administered gastrointestinal symptom questionnaires are extremely useful for identifying symptoms beyond the chief complaint (3). In this case, a combination of tools—including the GSRS, Izumo Scale, and FSSG—enabled efficient diagnosis.

In cases of FD coexisting with IBS or GERD, polypharmacy should be avoided. It is essential to consider drug interactions and dosing frequency when selecting medications. GERD has traditionally been classified into *reflux esophagitis (RE)* and *nonerosive reflux disease (NERD)* based on the presence or absence of mucosal erosions at the gastroesophageal junction (4). However, recent classifications have expanded to include four subtypes: RE, NERD, reflux hypersensitivity, and functional heartburn. While proton pump inhibitors remain the mainstay of treatment, in refractory cases, psychotropic agents and neuromodulators have also been reported as effective.

3 Case Presentation 3: Functional Dyspepsia with Coexisting Functional Somatic Syndromes

Among patients with *functional gastrointestinal disorders (FGIDs)* (5), it is clinically common to observe comorbid functional disorders outside the gastrointestinal system. These conditions are collectively referred to as *functional somatic syndromes (FSS)* (see Table 84.1).

3.1 Case Summary

- *Patient*: A 56-year-old male
- *Chief complaints*: Postprandial upper abdominal discomfort, intermittent epigastric pain, and occipital to vertex headache
- *History of present illness*: For the past five years, the patient had experienced intermittent dull occipital headaches in the evening, which were left untreated. In the spring of the current year, he began experiencing postprandial

Table 84.1 Overview of functional somatic syndromes (FSS)

Medical specialty	Syndrome
Gastroenterology	Functional gastrointestinal disorders (e.g., functional dyspepsia and irritable bowel syndrome)
Gynecology	Chronic pelvic pain and menstrual irregularities
Rheumatology/ collagen diseases	Fibromyalgia syndrome
Cardiology	Noncardiac chest pain
Endocrinology	Functional hyperthermia (psychogenic fever)
Cardiovascular medicine	Orthostatic dysregulation
Orthopedics	Chronic low back pain syndrome
Neurology	Chronic functional headache (e.g., migraine, tension-type headache)
Others	Chronic fatigue syndrome and globus sensation

upper abdominal discomfort. His headaches also intensified, occasionally becoming severe and extending to the vertex. He underwent a comprehensive evaluation at the internal medicine and gastroenterology departments of another hospital, but no gross abnormalities were detected. He was subsequently referred to the psychosomatic medicine outpatient clinic in June of this year.

- *Physical examination*: Mild epigastric distension with slight tenderness and normal bowel sounds
- *Gastrointestinal Symptom Rating Scale (GSRS)*: Abdominal bloating 6, nausea 5, fasting epigastric pain 3, and abdominal pain 3
- *Izumo Scale*: Heartburn 0/1/0, abdominal pain 2/1/3, stomach heaviness 4/4/4, constipation 1/0/0, and diarrhea 1/1/0
- *Frequency Scale for the Symptoms of GERD (FSSG)*: Acid reflux-related symptoms 7/28 and dysmotility symptoms 15/28
- *(Headache assessment omitted)*

3.2 Psychosocial Background

The patient is the youngest of three brothers. He was raised in a tolerant household and lived in the Hokuriku region until junior high school. Following his father's job transfer, the family relocated. He attended a commercial high school and later enrolled in a private university's commerce department. After graduation, he joined a general trading company but left at age 30 due to conflicts with his supervisor. He then worked in sales, where he was subjected to long working hours under a quota system, which imposed significant psychological stress. From his late 40s, he began experiencing intermittent symptoms such as shoulder stiffness and back pain and from his 50s occasional headaches accompanied by dizziness.

3.3 Clinical Course

The patient was diagnosed with *functional dyspepsia (FD)*. For pharmacological treatment, the acid-suppressive agent *famotidine* was selected. Regarding his headaches, a diagnosis of *tension-type headache (TTH)* with superimposed migraine features was made, and he was diagnosed with mixed-type headache (6). To alleviate symptoms, low-dose *amitriptyline* and *propranolol* were prescribed at bedtime. As a result, upper abdominal pain became intermittent, and headaches showed partial improvement, though symptoms persisted.

To further address gastrointestinal symptoms, *acotiamide* was added to regulate gastrointestinal function. Additionally, a medical certificate was issued requesting workplace accommodations, including adjustments to working hours and job responsibilities. These changes led to the implementation of flexible working hours and the avoidance of overtime. Following these environmental modifications, both headache and abdominal symptoms nearly resolved. On day 290 after the initial consultation, the patient was referred back to a local clinic for continued medication management, and care at our department was concluded.

3.4 Discussion

In this case, the patient presented with mixed headache symptoms, including epigastric pain syndrome and postprandial dyspepsia syndrome as FD, as well as TTH and migraine. The association between headache and functional gastrointestinal disorders has been observed previously and is commonly reported. FGID is often accompanied by mind-body relations, it is important to conduct a detailed interview about the patient's living environment at the initial consultation and to carefully inquire about changes in abdominal symptoms during subsequent follow-up consultations. At the same time, it is important to be aware of the possibility of functional somatic syndrome (FSS) and to plan treatment accordingly, seeking the help of specialists in relevant fields as needed.

4 Case Presentation 4: Differentiating Functional Dyspepsia from *Helicobacter pylori*-Associated Dyspepsia

In recent years, *Helicobacter pylori (H. pylori)*-associated gastric lesions, such as peptic ulcers and gastritis, have been recognized under national health insurance coverage in Japan, making eradication therapy an approved treatment. Clinically, however, dyspeptic symptoms resembling *functional dyspepsia (FD)* are frequently observed in patients infected with *H. pylori*. This clinical entity has led to the establishment of the concept of *H. pylori-associated dyspepsia (HpD)*. Due to differences in treatment strategies, HpD is considered pathophysiologically distinct from FD. Histologically, HpD is characterized by microscopic inflammation of the gastric mucosa, including eosinophilic infiltration, triggered by exposure to gastric acid or dietary antigens in the presence of *H. pylori*. This inflammation is thought to contribute to gastric motility disorders and visceral hypersensitivity.

4.1 Case Summary

- *Patient*: A 75-year-old female, unemployed
- *Chief complaints*: Epigastric burning and pain, postprandial nausea, and diarrhea
- *History of present illness*: Since July, the patient developed sudden onset of epigastric burning and pain, accompanied by multiple episodes of diarrhea per day. She was referred to the gastroenterology department of a university hospital by a local clinic and underwent inpatient evaluation. Upper gastrointestinal endoscopy revealed only mild gastritis. In September, she visited another hospital's gastroenterology department, where medication adjustments were made, but her symptoms persisted. In November of the same year, she was referred to the psychosomatic medicine outpatient clinic due to suspected psychogenic etiology.
- *Past medical history*: Intracerebral hemorrhage (no residual deficits)
- *Family history*: Father, angina pectoris; mother, hypertension, and chronic renal failure
- *Lifestyle history*: Nonsmoker, occasional alcohol consumption
- *Psychosocial background*: Second of four siblings, born to two schoolteachers. The family returned from Taiwan after World War II. She had good relationships with her siblings. From elementary through high school, she experienced mild social anxiety but was diligent. After graduating high school, she worked as an office clerk and later attended a dressmaking school at age 20. She married her current husband, who works in the printing industry. Although they moved frequently, they had one son and one daughter. The marital relationship was good, but in recent years, caregiving responsibilities increased due to her husband's diabetes and emphysema.

4.2 Physical Examination

No significant findings.

- *GSRS*: Heartburn 5, abdominal bloating 5, fasting epigastric pain 4, nausea 4, abdominal pain 4, diarrhea 4, loose stools 4, and epigastric discomfort 4
- *Izumo Scale*: Heartburn 2/3/3, abdominal pain 2/4/5, stomach heaviness 2/3/2, diarrhea 5/4/3, and constipation 4/2/1
- *FSSG*: Acid reflux 15/28 and dysmotility 20/28

4.3 Clinical Course

As several years had passed since her last upper gastrointestinal endoscopy, both upper and lower endoscopic evaluations were repeated at the psychosomatic medicine clinic. Findings were limited to C-III grade (severe) atrophic gastritis. During endoscopy, biopsy and culture testing for *H. pylori* were performed, yielding positive results. Based on these findings, HpD was suspected, and eradication therapy was initiated using a combination of *lansoprazole*, *amoxicillin*, and *clarithromycin*. Following a single course of treatment, *H. pylori* was eradicated. Posttreat ment, her abdominal bloating and nausea improved; however, diarrhea—likely stress-related—persisted.

To address environmental stressors, discussions were held regarding her caregiving responsibilities. Adjustments were made to her husband's care plan, including changes to his long-term care certification and the introduction of public support services. These interventions led to gradual improvement in her lower abdominal symptoms. She is currently under observation with a regimen of proton pump inhibitors and gastrointestinal motility regulators.

4.4 Discussion

This case represents a comorbidity of *H. pylori-associated dyspepsia (HpD)* and *irritable bowel syndrome (IBS)*. The differential diagnosis between HpD and FD is based not only on the presence of *H. pylori* infection but also on the clinical response to eradication therapy (7–9). In this case, *H. pylori* infection had not been previously identified. Upon detection, eradication therapy was administered, resulting in improvement of upper abdominal symptoms. However, lower abdominal symptoms persisted.

As discussed in the previous case, FD and IBS frequently coexist. However, it is important to recognize that upper abdominal symptoms in patients with IBS are not always indicative of FD. In *H. pylori*-positive patients with upper abdominal symptoms and no organic disease, if symptoms do not resolve after successful eradication, HpD should be ruled out, and a diagnosis of FD coexisting with asymptomatic *H. pylori* infection should be considered. Based on the association between upper abdominal symptoms and HP eradication therapy in FGID, it is necessary to accurately understand the course and condition of the disease and to flexibly perform treatment and diagnosis.

Take-Home Message

In FGIDs, where psychosomatic correlations are common, it is essential to understand the frequent overlap among FD, IBS, psychiatric disorders such as anxiety and depression, and other *functional somatic syndromes (FSS)*. At the initial consultation, comprehensive interviews should assess gastrointestinal symptoms, psychological distress, and the presence of nongastrointestinal functional disorders. In cases of upper abdominal symptoms, *H. pylori* infection should also be considered in the differential diagnosis.

Furthermore, careful assessment of the patient's living environment is crucial. At each follow-up visit, physical examination of the abdomen and detailed evaluation of symptom progression or remission should be conducted. Such a proactive and attentive approach by healthcare providers is key to successful treatment outcomes.

Competing Interests The author(s) has no competing interests to declare that are relevant to the content of this manuscript.

References

1. Japanese Society of Gastroenterology. Clinical practice guidelines for functional gastrointestinal disorders 2021 – Functional Dyspepsia (FD), Revised 2nd edn. 2021; pp. 57–8, 61–3. (in Japanese).
2. Tominaga K, et al. Rikkunshito simultaneously improves dyspepsia correlated with anxiety in patients with functional dyspepsia (the DREAM study). Neurogastroenterol Motil. 2018;30:e13319.
3. Palsson OS, et al. Development and validation of the Rome IV diagnostic questionnaire for adults. Gastroenterology. 2016;150:1481–91.
4. Ohara S, et al. Survey on the prevalence of GERD and FD based on the Montreal definition and the Rome III criteria among patients presenting with epigastric symptoms in Japan. J Gastroenterol. 2011;46:603–11.
5. Afari N, et al. Psychological trauma and functional somatic syndromes: a systematic review and meta-analysis. Psychosom Med. 2014;76:2–11.
6. Aurora SK, et al. A link between gastrointestinal disorders and migraine: insights into the gut-brain connection. Headache. 2021;61:576–89.
7. Japanese Society for *Helicobacter* Research, Guideline Committee. Guidelines for the Diagnosis

and Treatment of *H. pylori* Infection 2016, Revised Edition. Sentan Igakusha; 2016. (in Japanese).
8. Zhao B, et al. Efficacy of *Helicobacter pylori* eradication therapy on functional dyspepsia: a meta-analysis of randomized controlled studies with 12-month follow-up. J Clin Gastroenterol. 2014;48:241–7.
9. Suzuki H, et al. What is the difference between *Helicobacter pylori*-associated dyspepsia and functional dyspepsia? J Neurogastroenterol Motil. 2011;17:124–30.

85 Case Discussion, Psychotherapy (Hypnotherapy)

Yoshikazu Fukui

Abstract

Functional gastrointestinal disorders (FGIDs), including irritable bowel syndrome (IBS), often show limited response to standard medical treatments, making psychotherapy an important option. Gut-directed hypnotherapy (GDH) has established efficacy, yet treatment-resistant cases remain. We present a case of a woman in her 40s with diarrhea-predominant IBS unresponsive to pharmacotherapy. Initial GDH following the North Carolina Protocol led to partial improvement but persistent anxiety. Stabilization strategies such as the Extended Container Technique and autonomic regulation were introduced, followed by resource development. As traumatic memories appeared relevant, trauma-focused approaches including eye movement desensitization and reprocessing (EMDR) and ego state therapy were integrated. Symptom remission was achieved, with long-term resolution of IBS symptoms despite minor anxiety recurrence after treatment. This case illustrates how combining GDH with trauma-focused psychotherapy may benefit refractory IBS, consistent with evidence linking trauma to FGIDs. However, as evidence is limited, controlled studies are required. Clinically, careful psychoeducation and culturally sensitive introduction of hypnosis are essential in Japan, where negative perceptions of hypnosis persist. This report highlights the need for comprehensive, individualized approaches to psychotherapy for FGIDs.

Keywords

Functional gastrointestinal disorders (FGIDs) · Irritable bowel syndrome (IBS) · Gut-directed hypnotherapy (GDH) · Trauma-focused psychotherapy

1 Psychotherapy for Functional Gastrointestinal Disorders (FGIDs)

Notably, gut-directed hypnotherapy (GDH) has demonstrated specific efficacy in the treatment of FGIDs, in addition to evidence supporting the use of cognitive behavioral therapy (CBT), psychodynamic psychotherapy, and relaxation techniques. Based on these findings, clinical guidelines for prominent FGIDs such as irritable bowel syndrome (IBS) and functional dyspepsia (FD) recommend psychotherapy, including hypnotherapy, for patients unresponsive to standard treatments [1, 2].

Y. Fukui (✉)
Department of Human Sciences, Faculty of Letters, Konan University, Kobe, Japan
e-mail: yfukui@konan-u.ac.jp

H. Kaneko et al. (eds.), *Disorders of Gut-Brain Interaction*,
https://doi.org/10.1007/978-981-95-6974-8_85

Efficacy research on GDH was pioneered by the so-called Manchester approach [3]. This method includes progressive relaxation, ego strengthening, self-hypnosis practice, and gut-directed therapeutic suggestions aimed at normalizing gut function and enhancing self-control. Many efficacy studies have utilized this approach or its derivatives.

Recently, the North Carolina Protocol (North Carolina Hypnosis Treatment Protocol for IBS: NCP) has shown remarkable results [4, 5]. This comprehensive approach offers a balanced integration of elements such as distraction, ego strengthening, and desensitization. It is distinctive in that it is effective across all IBS subtypes and applicable to treatment-resistant cases, regardless of the patient's hypnotic susceptibility.

In Japan, Fukui [6] has provided detailed accounts of the practical application and challenges of hypnotherapy for IBS, while Kaneko and Fukui [7] have described the application of psychotherapy for FD.

However, in Japan, there are very few case studies and no domestically generated evidence-based research on psychotherapy for FGIDs [8, 9]. As a result, both patients and clinicians often lack a clear picture of the treatment process, which is thought to be one factor contributing to low accessibility.

Therefore, I present a case of treatment-resistant diarrhea-predominant IBS which is not only a standard GDH but also trauma-focused psychotherapy as combined in a more comprehensive approach, and I consider its application and challenges.

2 Case Presentation (Diarrhea-Predominant IBS)

Client: Female in her 40s, working in the social welfare sector.

Chief complaints: Diarrhea, abdominal pain, compulsive defecation behavior, and anxiety

History of present illness:

Three years prior, the client divorced her husband due to domestic violence (DV) and subsequently underwent mediation over child custody. She then took a job in the social welfare sector. Approximately 1 year ago, following a conflict with one of her colleagues, she developed abdominal pain and diarrhea. She visited a local clinic and was prescribed gastrointestinal medications for 2 months, but her symptoms did not improve. She was then referred to a university hospital, where she was diagnosed with diarrhea-predominant *irritable bowel syndrome (IBS)*. Due to anxiety about access to toilets, she had difficulty commuting by train and instead began cycling 60 min each way to work. During her commute, she compulsively used restrooms at several parks and convenience stores. She was referred to a psychosomatic medicine clinic by her local physician. After 1 month of treatment with anxiolytics and antidepressants, which proved ineffective, she discontinued the medication on her own. Psychotherapy was deemed appropriate, and she was referred to the author for treatment.

Therapeutic Structure:

Conducted at a private practice in clinical psychology. The initial session lasted 80 min, and the 2nd and 13th sessions were 50 min each. All other sessions were 100 min in duration, with the client attending once every 1–2 weeks.

3 Interview Progress

During the initial session, the client appeared completely exhausted. I obtained a history of her current symptoms and present illness. She spoke quickly, but her content was circuitous and verbose. She attempted to discuss workplace conflicts and DV from her husband, but due to concerns about symptom exacerbation from traumatic memory activation, I often had to interrupt after explaining my reasons for doing so.

In the second session, psychoeducation was provided on basic knowledge about IBS and the risks of avoidance conditioning from compulsive defecation. The client listened attentively while taking notes. At the end of the session, I explained the evidence for and applicability of GDH and obtained her consent to proceed.

In the third session, GDH was introduced, and the aforementioned standard NCP was implemented. The content was recorded on the client's smartphone, and she was assigned the homework of listening to it repeatedly at home before the next session.

In the fourth session, the subjective distress level of her overall symptoms decreased from 10 to 8 on a scale of 0–10, but her anxiety about possible defecation failures increased. Therefore, the extended container technique (ECT) was introduced for anxiety management [10]. This technique, developed to stabilize symptoms and daily functioning during the preparation phase of trauma care, involves imagining wrapping stress, worries, symptoms, and memories in cloth, placing them in a box, and storing them in a safe place. Case reports have shown stabilization effects [11], and randomized controlled trials (RCTs) have reported psychological effects such as decentering and increased tolerance for ambiguity [12]. After practicing the skill of temporarily setting aside anxiety with ECT, I added an original autonomic nervous system regulation protocol [6] NCP. This was recorded and assigned as homework along with ECT.

In the fifth session, the distress level decreased to 5. She became able to manage her anxiety to some extent, and the frequency and intensity of abdominal pain and diarrhea decreased. Using ECT, distressing memories related to DV and court proceedings were contained. The same homework as the previous session was assigned.

In the sixth session, the distress level decreased to 3. The frequency of diarrhea and preemptive defecation decreased, and workplace calmness increased. Memories of the conflict with the colleague that triggered the symptoms were contained using ECT. The same homework as the previous session was assigned.

In the seventh session, the subjective distress level decreased to 2. Abdominal pain and diarrhea symptoms markedly reduced, and the client expressed a desire to return to commuting by train. When asked about the qualities she considered necessary, she responded, "confidence." Therefore, resource development and installation (RDI) was introduced [13]. This procedure, used in the preparation phase of trauma-focused psychotherapy EMDR (eye movement desensitization and reprocessing) [14], involves activating and utilizing past experiences of confidence. Additionally, further ego strengthening and mental rehearsal for commuting by train were incorporated into the NCP. This exercise was recorded and assigned as homework.

In the eighth session, the subjective distress level decreased to 1, and IBS symptoms had nearly disappeared. It was confirmed that she could commute by train without any difficulties. However, she experienced mild abdominal pain several times. Upon reviewing her developmental history, she revealed extreme fear of her father, who had been violent toward her mother during her childhood. She recalled being severely reprimanded by her father for missing school due to abdominal pain, which resulted in her mother being beaten (she had no history of physical abuse herself). Additionally, during high school, she developed IBS-like symptoms (undiagnosed) following severe reprimands from a male advisor in the brass band, resulting in school absenteeism for about a month and a half, after which the symptoms remitted spontaneously. Therefore, the background factors of IBS were explained, and consent for trauma-focused psychotherapy was obtained. The same homework as the previous session was assigned.

In the ninth session, the subjective level of distress rose to 1.5, and both the frequency and intensity of abdominal pain increased slightly. Therefore, EMDR was introduced for the previously described episodes. During the process of memory reprocessing, the client reported hearing a voice inside her head saying, “It is your fault that your mother was beaten.” This was interpreted as an ego state (a facet of the self corresponding to a latent and fragmented personality) [15], and EMDR reprocessing was suspended in order to implement ego state therapy [16]. When the true intention of this ego state was questioned, it responded in the appearance and voice of her father: “If I do not keep watch over her like this, she will end up failing.” When the therapist acknowledged this role by saying, "So you have been protecting A during her childhood. Thank you for taking on such a difficult role," its stance softened, and it explained, "If this child were to do something wrong, the mother would suffer terribly, so I have been keeping watch here to prevent that." The therapist then asked, "You are not her real father, are you? If you were truly her father, you would not do things like prevent her mother from being beaten." At this point, the ego state transformed into the figure of a child resembling the client's younger self and said, "Because I wanted to protect my mother, I borrowed my father's image and have been doing my best to keep this child from failing." After sufficient acknowledgment from the therapist, the following question was posed as a cognitive interweave: "But in that situation, who truly needed to be protected—your mother, or you as the young child?" After a moment of silence, the ego state whispered, "Me?" and the client reported breaking down in tears. Adult A was then asked to hug the child ego state, providing protection and support. Once the child ego state calmed down, arrangements were made for it to be placed in an imagined safe room under the care of another nurturing ego state, after which reprocessing of the initial traumatic memory resumed. The client expressed what she had wanted to say to her parents at the time, and reprocessing of that scene was nearly completed. However, associations then extended to another old memory of being threatened by her father. This memory was contained using ECT, and the procedure was discontinued midway.

In the tenth session, the subjective distress level decreased to 0.5, and abdominal pain occurred only once. The distress level of the original event handled in the previous session was 0, so EMDR was applied to the newly emerged memory, completing its reprocessing (*details omitted for brevity*). Additionally, reprocessing of the high school memory was completed.

In the 11th session, the subjective distress level remained at 0.5, so EMDR was applied to representative memories of DV from her husband, completing their reprocessing.

In the 12th session, the subjective distress level decreased to 0, and IBS symptoms completely disappeared. The client expressed lingering resentment toward a former colleague, so interpersonal skills deficits were pointed out, and then specific coping skills were provided by the therapist.

In the 13th session, the client reported that IBS symptoms remained absent and that her adjustment at work had improved. The remaining time was spent reinforcing positive changes. The client was advised to contact the therapist in case of recurrence, and treatment was concluded. She did not return for further follow-up. Approximately 5 months later, the client experienced anxiety after seeing her ex-husband at a train station and visited the psychosomatic medicine clinic that had referred her the following day. She was prescribed anxiolytics on an as-needed basis, but no recurrence of IBS symptoms was confirmed. No further follow-up visits were conducted.

4 Discussion

This case was considered to represent treatment-resistant IBS, unresponsive to standard treatments. Gut-directed hypnotherapy GDH was chosen as the initial psychotherapeutic approach because it places relatively fewer demands on patient engagement and adherence than CBT—a consideration particularly important for patients already exhausted by maladaptive coping with persistent symptoms.

Initial improvement with standard GDH was modest, and the patient exhibited marked anxiety symptoms. Therefore, stabilization interventions were introduced. In addition, the GDH protocol was augmented by incorporating a component targeting autonomic nervous system regulation—not merely promoting parasympathetic dominance through relaxation but with the aim of optimizing the function of both sympathetic and parasympathetic systems. This modification appeared to facilitate progress; however, because both interventions were implemented simultaneously, it remains unclear which effect was responsible. It is hypothesized that stabilization enhanced the patient's sense of self-regulation over stress and anxiety, whereas autonomic regulation directly improved physical reactivity. As symptoms did not fully resolve, trauma-focused reprocessing was initiated to address childhood memories suspected to underlie the condition. The Clinical Practice Guidelines for Functional Gastrointestinal Disorders (FGIDs) [1, 2] also suggest that traumatic experiences may contribute to FGIDs, and accumulating evidence [17, 18] further supports this association. Thus, the introduction of trauma-focused psychotherapy represents a logical, evidence-informed step. In this case, complete remission of IBS symptoms was achieved following trauma memory reprocessing. Based on this and other clinical experiences, trauma-focused approaches may represent promising adjunctive strategies for treatment-resistant IBS. However, to date, no established evidence supports the efficacy of trauma-focused psychotherapy in IBS, and further research is needed before such approaches can be incorporated into standard treatment guidelines. In this case, psychoeducation and resource activation also contributed to improved social functioning. The IBS guidelines [1] highlight heightened stress reactivity, suggesting that comprehensive stress management may be beneficial. Incorporating CBT elements into GDH may further enhance outcomes.

It is worth noting that only a limited portion of the patient's trauma history was addressed. The brief resurgence of anxiety after encountering her ex-husband following termination of therapy is likely attributable to the activation of unresolved trauma memories. While the treatment was sufficient from an IBS perspective, it may have been incomplete as a course of psychotherapy. Providing additional sessions to promote broader psychosocial adaptation might have been appropriate.

5 Challenges in Psychotherapy for FGIDs

This report has focused primarily on GDH as a psychotherapeutic intervention for FGIDs. However, hypnotherapy is a modality that remains difficult to evaluate. Globally, the prevailing view is that hypnosis is a technique for enhancing suggestibility, serving primarily to amplify the effects of interventions administered during the hypnotic state [19]. Therefore, the efficacy of hypnotherapy depends largely on the content of the interventions administered under hypnosis. For example, if symptom improvement occurs after relaxation conducted under hypnosis, it is difficult to determine whether the effect is attributable to hypnosis itself or to the relaxation component. Clarifying the psychophysiological mechanisms through which hypnosis contributes to symptom improvement is essential. Recent models have evolved from the *brain-gut interaction* to the more comprehensive *brain-gut-microbiome interaction* [20], offering a broader explanatory framework. Positioning GDH within this model may facilitate further mechanistic research.

Another challenge is the limited accessibility of psychotherapy—particularly hypnotherapy—for the general population. Addressing this issue requires not only increased awareness among clinicians but also innovations such as shorter treatment durations and group-based formats. Recently, mobile app-based GDH interventions for IBS have been explored [21], representing a promising area for future development.

Take-Home Message
In Japan, negative perceptions surrounding hypnosis may lead some clients to reject treatment solely based on the term. When introducing GDH, clinicians must provide careful and accurate explanations to mitigate such resistance.

In addition, hypnosis should not be viewed as a panacea. As noted, it functions as an amplifier of other interventions. If a therapeutic goal cannot be achieved without hypnosis, it is unlikely to be achieved with it. To maximize treatment efficacy, clinicians must thoroughly understand the content and function of each GDH component before applying it.

With these considerations in mind, clinicians are encouraged to actively explore the use of GDH in the treatment of FGIDs.

Competing Interests The author(s) has no competing interests to declare that are relevant to the content of this manuscript.

References

1. Japanese Society of Gastroenterology. Clinical Practice Guidelines for Functional Gastrointestinal Disorders 2020, Revised 2nd Edition – Irritable Bowel Syndrome (IBS). (in Japanese).
2. Japanese Society of Gastroenterology. Clinical Practice Guidelines for Functional Gastrointestinal Disorders 2021, Revised 2nd Edition – Functional Dyspepsia (FD). (in Japanese).
3. Whorwell PJ, et al. Hypnotherapy in severe irritable bowel syndrome: further experience. Gut. 1987;28:423–5.
4. Palsson OS. Standardized hypnosis treatment for irritable bowel syndrome: The North Carolina protocol. Int J Clin Exp Hypn. 2006;54:51–64.
5. Palsson OS, Whitehead WE. Hypnosis and guided imagery treatment for gastrointestinal disorders: experience with scripted protocols developed at the University of North Carolina. Am J Clin Hypn. 2015;58:5–21.
6. Fukui Y. Practical application and challenges of hypnotherapy for irritable bowel syndrome (IBS) in Japan. Jpn J Psych Med. 2021;61:347–53. (in Japanese).
7. Kaneko H, et al. Expected developments in the treatment of functional dyspepsia: focus on psychosomatic approaches. J Jpn Soc Gastroenterol. 2016;113:947–58. (in Japanese).
8. Yokoyama A. A case of diarrhea-predominant IBS effectively treated with a single session of age regression hypnotherapy. Jpn J Psych Med. 2019;59:251–7. (in Japanese).
9. Fujita S, et al. A case of paralytic ileus after surgery effectively treated with hypnotherapy. J Clin Hyp. 2015;16:43–52. (in Japanese).
10. Fukui Y. Expansion and application of the container exercise in EMDR: practical use of the three-layer containment model. In: Proceedings of the 11th annual meeting of the Japan EMDR association; 2016. p. 16. (in Japanese).
11. Kajiwara T, et al. A case of panic disorder treated with stabilization techniques. In: Proceedings of the 2nd joint meeting of Japanese Psychosomatic Medicine Societies/60th Annual Meeting of the Japanese Society of Psychosomatic Medicine; 2019. p. 287. (in Japanese).
12. Ueda A, et al. Stress-reducing effects of the extended container technique: an intervention study targeting university students. In: Proceedings of the 64th Annual Meeting of the Japanese Society of Psychosomatic Medicine; 2023. p. 175. (in Japanese).
13. Korn DL, Leeds AM. Preliminary evidence of efficacy for EMDR resource development and installation in the stabilization phase of treatment of complex posttraumatic stress disorder. J Clin Psychol. 2002;58:1465–87.
14. Shapiro F. Eye movement desensitization and reprocessing: basic principles, protocols, and procedures. 2nd ed. Guilford Press; 2001. (Japanese translation supervised by Masaya Ichii: EMDR: A Psychotherapy for Processing Traumatic Memories. Nihon Hyoronsha; 2004).
15. Fukui Y. Ego state therapy. In: Matsushita M, editor. Somatic symptom disorders, dissociative disorders, psychosomatic disorders, and eating disorders; 2021. p. 165–8. (in Japanese).
16. Watkins JG, Watkins HH. Ego states: theory and therapy. W.W. Norton; 1997. (Japanese translation supervised by Yoshikazu Fukui et al.: Ego State Therapy: Theory and Practice. Kongō Shuppan; 2019).
17. Melchior C, et al. Relationship between abuse history and gastrointestinal and extraintestinal symptom severity in irritable bowel syndrome. Psychosom Med. 2022;84:1021–33.
18. Kearney DJ. Prevalence of gastrointestinal symptoms and irritable bowel syndrome among individuals with symptomatic posttraumatic stress disorder. J Clin Gastroenterol. 2022;56:592–6.
19. Takaishi N, et al. Contemporary hypnosis: clinical, theoretical, and empirical foundations. Kongō Shuppan; 2012. (in Japanese).
20. Mayer EA, et al. The neurobiology of irritable bowel syndrome. Mol Psychiatry. 2023;28:1451–65.
21. Peters SL, et al. Smartphone app-delivered gut-directed hypnotherapy improves symptoms of self-reported irritable bowel syndrome: a retrospective evaluation. Neurogastroenterol Motil. 2023;35:e14533.

86 Topics, Medical Remuneration for Psychosomatic Therapy

Mikihiko Fukunaga

Abstract

Psychological interventions that require specific skills and longer-than-usual consultation times are effective in treating functional gastrointestinal disorders. These interventions qualify for reimbursement as psychosomatic therapy. Reimbursable psychosomatic therapy is defined as a treatment method for psychosomatic patients that clarifies the relationship between physical illness and psychological and social factors. The therapy aims to improve symptoms or facilitate recovery from illness by exerting a psychological influence on the patient. Therefore, when billing for psychosomatic therapy, the medical record must document the assessment of mind-body correlations, the interventions performed, and their effects.

Keywords

Psychosomatic therapy · Psychosomatic disease · Psychotherapy · Remuneration · Health insurance system

A report indicates that 33% of outpatients visiting general medicine departments at Japanese university hospitals present with functional disorders, and among these, 47% are considered to have psychosocial issues [1]. In many cases, appropriate responses by physicians can alleviate patients' anxiety regarding their symptoms, thereby resolving the issue. However, a certain proportion of patients require intervention targeting psychosocial factors.

As discussed in Chap. 77—psychological interventions can be effective in the management of functional gastrointestinal disorders (FGIDs). However, such interventions typically require longer consultation times than standard medical care. For these cases, medical remuneration can be obtained under the national health insurance system for psychosomatic therapy. This section outlines what constitutes reimbursable psychosomatic therapy and under what circumstances it should be claimed *in Japan*.

According to the Ministry of Health, Labour and Welfare's Medical Fee Schedule [2], psychosomatic therapy is listed under Section 8, "Specialized Psychiatric Therapies," Item I004 (Table 86.1). Further details regarding the calculation of fees are provided in the accompanying notification [3] (Table 86.2), which will be explained below.

In Item 1 of the notification, psychosomatic therapy is defined as follows: "Psychosomatic therapy refers to a treatment method for patients

M. Fukunaga (✉)
Department of Psychosomatic Medicine, Naniwa Ikuno Hospital, Osaka, Japan
e-mail: fukunagam@hospynkh.jp

H. Kaneko et al. (eds.), *Disorders of Gut-Brain Interaction*,
https://doi.org/10.1007/978-981-95-6974-8_86

Table 86.1 Medical fee schedule for psychosomatic therapy (I004)

I004 psychosomatic therapy (per session)
1. Hospitalized patients: 150 points
2. Nonhospitalized patients:
a. Initial consultation: 110 points
b. Follow-up consultation: 80 points

Notes:
1. This therapy may be reimbursed even at medical institutions that are not officially designated as psychiatric facilities
2. On the day when the initial consultation fee listed under category code A000 is claimed, psychosomatic therapy may only be reimbursed if the consultation exceeds 30 min in duration
3. For hospitalized patients, reimbursement is limited to twice weekly during the first four weeks from the date of admission and once weekly thereafter
4. For nonhospitalized patients, reimbursement is limited to twice weekly during the first four weeks from the date of the initial consultation and once weekly thereafter
5. For patients under 20 years of age, an additional 200% of the designated point value is added to the base reimbursement
6. Editor's note: One point is equivalent to 10 Japanese yen. Under the national health insurance system, 70% of the cost is covered, and the patient's out-of-pocket share is 30%. As of March 2026, 1 U.S. dollar is approximately 155 yen. Therefore, when a patient receives an initial psychosomatic medical therapy by a doctor specialist lasting 30 minutes or longer, the additional out-of-pocket cost is approximately 3 U.S. dollars

with psychosomatic disorders that, based on a structured treatment plan, clarifies the relationship between physical illness and psychological/social factors, and aims to improve symptoms or facilitate recovery from illness by exerting psychological influence on the patient." Specific modalities include autogenic training, counseling, behavioral therapy, hypnotherapy, biofeedback therapy, transactional analysis, Gestalt therapy, bioenergetic therapy, Morita therapy, fasting therapy, general psychotherapy, and simplified psychoanalytic therapy.

However, among these, counseling and general psychotherapy lack clearly defined procedures, making it difficult to distinguish them from routine clinical practice. The critical point lies not in the specific modalities listed but in the earlier definition: "a treatment method that aims to improve symptoms or facilitate recovery

Table 86.2 Details regarding the medical fee schedule for physicians [2]

I004 psychosomatic therapy
(1) Psychosomatic therapy refers to a treatment method for patients with psychosomatic disorders, in which, based on a defined treatment plan, the relationship between physical illness and psychological or social factors is clarified, and psychological interventions are applied to the patient to promote symptom improvement or recovery from illness. This psychosomatic therapy includes autogenic training, counseling, behavioral therapy, hypnotherapy, biofeedback therapy, transactional analysis, Gestalt therapy, bioenergetic therapy, Morita therapy, fasting therapy, general psychotherapy, and brief psychoanalytic therapy
(2) Psychosomatic therapy is reimbursable only when performed by a physician who is proficient in the therapy
(3) Psychosomatic therapy may be reimbursed at the initial consultation (including the initial consultation as defined in the proviso of Note 3 under category code "A000") only if the consultation time exceeds 30 min. In this context, consultation time refers to the time the physician personally spends on patient interviews, physical examinations (inspection, auscultation, percussion, and palpation), and the psychosomatic therapy itself. Time spent on other medical services is not included. When claiming reimbursement for psychosomatic therapy at the initial consultation, the duration of the consultation must be recorded in the remarks column of the medical fee statement
(4) When claiming reimbursement for psychosomatic therapy, the diagnosis field of the medical fee statement must include the name of the physical illness followed by "(psychosomatic disorder)."
Example: "Gastric ulcer (psychosomatic disorder)"
(5) When psychosomatic therapy is performed, its key elements must be recorded in the medical record
(6) The handling of the date of admission and the hospitalization period shall follow the same rules as those applied to the basic hospitalization fee
(7) The additional reimbursement specified in Note 5 shall be applied when psychosomatic therapy is provided to patients under 20 years of age, in coordination with child consultation centers or similar institutions, and with appropriate guidance provided to guardians or caregivers
(8) Psychosomatic therapy cannot be claimed for patients who are already receiving reimbursement under category code "I001" (Inpatient Psychiatric Therapy), "I002" (Outpatient/Home Psychiatric Therapy), or "I003" (Standard Psychoanalytic Therapy)

from illness by clarifying the relationship between physical illness and psychological/

social factors and exerting psychological influence on the patient."

The distinction from standard medical care lies in two essential criteria: (1) clarifying the relationship between physical illness and psychological/social factors and (2) aiming to improve symptoms or facilitate recovery through psychological influence. In other words, if a physician can assess the psychosomatic correlation and provide therapeutic intervention with a reasonable expectation of efficacy, the treatment qualifies as psychosomatic therapy. Therefore, regardless of the specific method used, documentation in the medical record must include the psychosomatic assessment, the therapeutic intervention, and its anticipated or observed effects.

Item 2 of the notification states that "psychosomatic therapy must be performed by a physician proficient in the therapy." Although currently categorized under psychiatric therapies, any physician may claim reimbursement. Physicians treating FGIDs are typically gastroenterologists, general internists, general practitioners, or psychosomatic medicine specialists. A "physician proficient in psychosomatic therapy," as defined earlier, is one who can assess psychosomatic correlations and provide effective therapeutic interventions.

While all physicians are increasingly receiving education on psychological aspects of patient care, the multifactorial nature of psychosomatic correlations makes assessment complex. A deep understanding and insight into psychological and social dimensions are essential. Moreover, determining the appropriateness and effectiveness of therapeutic interventions requires adequate training and supervision. Although board certification in psychosomatic medicine is not mandatory, physicians must have received supervised training in psychosomatic therapy.

Item 3 pertains to the duration of the initial consultation. To claim reimbursement for psychosomatic therapy at the initial visit, the combined time spent on history-taking, physical examination, and psychosomatic therapy must exceed 30 min. In general internal medicine or gastroenterology outpatient settings, initial consultations rarely exceed 30 min. However, when psychosomatic assessment and therapeutic intervention are included, it is inevitable that the consultation will exceed this duration. The initial visit is crucial for establishing a trusting physician-patient relationship, which forms the foundation for effective psychological intervention. Therefore, the 30-min requirement is reasonable. Whether the reimbursement is adequate for the expertise and time involved is a separate issue.

Item 4 addresses the documentation of diagnoses. When claiming psychosomatic therapy, the physical diagnosis must be followed by the term "(psychosomatic disorder)." This applies to FGIDs as well. For example, "functional dyspepsia (psychosomatic disorder)" should be recorded. Even if the clinical presentation resembles psychiatric diagnoses such as somatic symptom disorder, it is inappropriate to document "somatic symptom disorder (psychosomatic disorder)" or "somatoform disorder (psychosomatic disorder)." While comorbid diagnoses may be listed, it is essential to append "(psychosomatic disorder)" to the physical diagnosis.

Item 5 reiterates the requirement for documentation in the medical record, as discussed in Item 1.

Item 6 concerns the handling of hospitalization dates and duration, which does not require further explanation here.

Item 7 states that when psychosomatic therapy is provided to patients under 20 years of age, a 200% increase in reimbursement is permitted. This reflects the importance of psychosomatic therapy in younger populations and emphasizes not only direct intervention with the patient but also collaboration with child welfare agencies and appropriate guidance for guardians. Interventions targeting the broader system surrounding the young patient, including caregivers, are time- and labor-intensive.

Item 8 states that psychosomatic therapy cannot be claimed concurrently with inpatient psychiatric therapy, outpatient/home psychiatric therapy, or standard psychoanalytic therapy. Although the coexistence of psychiatric diagnoses and physical illnesses (psychosomatic disorders) is logically possible, the rationale appears to be that these interventions are not typically conducted separately in practice. Therefore, only the higher-value psychiatric therapy is reimbursed. However, it is important to note that inpatient and outpatient psychiatric therapies can only be claimed at facilities officially designated as psychiatric institutions.

Summary

This section has outlined the requirements for the application of psychosomatic therapy. It should now be clear that physicians eligible to provide this therapy must possess substantial expertise in the diagnosis and management of psychosomatic disorders.

Finally, we will briefly address the actual reimbursement for psychosomatic therapy, which is granted under these stringent criteria. As shown in Table 86.1, for hospitalized patients, reimbursement of 150 points is approved for psychosomatic therapy administered twice weekly during the initial four weeks and once weekly thereafter. For outpatients, if the aforementioned criteria are met, reimbursement is set at 110 points for the initial consultation and 80 points for follow-up visits. For patients under 20 years of age, the reimbursement is tripled. However, both the Japanese Society of Psychosomatic Medicine and the Japanese Society of Psychosomatic Internal Medicine argue that the reimbursement for patients aged 20 and older is disproportionately low given the strict requirements.

It is the physician's professional responsibility to provide comprehensive care—drawing on knowledge of the gut-brain axis and delivering therapeutic interventions that address both psychological and somatic aspects—through extended consultation times. Nevertheless, the current reimbursement structure may undermine physician motivation. It is hoped that, in the near future, patients aged 20 and older will receive reimbursement equivalent to that of younger patients.

[Author's note: As of 2025, medical institutions in Japan receive reimbursement approximately ten times the official insurance point value. The patient's copayment rate ranges from 0% to 30%, depending on factors such as age, income level, financial status of the patient or their family, and government subsidies (e.g., public assistance). Accordingly, for an adult receiving an initial consultation with psychosomatic therapy, the typical out-of-pocket cost for the psychosomatic therapy add-on fee is approximately 330 yen.]

Take-Home Message

The coexistence of psychiatric diagnoses and somatic illnesses (i.e., psychosomatic disorders) is logically consistent. In clinical practice, comorbid depression and anxiety disorders are frequently observed in patients with functional gastrointestinal disorders (FGIDs). When such psychiatric conditions fall within the scope of the physician's expertise, the psychosomatic medicine specialist is expected to manage both the psychological and somatic aspects in an integrated manner.

It is important to reiterate that unless the medical facility is officially designated as a psychiatric institution, treatment of depression or anxiety disorders in addition to somatic illnesses will still be reimbursed under the category of psychosomatic therapy.

Competing Interests The author(s) has no competing interests to declare that are relevant to the content of this manuscript.

References

1. Nishiyama J, et al. Characteristics of outpatients with functional somatic syndromes at a university hospital's general medicine clinic. J Gen Fam Med. 2022;23:268–74.
2. Ministry of Health, Labour and Welfare. Medical Fee Schedule for Physicians. (in Japanese). https://www.mhlw.go.jp/content/12404000/000907834.pdf.
3. Ministry of Health, Labour and Welfare. Details regarding the medical fee schedule for physicians. (in Japanese). https://www.mhlw.go.jp/file/06-Seisakujouhou-12400000-Hokenkyoku/0000205632.pdf.

Topics, Patient Satisfaction Focused Medical Care

87

Sayuri Yamamoto and Kunio Kasugai

Abstract

Functional gastrointestinal disorders (FGIDS) have been renamed disorders of gut-brain interaction (DGBI) to reduce the associated stigma. The main goal of treatment is to improve symptoms to a patient's satisfaction, emphasizing the importance of a strong patient-physician relationship.

Initial management should focus on explanation and reassurance, which helps patients understand their condition and can even enhance the placebo effect. A multidimensional approach is essential, addressing not only symptoms but also psychological factors and lifestyle.

Psychological therapies, such as cognitive behavioral therapy (CBT) and hypnotherapy, are effective complements to medication. Lifestyle modifications, including diet and stress management, also play a key role.

Since conditions like functional dyspepsia (FD) and irritable bowel syndrome (IBS) frequently overlap, healthcare providers need to recognize this to ensure comprehensive care. Continuous patient education about the gut-brain axis and a collaborative approach involving nurses and psychologists and other medical staff such as a multidisciplinary teamwork is vital for long-term success.

Keywords

Disorders of gut-brain interaction (DGBI) · Stigma · Patients' satisfaction · Patient-physician relationship · Explanation and reassurance · Cognitive behavioral therapy · Hypnotherapy · Comprehensive care · Gut-brain axis · Multidisciplinary teamwork

Functional gastrointestinal disorders (FGIDs) were redefined in the 2016 Rome IV criteria as disorders of gut-brain interaction (DGBI). This redefinition emphasizes the concept of stigma, which is defined as a "social devaluation or discrimination based on negative stereotypes" or "an attribute that severely damages credibility." In the treatment of DGBI, such negative interactions serve as significant barriers to care [1]. Although DGBI are characterized by severe symptoms, the absence of identifiable organic pathology often leads to mutual stigmatization between patients and physicians. To mitigate this,

S. Yamamoto (✉)
Department of General Medicine & Gastroenterology, Aichi Medical University, Nagakute, Japan
e-mail: yuri3337@aichi-med-u.ac.jp

K. Kasugai
Department of Gastroenterology, Aichi Medical University, Nagakute, Japan
e-mail: kuku3487@aichi-med-u.ac.jp

H. Kaneko et al. (eds.), *Disorders of Gut-Brain Interaction*,
https://doi.org/10.1007/978-981-95-6974-8_87

the Rome Committee replaced the term "disorder" with "interaction" to avoid negative connotations and enhance patient understanding.

The 2018 Rome IV Working Team Report emphasized the importance of pharmacotherapy following the establishment of a strong patient-physician relationship [2], asserting that patient satisfaction is the most critical outcome in DGBI treatment. This section discusses the therapeutic goals of DGBI, nonpharmacological treatment strategies, and the rationale for their prioritization.

1 Therapeutic Goals

According to the *Clinical Practice Guidelines for Functional Gastrointestinal Disorders 2021, Revised 2nd Edition*, the treatment goal for functional dyspepsia (FD) is "symptom improvement that satisfies the patient," in the absence of organic lesions or biochemical abnormalities. While the *Clinical Practice Guidelines for Functional Gastrointestinal Disorders 2020, Revised 2nd Edition* for Irritable Bowel Syndrome (IBS), do not explicitly define treatment goals, the Rome IV criteria emphasize the importance of the patient-physician relationship [3].

2 Explanation, Reassurance, and the Patient-Physician Relationship

Initial management should prioritize explanation and reassurance. The FD guidelines recommend these steps prior to initiating first-line pharmacotherapy, while the IBS guidelines stress the importance of explaining the pathophysiology in terms the patient can understand. Clarifying the nature of DGBI as functional gastrointestinal disturbances and assuring patients that these conditions do not affect life expectancy can significantly alleviate symptoms. Even in the absence of abnormal test results or symptom improvement, a strong therapeutic alliance, combined with thorough explanation and reassurance, can enhance placebo effects. Meta-analyses report an average placebo response rate of 56%.

Table 87.1 Guidelines for building a therapeutic relationship with patients

1. Actively listen to determine whether the patient understands the concept of DGBI
2. Provide a complete and accurate explanation of the disorder
3. Identify and address what the patient is struggling with and what they expect from treatment
4. Set realistic and consistent treatment goals
5. Involve the patient in treatment decision-making
6. Establish a long-term perspective for care

Adapted from Drossman et al. [5]

Understanding the patient's complaints and behavioral tendencies is essential. Patients often expect a prompt diagnosis and immediate symptom relief, and they have a strong desire to escape pain. It is also important to address chronic or recurrent symptoms where the possibility of a cure is unclear [4]. Following the therapeutic relationship model proposed by Douglas Drossman, founder of the Rome Committee (see Table 87.1), can reduce doctor-shopping behavior and unnecessary surgeries, which are 1.5–3 times more common in DGBI patients compared to those without DGBI [4].

3 Multidimensional Approach

DGBI treatment requires a multidimensional approach (see Table 87.2). This includes addressing the patient-physician relationship, symptom severity, and the presence and combination of psychosocial comorbidities. A comprehensive strategy improves patient satisfaction.

Table 87.2 Multidimensional clinical profile (MDCP): algorithm for classifying IBS patients

MDCP category	How to determine	Example
A: Rome criteria diagnosis	Diagnose based on Rome IV criteria [7]	Recurrent abdominal pain, on average, at least one day per week in the last three months, associated with ≥2 of the following: related to defecation, associated with a change in stool frequency, or stool form. Criteria must be fulfilled for the last three months with symptom onset at least six months prior
B: Clinical modifiers	Assess clinical symptoms, physical signs, test results, and physiological findings	IBS-C: >25% of bowel movements (BM) are Bristol Stool Form Scale (BSFS) types 1–2 and <25% are types 6–7. IBS-D: >25% are BSFS 6–7 and <25% are BSFS 1–2. IBS-M: >25% are both BSFS 1–2 and 6–7. IBS-U: Meets IBS criteria but does not fit into the above subtypes
C: Impact on daily life	Ask the patient: "Overall, how much do your symptoms interfere with your daily life (work, school, social activities, self-care, concentration, performance)?"	None, mild, moderate, or severe
D: Psychosocial modifiers	Even nonmental health professionals can assess psychiatric diagnoses or social impact based on patient reports. Validated tools such as DSM-5 criteria or the Hospital Anxiety and Depression Scale (HADS) may be used	Anxiety disorders, major depressive disorder, PTSD, and somatic symptom disorder
E: Physiological features and biomarkers	Consider physiological tests and imaging relevant to the Rome diagnosis and its subtypes	Lactose tolerance test in IBS-D patients suspected of lactose intolerance

Adapted from Lin et al. [6]
Abbreviations: *DSM* Diagnostic and Statistical Manual of Mental Disorders, *IBS* Irritable bowel syndrome; *IBS-C* Constipation-predominant IBS, *IBS-D* Diarrhea-predominant IBS, *IBS-M* Mixed-type IBS, *IBS-U* Unclassified IBS, *FGID* Functional gastrointestinal disorder, *MDCP* Multidimensional clinical profile, *BM* Bowel movement, *BSFS* Bristol Stool Form Scale

4 Comorbid Psychiatric Disorders

A study using the Rome III psychosocial alarm symptom questionnaire found that 63.8% of FGID patients had some form of psychosocial issue, with the most common being coping difficulties (51.1%), followed by depression (23.4%) and anxiety (17.0%). Additionally, 20.2% reported severe somatic pain, and 14.9% experienced significant impairment in daily life due to gastrointestinal symptoms. Psychiatric and psychosomatic disorders such as depression and anxiety are frequently comorbid in DGBI patients, and in some cases, gastrointestinal symptoms may be manifestations of these conditions.

5 Psychological and Behavioral Therapies

Psychological and behavioral therapies act on the executive regions of the prefrontal cortex and support the effects of medications targeting deeper brain structures [8]. Cognitive behavioral therapy (CBT) helps reduce maladaptive thoughts, enhance a sense of control, and restructure responses to perceived threats. These neural changes significantly reduce pain, improve psychological well-being, and enhance gastrointestinal function. Randomized controlled trials have demonstrated that CBT is effective as an adjunct to pharmacotherapy for FGID symptoms [9]. Other well-studied interventions include hypnotherapy [10] and mindfulness meditation [11]. The most significant moderate improvements were observed in abdominal pain intensity, IBS symptom severity, quality of life, anxiety, depression, and daily functioning. CBT showed significant short-term symptom improvement [9], while hypnotherapy demonstrated long-term efficacy [12]. Comprehensive self-management interventions combining CBT, relaxation, and dietary therapy were effective for both short- and long-term (12-month) managements of IBS [10]. In Western countries, the number of nurses and clinical psychologists involved in treating gastrointestinal symptoms of IBS and other DGBI is increasing. In Japan, interdisciplinary pain management strategies involving pain medicine specialists may also contribute to long-term management of chronic pain [13–15].

6 Virtual Care

Virtual care refers to medical consultations and therapeutic support conducted remotely via webcam or communication applications in environments with adequate internet infrastructure. This setup enables more personalized and detailed care, even without in-person interaction.

There is growing evidence that virtual care, utilizing Internet-based and mobile digital platforms, may serve as an effective treatment option for patients with DGBI. Nurse-led virtual hypnotherapy has also been reported to be beneficial in improving symptoms of IBS.

7 Health-Related Quality of Life and Overlap

In clinical research, measurement tools such as the SF-36, Sickness Impact Profile, and disease specific questionary such as IBS-QOL and Nepean Dyspepsia Index are used to assess health-related quality of life (QOL). These tools help identify risk factors and disease variables that significantly impact outcomes, enabling physicians to evaluate disease burden and measure clinical predictors. Psychosocial stress is associated with exacerbation of FD symptoms and inflammation. The Rome IV Foundation Global Epidemiology Study (RFGES) examined the prevalence, overlap, and QOL impact of 22 kinds of DGBI across 54,127 individuals in 26 countries on 6 continents. Individuals with one or more DGBI had significantly lower QOL than those without, and QOL declined progressively with the number of overlapping DGBI. Although 64% of patients had overlapping FD and IBS, only 23% had documentation of this overlap in their medical records, indicating low awareness among healthcare providers [16]. FD and IBS are among the most prevalent and frequently cooccurring DGBI.

8 Lifestyle Modification and Psychotherapy

Although academic evidence is limited, lifestyle guidance remains important. Studies have linked irregular lifestyles, stress, and depressive tendencies to the onset of dyspeptic symptoms. Dietary recommendations include avoiding overeating, rapid eating, irregular meals, excessive spices, and high-fat foods. Regular exercise, structured daily routines, shared mealtimes, stress management, and enjoyable interactions with family and friends are also beneficial.

9 Patient Perception, Acceptance, and Stigma

Despite DGBIs being disorders of gut-brain interaction, patients may perceive prescriptions for neuromodulators as treatment for psychiatric illness. Clinicians must clearly explain the therapeutic value of such treatments and the negative impact of societal stigma. Without mutual understanding, patients may refuse medication or report exaggerated side effects due to anxiety unrelated to the drug itself.

10 Educating Patients About Symptom Understanding

Patients benefit from a detailed understanding of their symptoms. Physicians should assess the patient's knowledge level and provide repeated, tailored information. Patients often seek confirmation that their symptoms are real and want to understand their cause. For example, if a patient expresses concern about a missed diagnosis of FD, the physician might respond, "No organic abnormalities were found on testing, and your symptoms align with the Rome criteria for a functional disorder. Let's remain vigilant for any new developments." If a patient asks, "Could my diarrhea be due to an infection?" the physician might explain, "There is no evidence of infection. You may have post-infectious IBS, which is similar to phantom limb syndrome—where sensations persist even after a limb is lost. Medications that reduce nerve sensitivity can be effective in managing your symptoms." E-Learning platforms utilizing information technology and online support groups for patients and their families can also contribute to a better understanding of the condition. Therefore, these tools should be appropriately utilized.

11 Explaining the Physiological Basis of the Gut-Brain Axis

Chronic abdominal pain often results from dysregulation of the gut-brain axis. Increased neural signaling from the gastrointestinal tract (visceral hypersensitivity) or spinal cord (central hypersensitivity) and the brain's ability to control those nerve signals (disinhibition) are the main issues. This imbalance—heightened gut signaling and reduced central modulation—leads to chronic pain. Such symptoms can induce anxiety and depression, lowering pain thresholds and worsening symptoms. Acknowledging both physical and psychological distress within the patient-physician relationship contributes to pain relief.

12 Conclusion

The treatment of functional gastrointestinal disorders begins with attentive listening to the patient's concerns and requires a multidimensional approach to establish a strong patient-physician relationship. Both patients and healthcare providers must understand and work to eliminate the stigma associated with DGBIs. These comprehensive efforts must be closely integrated into patients' daily lives and require sustained commitment. Recent advances in telemedicine, IT-based interventions, and team-based care involving medical staff have enabled more efficient and effective treatment, ultimately enhancing patient satisfaction.

Take-Home Message
When treating patients with disorders of gut-brain interaction (DGBI), it is essential to explain thoroughly that symptoms are present despite the absence of organic disease. This explanation must continue until the patient fully understands the nature of their condition. During this process, it is critical to avoid reinforcing stigma. Communicating a message such as "I deeply and sincerely understand your symptoms" can contribute significantly to symptom relief. Collaboration with medical staff such as nurses and clinical psychologists and other medical staff as a multidisciplinary teamwork is also vital.

Competing Interests The author(s) has no competing interests to declare that are relevant to the content of this manuscript.

References

1. Feingold J, et al. Deconstructing stigma as a barrier to treating DGBI: lessons for clinicians. Neurogastroenterol Motil. 2021;33:e14080.
2. Drossman DA, et al. AGA technical review on the diagnosis and treatment of DGBI. Gastroenterology. 2018;154(4):1140–1171.e1.

3. Van Oudenhove L, et al. Biopsychosocial aspects of functional gastrointestinal disorders. Gastroenterology. 2016;
4. Drossman DA. The physician-patient relationship in FGIDs. Ann Intern Med. 1995;123:688–97.
5. Drossman DA, et al. AGA clinical practice update on the role of the biopsychosocial model in the management of DGBI. Gastroenterology. 2021;161:1670–88.
6. Lin LD, et al. Multidimensional clinical profile in IBS: a new approach. Am J Gastroenterol. 2018;113:453–6.
7. Mearin F, et al. Rome IV diagnostic criteria for FGIDs. Gastroenterology. 2016;150:1393–407.
8. Mayberg HS, et al. Deep brain stimulation for treatment-resistant depression. Am J Psychiatry. 1999;156:675–82.
9. Ford AC, et al. Efficacy of psychological therapies for IBS: systematic review and meta-analysis. Am J Gastroenterol. 2014;109:1350–65; quiz 1366.
10. Lee HH, et al. Hypnotherapy for IBS: a meta-analysis. J Neurogastroenterol Motil. 2014;20:152–62.
11. Aucoin M, et al. Mindfulness-based therapies in FGIDs. Evid Based Complement Alternat Med. 2014;2014:140724.
12. Lindfors P, et al. Long-term effects of hypnotherapy in IBS. Scand J Gastroenterol. 2012;47:414–20.
13. Zia JK, et al. Interdisciplinary care for chronic abdominal pain. Clin Gastroenterol Hepatol. 2016;14:212–219.e1–2.
14. Kamper J S, et al. Multidisciplinary biopsychosocial rehabilitation for chronic low back pain. Cochrane Database Syst Rev. 2014;(9)
15. Ushida T. Interdisciplinary pain management in Japan. J Orthop Sci. 2015;20:958–66.
16. Sperber AD, et al. The global burden of DGBIs: Rome Foundation Global Epidemiology Study. Clin Gastroenterol Hepatol. 2022;20:e945–56.

Part XI

New Perspectives on Disorders of Gut-Brain Interaction

Forgotten GI Hormones: What Gastrone Teaches Us/A New Perspective on DGBI

88

Michio Hongo

Abstract

Functional gastrointestinal disorders (FGIDs) or disorders of gut-brain interaction (DGBI) are functional gastrointestinal disorders (FGIDs), currently classified as disorders of gut-brain interaction (DGBIs), and are distinct clinical entities from gastrointestinal motility disorders (GIMDs). Nonetheless, motility abnormalities are frequently observed in FGID, often leading to diagnostic ambiguity. An important dimension in understanding these conditions is the role of gastrointestinal hormones, whose study began in the early twentieth century with the identification of secretin and gastrin. Subsequent discoveries in the 1930s included gastrone and enterogastrone, both inhibitory to gastric acid secretion and motility, and incretin, which augments insulin secretion. In the 1970s, gastric inhibitory polypeptide (GIP) was isolated, later redefined as glucose-dependent insulinotropic peptide following recognition of its incretin activity. Glucagon-like peptide-1 (GLP-1), initially considered synonymous with enterogastrone, was subsequently identified as a key regulator of gastrointestinal function. Postprandial physiology encompasses both gastrointestinal and metabolic processes. Ingestion stimulates gastrin-mediated gastric digestion, followed by the release of intestinal hormones such as secretin and cholecystokinin (CCK), which facilitate further digestion. GIP and GLP-1 enhance insulin secretion, thereby lowering postprandial glycemia and modulating gastrointestinal motility. Together with CCK, they also act centrally to suppress appetite. Dysregulation of these pathways may contribute to postprandial discomfort, dysmotility, and other negative gastrointestinal symptoms. Understanding these mechanisms offers important insights into the pathophysiology of DGBI.

Keywords

Disorders of gut-brain interaction (DGBI) · Functional gastrointestinal disorders (FGIDs) · Gastrointestinal motility disorders (GIMDs) · Functional dyspepsia · Gastrone · Enterogastrone · Gastric inhibitory polypeptide/glucose-dependent insulinotropic peptide (GIP) · Glucagon-like peptide-1 (GLP-1)

1 Introduction: Establishing the Concept of FGID/DGBI

Functional gastrointestinal disorders (FGIDs) emerged in the late 1980s to describe symptom-based syndromes undetectable through conven-

M. Hongo (✉)
Tohoku University, Sendai, Japan
e-mail: michio.hongo.a2@tohoku.ac.jp

H. Kaneko et al. (eds.), *Disorders of Gut-Brain Interaction*,
https://doi.org/10.1007/978-981-95-6974-8_88

tional diagnostic imaging, and abnormal gastrointestinal motility has long been considered a major contributing factor. Therefore gastrointestinal motility studies have played an important role in investigating symptoms that cannot be detected through conventional imaging studies. Consequently, FGIDs are sometimes mistakenly equated with gastrointestinal motility disorders (GIMDs).

In the late 1980s, an international group of researchers began focusing on nonulcer dyspepsia (NUD) and irritable bowel syndrome (IBS) as representative examples of functional gastrointestinal disorders, characterized by the absence of morphological abnormalities on radiological or endoscopic examination. The first major initiative took place in 1988 in Rome, in conjunction with the International Congress of Gastroenterology, and consensus reports on NUD and IBS were subsequently published [1–3].

To further develop these concepts, a landmark book titled *The Functional Gastrointestinal Disorder* was published in 1994 [4]. This work served as the foundation for the first Rome classification, now referred to as Rome I. Key figures in these efforts included D.A. Drossman, N.J. Talley, J.G. Thompson, and A. Torsoli.

In 1998, during the United European Gastroenterology Week held in Rome, the same group reconvened to re-valuate the concept of FGIDs. This led to the publication of Rome II in a 1999 special issue of Gut [5], followed by the publication of a corresponding book in 2000 [6]. Since then, the research community has continued to grow, becoming increasingly international and multidisciplinary. The scope of the Rome criteria has also expanded, with the announcement of Rome V expected in 2026.

One of the most notable developments in the Rome process has been the evolution of the term "functional." Rather than being narrowly defined by motility abnormalities, the Rome Committee emphasized the role of visceral hypersensitivity and gut-brain interactions. This shift was reflected in Rome III [7], which introduced the concept of disorders of gut-brain interaction (DGBI) as a broader and more integrative framework.

In response to this conceptual shift, an international group led by D. Wingate proposed a new classification system specifically for gastrointestinal motility disorders (GIMDs), published in 2002 [8]. However, confusion between the concepts of FGIDs/DGBI and GIMD has persisted—both within the Rome classification and among many researchers. Even in the Rome IV era [9], D.A. Drossman reaffirmed the emphasis on the DGBI framework. Ironically, the Rome Commission included opioid-induced constipation—clearly a motility disorder—under the DGBI umbrella.

Given this background, I believe that this book's renewed focus on disseminating the concept of FGIDs/DGBI will make a significant contribution to advancing research in this field and to promoting more appropriate clinical approaches. In this context, I would like to highlight the importance of viewing FGIDs and DGBI as distinct from GIMDs.

2 History of Gastrointestinal Hormone Research

The digestive tract is the first organ to have evolved in animals. As the organ responsible for nutrient intake, it forms the foundation of metabolic control in living organisms. Its functions are regulated by both neuroendocrine development during embryogenesis and later by the central nervous system. These functions include transporting ingested food to the appropriate locations, secreting digestive enzymes, mixing them with food, absorbing nutrients, and eliminating foreign substances, waste products, and unabsorbed residues—all of which are essential to sustaining metabolism.

Moreover, the gastrointestinal mucosa is in direct contact with the external biological environment, such as ingested food and intestinal microbiota. Thus, the regulation of the intestinal luminal microbial environment is also a crucial gastrointestinal function.

To carry out these diverse tasks, the gastrointestinal endocrine system has evolved with a highly purposeful architecture. In fact, two of the earliest discovered endocrine hormones were secretin [10] and gastrin [11]. Secretin is secreted by S cells in response to duodenal acidification caused by gastric acid entering the duodenum. It stimulates the pancreas to secrete bicarbonate to neutralize the acid. Gastrin, secreted by G cells in the gastric antrum in response to decreased acidity and protein stimulation from food intake, promotes hydrochloric acid secretion by parietal cells, thereby enhancing proteolytic enzyme activation and food digestion.

Research on gastrointestinal hormones accelerated with the discoveries of CCK, GIP, and VIP, leading to a surge of interest in the 1970s. However, this early research was often fragmented and lacked an integrative framework.

In contrast, I.P. Pavlov had already established the theory of conditioned reflexes in the early 1900s [12, 13], demonstrating that gastric acid secretion is regulated by vagal innervation. As a result, gastrointestinal physiology research shifted its focus toward neural control mechanisms, and hormone-based research did not form a major movement during this time. Endocrine research took a new direction following the discovery of insulin by Banting and Best in 1921 [14].

Although Bayliss and Starling's secretin was initially a crude extract from duodenal mucosa, further biochemical analysis followed. In 1930, Takao Kosaka and colleagues from the Department of Physiology at Kyowa Medical College in Beijing discovered a strong gastric acid secretion inhibitor, later termed gastrone, in mucosal extracts after intestinal fat perfusion. They also identified a similar factor in the ileal mucosa called enterogastrone [15, 16]. Around the same time, LaBarre et al. in Belgium discovered an insulin-stimulating factor, later termed incretin, in duodenal mucosal extracts [17].

Despite these discoveries, gastrointestinal hormone research remained relatively stagnant until the development of radioimmunoassay (RIA) for insulin by Berson and Yalow in 1959 [18]. Within this renewed context, J.C. Brown in Canada identified motilin, a hormone that promotes gastrointestinal motility, as well as gastric inhibitory peptide (GIP), which suppresses gastric acid secretion [19, 20].

The study of motilin became closely associated with research led by Dr. Ito at Gunma University. This group clarified the role of gastrointestinal motility during fasting, establishing Japan's leadership in motility research [21].

Initially, Brown named GIP for its gastric acid inhibitory properties based on duodenal mucosal extracts. However, subsequent research confirmed that this same peptide also exhibited the incretin effect described earlier by LaBarre et al. As a result, GIP was redefined as glucose-dependent insulinotropic peptide [22, 23]. In other words, it was revealed that the hormone known as incretin and the hormone inhibiting gastric motility were, in fact, the same substance. Following the name change, GIP became widely known for its incretin function, and its role as a gastric inhibitory hormone has since received less attention.

3 Purposefulness of Gastrointestinal Function Control

Animals, particularly mammals, consume food when nutritional needs arise and cease eating once those needs are met. Just as gastrointestinal motility is regulated after food intake, feeding behavior itself is also controlled by specific physiological mechanisms. Gastrointestinal hormones secreted by the mucosa play a key role in mediating this control. Understanding these mechanisms may significantly contribute to clarifying the pathophysiology of disorders of gut-brain interaction (DGBI) (Fig. 88.1).

Although a detailed discussion of postprandial hormone dynamics is beyond the scope of this section, the general sequence is as follows: After feeding, gastrin is secreted from gastric G cells, somatostatin from D cells in the stomach and small intestine, secretin from duodenal S cells, cholecystokinin (CCK) from I cells, gastric inhibitory peptide (GIP) from K cells, and glucagon-like peptide-1 (GLP-1) from L cells in the distal ileum. The initial stage involves the promotion of digestion. However, hormones such as secretin, GIP, vasoactive intestinal peptide (VIP), GLP-1, and somatostatin act to suppress gastric acid secretion, inhibit gastrointestinal

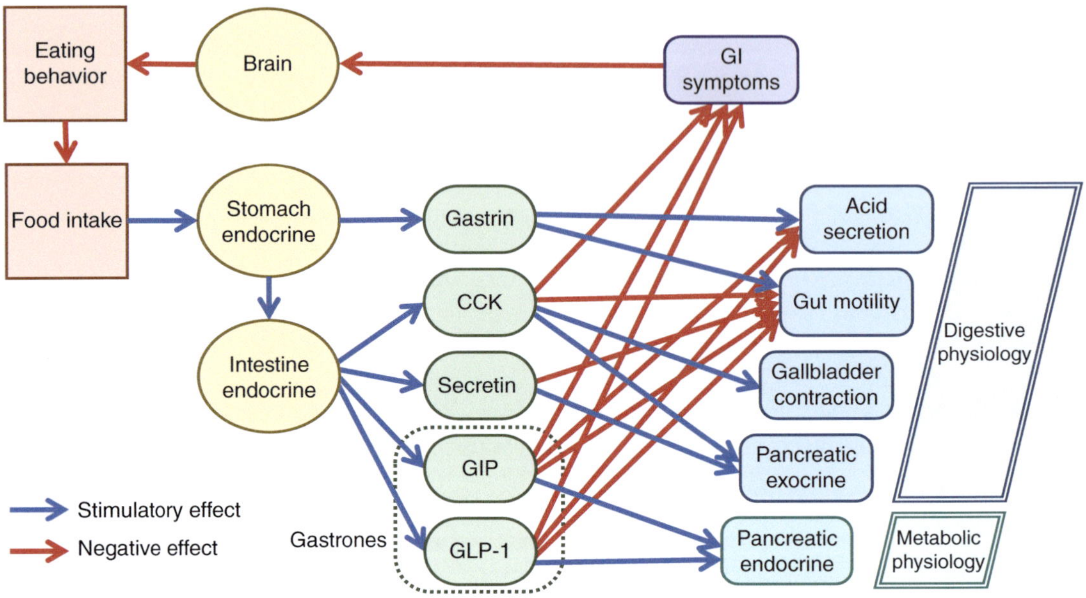

Fig. 88.1 Digestive and metabolic physiology after food intake. Serial gut hormone release after food intake control digestive physiology and metabolic physiology. After an adequate amount of food intake, eating behavior is suppressed by the serial gut hormones secretion. Gastrones, GIP and GLP-1, slow gut motility, along with generating gastrointestinal symptoms to modulate eating behavior. Stronger stimulation may induce uncomfortable symptoms such as nausea/vomiting

motility, and regulate feeding behavior—each with varying degrees of influence.

GIP and GLP-1, in particular, act as incretins that not only stimulate insulin secretion but also contribute to the inhibition of gastrointestinal activity and feeding behavior. In other words, with the initiation of nutrient influx into the duodenum, the body begins suppressing further food intake through mechanisms such as reduced acid secretion and motility, while GIP helps prevent excessive postprandial hyperglycemia.

When nutrient intake is excessive, carbohydrates may overflow into the distal ileum, stimulating GLP-1 secretion. GLP-1 promotes satiety, bloating, and nausea—subjective symptoms that serve to suppress further intake. Concurrently, it inhibits gastric acid secretion and gastric motility (digestive regulation) and limits insulin secretion to prevent a further rise in blood glucose (metabolic regulation). Thus, this orchestrated response can be interpreted as a highly appropriate and integrated defense against overnutrition, including slowed nutrient absorption, behavioral deterrents to additional food intake, and metabolic suppression of glycemic rise.

Once the stomach is emptied, the duodenum is exposed to strong acidic stimuli, triggering motilin secretion. This initiates the fasting pattern of gastrointestinal motility, known as the interdigestive migrating complex (IMC), particularly its phase III—characterized by strong peristaltic contractions. This phase serves to clear residual, nondigestible material and helps regulate the bacterial environment in the upper gastrointestinal tract. It is also considered a physiological preparation for the next meal. Subjectively, this state is associated with the sensation of "hunger," which aligns with the occurrence of phase III contractions.

While ghrelin is known to have appetite-stimulating properties, the exact regulatory mechanisms of its secretion remain incompletely understood.

4 Eating Behavior and Associated Digestive Symptoms

GLP-1 receptor agonists, initially introduced as incretin-based therapies for diabetes, have garnered significant attention for their dual role in enhancing insulin secretion and suppressing appetite. Their effects on both glycemic control and feeding behavior highlight their physiological relevance beyond glucose metabolism. From the digestive perspective, hormones such as GIP, GLP-1, gastrone, and enterogastrone have been shown to suppress gastric acid secretion, reduce gastric motility, and modulate feeding behavior. Metabolically, they act as incretins, enhancing insulin secretion. This interplay may be interpreted as an ecological defense mechanism against overnutrition.

The phenomenon commonly referred to as "appetite suppression" should be more precisely understood as the inhibition of eating behavior, which may be accompanied by a loss of appetite or upper abdominal discomfort. The sensation of satiety following a meal is likely regulated by gastrointestinal hormones that inhibit further food intake and facilitate digestion of ingested nutrients. While satiety is often associated with positive reward system activation in the brain, the absence of this positive feedback can instead manifest as nausea, vomiting, or postprandial discomfort—alternative mechanisms for suppressing eating behavior.

Conversely, malnutrition may lead to increased ghrelin secretion and enhanced appetite. Acute starvation induces hunger, though the precise pathophysiological mechanisms remain unclear. The involvement of the brain's reward system may help explain the difference between functional satiety and pathological postprandial symptoms—such as bloating or discomfort—as well as the distinction between appetite-driven hunger and nonappetite-induced hunger. This could also clarify the role of psychological and affective factors in disorders of gut-brain interaction (DGBI).

When gastrointestinal hormones are considered as mediators of symptom development in DGBI, it becomes clearer that DGBI represents a fundamentally different concept from gastrointestinal motility disorders (GIMD). This distinction may pave the way for new avenues of research in the field.

5 Clinical Use of GLP-1 Receptor Agonists/"Gastrone Effect"

In 2010, the first GLP-1 receptor agonist was approved for clinical use as a type 2 diabetes medication in both the United States and Japan. Since then, several formulations have been approved. Given their weight loss effects, these medications were subsequently developed as treatments for obesity, receiving insurance coverage in the United States in 2014 and in Japan in 2023. Not all GLP-1 agonists have been approved for obesity treatment, and even the approved drugs have strict criteria for their use. Notably, these compounds induce weight loss through appetite suppression, with approximately one-quarter of patients receiving GLP-1 receptor agonist treatment experiencing symptoms such as nausea, vomiting, epigastric discomfort, constipation, diarrhea, or related dyspepsia symptoms, as well as delayed gastric emptying effects [24]. This is a reflection of incretin effect of GLP-a receptor agonist accompanies "gastrone effect." These "gastrone effect" overlap with those of functional dyspepsia, suggesting that these gastrointestinal hormones may play a key role in the pathophysiology of functional dyspepsia or DGBI, warranting consideration in the context of these conditions.

6 Conclusion

In the early 1930s, Japanese physiologist Takao Kosaka and his colleagues discovered gastrone and enterogastrone—hormones that were later found to correspond to gastric inhibitory peptide (GIP) and subsequently renamed glucose-dependent insulinotropic peptide. Due to their incretin effect, GIP/GLP-1 receptor agonists have been employed not only in the treatment of diabetes but also—as approved in the United States—for appetite suppression and obesity management.

Researchers of functional gastrointestinal disorders (FGIDs) and disorders of gut-brain interaction (DGBI) must revisit the physiological role of gastrones. These hormones, secreted in response to excessive nutrient intake, have important regulatory effects on gastrointestinal function, feeding behavior, and glucose metabolism. The recent attention surrounding GLP-1 receptor agonists and their appetite-suppressing properties reminds us that these same mechanisms may also contribute to the development of unpleasant gastrointestinal symptoms.

Building on the legacy of Takao Kosaka, the discoverer of gastrone and enterogastrone, and Zen Ito, who laid the foundation for neurogastroenterology in Japan, we hope to witness a new era of neurogastroenterological research emerging from Japan.

Competing Interests The author(s) has no competing interests to declare that are relevant to the content of this manuscript.

References

1. Torsoli A, Corazziari E. The WTR's, the Delphic Oracle and the Roman conclaves. Gastroenterol Int. 1991;4:44–5.
2. Talley NJ, et al. Functional dyspepsia: a classification with guidelines for diagnosis and management. Gastroenterol Int. 1991;4:145–60.
3. Tompson WG, et al. Functional bowel disease and functional abdominal pain. Gastroentrol Int. 1992;5:75–91.
4. Drossman DA, et al., editors. The functional gastrointestinal disorders: diagnosis, pathophysiology and treatment. 1st ed. McLean: Degnon Associates; 1994.
5. Drossman DA. The functional gastrointestinal disorders and the Rome II process. Gut. 1999;45(suppl 2):II1-5.
6. Drossman DA. Rome II: the functional gastrointestinal disorders: diagnosis, pathophysiology, and treatment: a multinational consensus. Degnon Associates Inc; 2000.
7. Drossman DA, et al. Rome III: the functional gastrointestinal disorders. 3rd ed. Degnon Associates, Inc; 2006.
8. Wingate D, et al. Disorders of gastrointestinal motility: towards a new classification 1. J Gastroenterol Hepatol. 2002;17:S1–S14.
9. Drossman DA, Hasler WL. Rome IV – functional GI disorders: disorders of gut-brain interaction. Gastroenterology. 2016;150:1257–61.
10. Bayliss W, Starling E. The mechanism of pancreatic secretion. J Physiol (London). 1902;28:325–52.
11. Edkins JS, Cantab MB. On the chemical mechanism of gastric secretion. Lancet. 1905;166(4272):156.
12. Pavlov IP. The scientific investigation of the psychical faculties or processes in the higher animals. Science. 1906;24:613–9.
13. Pavlov IP. Conditioned reflexes: an investigation of the physiological activity of the cerebral cortex. London: Oxford University Press; 1927.
14. Banting FG, et al. The effect of pancreatic extract (insulin) on normal rabbits. Am J Physiol-Legacy Content. 1922;62:162–76.
15. Kosaka T, Lim RKS. Demonstration of the humoral agent in fat inhibition of gastric secretion. Proc Soc Exp Biol Med. 1930;27:890–1.
16. Kosaka T, et al. On the mechanism of the inhibition of gastric secretion by fat. A gastric-inhibitory agent obtained from the intestinal mucosa. Chin J Physiol. 1932;6:107–28.
17. La Barre J. On the possibilities of diabetes treatment with incretin. Bull Acad R Med Belg. 1932;12:620–34.
18. Yalow RS, Berson SA. Immunoassay of endogenous plasma insulin in man. J Clin Invest. 1960;39:1157–75.
19. Brown JC. Presence of a gastric motor-stimulating property in duodenal extracts. Gastroenterology. 1967;52:225–9.
20. Brown JC. A gastric inhibitory polypeptide. I. The amino acid composition and the tryptic peptides. Can J Biochem. 1971;49:255–61.
21. Itoh Z, et al. Changes in plasma motilin concentration and gastrointestinal contractile activity in conscious dogs. Am J Dig Dis. 1978;23:929–35.
22. Dupre J, et al. Stimulation of insulin secretion by gastric inhibitory polypeptide in man. J Clin Endocrinol Metab. 1973;37:826–8.
23. Brown JC, et al. Physiology and pathophysiology of GIP. In: Gastrointestinal hormones and pathology of the digestive system; 1978. p. 169–71.
24. Chang MG, et al. A scoping review of GLP-1 receptor agonists: are they associated with increased gastric contents, regurgitation, and aspiration events? J Clin Med. 2024;13:6336.

Appendices: The Path to Expertise: Pursuing a Career as a Medical Specialist

Toshimi Chiba

Abstract

"The Path to Expertise: Pursuing a Career as a Medical Specialist" is designed to deepen understanding of the important points in each chapter and diseases by reviewing knowledge in the form of questions, answers, and explanations. Questions have been created for each chapter, esophagus, stomach and duodenum, small bowel and colon, rectum and anus, and clinical practice, followed by answers and explanations. This chapter presents 21 questions. This chapter provides answers and explanations to promote understanding of the 21 questions in the previous chapter.

Keywords

Questions · Answers and explanation · Esophagus · Stomach and duodenum · Small bowel and colon · Rectum and anus · Clinical practice

Questions

1. Esophagus

Q1-1. Esophageal Motility Test

(1) **Which of the following statements regarding esophageal manometry is *incorrect*? Select one.**

(a) Esophageal motility disorders cannot be detected without performing esophageal manometry.

(b) There are two main systems for measuring esophageal pressure: the water-perfused system and the intraluminal transducer system.

(c) In high-resolution manometry (HRM), the sleeve sensor cannot be used; however, the e-sleeve function allows for continuous measurement of the esophagogastric junction pressure.

T. Chiba
Division of Internal Medicine, Department of Oral Medicine, Iwate Medical University, Morioka, Japan
e-mail: toschiba@iwate-med.ac.jp

H. Kaneko et al. (eds.), *Disorders of Gut-Brain Interaction*,
https://doi.org/10.1007/978-981-95-6974-8

(d) In the Chicago Classification, the integrated relaxation pressure (IRP) is a parameter used to evaluate swallow-related relaxation of the esophagogastric junction.
(e) In the Chicago Classification, the distal contractile integral (DCI) is used to assess the contractile vigor of primary peristalsis.

(2) **Which of the following statements regarding high-resolution impedance manometry (HRIM) is *incorrect*? Select one.**
(a) It is useful for evaluating esophagogastric junction outflow obstruction.
(b) It is useful for assessing rumination syndrome and excessive supragastric belching.
(c) Esophageal distensibility can be evaluated using HRIM.
(d) Distilled water is swallowed during HRIM.
(e) It is not useful for evaluating swallowing function in the pharynx.

(3) **Which of the following statements regarding esophagram is correct? Select two.**
(a) Esophagram does not allow for quantitative evaluation.
(b) High-resolution manometry (HRM) is more useful than esophagram for evaluating the subtype of esophageal achalasia.
(c) Nonachalasia esophageal motility disorders cannot be detected by esophagram.
(d) The diagnostic sensitivity of esophagram increases when solid food is used in addition to liquid barium.
(e) Timed barium esophagram is useful for evaluating the therapeutic efficacy in esophageal achalasia.

Refer to Part II—Esophagus, Basic Edition, Chaps. 4, 5, 6 and 7: Esophageal Motility Test

Q1-2 Functional Esophageal Disorders

Which of the following statements regarding functional esophageal disorders is *incorrect*? Select one.
(a) The diagnosis of functional heartburn is characterized by specific findings on high-resolution esophageal manometry.
(b) Functional heartburn and reflux hypersensitivity can be differentiated using esophageal pH monitoring or esophageal impedance-pH monitoring.
(c) Common causes of noncardiac chest pain (NCCP) include gastroesophageal reflux disease (GERD), esophageal motility disorders, and anxiety disorders.
(d) Esophageal motility disorders are frequently observed in patients with PPI-refractory globus sensation.
(e) In the diagnosis of functional dysphagia, it is important to exclude GERD and eosinophilic esophagitis.

Refer to Part III—Esophagus, Practical Edition, Chap. 16—Case Discussion: Heartburn.

Q1-3 Non-erosive Reflux Disease (NERD)

(1) **Which of the following statements regarding the diagnosis and characteristics of nonerosive reflux disease (NERD) are correct? Select two.**
(a) No esophageal mucosal injury is observed on endoscopic examination.
(b) Proton pump inhibitors (PPIs) are effective in the majority of patients.
(c) Twenty-four-hour reflux monitoring is essential for diagnosis.
(d) Reflux symptoms are generally mild.
(e) Definitions vary across reports and publications, necessitating careful interpretation.

(2) **Which of the following statements regarding the management of NERD are correct? Select two.**
(a) Vonoprazan is the first-line treatment.
(b) In some cases, cognitive behavioral therapy should be considered over pharmacological therapy.
(c) If acid-suppressive therapy is ineffective, the condition should be deemed psychogenic, and referral to psychoso-

matic or psychiatric care should be strongly recommended.
(d) Management should consider the potential coexistence of other functional gastrointestinal disorders (FGIDs), such as functional dyspepsia (FD) and irritable bowel syndrome (IBS).
(e) For evaluating treatment efficacy, endoscopic or reflux monitoring findings should be prioritized over symptom assessment.

Refer to Part III—Esophagus, Practical Edition Chap. 12—Diagnosis and Treatment of Motility Disorder: Non-erosive Reflux Disease (including reflux hypersensitivity).

Q1-4 Achalasia

Which of the following statements regarding achalasia is correct? Select one.
(a) Impaired relaxation of the lower esophageal sphincter is observed, but peristalsis of the esophageal body remains normal.
(b) It predominantly affects younger individuals and does not occur in the elderly.
(c) High-resolution esophageal manometry classifies achalasia into three subtypes.
(d) High-resolution esophageal manometry confirms the diagnosis in all cases.
(e) Peroral endoscopic myotomy (POEM) is not indicated for Type III achalasia.

Refer to Part III—Esophagus, Practical Edition, Chap. 13—Diagnosis and Treatment of Motility Disorder, Achalasia

2. Stomach and Duodenum

Q2-1 Gastroduodenal Motility Test

Which of the following tests can evaluate both gastric accommodation and gastric emptying? Select two.
(a) Electrogastrography
(b) Water load test
(c) Transabdominal ultrasonography
(d) Barostat testing
(e) Gastric scintigraphy

Refer to Part IV—S*tomach and duodenum, Basic Edition,* Chap. 23, 24, 25 and 26—Gastroduodenal Motility Test.

Q2-2 Functional Dyspepsia (FD)

Which of the following cases presenting with postprandial fullness and epigastric pain *cannot be diagnosed* as functional dyspepsia (FD)? Select two.
(a) Postgastrectomy
(b) History of depression
(c) Erosive gastritis
(d) Use of nonsteroidal antiinflammatory drugs (NSAIDs)
(e) Alternating diarrhea and constipation

*Refer to Par*t V—Stom*ach and duodenum, Practical Edition, Chap.* 28—Diagnosis and Treatment of DGBI: Functional Dyspepsia.

Q2-3 Functional Gastroduodenal Disorders

Which of the following statements regarding excessive supragastric belching are correct? Select two.
(a) It involves frequent expulsion of gas stored in the gastric fundus.
(b) It is characterized by belching during conversation.
(c) Cognitive behavioral therapy is effective.
(d) It is associated with transient lower esophageal sphincter relaxation.
(e) Esophageal impedance testing is useful for diagnosis.

Refer to Part V—Stoma*ch and duodenum, Practical Edition,* Chap. 29—Diagnosis and Treatment of DGBI: Belching Disorders.

Q2-4 Gastroparesis

Which of the following statements regarding gastroparesis are correct? Select two.

(a) "Early satiety" is not included among the symptoms of gastroparesis.
(b) Unlike gastroparesis, symptoms such as "nausea" and "vomiting" are uncommon in functional dyspepsia (FD).
(c) The two major causes of gastroparesis are diabetes mellitus and Parkinson's disease.
(d) The term "gastroparesis" is frequently used in countries outside Japan, particularly in other parts of Asia.
(e) Demonstrating delayed gastric emptying is essential for the diagnosis of gastroparesis.

Refer to Part V— Stomach a*nd duodenum, Practical Edition,* Chap. 32—Diagnosis and Treatment of Motility Disorder: Gastroparesis.

3. Small Bowel and Colon

Q3-1 Small Bowel and Colonic Motility Test

Which of the following statements regarding cine-MRI is *incorrect*? Select two.

(a) Intestinal fluid appears as a low-intensity signal.
(b) Peristalsis is evaluated using axial slices.
(c) In chronic intestinal pseudoobstruction (CIPO), the contraction rate is significantly reduced compared to healthy individuals.
(d) Cine-MRI is widely applied in clinical practice outside the gastrointestinal field, such as in cardiovascular medicine.
(e) Compared to gastrointestinal manometry, cine-MRI is less invasive for patients.

Refer to Part VI—Small b*owel and colon, Basic Edition,* Chap. 41—Small Bowel and Colonic Motility Test, Cine-MRI.

Q3-2 Irritable Bowel Syndrome (IBS)

(1) **A 25-year-old woman presents with abdominal pain and sudden urgency to defecate. The pain is dull, lasts about 60 minutes, and occurs approximately six days per month. The pain often improves after defecation. On days with severe pain, frequency of bowel movement increases from once to four times per day, and stool consistency changes to loose stools. She also reports abdominal discomfort, abdominal bloating, borborygmi, and a sensation of incomplete evacuation. On normal days, 90% of her stools are sausage-shaped and approximately 35 mm in diameter. On symptomatic days, 45% of stools are loose, and 30% begin as pellet-like stools. Urinalysis, blood chemistry, and colonoscopy show normal. What is the most appropriate diagnosis? Select one.**
(a) Centrally mediated abdominal pain syndrome
(b) Irritable bowel syndrome with predominant diarrhea (IBS-D)
(c) Irritable bowel syndrome with predominant constipation (IBS-C)
(d) Irritable bowel syndrome with mixed bowel habits (IBS-M)
(e) Irritable bowel syndrome unclassified (IBS-U)

(2) **Which of the following medications is most appropriate for the above patient? Select one.**
(a) Mosapride
(b) Elobixibat
(c) Tramadol
(d) Pentazocine
(e) Trimebutine

Refer to Part VII Small bow*el and colon, Practical Edition,* Chap. 44—Diagnosis and Treatment of DGBI: Irritable Bowel Syndrome.

Q3-3 Functional Bowel Disorders

Which of the following statements regarding pharmacological treatment for constipation in patients with functional bowel disorders is correct? Select two.

(a) In patients consistently presenting with hard stools, the dosage of probiotics should be reduced.

(b) In patients with renal dysfunction, the dosage of magnesium oxide should be reduced.
(c) Lubiprostone should be used as the first-line treatment in pregnant women.
(d) In patients with IBS-C, linaclotide is expected to alleviate abdominal pain.
(e) Daikenchuto contains rhubarb and should not be used long term.
(f) Elobixibat is classified as a mucosal epithelial function-modifying agent.

Refer to Part VII Small *Bowel and Colon, Practical Edition,* Chap. 45—Diagnosis and Treatment of DGBI: Functional Constipation.

Q3-4 Pseudo-obstruction and Megacolon

Which of the following statements regarding chronic megacolon is *incorrect*? Select one.
(a) When unexplained abdominal bloating persists for more than six months, this condition should be considered in the differential diagnosis.
(b) CT or plain abdominal radiography is useful for diagnosis.
(c) When surgical treatment is indicated, total colectomy is recommended.
(d) Oral polyethylene glycol is effective.
(e) Patients should be advised to increase dietary fiber intake to improve constipation.

Refer to Part VII *Small Bowel and Colon, Practical Edition,* Chap. 49—Diagnosis and Treatment of Motility Disorder: Megacolon

4. Anorectum

Q4-1 Anorectal Function Test

(1) **Which of the following disease-test combinations is *incorrect*? Select one.**
(a) Fecal incontinence—anorectal manometry
(b) Fecal incontinence—anal ultrasound
(c) Paradoxical contraction—defecography
(d) Neuropathy—pudendal nerve terminal motor latency
(e) Rectocele—breath hydrogen test

(2) **Which of the following disease-severity assessment combinations is *incorrect*? Select one.**
(a) Cleveland Clinic Florida Constipation Scoring System—constipation
(b) Cleveland Clinic Florida Fecal Incontinence Score—fecal incontinence
(c) Fecal Incontinence Severity Index (FISI)—fecal incontinence
(d) Low Anterior Resection Syndrome Score—postoperative rectal dysfunction
(e) Obstructed Defecation Syndrome Score—slow transit constipation

(3) **Which of the following tests for fecal incontinence is *incorrect*? Select one.**
(a) Anoscopy
(b) Anorectal manometry
(c) Transanal ultrasonography
(d) Anal electrical sensory testing
(e) Rectal balloon sensory testing

(4) **Defecography Findings**
A 70-year-old woman presents with a chief complaint of difficult defecation. A defecography image taken during straining is shown in Figure 1.

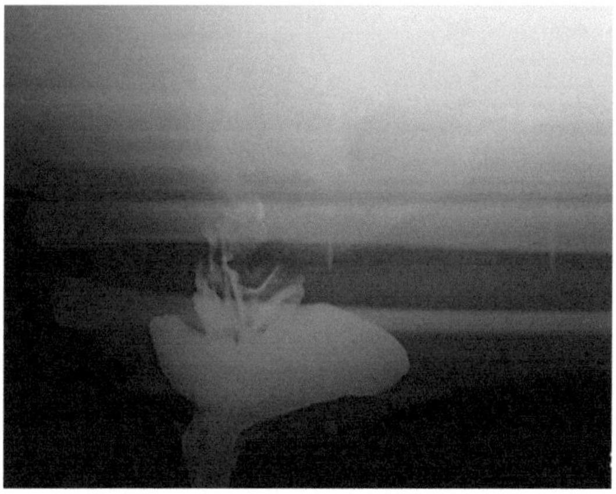

Which of the following findings are correct? Select two.
(a) Enterocele
(b) Rectocele
(c) Rectal intussusception
(d) Paradoxical contraction
(e) External anal sphincter injury

(5) **Interpretation of Defecography**

Regarding the defecography image shown in Figure 2, which of the following statements are correct? Select two.

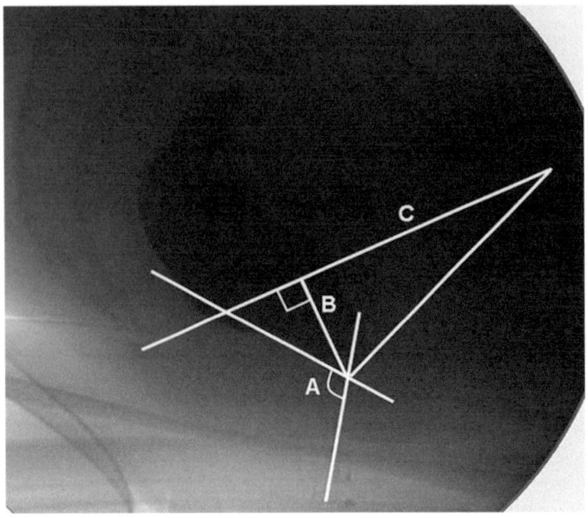

(a) A represents the anorectal angle.
(b) B represents the length of the anal canal.
(c) C is the line connecting the pubic symphysis and the tip of the coccyx.
(d) In normal cases, the value of A decreases during straining compared to resting.
(e) In normal cases, the value of B decreases during straining compared to resting.

Refer to Part VIII *Anorectum, Basic Edition,* Chaps. 58, 59, 60, 61, 62 and 63—Anorectal Function Test.

Q4-2 Fecal Incontinence

Which of the following statements regarding the pathophysiology of fecal incontinence is correct? Select one.

(a) In the 2017 edition of Japanese Practice Guidelines for Fecal Incontinence, fecal incontinence is defined as "involuntary loss of feces."
(b) The characteristic symptom of fecal incontinence due to internal anal sphincter dysfunction is urge fecal incontinence.
(c) The characteristic symptom of fecal incontinence due to rectal fecal impaction is passive fecal incontinence.
(d) The scoring system used to subjectively evaluate resting anal tone and voluntary anal sphincter contraction during digital rectoanal examination is the Cleveland Clinic Florida Fecal Incontinence Score.
(e) As of January 2023, transanal irrigation is covered by insurance for the management of low anterior resection syndrome, a defecation disorder following rectal resection.

*Refer to Part IX Anorectu*m, Pr*actical Edition,* Chap. 64—Diagnosis and Treatment of DGBI: Fecal Incontinence.

Q4-3 Functional Anorectal Pain

(1) **Which of the following *does not* meet the diagnostic criteria for levator ani syndrome? Select one.**
(a) Chronic or recurrent rectal pain
(b) Pain lasting more than 30 minutes
(c) Absence of tenderness on traction of the puborectalis muscle
(d) Exclusion of organic diseases causing rectal pain
(e) Symptoms present for at least six months, with diagnostic criteria met in the most recent three months

(2) **Which of the following statements regarding rectocele is *incorrect*? Select one.**
(a) The anterior rectal wall protrudes toward the posterior vaginal wall.
(b) It is caused by weakening of the rectovaginal septum.
(c) Symptoms include difficult defecation and a sensation of incomplete evacuation.
(d) Diagnosis can be made by hooking the anterior rectal wall with a finger during rectal examination
(e) Surgical treatment should be the first-line approach.

Refer to Part IX Anore*ctum, Practical Edition,* Chap. 65—Diagnosis and Treatment of DGBI: Functional Anorectal Pain.

Q4-4 Functional Defecation Disorders

Which of the following is *not* an appropriate test for diagnosing dyssynergic defecation? Select one.

(a) Endoanal ultrasonography
(b) Anorectal manometry
(c) Defecography
(d) Anal surface electromyography (EMG)
(e) Balloon expulsion test

Refer to Part IX Ano*rectum, Practical Edition,* Chap. 66—Diagnosis and Treatment of DGBI: Functional Defecation Disorders, Dyssynergic defecation.

Q4-5 Anorectal Dysfunction due to Organic Disease

Which of the following statements regarding rectal prolapse is correct? Select two.

(a) A shallow Douglas' pouch and rectovesical pouch are anatomical features.
(b) Defecography is useful for diagnosing rectal intussusception.
(c) The recurrence rate after transabdominal surgery is higher than that after transperineal surgery.
(d) The Delorme procedure is a representative transabdominal surgical technique.
(e) The Wells procedure involves posterior rectopexy.

Refer to Part IX Anorectum, Practical Edition, Chap. 69—Diagnosis and Treatment of Anorectal Dysfunction Due to Organic Disease, Rectal Prolapse

5. Practical Treatment

Q5-1 Scientific Basis of "Illness Begins in the Mind"

Which receptor is involved in the vagal cholinergic antiinflammatory pathway, which supports the concept that "illness begins in the mind"? Select one.

(a) β_2-Adrenergic receptor
(b) H_2 histamine receptor
(c) α7 Nicotinic acetylcholine receptor (α7Ach receptor)
(d) 5-HT_3 receptor
(e) Cannabinoid CB_2 receptor

Refer to Part X Practic*al Treatment,* Chap. 76—The Science of "Illness Begins in the Mind."

Q5-2 Explore Issues with Psychosomatic Medicine Treatment

Which of the following statements is *incorrect*? Select one.

(a) The prognosis of functional gastrointestinal disorders (FGIDs) is generally favorable.
(b) Longer consultation times do not necessarily lead to better treatment outcomes in FGIDs.
(c) Multidisciplinary collaboration may be necessary in the management of FGIDs.
(d) The sole treatment goal for FGIDs is complete symptom resolution.
(e) Understanding the patient's explanatory model is helpful in treatment.

*Refer to Part X Prac*tical *Treatment,* Chap. 77—Explore Issues with Psychosomatic Medicine Treatment.

Q5-3 Estimating Gastrointestinal Function Through Abdominal Examination

A teenage male presents with abdominal bloating without abdominal pain. He has had infrequent bowel movements since early childhood and has never received treatment for constipation. He does not experience the urge to defecate. Which of the following physical findings are likely? (multiple answers allowed)

(a) Visual inspection reveals distension primarily in the lower abdomen.
(b) Auscultation reveals hyperactive bowel sounds.
(c) Auscultation reveals hypoactive bowel sounds.
(d) Percussion reveals tympany throughout the abdomen.
(e) Palpation reveals a firm mass in the lower abdomen.

Refer to Part X Prac*tical Treatment,* Chap. 78—Physical Findings in the Abdomen: Physical Findings.

Q5-4 Practice of Family Medicine

(1) **Which of the following statements regarding the role of family physicians in the management of FGIDs is correct? Select one.**
- (a) Since patients with FGIDs often engage in doctor shopping, prompt referral to psychiatry is recommended.
- (b) Because precise diagnosis requires advanced testing, referral to a gastroenterologist is essential.
- (c) Family physicians play a significant role in diagnosis and treatment and should be well versed in FGID management.
- (d) Although Kampo medicine is used in FGID treatment, it lacks sufficient evidence and is not included in treatment guidelines.
- (e) Most patients presenting with epigastric pain to family physicians have organic gastrointestinal diseases, so there are few opportunities to refer them to other specialists.

(2) **Which of the following statements regarding Kampo therapy for functional dyspepsia (FD) are correct? Select three.**
- (a) The treatment flowchart of the Japanese Society of Gastroenterology lists rikkunshito as a first-line therapy.
- (b) If rikkunshito is ineffective, no alternative Kampo options are available.
- (c) FD can be subtyped in Kampo medicine into "Qi deficiency" and "Qi stagnation" types; the former responds to rikkunshito, while the latter may benefit from bukuryoin or daisaikoto.
- (d) Upper gastrointestinal endoscopy is essential for Kampo subtyping.
- (e) Esophageal anisakiasis may present with symptoms resembling gastroesophageal reflux disease (GERD) or functional dyspepsia (FD), unlike gastric anisakiasis.

Refer to Part X Prac*tical Treatment,* Chap. 82—Practice of Family Medicine.

Answers and Explanation

1: Esophagus

A1-1 Esophageal Motility Test

(1) **Correct Answer: a**
- **a. Incorrect.** In addition to esophageal manometry, esophageal motility disorders can sometimes be detected using esophagram or esophagogastroduodenoscopy.
- **b. Correct.** Two main systems are used to measure esophageal pressure: the water-perfused system and the intraluminal transducer system. High-resolution manometry systems such as ManoScan™ and the Starlet® utilize the intraluminal transducer system.
- **c. Correct.** A sleeve sensor has been used for continuously measuring the esophagogastric junction pressure since the location of the esophagogastric junction changes with respiration. The e-sleeve function in intraluminal transducer systems also allows continuous measurement of the esophagogastric junction pressure.
- **d. Correct.** The integrated relaxation pressure (IRP) is a parameter used to evaluate swallow-related relaxation of the esophagogastric junction.
- **e. Correct.** The distal contractile integral (DCI) is a parameter used to assess the contractile vigor of primary peristalsis.

(2) **Correct Answer: d**
- **a. Correct.** High-resolution impedance manometry (HRIM) is useful for evaluating esophagogastric junction outflow obstruction.
- **b. Correct.** HRIM is also useful in evaluating rumination syndrome and excessive supragastric belching.
- **c. Correct.** HRIM can calculate cross-sectional area from pressure and impedance values, allowing assessment of esophageal distensibility.

- **d. Incorrect.** Impedance values cannot be accurately assessed with distilled water swallows; therefore, electrolyte solutions such as diluted saline should be used.
- **e. Correct.** HRIM is also useful for evaluating swallowing function in the pharynx.

(3) **Correct Answers: d, e**

- **a. Incorrect.** Quantitative evaluation is possible with esophagram using the timed barium esophagram.
- **b. Incorrect.** For evaluating the diameter or shape of the esophagus in achalasia, esophagogram is more useful than manometry.
- **c. Incorrect.** Disorders such as esophagogastric junction outflow obstruction and diffuse esophageal spasm can also be detected by esophagram.
- **d. Correct.** Using solid food in addition to liquid barium during esophagram increases diagnostic yield.
- **e. Correct.** The timed barium esophagram is useful for evaluating treatment outcomes in esophageal achalasia.

A1-2 Functional Esophageal Disorders

Correct Answer: a

- **a. Incorrect.** Functional heartburn does not show abnormalities in esophageal motility including primary peristalsis on high-resolution manometry (HRM) and/or high-resolution impedance manometry (HRIM).
- **b. Correct.** Esophageal manometry is performed to confirm normal esophageal motility, followed by a 24-hour multichannel intraluminal impedance-pH (MII-pH) monitoring to calculate the symptom index (SI) and symptom association probability (SAP). SI is defined as positive if the proportion of symptoms caused by reflux accounts for 50% or more of the total number of symptoms over 24 hours. SAP is calculated based on the results of the MII-pH monitoring to determine the relationship between symptom and reflux, with a positive result if the probability is 95% or higher. Functional heartburn is diagnosed when both SI and SAP are negative, while reflux hypersensitivity is diagnosed when either SI or SAP is positive.
- **c. Correct.** Noncardiac chest pain (NCCP) includes GERD, esophageal motility disorders, and anxiety disorders such as panic disorder, which are common in daily clinical practice.
- **d. Correct.** In patients with PPI-refractory globus sensation, elevated upper esophageal sphincter (UES) pressure is frequently observed, suggesting a relationship between symptoms and elevated UES pressure.
- **e. Correct.** The diagnosis of functional dysphagia requires exclusion of organic diseases through an upper GI endoscopy, as well as the exclusion of esophageal motility disorders through esophageal manometry and pH monitoring.

A1-3 Non-erosive Reflux Disease (NERD)

(1) **Correct Answers: a, e**

- **a. Correct.** A broad definition of NERD includes patients with reflux symptoms but no mucosal injury on endoscopy. However, if the patient is taking acid-suppressive therapy, mucosal healing may mask findings.
- **b. Incorrect.** Only about half of patients with broadly defined NERD respond to PPIs; the rest are considered PPI refractory.
- **c. Incorrect.** Reflux monitoring is not essential for diagnosing broadly defined NERD, though it is required for the narrow definition under Rome IV criteria.
- **d. Incorrect.** There is no correlation between symptom severity and mucosal

injury. Some patients with reflux esophagitis do not report symptoms.

- **e. Correct.** Broadly defined NERD includes patients with reflux symptoms and no mucosal injury. Narrowly defined NERD also requires evidence of pathological acid reflux on monitoring.

(2) **Correct Answers: b, d**

- **a. Incorrect.** Evidence regarding the comparative efficacy of vonoprazan versus PPIs in treating NERD is inconclusive, as findings across studies have been inconsistent. Moreover, vonoprazan is not approved for NERD in Japan.
- **b. Correct.** Behavioral disorders such as supragastric belching and rumination syndrome are common in PPI/vonoprazan-refractory cases and may respond better to cognitive behavioral therapy than to acid suppression.
- **c. Incorrect.** Lack of response to acid suppression does not automatically indicate a psychogenic cause. Further evaluation with impedance-pH monitoring is recommended.
- **d. Correct.** FGIDs often coexist, and treatment should be tailored to the individual's symptom profile.
- **e. Incorrect.** Except in cases of pathological acid reflux, NERD does not significantly affect prognosis. Treatment should focus on symptom relief and quality of life (patient-reported outcomes).

A1-4 Achalasia

Correct Answer: c

- **a. Incorrect.** Achalasia is characterized by impaired relaxation of the lower esophageal sphincter and absence of peristalsis in the esophageal body. If some peristaltic activity is observed, the condition may be classified as Esophagogastric Junction Outflow Obstruction (EGJOO).
- **b. Incorrect.** Achalasia has no gender differences and can occur in all age groups, with a peak incidence between 30 and 60 years. In elderly patients, pseudoachalasia due to malignancy or paraneoplastic syndromes must be considered.
- **c. Correct.** High-resolution esophageal manometry classifies achalasia into three subtypes: types I, II, and III.
- **d. Incorrect.** The integrated relaxation pressure (IRP) is used to assess lower esophageal sphincter relaxation. In cases where the IRP is high but peristaltic waves (partial) are observed in the esophageal body, or where there is 100% failed peristalsis but the IRP is within the normal range, the diagnosis is inconclusive achalasia, and additional diagnostic tests such as a timed barium esophagram (TBE) or functional luminal imaging probe (FLIP) are required.
- **e. Incorrect.** Type III achalasia is characterized by premature contractions of the esophageal body in 20% or more of swallows. Peroral endoscopic myotomy (POEM) is particularly effective for this type III achalasia due to its ability to extend the myotomy length as needed. This results in improved treatment outcomes compared to endoscopic balloon dilation.

2: Stomach and Duodenum

A2-1 Gastroduodenal Motility Test

Correct Answers: c, e

- **a. Incorrect.** Electrogastrography (EGG) measures gastric electrical activity from the body surface. While abnormalities are reported in about half of functional dyspepsia (FD) patients, it does not assess both accommodation and emptying.
- **b. Incorrect.** The water load test evaluates gastric accommodation and visceral sensitivity but is limited by patient burden and variability.
- **c. Correct.** Transabdominal ultrasonography can assess both gastric accommodation and emptying by measuring changes in the cross-sectional area of the gastric antrum before and after a test meal.

- **d. Incorrect.** The barostat test evaluates gastric accommodation and visceral sensitivity but is invasive and not commonly used in clinical practice.
- **e. Correct.** Gastric scintigraphy is the gold standard for assessing gastric motility, including emptying and accommodation, using radiolabeled meals.

A2-2 Functional Dyspepsia (FD)

Correct Answers: b, c, e

- **a. Incorrect.** Postgastrectomy patients cannot be diagnosed with FD, as it is a functional disorder requiring an intact anatomy.
- **b. Correct.** FD often coexists with psychiatric conditions such as anxiety and depression.
- **c. Correct.** Mild endoscopic findings such as erosive gastritis do not exclude FD.
- **d. Incorrect.** NSAID use suggests drug-induced symptoms rather than FD.
- **e. Correct.** Alternating diarrhea and constipation are IBS symptoms, but FD and IBS frequently coexist.

A2-3 Functional Gastroduodenal Disorders

Correct Answers: c, e

- **a. Incorrect.** Frequent expulsion of gas from the gastric fundus is characteristic of gastric belching, not supragastric belching.
- **b. Incorrect.** Supragastric belching typically does not occur during conversation.
- **c. Correct.** Cognitive behavioral therapy, including diaphragmatic breathing, is effective for excessive supragastric belching.
- **d. Incorrect.** Transient lower esophageal sphincter relaxation is associated with gastric belching, not supragastric belching.
- **e. Correct.** Esophageal impedance testing can differentiate between gastric belching, supragastric belching, and aerophagia based on impedance patterns.

A2-4 Gastroparesis

Correct Answers: b, e

- **a. Incorrect.** Gastroparesis causes symptoms such as early satiety, postprandial fullness, nausea, vomiting, belching, and abdominal pain.
- **b. Correct.** Unlike FD, nausea and vomiting are more common in gastroparesis.
- **c. Incorrect.** The most common causes of gastroparesis are diabetes mellitus and idiopathic (unknown) causes.
- **d. Incorrect.** The term "gastroparesis" is rarely used in other Asian countries, including Japan.

e. Correct. Demonstrating delayed gastric emptying using solid meal testing is essential for diagnosing gastroparesis.

3: Small Bowel and Colon

A3-1 Small Bowel and Colonic Motility Test

Correct Answers: c, d, e

- **a. Incorrect.** On T2-weighted MRI, intestinal fluid appears as a high-intensity signal.
- **b. Incorrect.** Cine-MRI evaluates peristalsis using coronal slices, not axial.
- **c. Correct.** In chronic intestinal pseudo-obstruction (CIPO), small intestinal contraction rates drop below 20%, compared to over 70% in healthy individuals.
- **d. Correct.** Cine-MRI is also widely used in cardiovascular imaging.
- **e. Correct.** Cine-MRI is noninvasive and less burdensome than manometry, which requires catheter insertion.

A3-2 Irritable Bowel Syndrome (IBS)

(1) **Correct Answer: d**

- **a. Incorrect.** Centrally mediated abdominal pain syndrome involves persistent pain unrelated to physiological stimuli.
- **b. Incorrect.** IBS-D is defined by >25% loose/watery stools and <25% hard stools on symptomatic days.

- **c. Incorrect.** IBS-C is defined by >25% hard stools and <25% loose stools.
- **d. Correct.** IBS-M is defined by >25% loose/watery stools and >25% hard stools on symptomatic days.
- **e. Incorrect.** Unclassified IBS includes patients with <25% of both stool types.

(2) **Correct Answer: e**

- **a. Incorrect.** Mosapride is more appropriate for IBS-C due to its prokinetic effects.
- **b. Incorrect.** Elobixibat is indicated for functional constipation.
- **c. Incorrect.** Tramadol is an opioid and may worsen symptoms or cause narcotic bowel syndrome.
- **d. Incorrect.** Pentazocine is also an opioid with similar risks to tramadol.
- **e. Correct.** Trimebutine is effective across all IBS subtypes.

A3-3 Functional Bowel Disorders

Correct Answers: b, d

This question addresses pharmacological treatments for constipation.

- **a. Incorrect.** Although probiotics are not covered by insurance in Japan for chronic constipation, they have been shown to improve gut dysbiosis and alleviate several symptoms, including stool form and frequency.
- **b. Correct.** In patients with renal dysfunction, magnesium oxide can lead to hypermagnesemia. Therefore, serum magnesium levels should be monitored, and alternative treatments considered in severe renal failure.
- **c. Incorrect.** Animal studies have shown an increased risk of miscarriage and preterm labor with lubiprostone. It is contraindicated in pregnant women or those who may be pregnant.
- **d. Correct.** Linaclotide, a guanylate cyclase-C receptor agonist, increases intracellular cGMP in intestinal epithelial cells, which reduces visceral hypersensitivity and promotes bowel movements. It is effective in relieving abdominal pain in patients with IBS-C.
- **e. Incorrect.** Daikenchuto does not contain rhubarb (daio) which may lead to tolerance and dependence. Alternatively, it contains Japanese pepper (sansho) which promotes gastrointestinal motility, thereby improving bowel movements and abdominal bloating, and can be used long-term.
- **f. Incorrect.** Elobixibat is a bile acid transporter inhibitor, not a mucosal epithelial function-modifying agent. By partially inhibiting the reabsorption of bile acids at the terminal ileum, the flow of bile acids to the colon is increased, thereby promoting colonic motility and secretion.

A3-4 Pseudo-obstruction and Megacolon

Correct Answer: e

- **a. Correct.** Chronic megacolon cannot be diagnosed based on symptoms alone, as it does not present specific symptoms. Chronic megacolon should be considered in the differential diagnosis of unexplained abdominal bloating.
- **b. Correct.** Radiological imaging is essential to confirm pathological colonic dilation and rule out organic causes.
- **c. Correct.** Total colectomy is the most recommended surgical treatment. Segmental resection often leads to recurrence in the remaining colon.
- **d. Correct.** Osmotic laxatives such as polyethylene glycol are effective for defecation control. Other options include probiotics and enemas.

e. Incorrect. High-fiber diets often worsen symptoms by increasing stool volume. A low-residue diet is recommended.

4: Anorectum

A4-1 Anorectal Function Test

(1) **Correct Answer: e**

- **a–d. Correct.** All listed tests are appropriate for their respective conditions.
- **e. Incorrect.** Breath hydrogen testing is used to assess intestinal transit time, not

for diagnosing rectocele. Defecography is the appropriate test for rectocele.

(2) **Correct Answer: e**
- **a–d. Correct.** These scoring systems are appropriately matched to their respective conditions.
- **e. Incorrect.** The Obstructed Defecation Syndrome Score is used for evaluating difficult defecation, not slow transit constipation.

(3) **Correct Answer: a**
- **a. Incorrect.** Anoscopy provides limited information for fecal incontinence. More informative tests include defecography and digital rectal examination.
- **b–e. Correct.** These are all appropriate tests for evaluating fecal incontinence.

(4) **Correct Answers: b, c**
- **a, d, e. Incorrect.** These findings cannot be confirmed from the image.
- **b. Correct.** The image shows a rectocele.
- **c. Correct.** The image also shows rectal intussusception.

(5) **Correct Answers: a, c**
- **a. Correct.** A represents the anorectal angle.
- **b. Incorrect.** Anal canal length is not typically assessed via defecography.
- **c. Correct.** C is the line connecting the pubic symphysis and the tip of the coccyx.
- **d. Incorrect.** The anorectal angle typically increases (becomes more obtuse) during straining.
- **e. Incorrect.** The anal canal length usually increases during straining.

A4-2 Fecal Incontinence

Correct Answer: c
- **a. Incorrect.** The 2017 edition of Japanese Guidelines define fecal incontinence as "involuntary or uncontrollable loss of feces from the anus," encompassing both urge and passive types. The definition "involuntary loss of feces" comes from a different source.
- **b. Incorrect.** Internal anal sphincter dysfunction typically causes passive fecal incontinence, not urge fecal incontinence.
- **c. Correct.** Rectal fecal impaction causes passive fecal incontinence as the mechanism of overflow incontinence. It often occurs even during sleep in the supine position.
- **d. Incorrect.** The scoring system used to subjectively evaluate resting anal tone and voluntary anal sphincter contraction during digital rectoanal examination is DRESS (Digital Rectal Examination Scoring System), not the Cleveland Clinic Florida Fecal Incontinence Score (CCFIS), which is a score to assess the severity of fecal incontinence.
- **e. Incorrect.** As of January 2023, transanal irrigation is not covered by insurance for low anterior resection syndrome in Japan, despite its reported effectiveness.

A4-3 Functional Anorectal Pain

(1) **Correct Answer: c**
- **c. Incorrect.** In levator ani syndrome, tenderness on traction of the puborectalis muscle is a key diagnostic criterion. The absence of such tenderness suggests nonspecific anorectal pain, which must be differentiated from levator ani syndrome.

(2) **Correct Answer: e**
- **e. Correct.** Even if a rectocele is present, treatment is not indicated in asymptomatic cases. When symptoms are present, conservative management such as bowel habit training and laxatives should be initiated. Surgical intervention is considered only if conservative therapy fails.

A4-4 Functional Defecation Disorders

Correct Answer: a
- **a. Correct.** Endoanal ultrasonography is used to detect structural abnormalities of the anal sphincter and is primarily applied in the evaluation of fecal incontinence.
- **b. Incorrect.** Anorectal manometry measures rectal pressure during straining to detect the presence of dyssynergic defecation.
- **c. Incorrect.** A defecography examination can diagnose dyssynergic defecation based

on the presence or absence of difficulty in passing simulated stool or paradoxical contraction of the puborectalis muscle during straining.

- **d. Incorrect.** Anal surface electromyography can detect dyssynergic defecation between abdominal pressure and anal contraction in the same way as anorectal manometry.
- **e. Incorrect.** Balloon expulsion test has high specificity for dyssynergic defecation.

A4-5 Anorectal Dysfunction Due to Organic Disease

Correct Answers: b, e

- **a. Incorrect.** Anatomical features of rectal prolapse include a deep Douglas' pouch or rectovesical pouch, elongated sigmoid colon, stretched rectal mesentery, perineal descent, and widened anal sphincter.
- **b. Correct.** Rectal intussusception may not be visible on physical examination and often requires defecography for diagnosis.
- **c. Incorrect.** The recurrence rate after transabdominal surgery is significantly lower than that of transperineal surgery.
- **d. Incorrect.** The Delorme procedure is a representative transperineal surgery, not transabdominal. It involves mucosal resection and plication of the muscular layer.

e. Correct. The Wells procedure involves posterior rectopexy, in contrast to the Ripstein procedure, which uses anterior fixation.

5: Practical Treatment

A5-1 Scientific Basis of "Illness Begins in the Mind"

Correct Answer: c

- **c. Correct.** The α7 nicotinic acetylcholine receptor (α7Ach receptor) is involved in the vagal cholinergic antiinflammatory pathway. Stimulation of the vagus nerve activates this receptor on splenic macrophages, suppressing the production of inflammatory cytokines such as TNF-α, thereby exerting systemic antiinflammatory effects.

Key References

- Borovikova et al. Vagus nerve stimulation attenuates the systemic inflammatory response to endotoxin. Nature. 2000; 405(6785): 458–462.
- Huston et al. Splenectomy inactivates the cholinergic anti-inflammatory pathway during lethal endotoxemia and polymicrobial sepsis. J Exp Med. 2006; 203(7): 1623–1628.

A5-2 Explore Issues with Psychosomatic Therapy

Correct Answer: d

- **d. Incorrect.** The treatment goals for functional gastrointestinal disorders (FGIDs) include not only complete symptom resolution but also symptom improvement, patient satisfaction, and restoration of social functioning. Multidisciplinary collaboration is often necessary. Although some studies suggest increased mortality in patients with chronic constipation, the overall prognosis for FGIDs is generally favorable. That may also be related to the decline in treatment motivation among healthcare professionals.

A5-3 Estimating Gastrointestinal Function Through Abdominal Examination

Correct Answers: c, d, e

This case describes a young male with constipation since early childhood, likely due to rectal hyposensitivity, leading to rectal-type constipation. Avoidance of defecation due to pain or discomfort in early childhood can result in diminished rectal sensation and loss of the rectoanal reflex, leading to absence of the urge to defecate. Despite significant fecal retention, abdominal pain is often absent. Imaging reveals a large fecal mass extending from the rectum to above the umbilicus, with copious stool and gas throughout the colon (Figure 3).

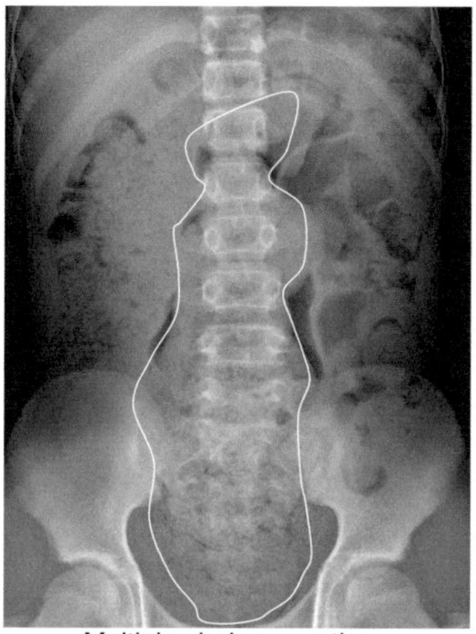

Multiple choice question
"A massive fecal impaction is observed from the rectum up to above the umbilicus. Large amounts of stool and gas are also noted in the colon."

- **a. Incorrect.** Distension primarily in the lower abdomen on inspection is more characteristic of universal mesentery. In rectal-type constipation, fecal retention is widespread throughout the colon.
- **b. Incorrect.** With loss of the rectoanal reflex and reduced peristalsis, bowel sounds are typically diminished.
- **c. Correct.** Bowel sounds are often hypoactive due to reduced motility.
- **d. Correct.** Percussion often reveals tympany throughout the abdomen due to gas accumulation along with fecal retention.
- **e. Correct.** Palpation may detect a large, firm fecal mass in the rectum, which has often been retained for an extended period.

A5-4 Practice of Family Medicine

(1) **Correct Answer: c**

- **a. Incorrect.** Family physicians should aim to prevent doctor shopping by building trust and continuity of care. Psychiatric referral may be necessary in cases with strong psychosomatic involvement, but not as a first step.
- **b. Incorrect.** Western guidelines recommend diagnosing FGIDs based on detailed history, physical examination, and minimal testing, reserving specialist referral for cases with alarm features or treatment resistant.
- **c. Correct.** Family physicians play a central role in the diagnosis and management of FGIDs and should be well versed in their evaluation and treatment.
- **d. Incorrect.** Rikkunshito is listed as a first-line treatment in Japan's clinical algorithm for functional dyspepsia (FD).
- **e. Incorrect.** Patients presenting with epigastric pain may have serious conditions such as aortic dissection, myocardial infarction, pulmonary embolism, appendicitis, herpes zoster, pregnancy, or anxiety disorders, requiring careful differential diagnosis.

(2) **Correct Answers: a, c, e**

- **a. Correct.** Rikkunshito is explicitly listed as a first-line treatment in the Japanese Society of Gastroenterology's treatment flowchart for FD.

- **b. Incorrect.** The flowchart for FD also includes other Kampo medicines as second-line options if rikkunshito is ineffective.
- **c. Correct.** Kampo medicine classifies FD into subtypes such as "Qi deficiency" and "Qi stagnation." Rikkunshito is used for the former, while bukuryoin or dai-saikoto may be used for the latter.
- **d. Incorrect.** Kampo subtyping can be performed using diagnostic criteria for Qi deficiency and Qi stagnation, without requiring endoscopy.
- **e. Correct.** Esophageal anisakiasis may mimic symptoms of GERD or FD, unlike gastric anisakiasis, which presents more acutely.

Competing Interests The author(s) has no competing interests to declare that are relevant to the content of this manuscript.

Index

H. Kaneko et al. (eds.), *Disorders of Gut-Brain Interaction*,
https://doi.org/10.1007/978-981-95-6974-8

C

D

E

MIX
Papier aus verantwortungsvollen Quellen
Paper from responsible sources
FSC® C105338

If you have any concerns about our products,
you can contact us on
ProductSafety@springernature.com

In case Publisher is established outside the EU,
the EU authorized representative is:
Springer Nature Customer Service Center GmbH
Europaplatz 3, 69115 Heidelberg, Germany

Printed by Libri Plureos GmbH
in Hamburg, Germany